Fundamentals of
Pharmacognosy
and Phytotherapy

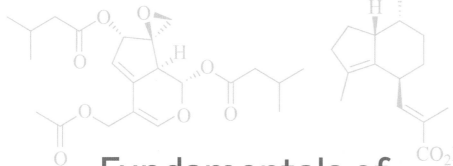

Fourth Edition

Fundamentals of
Pharmacognosy
and Phytotherapy

Michael Heinrich, Dr rer nat habil
MA(WSU) Dipl. Biol. FLS

Professor of Ethnopharmacology and Pharmacognosy and Head of
the Centre for Pharma & Bio Chemistry, School of Pharmacy,
University of London, UK; Yushan Fellow,
Chinese Medicine Research Center, and Department of
Pharmaceutical Sciences and Chinese Medicine Resources,
College of Chinese Medicine, China Medical University,
Taichung City, Taiwan.

Joanne Barnes, BPharm(Hons) PhD
MPS RegPharmNZ FISoP FLS

Professor in Herbal Medicines, School of Pharmacy,
University of Auckland, Auckland, New Zealand

José M Prieto-Garcia, MPharm PhD
MRSC FLS FHEA

Associate Professor in Natural Products and Phytochemistry,
Liverpool John Moores University, UK

Simon Gibbons, BSc MRSC CChem
PhD FLS

Professor of Natural Product Chemistry,
University of East Anglia School of Pharmacy, UK

Elizabeth M Williamson, BSc
(Pharm) PhD FLS

Emerita Professor of Pharmacy, School of Pharmacy,
University of Reading, UK; former Editor-in-Chief—now a Senior
Editor of *Phytotherapy Research*; Member of the Herbal Drugs
Committees for *The British Pharmacopoeia*

Forewords by

A Douglas Kinghorn, BPharm MSc PhD DSc
FRPharmS FAAAS FAAPS FLS FSP

Professor and Jack L. Beal Chair of Natural Products Chemistry
and Pharmacognosy, College of Pharmacy, The Ohio State University,
Columbus, OH, USA

Mark Blumenthal, BA ND (hon causa)
PhD (hon causa)

Founder and Executive Director, American Botanical Council;
Editor-in-Chief, *HerbalGram* and *HerbClip*; Founder and Director,
ABC-AHP-NCNPR Botanical Adulterants Program,
Austin, TX, USA

ELSEVIER

First edition 2004
Second edition 2012
Third edition 2018
The rights of Michael Heinrich, Joanne Barnes, José M Prieto-Garcia, Simon Gibbons, Elizabeth M Williamson to be identified as authors of this work have been asserted by them in accordance with the Copyright, Designs and Patents Act 1988.

Notices

Practitioners and researchers must always rely on their own experience and knowledge in evaluating and using any information, methods, compounds or experiments described herein. Because of rapid advances in the medical sciences, in particular, independent verification of diagnoses and drug dosages should be made. To the fullest extent of the law, no responsibility is assumed by Elsevier, authors, editors or contributors for any injury and/or damage to persons or property as a matter of products liability, negligence or otherwise, or from any use or operation of any methods, products, instructions, or ideas contained in the material herein.

ISBN: 978-0-323-83434-6

Content Strategist: Alex Mortimer
Content Project Manager: Supriya Barua Kumar
Design: Renee Duenow
Marketing Manager: Deborah Watkins

Printed in India

Last digit is the print number: 9   8   7   6   5   4   3   2   1

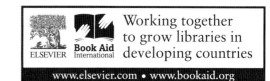

CONTENTS

Drugs derived from organisms continue to be of importance globally for the treatment and prevention of many diseases. Pharmacognosy, which is defined in this book as 'the science of biogenic or nature-derived pharmaceuticals and poisons', has been an established pharmaceutical science taught in institutions of pharmacy education for well over a hundred years.

The subject area has changed considerably since its initiation with its first mention in 1811, having metamorphosed from a largely descriptive botanical and mycological field from the late 19th century to the mid-20th century, to having much more of a chemical and biological focus within approximately the last 60 years. Today, pharmacognosy embraces the scientific study of mainly small-molecule organic compounds from plants, animals and microbes, of both terrestrial and marine origin. It has been estimated that almost 50% of new drugs introduced into medicine in Western countries over the last 75 years either were obtained directly from an ever more diverse range of organisms or were otherwise derived from natural products. Even in an age of biotechnology, computer chemistry and refinements in chemical synthesis, there continues to be a steady stream of new 'single chemical entity' natural product-derived drugs approved by the US Food and Drug Administration (FDA). Most of the new natural product-derived drugs that have reached the market over the last 20 years have been obtained from terrestrial microbe sources, but there are several other examples of both higher plant and marine animal origin. Two very recent plant-derived FDA-approved drugs are cocaine hydrochloride, as a nasal local anaesthetic, and artesunate, to treat severe malaria. In the United States, two 'botanical drug products' (sinecatechins from green tea—*Camellia sinensis* (L.) Kuntze, and crofelemer from *Croton lechleri* Müll.Arg.) have received official approval within the last 15 years. Natural products continue to be widely utilised as laboratory probes for many different targets to help better understand cellular processes.

Pharmacognosy has evolved relatively recently to include the topics of phytotherapy and nutraceuticals. Also, the teaching of pharmacognosy has become more relevant than previously over the last 30 years, as a result of a substantially increased use of herbal remedies (phytomedicines) by the public, particularly in Europe, North America and Australasia. If the United States is taken as an example, community pharmacists have to deal with the availability of a rather bewildering array of thousands of 'botanical dietary supplement' products, of which many were introduced soon after the passage of the Dietary Supplement Health and Education Act of 1994. There are now many publications in the biomedical literature describing the biological properties and mechanistic parameters of purified constituents of dietary supplements of natural origin. Therefore societal interest in pharmacognosy is likely to increase in the future as the biochemical role of phytomedicines, nutraceuticals and drugs of natural origin in general becomes more clearly defined.

The Fourth Edition of this volume, *Fundamentals of Pharmacognosy and Phytotherapy*, by Michael Heinrich, Joanne Barnes, José M Prieto-Garcia, Simon Gibbons and Elizabeth M Williamson, aims to provide a contemporary perspective of natural product drugs providing an introduction into this field. The book is organised into two major parts, 'Fundamentals of Pharmacognosy' (Part A) and 'Important Plant Medicines' (Part B). Part A is divided into four sections, dealing, in turn, with: an overview of pharmacognosy and phytotherapy; an introduction to natural products; herbal medicinal products; and natural products in traditional, complementary and alternative medicine. Part B provides coverage of the use of phytomedicines in various therapeutic categories, affecting, respectively: digestive and liver disorders; cardiovascular disease and related conditions; weight loss; upper respiratory disorders; nervous system disorders; musculoskeletal disorders; female hormonal imbalance, pregnancy, childbirth and nursing; male hormonal and reproductive disorders; nutraceuticals and natural products used to support health; and topical phytotherapy. Some of these categories are new for this Fourth Edition of the book. There is also a helpful Annex, with listings on herbal drugs with pharmacopoeial standards, in addition to relevant Latin pharmaceutical names and English common names.

This comprehensive pharmacognosy textbook integrates very effectively the various traditional elements of pharmacognosy and phytotherapy. The five talented co-authors have been successful in this endeavour in large part because they have contributed their collective and complementary technical expertise in several diverse areas, including ethnobotany and ethnopharmacology, classical botanical pharmacognosy, natural product and analytical chemistry, phytochemistry, phytotherapy and clinical pharmacy.

This new edition may be recommended highly for purchase by undergraduate and professional doctoral students in pharmacy, as well as beginning graduate students in programmes in the pharmaceutical sciences and related areas. It will also be of great interest for use in continuing education courses for pharmacists, dentists, nurses and physicians. In addition, those with a scientific interest in herbalism and traditional medicine and nutrition will find the content of value. Moreover, this book will serve as a reliable source of information on natural product drugs for the interested lay reader. The previous editions of *Fundamentals of Pharmacognosy and Phytotherapy* have proven to be very highly regarded by readers. This updated and partially reorganised volume should be welcomed especially by educators of future pharmacists and of other healthcare professionals.

Prof. A. Douglas Kinghorn
Columbus, OH, USA

Significant changes in the global market for herbal remedies and phytomedicinal and other natural products have occurred since the writing of the foreword for the third edition of this book in 2017. Consumer attitudes have shifted due to a variety of factors, noted below. The markets in most countries abound with myriads of natural product formulations from medicinal plants (teas, capsules, tablets, extracts, cosmetics, etc.), as well as plant-based 'functional foods', beneficial fungi and related natural products. Many are sold as 'traditional herbal medicinal products' or 'food supplements' in the United Kingdom and European Union, 'dietary supplements' in the United States and other countries, and 'natural health products' as they are regulated as a class of medicines in Canada.

The most obvious health-related event is the global pandemic caused by the SARS-CoV-2 virus or COVID-19 illness, which has had an enormous impact on consumer attitudes on public health issues, personal health and self-care, and many related aspects of modern life.

To a lesser extent, but just as compelling an issue to a growing number of informed and motivated consumers, are mounting concerns about the climate crisis and needs for governments, nonprofit organisations and NGOs, private businesses and consumers to take actions that promote sustainable and regenerative practices in all aspects of business, government activity, and daily lifestyle, including, but not limited to, healthcare and self-care.

While consumer interest in and use of herbs, teas, medicinal plants, phytomedicines, plant-derived ingredients and so-called 'nutraceuticals' has been growing worldwide over the past four-plus decades, the recent COVID pandemic has had a marked effect on consumers' attitudes related to healthcare and self-care, particularly with respect to issues related to immune system function, sleep, anxiety and other conditions that have become priorities for millions of consumers in many countries. The rate of increase in the purchase of herbal and non-herbal dietary supplements in 2020 and 2021, i.e. during the so-called 'lockdown' periods of the pandemic, increased significantly over the previous years, reflecting this increased consumer demand. For example, in the United States, where econometric retail market data are readily available, retail sales of botanical dietary supplements in 2020 increased by an unprecedented 17.3% over sales in 2019. In the US market, retail sales of herbs and other plant-based dietary supplements in 2020 reached almost US$11.26 billion (up markedly from ca. $7B in 2015)—a new record for sales in the United States. These sales data do not reflect similar growth in other countries, nor do they reflect the additional sales volume related to the use of herbal teas or the growing use of botanical ingredients in cosmetics and, more recently, in conventional foods, e.g. nutrition bars, beverages like 'smoothies', etc.

The rise in consumer demand for natural health products continues to spark interest in the academic and scientific domains. Scientific and clinical research on the chemistry, pharmacology, toxicology and clinical applications of medicinal plants and related natural products has accelerated at a fairly significant rate, although it is difficult to obtain reliable metrics on this growth. The increase of publications on phytomedicinal research increased almost 700% in a 30-year period from 1977 to 2007, and if such growth in research publications were measured today (2022), the rate of the continued increase might be as much, or perhaps even higher.

Accordingly, as before, the corresponding need for reliable professional educational materials on these increasingly popular natural products, and the growing body of scientific/clinical research on them, has never been more compelling.

Pharmacognosy is the study of medicines of natural origin, whether they are derived from plants, bacteria, fungi or animals. Many modern drugs are derived directly from plants—a truism that is commonly known among pharmacists, physicians, researchers and even many educated consumers. Classic examples include the still-employed cardiac drug digoxin (from the toxic foxglove plant, *Digitalis purpurea* and *D. lanata*), the antiinflammatory drug colchicine (from the also toxic Mediterranean autumn crocus, *Colchicum autumnale*) and the analgesic and anodyne opiates—codeine and morphine—from the opium poppy (*Papaver somniferum*). The latter (morphine) is the very first plant-based drug (isolated in 1804). In relatively rapid succession, in the early 19th century other plant-derived single-chemical entity drugs were isolated from their plant sources: strychnine (from *Strychnos nux-vomica*), the antimalarial quinine (from the South American cinchona bark, *Cinchona officinalis*) and numerous others, giving rise to the modern pharmaceutical industry.

In recent years there has been some debate among researchers as to whether the search for new pharmaceutical drugs from plants is a worthwhile endeavour. Chemists normally prefer the purity of single-chemical entity (SCE) drugs, whether natural or synthetic, and chemical synthesis has often been the preferred route of discovery, when appropriate, usually due to the lower cost and chemical simplicity of SCEs, i.e. when compared to the chemically complex botanical materials—roots, leaves, barks, flowers, seeds, etc., and their increasingly wide array of various types of extracts.

Investigations into the long history of the use of medicinal plants in indigenous cultures—the sciences of ethnobotany and ethnopharmacology—have often produced excellent leads for the development of new medicines. Although now dated, the most-cited study of this process was conducted by the late research pharmacognosist Norman R. Farnsworth at the University of Illinois-Chicago and colleagues, published by the World Health Organization in 1985, in which 119 modern plant-derived drugs were listed (including, of course, all those mentioned above). Not surprisingly, the modern applications of 74% of these drugs correlated directly with the historical, traditional ethnobotanical uses of their source plants.

Lest anyone think that the ethnobotanical approach to drug discovery is an archaic and/or futile endeavour, one only need review the blockbuster news in the medical plant community in 2015 that Chinese researchers were granted the Nobel Prize in Physiology or Medicine for discovery of the highly successful antimalarial drug artemisinin, derived from the traditional Chinese herb *quinghao* (*Artemisia annua*, sometimes referred to as sweet wormwood). Traditional uses of this plant for reducing intermittent fevers led to its being investigated by Chinese scientists in the 1970s when seeking leads for the development of a new antimalarial drug.

Further interest is generated by the development and official US government approval of two new plant-derived chemically complex medicines, a tannin-rich extract of green tea (*Camellia sinensis*) in an ointment for the topical treatment of human papilloma virus and crofelemer, an oligomeric proanthocyanidin-rich extract of the exudate of the bark of a South American tree sangre de drago (*Croton lechleri*, dragon's blood) for symptomatic relief of diarrhoea in patients with HIV/AIDS on antiretroviral therapy. (And, in 2021 crofelemer received conditional US government approval for chemotherapy-induced diarrhoea in dogs, thereby extending phytomedicinal research benefits to veterinary applications for companion animals.) Approval of additional new chemically complex plant-derived medicines is most likely inevitable and may constitute a new era in pharmacy and medicine.

As noted, medicinal plants have played and will continue to play a significant role in the development of modern medicines and will continue to be used by the public as self-selected remedies and supplements. Correspondingly, a growing number of licensed health professionals also recommend or prescribe medicinal plant-based supplements and related natural products.

What should be immediately clear from examining a list of top-selling herbs (at least as it represents consumer demand in the United States) is the presence of many botanicals that have a long history of food use, either as spices and food flavourings and/or as conventional foods.

Popular spices such as turmeric root and rhizome (*Curcuma longa*), one of the top-selling supplements in the United States in the natural food store channel for the past decade, garlic (*Allium sativum*), ginger (*Zingiber officinale*) and red pepper (*Capsicum annuum*) are used by consumers for a variety of traditional and clinically documented health benefits. Conventional foods, such as cranberry (*Vaccinium macrocarpon*), bilberry (*Vaccinium myrtillus*, an anthocyanin-rich type of blueberry), pomegranate (*Punica granatum*), soy (*Glycine max*) and/or their extracts, have gained significant popularity as dietary/food supplements and phytomedicines in various countries, again based on the growing amount of clinical research demonstrating their obvious safety, as well as their activity/efficacy in published clinical trials.

This brings a relatively new spectrum of plants to the pharmacognosist for study of their chemistry, pharmacology, toxicology and various ways that these substances in raw, dried, powdered form, or as extracts (and essential oils) can be formulated for optimal consumption by a growing consumer base interested in safe, effective, reliable natural products.

With the increased acceptance of the health-promoting benefits of many food items, one can forecast that future pharmacognosy educational materials will recognise the field of nutritional biochemistry as an equally important area of research. The growing trend of 'food as medicine' is rife with opportunities for pharmacists, physicians and dietitians/nutritionists to share vitally important information for the benefit of health consumers. One can simply view the vastly growing body of scientific and clinical research on broccoli (*Brassica oleracea*) to see evidence of this.

While consumer demand for natural health products continues to grow and the market responds with an almost dizzying array of natural products, there has been growing concern by botanical experts regarding the quality and identity of botanical raw materials, extracts, and essential oils.

Quality issues related to herbal ingredients have come under increased scrutiny due to growing reports of problems related to the adulteration of the raw materials, extracts or essential oils with undisclosed lower-cost ingredients. While adulteration with another plant can be a result of accidental misidentification of the plant in the field or in processing and/or inadequate training of harvesting and processing personnel, reliable reports continue to confirm the highly lamentable practice of intentional adulteration of botanical materials used as ingredients in consumer products meant for health effects, e.g. dietary/food supplements. Adulterated botanical materials are also found in cosmetic products and other items for topical use, as well as in household products.

There are generally two areas of primary concern when it comes to medicinal plant quality: (1) identity and authenticity, and (2) purity. With respect to the former, the first priority in any effective quality-control system for herbs and medicinal plants is ensuring the proper identity of the raw plant material, whether it is to be used as simply raw material for a consumer product (e.g. a herbal tea or capsule containing dry, powdered herb material), or whether it is to be used as the starting material for the creation of a botanical extract (made with one or more solvents) or distilled into an essential oil. The second priority of purity deals with ensuring that the raw material does not contain any excessive levels of other plant materials—official pharmacopoeias usually allow up to 2% of foreign organic material in herbal starting materials used for medicinal purposes—excessive levels of pesticides or other agricultural chemicals, or excessive levels of heavy metals (often derived from soil or water), and that there is no excessive microbial contamination (that it is contained to a specified allowable level).

Adulteration of foods, spices, botanical drugs and medicinal products is not a recent phenomenon. The problem of substitution of such botanical materials and finished products with undisclosed lower-cost materials and/or dilution with such ingredients has been documented as far back as 2000 years, and probably even earlier. It was for this reason that the first pharmacopoeia was initiated in the late 15th century:—to compile methods to ensure the proper botanical identity of herbal drugs and to detect known adulterants.

As a section of this book demonstrates, botanical authentication is a necessary first step in any robust and effective quality-control system used in the various areas of the supply chain and manufacturing in the botanical industry. Plant species identification and authentication is conducted using various techniques—macroscopic and organoleptic, microscopic, chemical and genetic. Industry and non-profit groups continually offer training programmes on these techniques to serve the increasingly specialised quality-control needs of the global botanical industry. Accordingly, there is a growing need in the burgeoning botanical industry for well-qualified technicians and scientists with adequate training in medicinal plant identity, authentication and other means of appropriate qualification, e.g. botanists, pharmacognosists, natural product chemists and others. This textbook presents is an excellent reference contributing to such education and training.

In 2010, the nonprofit American Botanical Council (www.herbalgram.org) teamed up with the nonprofit American Herbal Pharmacopoeia (https://herbal-ahp.org) and the National Center for Natural Product Research at the University of Mississippi (https://pharmacy.olemiss.edu/ncnpr/) to form the ABC-AHP-NCNPR Botanical Adulterants Prevention Program (BAPP) to assist responsible elements in the global botanical industry, as well as academic researchers and regulatory agencies, in properly authenticating and identifying botanical (and fungal) ingredients in global commerce and determine which might be subject to accidental or intentional adulteration (the latter being criminal fraud). Evidence from published reports in the peer-reviewed literature demonstrates that some adulterators produce fraudulent extracts that are intentionally designed to fool prevalent laboratory analytical methods—the types of adulteration that have been confirmed make this conclusion obvious. Based on the retail sales of herbal dietary supplements in the United States, with respect to the 22 top-selling herbs in the mainstream (food stores, drugstores, mass market retail stores) and natural (health and natural food stores) channels, between 45% and 64% of these top-selling herbal supplements sold in these two market channels, respectively, *are subject to adulteration* and such adulteration has been confirmed, although the *extent* of the adulteration on a per-herb basis is difficult to assess. To date, BAPP has published 73 extensively peer-reviewed documents documenting such adulteration and offering laboratory guidance on appropriate, fit-for-purpose analytical methods. (BAPP publications are freely accessible at https://www.herbalgram.org/resources/botanical-adulterants-prevention-program/.)

As suggested briefly above, in the past 5 years since the publication of the previous edition of this textbook, one of the key areas of dynamic change in the market for botanical therapeutic products is the rising consumer interest in issues related to climate change (more accurately referred to as the *climate crisis*), sustainable production of botanical ingredients, social and economic welfare of people in medicinal plant-producing areas, issues related to regenerative farming, and more. In recognition of this important and growing trend, in 2018 the nonprofit American Botanical Council launched the ABC Sustainable Herbs Program (SHP; https://sustainableherbsprogram.org/), with the intention to help consumers, practitioners, industry members, et al., answer the compelling question, 'Do you know where your herbs come from?' The video-centric SHP website contains numerous educational videos on various aspects of sustainable sourcing of wild and cultivated medicinal and aromatic plants (commonly referred to as MAPs). (Other international organisations, e.g. TRAFFIC and FairWild, have published reports on the sustainable harvesting and processing of MAPs.) One of the key messages of SHP to industry members and the public is that the term 'supply chain' is limited and outdated. A preferable term, at least in many instances, is 'value network'. This is more than merely a semantic shift; it is a shift in consciousness and scope. It represents the nonlinearity of the supply network and emphasises the importance of focusing on providing economic and social justice to the people involved in these networks.

While earlier pharmacognosy texts tended to be organised on a phytochemical basis (e.g. alkaloids, glycosides, tannins, etc.), this text takes the rational approach of organising the content based on a therapeutic and clinical basis—physiological systems upon which the natural medicines have their primary actions and uses (e.g. cardiovascular system, digestive system, nervous system, etc.). The authors, all experts in pharmacognosy, also provide essential and rational information for the appropriate use of medicinal plants and their products—phytomedicines—in therapy, especially as documented for their safety and therapeutic activity in published controlled clinical trials and practiced by licensed health professionals.

This fourth edition of a work that has gained significant prominence and respect as a leading textbook contains highly valuable and authoritative information for anyone who is a student of pharmacy and/or pharmacognosy. It is also a valuable reference for industry quality-control personnel, herbalists, natural product researchers and others in the health professionals who wish to learn about the growing popularity of MAPs and how natural botanical and fungal preparations can provide a growing range of safe and reliable health benefits for consumers worldwide.

Mark Blumenthal
Austin, Texas

PREFACE

The first edition of this unique book was published in 2004 and, today, almost 20 years on, the focus of the publication with this fourth edition has changed substantially. An innovative feature of the first edition was to bring together the scientific basis of medicinal-plant and natural-product research with a therapy-oriented introduction to the uses of medicinal plants and natural products in healthcare. The fourth edition upholds this approach through retaining content on traditional studies of the identification and quality of plant-based medicines: these aspects remain fundamental to understanding the therapeutic properties of natural products, and are intrinsic to their safety, including compatibility and interactions when used with prescribed drugs. This new edition also provides readers with an understanding of the role of natural products in the drug discovery process, the analysis and isolation of active molecules, and their structure elucidation, and these aspects are illustrated with chemical structures, chromatograms and spectra where appropriate.

In addition, the scope of this edition has been widened considerably. The book includes a new section on antiseptic and antibiotic natural products, and their potential role in reversing bacterial resistance and in providing alternatives to existing antibiotics. Antiviral agents are also given special consideration in the light of coronavirus infection and the predictable seasonal recurrence of influenza, as are agents used to combat the protozoal diseases still endemic in many parts of the world. New diagrams have been introduced to clarify the role of natural products and their mechanisms of action; this material is focused on phytochemicals but also includes other organisms (fungi, algae, bacteria), as the techniques used in their study are adapted from those used for medicinal plants. A new chapter on pharmacovigilance (safety monitoring) for herbal and other traditional medicines is included, because the science and practice of identifying adverse reactions associated with natural products are crucial to understanding their safety profile and ensuring they are used appropriately.

Traditional systems of medicine have produced many important drugs, and medicinal plant species originating from these systems continue to be important in their region of origin, as well as where they are introduced to new markets. In chapters covering these traditional medicine systems (organised according to geographical region or cultural background), their principles and philosophies are briefly introduced, and examples of significant medicinal species from these traditions are included in the form of new tables.

The revised and updated second part of the book gives an overview of the use of herbal medicines and pure natural substances, along with summaries of preclinical and clinical evidence; this content is, as in previous editions, organised by body systems (e.g. musculoskeletal system) or by areas of medical care (e.g. supportive therapies for stress, ageing, cancer and debility). Since healthcare incorporates preventive medicine, cancer chemoprevention is now included in the latter chapter as part of the spectrum of anticancer activity of natural products. The use of preventive and supportive therapies is also relevant for other areas of healthcare. For example, the COVID-19 pandemic has strained healthcare systems globally and demonstrated the importance of evidence-based approaches to self-care, including the use of plant-derived products.

Beyond specific additions and updates, general revisions have been applied throughout the new edition. Information for some older plant medicines has been truncated to allow inclusion of newer species, acknowledging that plant medicines are discovered, developed (and discarded) in the same way as other drugs. Naturally, references have been refreshed and many new ones added; the subject area is now so vast that we have provided further key references—mainly reviews, and official publications (such as national pharmacopoeias, World Health Organization guidance documents, standard reference works)—to enable rapid access to the relevant literature and support the content of each section.

As plant drugs originating from many different parts of the world are more widely introduced, the correct identification of the species intended for use becomes even more vitally important for the global market; confusion between traditional folklore or common names and synonyms, botanical species names (binomials) and terms used in trade can seriously compromise safety and efficacy. Pharmacopoeial names and definitions are used to specify exactly which plant species (in some cases, more than one may be acceptable), variety, and plant part used, and the method of processing required to comply with the drug monograph. These various names do not always follow a logical system, as they are used for different purposes. To aid understanding of botanical nomenclature, this edition includes a new annex as a reference guide to many of the most common medicinal plant species found in commerce. The examples provided originate from around the world, and all are included in the European and/or British Pharmacopoeia, and are used in Australasia; thus the list is a quick reference for checking whether quality standards are available internationally for a particular herbal drug.

In keeping with our original aim, we trust that this new edition will enable health professionals, particularly pharmacists, medical practitioners, nurses and others, as well as students and readers interested generally in pharmacognosy and phytotherapy, to gain a basic understanding of important aspects relating to the use of medicinal plants and other natural products. Beyond this, we hope this volume aids in the consideration of the potential benefits and harms of plant-based medicines, whether as part of regulatory processes or where health professionals provide advice to patients.

We are sincerely grateful to the publisher for its long-standing support and commitment to this publication. We particularly thank Alexandra Mortimer for her encouragement and editorial oversight, and Supriya Barua Kumar for her helpful and efficient in-house administration and editing, and Wendy Bibby for her meticulous checking of current botanical names and proof-reading for this book.

The 20-year period since the first edition has seen great change in pharmacognosy, and this book is testament to that. The enormous importance of medicinal plants, and of products derived from them, has increased, with a rapid rise in the use of herbal medicines also in countries which, in recent decades, had seen a decline. Such products are now even more vital, with humans enjoying a longer life span, yet still being challenged by new health problems.

Michael Heinrich
Joanne Barnes
Simon Gibbons,
José M Prieto-Garcia
Elizabeth M Williamson

PART A

Fundamentals of Pharmacognosy

1

Pharmacognosy and Phytotherapy

Importance of Plants in Modern Pharmacy and Medicine

Pharmacognosy (derived from *pharmakon*, 'remedy', and *cognosco*, 'knowledge') is the science of medicinal plants, which may be used therapeutically in different ways.

INTRODUCTION

There has been a considerable rise in interest and consumption of medicinal plants globally, with consumers wanting to treat minor health problems with a 'natural' remedy, optimise health and fitness, and combat signs and symptoms of ageing. Traditional medicine (TM) remains an important, and sometimes the only, form of healthcare in many parts of the world and is increasingly popular outside its ethnic or geographical origin, as with traditional Chinese medicine and Ayurveda.

Plants have yielded some of our most important drugs, and the development of modern drugs derived from natural products continues. Pure compounds, often isolated from 'poisonous' plants, are commonly used as conventional drugs, whereas herbal medicines and nutritional supplements are usually derived from more benign species.

Pharmacognosy encompasses a wealth of tradition and history and has evolved and diversified dramatically over the 20th and 21st centuries. The first edition of this text was conceived in a very different environment to the current situation. In 2004, we wished to explain—and justify to some extent—the use of plants in medicine to a readership of conventional healthcare students.

Since then, the acceptance of natural therapies has become more widespread and even embraced by doctors, nurses, pharmacists and counsellors in many clinical settings. TM and complementary/alternative medicine (CAM) therapists often work under professional, ethical guidelines and are aware of potential health conflicts. Our original, somewhat defensive approach to the role of plants in healthcare has thus evolved as research has substantiated some traditional claims and identified novel applications. The new edition recognises these changes while still providing an overview of how and which plant species are used in various healthcare settings. It is intended to inform anyone wishing to know more about the rich and sometimes nefarious history of medicinal plant use, the contribution of medicinal plants to the understanding of physiological processes, and their role in the treatment of disease and maintenance of health.

As with previous editions, Part A addresses fundamental concepts in pharmacognosy, the science supporting the use of medicinal plants, and specific applications of natural products as anticancer and antibacterial agents. In this new edition, the philosophical basis of some traditional, complementary and alternative systems of medicine has been condensed, as that information is widely available elsewhere. However, we now provide more detail on each tradition's important medicinal plant species. TM systems are now considered together in Chapter 16 to highlight the commonality of plants used globally for similar purposes, regardless of geographical origin. Many TM species have been scientifically investigated to a degree, although it is not always in the context of TM use. An overview of CAM is presented separately in Chapter 17. These therapies are not evidence-based, although some, such as aromatherapy, are widely accepted, with preclinical studies broadly supporting the benefits of the used essential oils.

Part B provides more details of the therapeutic use of specific medicinal plants, extracts, and phytochemicals widely used in conventional, herbal, complementary and alternative medicine, with their constituents, pharmacological actions and evidence base. This section is arranged in modern therapeutic categories with relevant traditional and historical use.

TYPES OF DRUGS DERIVED FROM PLANTS

Herbal Drugs

These are derived from specific plant parts and form the starting material for producing herbal medicines and extracts. They include, for example:
- **Aerial parts** of St John's wort, *Hypericum perforatum*, used for mild to moderately severe depression
- **Leaves** of *Ginkgo biloba,* used for cognitive deficiencies and memory impairment
- **Flowerheads** of chamomile, *Matricaria chamomilla*, used for mild gastrointestinal complaints and as a topical antiinflammatory
- **Buds** of clove, *Syzygium aromaticum,* used for digestive disorders and as a source of clove oil
- **Fruit** (pods) and leaves of senna, *Cassia* spp., used for constipation
- **Roots** of devil's claw, *Harpagophytum procumbens*, used for rheumatic pain
- **Bark** of willow, *Salix* spp., used for inflammation
- **Seeds** of horse chestnut, *Aesculus hippocastanum*, used for improving venous circulation.

Herbal medicines may also be used as conventional drugs, but are more often considered to be part of complementary and alternative medicine.

Natural Products or Compounds Isolated From Nature

These are single chemical entities often used in licensed medicines. If produced synthetically, they are referred to as 'nature identical' (if that is the case) but were originally discovered from plants. Examples include:
- Morphine, from opium poppy (*Papaver somniferum*), used as an analgesic;
- Digoxin and other glycosides from foxglove (*Digitalis* spp.) are used to treat heart failure;
- Taxol, from the Pacific yew (*Taxus brevifolia*), is used as an anticancer treatment;
- Quinine, from *Cinchona* bark (*Cinchona* spp.), is used in the treatment of malaria;
- Galanthamine, from *Galanthus* and *Leucojum* species, is used for cognitive disorders.

Nutraceuticals and Functional Foods

Many foods are known to have beneficial effects on health. Examples include:

- Garlic, ginger, turmeric and many other herbs and spices;
- Anthocyanin- or flavonoid-containing plants, such as bilberries, cocoa and red wine;
- Carotenoid-containing plants, such as tomatoes, carrots and many other vegetables.

There are many reasons for the increased use of herbal medicines and nutraceuticals. These may range from the appeal of products from 'nature' and the perception that such products are 'safe' (or at least 'safer' than conventional medicines, which are often referred to derogatorily as 'drugs') to more complex reasons related to the philosophical views and religious beliefs of individuals.

Most purchases of herbal medicines and nutraceuticals are made on a self-selection basis from pharmacies, health-food stores, supermarkets, by mail order and via the Internet. **Usually, except for pharmacists, there is no requirement for a trained healthcare professional to be available on the premises to provide information and advice.** In any case, most herbal medicines can be sold or supplied without the involvement of a healthcare professional. Several studies have confirmed that many people do not seek professional advice before purchasing or using herbal medicines, even when purchased from a pharmacy. Instead, they tend to rely on their own knowledge or advice from friends, relatives or the popular media. Consumers who do seek professional advice (e.g. from their pharmacist or general practitioner) may find that their question(s) cannot be answered fully. This may be because the information simply is not available, but many healthcare professionals do not feel adequately informed about herbal medicines. This book attempts to redress that omission.

Herbal medicines are used for general health maintenance and treating symptoms of chronic diseases, including serious conditions such as cancer, HIV/AIDS, multiple sclerosis, asthma, rheumatoid arthritis and osteoarthritis. Older patients, pregnant and breastfeeding women, and children also take herbal medicines. The use of herbal medicines by patients who are already taking prescribed medicines is of further concern as there is the potential for drug–herb interactions, as discussed in Chapter 14.

In summary, many health professionals, especially pharmacists who sell herbal medicines, are likely to be asked for advice on such products or need to consider the implications of a patient's use or impact on their current treatment regimen. This book provides the background to using plants as medicines, with supporting scientific evidence where available.

Pharmacognosy and Its History: People, Plants and Natural Products

The history of pharmacy was for centuries identical to the history of pharmacognosy, or the study of **materia medica,** which were obtained from natural sources—mostly plants, but also minerals, animals and fungi. European traditions are particularly well known and have had a strong influence on modern pharmacognosy in the West, but almost all societies have well-established customs, some of which have hardly been studied at all. The study of these traditions not only provides insight into how the field has developed, but it is also a fascinating example of our ability to develop a diversity of cultural practices. The use of medicinal plants in Europe has been influenced by early European scholars, the concepts of lay people and, more recently, an influx of people and products from non-European traditions. This historical overview covers only Europe and the most well-known traditions of Asia: **traditional Chinese medicine** (TCM), **Ayurveda** and **Jamu.** TCM and Ayurveda will be discussed further in a separate chapter, because they are still used widely nowadays.

SOURCES OF INFORMATION

The sources available for understanding the history of medicinal (as well as nutritional and toxic) plant use are archaeological records and written documents. The desire to summarise information for future generations and to present the writings of the classical (mostly early Greek) scholars to a wider audience was the major stimulus for writing about medicinal plants. The traditions of Japan, India and China were also documented in many early manuscripts and books (Mazar, 1998; Waller, 1998). No written records are available for other regions of the world, either because they were never produced (e.g. in Australia, many parts of Africa and South America, some regions of Asia) or because documents were lost or destroyed by (especially European) invaders (e.g. in Meso-America). Therefore, for many parts of the world, the first written records are reports by early travellers who were sent by their respective feudal governments to explore the wealth of the New World. These people included missionaries, explorers, salesmen, researchers and, later, colonial officers. The information was important to European societies for several reasons, such as poisoned arrows posing a threat to explorers and settlers, as well as the prospect of finding new medicines.

Early Arabic and European Records

Humans have used plants, algae, and fungi for medicinal purposes in a multitude of ways spanning human evolution. Their selection has led to an enormous number of natural materials ('*materia medica*') used by cultures all over the world.

Medicinal mushrooms were found with the Austrian/Italian 'iceman' of the Alps of Ötztal (3300 BCE). Two walnut-sized objects were identified as the birch polypore (*Piptoporus betulinus* (Bull. ex Fr.) P. Karst. = *Fomitopsis betulina* (Bull.) B.K. Cui, M.L. Han & Y.C. Dai), a bracket fungus common in alpine and other cooler environments. This species contains toxic natural products, and one of its active constituents (agaric acid) is a very strong and effective purgative,

which leads to strong and short-lasting diarrhoea. It also has antibiotic effects against mycobacteria and toxic effects on diverse organisms (Capasso, 1998). Since the iceman also harboured eggs of the whipworm (*Trichuris trichiura*) in his gut, he may well have suffered from gastrointestinal cramps and anaemia. The finding of *P. betulinus* points to the possible treatment of gastrointestinal problems using these mushrooms. In addition, scarred cuts on the skin of the iceman might indicate the use of medicinal plants because the burning of herbs over an incision on the skin was a frequent practice in many ancient European cultures (Capasso, 1998).

THE DOCUMENTS OF SHANIDAR IV: The earliest documented record, which presumably relates to medicinal (or ritual) plants, dates from 60,000 BCE and was found in the grave of a Neanderthal man from Shanidar IV, an archaeologic site in Iraq. Pollen of several species of plants was discovered (Leroi-Gourhan, 1975; Lietava, 1992; Solecki, 1975):

Centaurea solstitialis L. (knapweed, Asteraceae).

Ephedra altissima Desf. (ephedra, Ephedraceae).

Achillea sp. (yarrow, Asteraceae).

Althea sp. (mallow, Malvaceae).

Muscari sp. (grape hyacinth, Liliaceae/Hyacinthaceae).

Senecio sp. (groundsel, Asteraceae).

These species were possibly laid on the ground and formed a carpet on which the dead were laid. These plants could have been of major cultural importance to the people of Shanidar IV. Whether they were used as medicine cannot be determined, but it seems likely. Currently, these species are important medicinal plants used for a range of indications. However, others have criticised these reports because:

1. Detailed archaeobotanical descriptions of the pollen were never published.
2. Normally, pollen does not survive well in the Near East.
3. There is good evidence that ants often hoard pollen in a similar context (Sommer, 1999).

Thus, although this may be a finding with no direct bearing on the culture of Shanidar, these species (or closely related ones from the same genus) are still important nowadays in the phytotherapy of Iraq and are also known from other cultural traditions. These species may well be typical for the Neanderthal people and may also be part of a tradition for which Shanidar IV represents the first available record.

Classical Arabic, Greek and Roman Records

The oldest written information in the European-Arabic traditions comes from the Sumerians and Akkadians of Mesopotamia, thus originating from the same area as the archaeological records of Shanidar IV. Similar documents have survived for millennia in Egypt. The Egyptians documented their knowledge (including medical and pharmaceutical) on papyrus, which is a sort of paper made from *Cyperus papyrus* L., an aquatic sedge (also called papyrus) found throughout southern Europe and northern Africa. The most important of these writings is the Ebers Papyrus, which originates from approximately 1500 BCE.

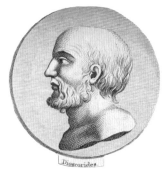

Fig. 2.1 Pedanius Dioscorides. (Reproduced with permission from The Wellcome Library, London.)

This document was reputedly found in a tomb and bought in 1873 by Georg Ebers, who deposited it at the University of Leipzig and 2 years later published a facsimile edition. The Ebers Papyrus is a medical handbook covering all sorts of illnesses and includes empiric and symbolic forms of treatment. The diagnostic precision documented in this text is impressive. Other papyri focus on recipes for pharmaceutical preparations (e.g. the so-called Berlin Papyrus).

Greek medicine has been the focus of historical pharmaceutical research for many decades. The Greek scholar Pedanius Dioscorides (Fig. 2.1) from Anarzabos (1st century BCE) is considered to be the 'father of [Western] medicine'. His works were a doctrine governing pharmaceutical and medical practice for more than 1500 years and heavily influenced European pharmacy. He was an excellent pharmacognosist and described more than 600 medicinal plants. Other Greek and Roman scholars were also influential in developing related fields of healthcare and the natural sciences. Hippocrates, a Greek medical doctor (ca. 460–375 BCE), came from the island of Kos and heavily influenced European medical traditions. He was the first of a series of (otherwise largely unknown) authors who produced the so-called *Corpus Hippocraticum* (a collection of works on medical practice). Importantly, the Hippocratic authors started to differentiate between food and medicine (cf. Totelin, 2015) and thus laid the foundation for one of the key differentiations of natural resources used by humans. The Graeco-Roman medical doctor Claudius Galen (Galenus) (CE 130–201) summarised the complex body of Graeco-Roman pharmacy and medicine, and his name survives in the pharmaceutical term 'galenical'. Pliny the Elder (CE 23 or 24–79, killed in Pompeii at the eruption of Vesuvius) was the first to produce a 'cosmography' (a detailed account) of natural history, which included cosmology, mineralogy, botany, zoology and medicinal products derived from plants and animals.

Classical Chinese Records

Written documents about medicinal plants are essential elements of many cultures of Asia. In China, India, Japan and Indonesia, writings pointing to a long tradition of plant use survive. In China, the field developed as an element of Taoist thought: followers tried to ensure a long life (or immortality) through meditation, special diets, medicinal plants, exercise and specific sexual practices. The most important work in this tradition is the *Shen nong ben cao jing* (the 'Drug treatise of the divine countryman'), which is now only available as part of later compilations (Waller, 1998). This 2200-year-old work provides the earliest treatise of Chinese medicine theory and is one of the four classical sources on Chinese traditional medicine, including 365 drugs, most of botanical origin. For each, the following information is provided:
• Geographical origin.

TABLE 2.1 Chinese Texts Which Include Sections on Medicine (After Waller, 1998)

Year	Author if Known	Title
200 BCE	Various	*Shen nong ben cao jing* (the drug treatise of the divine countryman)
2nd century	Zhang Zhongjing	*Shang han za bing lun* (about the various illnesses caused by cold damage)
6th century	Tao Hongjing	*Shen nong ben cao jingji zhu* (collected commentaries on *Shen nong ben cao jing*)
1082 (Song dynasty)	Tang Shenwei	*Jing shi zheng lei bei ji ben cao* (classified materia medica from historical classics for emergency)
10th to 11th centuries	Su Song	*Ben cao tu jing* (illustrated materia medica)
16th century	Li Shizhen	*Ben cao gang mu* (information about medicinal drugs: a monographic treatment)

• Optimum period for collection.
• Therapeutic properties.
• Forms of preparation and dose.

These scholarly ideas were passed on from master to student and modified and adapted over centuries of use. Unfortunately, in none of the cases do we have a surviving written record. Table 2.1 summarises some of the Chinese works that include important chapters on drugs.

In the 16th century the first systematic treatise on (herbal) drugs using a scientific method was produced. The *Ben Cao Gang Mu* ('Drugs', by Li Shizhen, 1518–1593) contains information about 1892 drugs (in 52 chapters), and more than 11,000 recipes are given in an appendix. The drugs are classified into 16 categories (e.g. herbs, cereals, vegetables, fruits). For each drug the following information is provided (Waller, 1998):
• Definition of the drug.
• Selected commentaries.
• Classification according to the four characteristics of temperatures and the five types of taste.
• Uses (detailed information on uses according to the criteria of Chinese medicine).
• Corrections of previous mistakes.
• Methods of preparing the drug.
• New features.
• Examples of recipes.

The recognition of the need to further develop the use of a plant, to correct earlier mistakes and include new information is particularly noteworthy. However, the numerous medicopharmaceutical traditions of the Chinese minorities were not included in these works, and we therefore have no historical records of their pharmacopoeias. Currently, TCM has become a medical system used in many countries, and the governments of the People's Republic of China and Taiwan actively promote it. However, there also are many concerns with regards to quality, therapeutic benefits, safety and appropriateness (Booker, 2015).

Other Asian Traditional Medicine

Overall, the written records on other Asian medicines are less comprehensive than for Chinese medicine. The oldest form of traditional Asian medicine is Ayurveda, which is basically Hindu in origin and which is a sort of art–science–philosophy of life. In this respect, it resembles TCM, and like TCM it has influenced the development of more practical, less esoteric forms of medicine, which are used for routine or minor illnesses in the home. Related types of medicine include Jamu, the traditional system of Indonesia, which will be described briefly later. All these forms of traditional medicine use herbs and minerals and have many features in common. Naturally, many plants are common to all systems and to various official drugs that were formerly (or still) included in the British Pharmacopoeia (BP), European Pharmacopoeia (Eur. Ph.) and US Pharmacopeia (USP).

Ayurveda

Ayurveda is arguably one of the most ancient of all recorded medicinal traditions. It is considered to be the origin of systemised medicine because ancient Hindu writings on medicine contain no references to foreign medicine, whereas Greek and Middle Eastern texts do refer to ideas and drugs of Indian origin. Dioscorides (who influenced Hippocrates) is thought to have taken many of his ideas from India, so it looks as though the first comprehensive medical knowledge originated there. The term 'Ayurveda' comes from *ayur* meaning 'life' and *veda* meaning 'knowledge' and is a later addition to Hindu sacred writing from 1200 BCE called the *Atharvaveda*. The first school to teach ayurvedic medicine was at the University of Banaras in 500 BCE, and the great Samhita (or encyclopaedia of medicine) was written. Seven hundred years later another great encyclopaedia was written, and these two together form the basis of Ayurveda. The living and the nonliving environment, including humans, is composed of the elements earth (*prithvi*), water (*jala*), fire (*tejas*), air (*vayu*) and space (*akasha*). For an understanding of these traditions, the concept of impurity and cleansing is also essential. Illness is the consequence of imbalance between the various elements and it is the goal of treatment to restore this balance.

Jamu

Indonesian traditional medicine, Jamu, is thought to have originated in the ancient palaces of Surakarta and Yogyakarta in central Java, from ancient Javanese cultural practices and also as a result of the influence of Chinese, Indian and Arabian medicine. Carvings at the temple of Borobudur dating back to CE 800–900 depict the use of *kalpataruh* leaves ('the tree that never dies') to make medicines. The Javanese influence spread to Bali as links were established, and in 1343 an army of the Majapahit kingdom of eastern Java was sent to subjugate the Balinese. Success was short-lived, and the Balinese retaliated, regaining their independence. After Islam was adopted in Java and the Majapahit Empire destroyed, many Javanese fled, mainly to Bali, taking with them their books, culture and customs, including medicine. In this way, Javanese traditions survived in Bali more or less intact, and the island remained relatively isolated until the conquest by the Dutch in 1906 and 1908. Other islands in the archipelago use Jamu with regional variations.

There are a few surviving records, but often those that do exist are closely guarded by healers or their families. They are considered to be sacred, and, for example, those in the palace at Yogyakarta are closed to outsiders. In Bali, medical knowledge was inscribed on *lontar* leaves (a type of palm) and in Java on paper. Consequently, they are often in poor condition and difficult to read. Two of the most important manuscripts—*Serat kawruh bab jampi-jampi* ('A treatise on all manner of cures') and *Serat Centhini* ('Book of Centhini')—are in the Surakarta Palace library. The former contains a total of 1734 formulae made from natural materials and indications as to their use. The *Serat Centhini* is an 18th century work of 12 volumes, and, although it contains much information and advice of a general nature and numerous folk tales, it is still an excellent account of medical treatment in ancient Java.

The status of Jamu started to improve ca. 1940 with the Second Congress of Indonesian Physicians, at which time it was decided that an in-depth study of traditional medicine was needed. A further impetus was the Japanese occupation of 1942–1944, when the Dai Nippon government set up the Indonesian Traditional Medicines Committee; another boost occurred during Indonesia's War of Independence, when orthodox medicine was in short supply. President Sukarno decreed that the nation should be self-supporting, so many people turned to the traditional remedies used by their ancestors (see Beers, 2001).

Jamu contains many elements of TCM, such as treating 'hot' illnesses with 'cold' remedies, and of Ayurveda, in which religious aspects and the use of massage are very important. Remedies from Indonesia such as clove (*Syzygium aromaticum*), nutmeg (*Myristica fragrans*), Java tea (*Orthosiphon stamineus* (=O. *aristatus*) and *Orthosiphon* spp.), jambul (*Eugenia jambolana*) and galangal (*Alpinia galanga*) are still used around the world as medicines or culinary spices.

Kampo

Kampo, or traditional Japanese medicine, is sometimes referred to as low-dose TCM. Until 1875 (when the medical examination for Japanese doctors became restricted to Western medicine), the Chinese system was the main form of medical practice in Japan, having arrived via Korea and been absorbed into native medicine. Exchange of scholars with China meant that religious and medical practices were virtually identical; for example, the medical system established in Japan in 701 was an exact copy of that of the T'ang dynasty in China. In the Nara period (710–783), when Buddhism became even more popular, medicine became extremely complex and included facets of Ayurveda as well as of Arabian medicine. Native medicine remained in the background and, after concerns that it would be subsumed into Chinese medicine, the compendium of Japanese medicine, *Daidoruijoho*, was compiled in 808 on the orders of the Emperor Heizei. In 894, official cultural exchange with China was halted, and native medicine was temporarily reinstated. However, knowledge gained from China continued to be assimilated, and in 984 the court physician Yasuyori Tamba compiled the *Ishinho*, which consisted of 30 scrolls detailing the medical knowledge of the Sui and T'ang dynasties. Although based entirely on Chinese medicine, it is still invaluable as a record of medicine as practised in Japan at that time.

In 1184, the framework began to change when a reformed system was introduced by Yorimoto Minamoto in which native medicine was included, and by 1574 Dosan Manase had set down all the elements of medical thought, which became a form of independent Japanese medicine during the Edo period. This resulted in Kampo, and it remained the main form of medicine until the introduction of Western medicine in 1771, by Genpaku Sugita. Although Sugita did not reject Kampo and advocated its use in his textbook *Keieiyawa*, it fell into decline because of a lack of evidence and an increasingly scholastic rather than empirical approach to treatment. Towards the end of the 19th century, despite important events such as the isolation of ephedrine (Fig. 2.2) by Nagayoshi Nagai, Kampo was still largely ignored by the Japanese medical establishment. However, by 1940, a university course on Kampo was instituted, and now most schools of medicine in Japan offer courses on traditional medicine integrated with Western medicine. In 1983, it was estimated that approximately 40% of Japanese clinicians were writing Kampo herbal prescriptions and current research in Japan and Korea continues to confirm the validity of many of its remedies (Takemi et al., 1985).

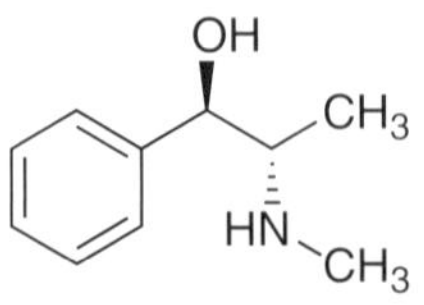

(−)-Ephedrine

Fig. 2.2 (−)-Ephedrine from *Ephedra* spp.

Medicine at the Centre of the Americas—Aztecs and Other Cultures

We have numerous written documents relating to the medicines used in Asia and Europe, but very little has been documented in writing for the Americas. Until 1492, American medicine was truly traditional, without links with the 'Old World'. Under Spanish rule, interest in plants known to Amerindians produced manifold contributions to the world's medicine and science.

The first written document dates from 1552 and is by Martín de la Cruz, the *Libellus de Medicinalibus Indorum Herbis* (Little Book of the Medicinal Herbs of the Indians). It is written in Nahuatl, the Aztec's language, and was translated into Latin by Juan Badiano. The book describes the medicinal properties of plants used in the highlands of Mexico with colour illustrations. This first illustrated and descriptive text on American traditional plant-based medicine gave rise to pioneering works on American medical botany, including Fray Bernadino de Sahagún's famous *Codex Florentino* (ca. 1570), and Francisco Hernandez's *'History of the Plants of New Spain'* (1571–1576), providing a basis for bioscientific assessment of the documented effects desired by the Aztecs. Similar compilations in the former Inca empire (De Acosta 1588, Monardes 1568) responded more to current medical interests in Europe. Over four centuries, plants from the Americas were heralded as potential panaceas. Quinine (from the bark of *Cinchona officinalis* L.) and D-tubocurarine (from arrow poisons), both derived from South American plants, changed medicine and world history (see Chapter 6).

The European Middle Ages and Arabia

After the conquest of the southern part of the Roman Empire by Arab troops, Greek medical texts were translated into Arabic and adapted to the needs of the Arabs. Many of the Greek texts survived only in Arab transcripts. Ibn Sina, or Avicenna from Afshana (980–1037), wrote a monumental treatise *Qânûn fi'l tibb* ('Canon of medicine'; ca. 1020), which was heavily influenced by Galen and which in turn influenced the scholastic traditions especially of southern Europe. This five-volume book remained the most influential work in the field of medicine and pharmacy for more than 500 years, together with direct interpretations of Dioscorides' work. Although many Arab scholars worked in eastern Arabia, Arab-dominated parts of Spain became a second centre for classical Arab medicine. An important early example is the *Umdat at-tabib* ('The medical references') by an unknown botanist from Seville. Similarly, the pharmacist, botanist and physician Ibn al-Baytar (1197–1248) systematically recorded Islamic physicians' contributions to medicine during the Middle Ages and, most importantly, approximately 300–400 new medicinal preparations from this period.

Thanks to the tolerant policies of the Arab administration, many of the most influential representatives of Arab scholarly traditions were Jews, including Maimonides (1135–1204) and Averroes (1126–1198). In Christian parts of Europe, the texts of the classical Greeks and Romans were copied from the Arabian records and annotated, often by monks. The Italian monastery of Monte Cassino is one of the earliest examples of such a tradition; others developed around the monasteries of Chartres (France) and St Gall (Switzerland).

A common element of all monasteries was a medicinal plant garden, which was used both for growing herbs to treat patients and to teach the younger generation about medicinal plants. The species included in these gardens were common to most monasteries, and many of the species are still important medicinal plants nowadays. Of particular interest is the *Capitulare de villis* of Charles the Great (Charlemagne, 747–814), who ordered that medicinal and other plants should be grown in the King's gardens and in monasteries and specifically listed 24 species. Walahfri(e)d Strabo (808 or 809–849), Abbot of the monastery of Reichenau (Lake Constance), deserves mention because of his *Liber de cultura hortum* ('Book on the growing of plants'), the first 'textbook' on (medical) botany, and the *Hortulus*, a Latin poem about the medical plants grown in the district. The *Hortulus* is not only famous as a piece of poetry but also as a vivid and excellent description of the appearance and virtues of medicinal plants. Table 2.2 lists the plants reported in the *Capitulare de villis* and in some other sources of the 10th and 11th centuries. Currently, many of these plants are still important medicinally or in other ways. Many are vegetables, fruits or other foods. The list shows not only the long tradition of medicinal plant use in Europe but also the importance of these resources to the state and religious powers during the Middle Ages. Although these were not necessarily of interest as scholarly writings, they were at least a practical resource.

A plan (which was not executed) for a medicinal herb garden for the Cloister of St Gall. (Switzerland), dating from the year 820, has been preserved and gives an account of the species that were to be grown in a cloister garden. In general, pharmacy and medicine were of minor importance in the European scholastic traditions, as shown for example by the fact that in the Monastery of St Gall there were only six books on medicine but 1000 on theology. Scholastic traditions, influenced by Greek-Arab medicine and philosophy, were practised in numerous European cloisters. The first medical centre of medieval Europe was established in Salerno, Italy, in the 12th century. Until 1130, before the Council of Clermont, the monks combined medical and theological work, but after this date only lay members of the monastery were permitted to practise medicine. Simultaneously, the first universities (Paris 1150, Bologna 1088, Oxford 1096, Monpellier 1180, Prague 1348) were founded which provided training in medicine.

The climax of medieval medicobotanical literature was reached in the 11th century with *De viribus herbarum* ('On the virtues of herbs') and *'De viridibus herbarium carmen'*, a poem by Macer floridus, presumed to be a pseudonym of Odo de Meung. In this educational poem, 65 medicinal plants and spices are presented. Other frequently cited sources are the descriptions of the medical virtues of plants by the Benedictine nun, early mysticist and abbess Hildegard of Bingen (1098–1179). In her works *Physica* and *Causae et curae* she included many remedies that were popularly used during the 12th century. Her writings also focus on prophetic and mystical topics. The works of both scholars are available only as later copies in other texts, which unfortunately gives a rather distorted idea of the originals because they are heavily reinterpreted.

Printed Reports in the European Tradition (16th Century)

For more than 1500 years the classical and most influential book in Europe had been Dioscorides' *De materia medica*. Until the Europeans' (re)invention of printing in the mid-15th century (by Gutenberg), texts were hand-written codices, which were used almost exclusively by the clergy and scholars in monasteries. A wider distribution of the information on medicinal plants in Europe began with the early herbals, which rapidly became very popular and which made the information about medicinal plants available in the languages of lay people. These were still strongly influenced by Graeco-Roman concepts, but during the 16th century many other sources began to have an influence (Table 2.3).

TABLE 2.2 Species of Plants Listed in the *Capitulare de villis*

Botanical Name[a]	Family	English Name	Geographic Origin
Achillea millefolium[b,c]	Asteraceae	Yarrow	Northern hemisphere
Agrimonia eupatoria[b,c]	Rosaceae	Agrimony	Europe, southeastern Asia
Allium ampeloprasum	Alliaceae	Leek	Western Mediterranean
Allium ascalonicum	Alliaceae	Shallot	Western Asia
Allium cepa	Alliaceae	Onion	Western Persia
Allium sativum	Alliaceae	Garlic	Southeastern Asia
Allium schoenoprasum	Alliaceae	Chives	Southern Europe
Althaea officinalis	Malvaceae	Marsh mallow	Eastern Mediterranean
Anethum graveolens	Apiaceae	Dill	Western Asia, southern Europe
Anthriscus cerefolium (L.) Hoffm.[b]	Poaceae	Chervil	Western Asia, southeastern Europe
Apium graveolens[b]	Apiaceae	Celery	Western Asia, southern Europe
Artemisia abrotanum[b]	Asteraceae	Southernwood, old man	Eastern Europe, western Asia
Artemisia absinthium[b,c]	Asteraceae	Wormwood	Europe, Asia
Beta vulgaris	Chenopodiaceae	Beetroot	Mediterranean and Northern Europe
Brassica oleracea var *acephala* DC	Brassicaceae	Kale, borecole	Mediterranean and Northern Europe
Brassica oleracea var. *gongylodes*	Brassicaceae	Kohlrabi	Mediterranean and Northern Europe
Castanea sativa Mill.	Fagaceae	Sweet chestnut	Southern Europe, Africa, southeastern Asia
Cichorium intybus	Asteraceae	Chicory	Europe, Asia
Coriandrum sativum	Apiaceae	Coriander	Southern Europe, Asia
Corylus avellana	Betulaceae	Hazel	Europe, Asia
Cucumis melo[b]	Cucurbitaceae	Melon	Africa, southern Asia
Cucumis sativus	Cucurbitaceae	Cucumber	Western India
Cuminum cyminum	Apiaceae	Cumin	Turkey, eastern Europe
Cydonia oblonga	Rosaceae	Quince	Western Asia
Ficus carica	Moraceae	Fig	Western Mediterranean
Foeniculum vulgare Mill.[b]	Apiacae	Fennel	Mediterranean
Iris x germanica[b]	Iridaceae	Iris	Southeastern Europe
Juglans regia	Juglandaceae	European walnut	Western Asia, eastern Europe
Juniperus sabina	Juniperaceae	Juniper	Alps, southern Europe
Lactuca sativa	Asteraceae	Lettuce	Western Asia, southern Europe
Lagenaria siceraria (Molina) Standl.[b]	Cucurbitaceae	Calabash, bottle gourd	Africa, Asia (America)
Laurus nobilis	Lauraceae	(Bay) laurel	Southeastern Europe, southwestern Asia
Lepidium sativum	Brassicaceae	Pepperwort	Orient
Levisticum officinale W.D.J. Koch[b]	Apiaceae	Lovage	Persia/Iran
Lilium candidum[b]	Liliaceae	Lily	Western Asia
Malus pumila (Mill.)	Rosaceae	Apple	Europe, western Asia
Malva neglecta Wallr.	Malvaceae	Mallow	Europe, Asia
Marrubium vulgare[b,c]	Lamiaceae	Horehound	Mediterranean
Mentha pulegium[b]	Lamiaceae	Pennyroyal	Mediterranean
Mentha spicata subsp. *spicata* (syn.: *Mentha crispa*)	Lamiaceae	True spearmint	Mediterranean
Mentha spp.[b]	Lamiaceae	Mint	Southern Europe, Mediterranean
Mespilus germanica	Rosaceae	Medlar	Southeastern Europe, western Asia
Morus nigra	Moraceae	Mulberry	Western Asia
Nepeta cataria[b]	Lamiaceae	Catnip	Eastern Mediterranean
Nigella sativa	Ranunculaceae	Nigella, black cumin	Western Asia, southern Europe
Papaver somniferum[b]	Papaveraceae	Opium poppy	Mediterranean
Pastinaca sativa	Apiaceae	Parsnip	Europe, Caucasus
Petroselinum crispum (Mill.) Fuss	Apiaceae	Parsley	Southeastern Europe, western Asia

Continued

TABLE 2.2   Species of Plants Listed in the *Capitulare de villis*—cont'd

Botanical Name[a]	Family	English Name	Geographic Origin
Prunus amygdalus Batch (=*P. dulcis* (Mill.) D.A.Webb)	Rosaceae	(Sweet) almond	Western Asia
Prunus avium (L.) L./*P. cerasus*	Rosaceae	Wild cherry, mazzard	Europe, Asia, Persia
Prunus domestica	Rosaceae	Plum	Western Asia
Prunus persica (L.) Batsch	Rosaceae	Peach	China
Pyrus communis	Rosaceae	Pear	Central and southern Europe, southwestern Asia
Raphanus raphanistrum subsp. *sativus* (L.) Domin (syn.: *Raphanus sativus*)[b]	Brassicaceae	Radish	Western Asia
Rosa gallica[b]	Rosaceae	French rose	Southern Europe
Rosmarinus officinalis	Lamiaceae	Rosemary	Mediterranean
Ruta graveolens[b]	Rutaceae	Rue	Southeastern Europe
Salvia officinalis[b]	Lamiaceae	Sage	Southeastern Europe, Mediterranean
Salvia sclarea[b]	Lamiaceae	Clary (sage)	Mediterranean
Satureja hortensis	Lamiaceae	Summer savoury	Western Mediterranean
Sorbus domestica	Rosaceae	Service tree	Central and southern Europe, southwestern Asia
Stachys officinalis (L.) Trevis. (*Betonica officinalis* L.)[b,c]	Lamiaceae	Betony	Western Europe, Mediterranean
Tanacetum balsamita[b]	Asteraceae	Balsamite, costmary	Southeastern Europe
Tanacetum vulgare	Asteraceae	Tansy	Europe, Caucasus

[a]Unless stated otherwise, the species was first and validly described by Carl von Linnaeus and the abbreviation is 'L.'
[b]Species listed by Walahfried Strabo in his *Hortulus* (information based on Vogellehner (1987)).
[c]Not in the *Capitulare de villis* but in other sources from the period.

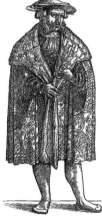

Fig. 2.3 Leonhard Fuchs. (Reproduced with permission from The University Library, Tübingen.)

Herbals were rapidly becoming available in various European languages, and in fact many later authors copied, translated and reinterpreted the earlier books. This was especially so for the woodcuts used for illustration (Fig. 2.4); these were often used in several editions or were copied. The herbals changed the role of European pharmacy and medicine and influenced contemporary orally transmitted popular medicine. Previously there had been two lines of practice: the herbal traditions of the monasteries and the popular tradition, which remains practically unknown. Books in European languages made scholastic information much more widely available, and it seems that the literate population was eager to learn about these medicopharmaceutical practices. These new books became the driving force of European 'phytotherapy', which developed rapidly over the following centuries.

The trade in botanical drugs increased during this period. From the East Indies came nutmeg (*M. fragrans* Houtt., Myristicaceae), already used by the Greeks as an aromatic and for treating gastrointestinal problems. Rhubarb (*Rheum palmatum* L. and *Rh. officinale* Baill., Polygonaceae) arrived in Europe from India in the 10th century and was used as a strong purgative. Another important change at this time was the discovery of healing plants with new properties, during the exploration and conquest of the 'New Worlds'—the Americas, as well as some regions of Asia and Africa. For example, 'guayacán' (*Guaiacum sanctum*, Zygophyllaceae), from Meso-America, was used against syphilis, despite its lack of any relevant pharmacological effects.

Nicolás Monardes was particularly important in the dissemination of knowledge about medicinal plants from the New World. His principal work, *Historia medicinal de las cosas que se traen de nuestras Indias Occidentales que sirven en medicina* ('Medical history of all those things which are brought from our Western India and may be used as medicines') was published in 1574. Some parts had appeared as early as ca. 1530. Another influential scholar during this period was Theophrastus Bombastus of Hohenheim, better known as Paracelsus (1493–1541). His importance lies less in the written record he left but more in his medical and pharmaceutical inventions and concepts. He rejected the established medical system and, after a fierce fight with the medical faculty of Basel in 1528, fled to Salzburg. According to some sources, he had publicly burned the 'Canon of medicine' by Avicenna. He introduced minerals into medical practice and called for the extraction of the active principle from animals, plants or minerals, a goal that was not achieved until the beginning of the 19th century (see later). He regarded the human body as a 'microcosm', with its substances and powers needing to be brought into harmony with the 'macrocosm' or universe. According to Paracelsus, healing was due to 'the power of life, which is only supported by the medical doctor and the medicine'.

TABLE 2.3   Examples of Early European Herbals from the 15th and 16th Centuries (Based on Leibrock-Plehn, 1992; Arber, 1938)

Year	Author	Title	Language
1478	Dioscorides	*De materia medica*	Latin
1481	Anon.	The Latin Herbarius	Latin
1485	Anon.	The German Herbarius (*Gart der Gesundheit*)	German
1525	Anon.	Herball (*Rycharde Banckes' Herball*)	English
1526 (ca.)	Anon.	*Le grand herbier en francoys*	French
1530	Otto Brunfels	*Herbarum vivae eicones ad naturae imitationem*	Latin
1530–1574	Nicolás Monardes	*Historia medicinal de las cosas que se traen de nuestras Indias Occidentales que sirven en medicina*	Spanish
1532	Otto Brunfels	*Contrafayt Kreüterbuch*	German
1533	Eucharius Rösslin/Adam Lonitzer (1946)	*Kreüterbuch von allen Erdtgewächs*	German
1534	Various	*Ogrod zdrowia* ('The garden of health')	Polish
1541	Conradus Gesnerus	*Historia plantarum et vires ex Dioscorides*	Latin
1542	Leonhard Fuchs (Fig. 2.3)	*De historia stirpium commentarii insignes*	Latin
1543	Leonhard Fuchs	*New Kreüterbuch*	German
1546	Hieronymus Bock	*Kreüterbuch*	German
1546	Dioskorides	*Kreüter Buch* (translated by J. Dantzen von Ast)	German
1548	William Turner	*Libellus de re herbaria novus, in quo herbarium*	Latin
1554	Remibertus Dodonaeus	*Cruÿterboeck*	Flemish
1554	Pietro A. Mattioli	*Commentarii, in libros sex pedacii Dioscoridis Anazarbi*	Latin/Italian
1560 (ca.)	(Pseudo) Albertus Magnus	*Ein neuer Albert Magnus*	German
1563	Garcia ab Horto (Orto/d'Orta)	*Orto/coloquios dos simples, e drogas he cousas medicinais da India* (Portuguese d'Orta; first published in Goa, India)	Portuguese
1576	Carolus Clusius	*Rariorum aliquot stirpium per hispanias observatarum historia*	Latin
1588	Jakob Theodor (Tabernae montanus)	*Neuw Kreüterbuch*	German
1596	Casparus Bauhinus	*Phytopinax*	Latin
1596	John Gerard	*General historie of plantes* (or The 'Herball')	English
1597	Antoine Constantin	*Brief traicté de la pharmacie provinciale…*	French

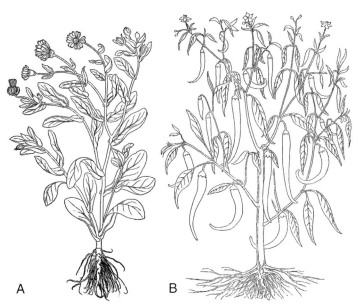

Fig. 2.4 Examples of early woodcuts: (A) marigold or Ringelblume (*Calendula officinalis* L.), one of the most important medicinal plants in historical and modern phytotherapy; (B) capsicum (chili pepper; *Capsicum frutescens* L.). (Reproduced with permission from The University Library, Tübingen.)

Although some of his ideas anticipated later ones, at the time they were largely rejected. The first pharmacopoeias were issued by autonomous cities and became legally binding documents on the composition, preparation and storage of pharmaceuticals.

> **THE FIRST PHARMACOPOEIAS:**
> - *Ricettario Fiorentino* (Florence, Italy), 1498.
> - *Pharmacopoeia of Nuremberg* (Frankonia, Germany) or *Pharmacorum omnium*, 1546.
> - *Pharmacopoeia Londiniensis* (UK), 1618, one of the most influential early pharmaceutical treatises.

These pharmacopoeias were mainly intended to bring some order into the many forms of preparation available at the time and the varying composition of medicines and to reduce the problems arising out of their variability.

Another development was the establishment of independent guilds specialising in the sale of medicinal plants, even though apothecaries had practiced this for centuries. In 1617, the Worshipful Society of Apothecaries was founded in London, and in 1673 it formed its own garden of medicinal plants, known today as the Chelsea Physic Garden (Minter, 2000). One of the most well-known English apothecaries (and astrologers) of the 17th century is Nicholas Culpeper (1616–1654), best known for his 'English physician'—more commonly called 'Culpeper's herbal'. This is the only herbal that rivals in popularity John Gerard's *General historie of plantes*, but his arrogant dismissal of orthodox practitioners made him very unpopular with many physicians. Culpeper describes plants that grow in Britain and which can be used to cure a person or to 'preserve one's body in health'. He is also known for his translation *A physicall directory* (from Latin into English) of the London Pharmacopoeia of 1618 published in 1649 (Arber, 1938).

MEDICAL HERBALISM

The use of medicinal plants was always an important part of the medical systems of the world, and Europe was no exception. Little is known about popular traditions in medieval and early modern Europe, and our knowledge starts with the availability of written (printed) records on medicinal plant use by common people. As pointed out by Griggs (1981: 88), a woman in the 17th century was a 'superwoman' capable of administering 'any wholesome receipts or medicines for the good of the family's health'. A typical example of such a remedy is foxglove (*Digitalis purpurea*), reportedly used by an English housewife to treat dropsy, and then more systematically by the physician William Withering (1741–1799; Fig. 2.5). Withering transformed the orally transmitted knowledge of British herbalism into a form of medicine that could be used by medical doctors. Prior to that, herbalism was more of a clinical practice interested in the patient's welfare and less of a systematic study of the virtues and chemical properties of medicinal plants.

European Pharmacognosy and Natural Product Chemistry in the 18th and 19th Centuries

In the 17th and 18th centuries, knowledge about plant-derived drugs expanded, but attempts to 'distillate' the active ingredients from plants were unsuccessful. The main outcome during this period was detailed observations on the clinical usefulness of medicinal products, which had been recorded in previous centuries or imported from non-European countries. The next main shift in emphasis came in the early 19th century, when it became clear that the pharmaceutical properties of plants are due to specific molecules that can be isolated and characterised. This led to the development of a field of research now called **natural product chemistry** or, specifically for plants, **phytochemistry**. Pure chemical entities were isolated and their structures elucidated. Some were then developed into medicines or chemically modified for medicinal use. Examples of such early pure drugs include:

- **Morphine** (Fig. 2.6), from opium poppy (*Papaver somniferum* L., Papaveraceae), was first identified by F.W. Sertürner of Germany (Fig. 2.7) in 1804 and chemically characterised in 1817 as an alkaloid. The full structure was established in 1923 by J.M. Gulland and R. Robinson in Manchester.

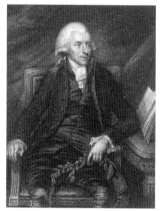

Fig. 2.5 William Withering. (Reproduced with permission from The Wellcome Library, London.)

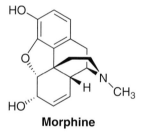

Morphine

Fig. 2.6 Morphine from opium poppy (*Papaver somniferum*).

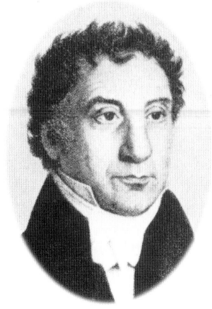

Fig. 2.7 F.W. Sertürner. (Reproduced with permission from Wood Library-Museum of Anesthesiology, Park Ridge, IL.)

- **Quinine** (Fig. 2.8), from cinchona bark (*Cinchona succirubra* Vahl and others), was first isolated by Pierre Joseph Pelletier and Joseph Bienaime Caventou of France in 1820; the structure was elucidated in the 1880s by various laboratories. Pelletier and Caventou were also instrumental in isolating many of the alkaloids mentioned later.
- **Salicin**, from willow bark (*Salix* spp., Salicaceae), was first isolated by Johannes Buchner in Germany. It was derivatised first (in 1838) by Rafaele Pirea (France) to yield salicylic acid, and later (1899) by the Bayer company, to yield acetylsalicylic acid, or **aspirin**—a compound that was previously known but which had not been exploited pharmaceutically (Fig. 2.9).

EXAMPLES OF PURE COMPOUNDS ISOLATED DURING THE EARLY 19TH CENTURY:

Atropine (1833), from belladonna (*Atropa belladonna* L., Solanaceae), was used at the time for asthma.

Caffeine (1821), from the coffee shrub (*Coffea arabica* L. and *C. canephora* Pierre ex A. Froehner, Rubiaceae); its structure was elucidated in 1882.

Coniine, a highly poisonous natural product, was first isolated in 1826 from hemlock (*Conium maculatum* L., Apiaceae). Its properties had been known for years (Socrates used hemlock to commit suicide), and it was the first alkaloid to have its structure elucidated (1870). Some years later it was synthesised (1889).

Emetine (1817), from ipecacuanha (*Carapichea ipecacuanha* (Brot.) L. Andersson, syn.: *Cephaelis ipecacuanha* (Brot.) Willd., Rubiaceae), was fully characterised as late as 1948 and used as an emetic as well as in cough medications.

Strychnine (1817), from *Strychnos* spp. (Loganiaceae), was used as a tonic and stimulant (Sneader, 1996).

In addition, early in the 19th century, the term 'pharmacognosy' was coined by the Austrian professor Johann Adam Schmidt (1759–1809) and was included in his posthumously published book *Lehrbuch der Materia Medica* (1811). This period thus saw the development of a well-defined scientific field of inquiry, which developed rapidly during the century.

One of the main achievements of 19th century science in the field of medicinal plants was the development of methods to study the pharmacological effects of compounds and extracts. The French physiologist

Claude Bernard (1813–1878), who conducted detailed studies on the pharmacological effects of plant extracts, must be considered one of the first scientists in this tradition. He was particularly interested in curare—a drug and arrow poison used by the American Indians of the Amazon and the focus of research of many explorers. The ethnobotanical story of curare is described further in Chapter 5 (von Humboldt, 1997).

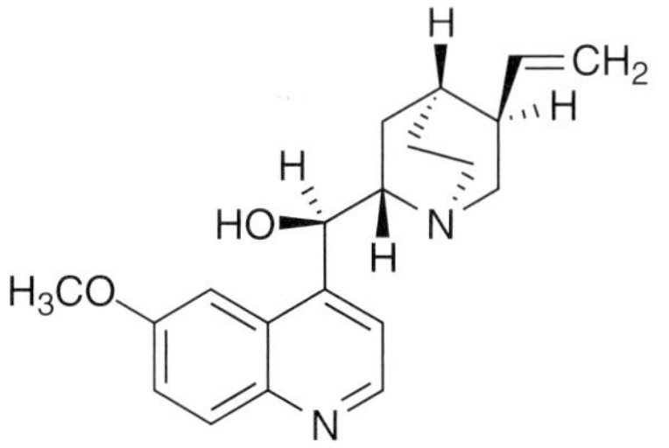

Bernard noted that, if curare was administered into living tissue directly, via an arrow or a poisoned instrument, it resulted in death more quickly and that death occurred more rapidly if dissolved curare was used rather than the dried toxin (Bernard, 1966:92). He was also able to demonstrate that the main cause of death was by muscular paralysis and that animals showed no signs of nervousness or pain. Further investigations showed that, if the blood flow in the hind leg of a frog was interrupted using a ligature (without affecting the innervation) and the curare was introduced via an injury of that limb, the limb retained mobility and the animal did not die (Bernard, 1966:95–96, 115 [orig. 1864]). One of the facts noted by all those who reported on curare is the lack of toxicity of the poison in the gastrointestinal tract, and, indeed, the Indians used curare both as a poison and as a remedy for the stomach.

Bernard went on to say:

> *In our physiological studies we were able to identify the effect of the American arrow poison curare as one on the nervous motoric element and subsequently to determine a mechanism which results in death, which is an inert ability of this poisoned substance, but do we have to stop here and have we reached the border which our current [19th century] science allows us to reach? I do not think so. One has to separate the active principle of curare from the foreign substances, with which it is mixed, and one also has to study which physical and chemical changes the toxic substance imprints onto the organic element [i.e. the body] in order to paralyse its activity.*
>
> **Bernard, 1966:121 (orig. 1864), translation MH**

Later, the botanical source of curare was identified as *Chondrodendron tomentosum* Ruiz & Pavon, the agent largely responsible for the pharmacological activity first isolated. It was found to be an alkaloid and named D-tubocurarine because of its source, 'tube curare', so-called because of the bamboo tubes used as storage containers. In 1947 the structure of this complex alkaloid, a bisbenzylisoquinoline, was finally established (Fig. 2.10). The story of this poison is one of the most fascinating examples of transforming a drug used in an indigenous culture into a medication and research tool, and, although D-tubocurarine is currently used less frequently for muscular relaxation during surgery, it has been used as a template for the development of newer and better drugs.

The 19th century thus saw the integration of ethnobotanical, pharmacological and phytochemical studies, a process that had taken many decades but which allowed the development of a new approach to the study and the pharmaceutical use of plants. Ultimately, herbal remedies became transformed into chemically defined drugs.

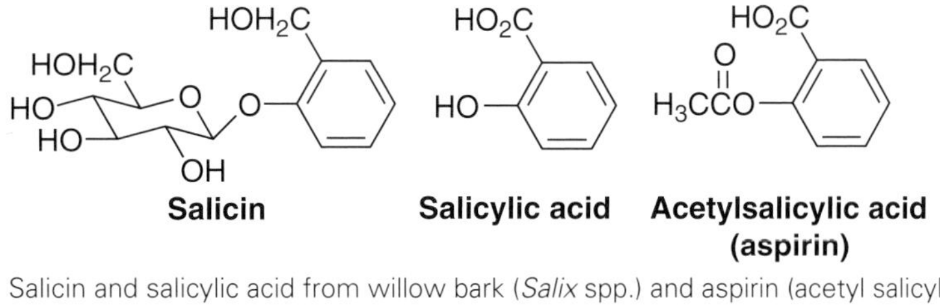

Fig. 2.8 Quinine from cinchona bark (*Cinchona succirubra*).

Salicin   Salicylic acid   Acetylsalicylic acid (aspirin)

Fig. 2.9 Salicin and salicylic acid from willow bark (*Salix* spp.) and aspirin (acetyl salicylic acid).

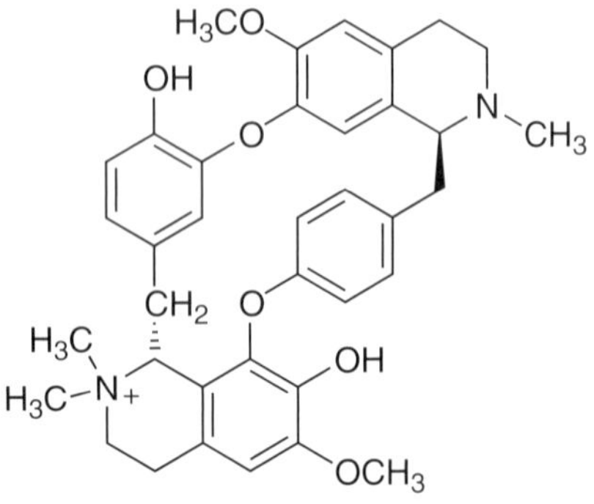

Tubocurarine

Fig. 2.10 D-tubocurarine from the American arrow poison curare.

The 20th Century

One of the most important events that influenced the use of medicinal plants in the Western world in the past century was the serendipitous discovery of the antibacterial properties of fungal metabolites such as benzylpenicillin, by Florey and Fleming in 1928 at St Mary's Hospital (London). These discoveries changed forever the perception, and use, of natural compounds from plants and fungi as medicines, by medical practitioners, scientists, and the lay public. Another important development came with the advent of synthetic chemistry in the field of pharmacy. Many of these studies involved compounds that were synthesised because of their potential as colouring material (Sneader, 1996). The first successful use of a synthetic compound as a chemotherapeutic agent was achieved by Paul Ehrlich in Germany (1854–1915); he successfully used methylene blue in the treatment of mild forms of malaria in 1891. Unfortunately, this finding could not be extended to the more severe forms of malaria common in the tropics. Many further studies on the therapeutic properties of dyes and of other synthetic compounds followed.

The latter part of the 20th century saw a rapid expansion in knowledge of secondary natural products, their biosynthesis and biological and pharmacological effects. A large number of natural products or their derivatives, including many anticancer agents (Taxol, the Vinca alkaloids; see Chapter 9), the antimalarial agent artemisinin and the antidementia medication galantamine, to name just a few, were introduced as medicines (Heinrich, 2010; Heinrich & Teoh, 2004; Newman & Cragg, 2012). Numerous examples of drugs that are natural products, their derivatives or a pharmacophore based on a natural product have been introduced. There is now a better understanding of the genetic basis of the reactions that give rise to such compounds and the biochemical (and in many cases genetic) basis of many important illnesses. This has opened up new opportunities and avenues for drug development. This culminated in 2015 with the Nobel Prize in Physiology or Medicine being awarded to Youyou Tu (2011), William C. Campbell and Satoshi Ōmura for their seminal contribution to the discovery and development of novel nature-derived medicines for treating parasitic diseases.

REFERENCES

Arber, A., 1938. Herbals. their origin and evolution. A chapter in the history of botany. Cambridge University Press, Cambridge.

Beers, S.-J., 2001. Jamu. the ancient art of indonesian herbal healing. Periplus Editions (HK) Ltd, Singapore.

Bernard, C., 1966. Physiologische Untersuchungen über einige amerikanische Gifte. Das Curare. In: Bernard, C., Mani, N. (Eds.), Ausgewählte Physiologische Schriften. Huber Verlag, Bern, pp. 84–133. [orig. French 1864].

Booker, A., 2015. Chinese medicine: contentions and global complexities. In: Heinrich, M., Jaeger, A.K. (Eds.), Ethnopharmacology. Wiley, Chichester.

Capasso, L., 1998. 5300 years ago, the ice man used natural laxatives and antibiotics. Lancet 352, 1894.

Griggs, B., 1981. Green pharmacy. A history of herbal medicine. Norman & Hobhouse, London.

Heinrich, M., 2010. Ethnopharmacology and drug development. In: Mander, L., Lui, H.-W. (Eds.), Comprehensive Natural Products II Chemistry and Biology. vol. 3. Elsevier, Oxford. pp. 351–338.

Heinrich, M., Leonti, M., Frei-Haller, B., 2014. A perspective on natural products research and ethnopharmacology in México. The eagle and the serpent on the prickly pear cactus. J. Nat. Prod. 77, 678–689.

Heinrich, M., Teoh, H.L., 2004. Galantamine from snowdrop – the development of a modern drug against Alzheimer's disease from local Caucasian knowledge. J. Ethnopharmacol. 92, 147–162.

Leibrock-Plehn, L., 1992. Hexenkräuter oder Arznei: Die Abtreibungsmittel im 16 und 17 Jahrhundert. Heidelberger Schriften zur Pharmazie- und Naturwissenschaftsgeschichte. Wissenschaftliche Verlagsgesellschaft, Stuttgart. Bd 6.

Leroi-Gourhan, A., 1975. The flowers found with Shanidar IV, a Neanderthal burial in Iraq. Science 190, 562–564.

Lietava, J., 1992. Medicinal plants in a middle paleolithic grave Shanidar IV. J. Ethnopharmacol. 35, 263–266.

Mazar, G., 1998. Ayurvedische Phytotherapie in Indien. Z. Phytother. 19, 269–274.

Minter, S., 2000. The apothecaries' garden. Sutton Publications, Stroud.

Newman, D.J., Cragg, G.M., 2012. Natural products as sources of new drugs over the 30 years from 1981 to 2010. J. Nat. Prod. 75, 311–335.

Sneader, W., 1996. Drug prototypes and their exploitation. Wiley, Chichester.

Solecki, R.S., 1975. Shanidar IV, a Neanderthal flower burial in northern Iraq. Science 190, 880–881.

Sommer, J.D., 1999. The Shanidar IV 'flower burial': a re-evaluation of Neanderthal burial ritual. Cambridge Archaeol. J. 9 (1), 127–137.

Takemi, T., Hasegawa, M., Kumagai, A., Otsuka, Y., 1985. Herbal medicine: kampo, past and present. Tsumura Juntendo Inc., Tokyo.

Totelin, L., 2015. When foods become remedies in ancient Greece: the curious case of garlic and other substances. J. Ethnopharmacol. 67, 30–37.

Tu, Y., 2011. The discovery of artemisinin (qinghaosu) and gifts from Chinese medicine. Nat. Med. 17, 1217–1220.

Vogellehner, D., 1987. Jardines et verges en Europe occidentale (VIII–XVIII siècles). Flaran 9, 11–40.

von Humboldt, A., 1997. Die Forschungsreise in den Tropen Amerikas. [Studienausgabe Bd 2, Teilband 3]. Wissenschaftliche Buchsgesellschaft, Darmstadt.

Waller, F., 1998. Phytotherapie der traditionellen chinesischen Medizin. Z. Phytother. 19, 77–89.

FURTHER READING

Adams, M., Berset, C., Kessler, M., Hamburger, M., 2009. Medicinal herbs for the treatment of rheumatic disorders – a survey of European herbals from the 16th and 17th century. J. Ethnopharmacol. 121, 343–359.

Burger, A., Wachter, H., 1998. Hunnius pharmazeutisches Wörterbuch, 8 Aufl. Walter de Gruyter, Berlin.

Harvey, A.L., Edrada-Ebel, R.A., Quinn, R.A., 2015. The re-emergence of natural products for drug discovery in the genomics era. Nat. Rev. Drug Discov. 14, 111–129.

SECTION 2

Plant drugs

3

General Principles of Botany: Morphology and Systematics

The chapters in this section provide a short introduction to the bioscientific basis for all aspects of the use of plants in pharmacy required for understanding herbal medicines and pure natural products.

The following case study shows not only that knowledge about medicinal plants is relevant, because pharmacy uses many pure natural products derived from plants, but also that pharmacists can and should advise patients about common medicinal plants.

A (HYPOTHETICAL) CASE STUDY BASED ON G. HATFIELD'S RESEARCH ABOUT THE USAGE OF MEDICINAL PLANTS IN NORFOLK: While you are working as a locum pharmacist, a patient informs you that his general practitioner is worried about unexplained low levels of potassium (hypokalaemia). Among other things, the patient is complaining of chronic constipation and requests several pharmaceuticals. He also reports that he uses a 'herbal tea', which he prepares from the plant he calls 'pick-a-cheese' and grows in his back garden. This tea helps him to overcome the problem of constipation.

How do you react? Is the patient using a little known, but unproblematic, herbal product? Further inquiry about the case tells you:
- 'Pick-a-cheese' may be a widely distributed garden plant and weed known also as 'common mallow', which has the botanical name of *Malva sylvestris*, or it may be some other botanical species known under the same common name.
- Upon your request, the patient brings you a branch of the plant and with the help of the scientific (botanical) literature you make a positive identification of this plant as *M. sylvestris*. The identification is based on the features of the plant (leaves, fruit, flowers) that you are able to observe.
- In checking the active constituents (especially polysaccharides) you come to the conclusion that the plant is unlikely to contribute to the symptoms as they were reported by the patient. The plant is widely used as a local food item (also, for example, in Mediterranean France) and as a household remedy. Toxic natural products seem to be absent. Therefore, the search for a cause of the hypokalaemia continues…

For further information on Norfolk country remedies readers are referred to Hatfield, G., 1994. Country Remedies. The Boydell Press, Woodbridge.

PLANTS AND DRUGS

Pharmacognosy is the study of medical products derived from our living environment, especially those derived from plants and fungi. From the botanical point of view, the first concern is how to define a pharmaceutical (or medical) plant-derived drug.

In the context of pharmacy a botanical drug is a product that is either:
- derived from a plant and transformed into a drug by drying certain plant parts, or sometimes the whole plant, or
- obtained from a plant, but no longer retains the structure of the plant or its organs and contains a complex mixture of biogenic compounds (e.g. fatty and essential oils, gums, resins, balms).

The term 'drug' is linguistically related to 'dry' and is presumably derived from the Middle Low German *droge* ('dry').

Isolated pure natural products such as the numerous pharmaceuticals used in pharmacy are thus not 'botanical drugs', but rather chemically defined drugs derived from nature. Botanical drugs are generally derived from specific plant organs of a plant species. The following plant organs are the most important, with the Latin name that is used, for example in international trade, in parentheses:
- Aerial parts or herb (herba).
- Leaf (folia).
- Flower (flos).
- Fruit (fructus).
- Bark (cortex).
- Root (radix).
- Rhizome (rhizoma).
- Bulb (bulbus).

A large majority of botanical drugs in current use is derived from leaves or aerial parts.

Botanically speaking, a plant-derived drug should be defined in terms of not only the species from which it is obtained, but also the plant part that is used to produce the dried product. Thus, a drug is considered to be adulterated if the wrong plant parts are included (e.g. aerial parts instead of leaves).

In the following sections of this chapter, a brief overview of botanical taxonomy is given, and then the higher plants are discussed on the basis of their main organs, function, morphology and anatomy. Since most of the pharmaceutical products derived from plants are from the higher plants (or Magnoliopsida), little reference is made here to other plants such as lichens, mosses or algae, or to mushrooms or microorganisms.

Microscopic characteristics play an important role in identifying a botanical drug. Although microscopy is now only rarely used in everyday pharmaceutical practice, there are a large number of features that allow the identification of botanical material. Since classical textbooks provide an extensive description of such features, microscopic identification is only occasionally discussed in this introductory textbook.

These days, drug identification is achieved using a combination of methods, including thin-layer chromatography, high-performance liquid chromatography and microscopic methods. In large (phyto-) pharmaceutical companies, near-infrared spectroscopy has become an essential tool.

TAXONOMY

The **species** is the principal unit within the study of **systematics**. Biological diversity is subdivided into greater than 500,000 discontinuous units (the botanical species) and greater than 2 million zoological species. The species is thus the basic unit for studying relationships among living organisms. Systematicists study the relationships between species.

Taxonomy is the science of naming organisms and their correct integration into the existing system of nomenclature. Each of these names is called a **taxon** (pl. taxa), which thus stands for any named taxonomic unit. In order to make this diversity easier to understand, it is structured into a series of highly hierarchical categories, which ideally should represent the natural relationship between all the taxa.

A species is generally characterised as having morphologically similar members and being able to inbreed. Since Carl Linnaeus, the names of species are given in binomial form: the first part of the name indicates the wider taxonomic group, the **genus**; the second part of the name is the **species**. Plant species must be reported in a taxonomically correct way and a wide range of Internet resources exists, including the 'Medicinal Plant Name Service' (https://www.kew.org/science/our-science/science-services/medicinal-plant-names-services) and the 'WFO Plant List' (https://wfoplantlist.org/plant-list).

In order to better understand biological diversity, the species are arranged into clusters of varying degrees of similarity, forming a hierarchy. The basic classification of the plant kingdom into divisions circumscribes the main groups of plants, including the following:
- Algae, including the green algae (Chlorophyta) and the red algae (Rhodophyta).
- Mosses (Bryophyta).
- Ferns (Pteridophyta).
- Seed-bearing plants (Spermatophyta).

As mentioned above, only a few algae, mosses and ferns have yielded pharmaceutically important products and will therefore only be discussed very cursorily.

The Importance of Taxonomy

The exact naming (taxonomy) and an understanding of the species' relationship to other species is an essential basis for pharmacognostical work. Only such endeavour allows the correct identification of a botanical drug, and consequently is the basis for further pharmacological, phytochemical, analytical or clinical studies.

MORPHOLOGY AND ANATOMY OF HIGHER PLANTS (SPERMATOPHYTA)

Flower

The flower (Fig. 3.1) is the essential reproductive organ of a plant. It is frequently very showy in order to attract pollinators, but in other instances the flowers are minute and difficult to distinguish from the neighbouring organs or from other flowers.

For an inexperienced observer, two characteristics of a flower are particularly noteworthy: their size and colour. Although these are often

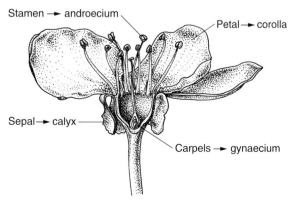

Fig. 3.1 Schematic line drawing of a flower.

> ### THE OPIUM POPPY, *PAPAVER SOMNIFERUM* L.
>
> **Binomial**: This is the genus and species names, plus the authority. Thus, in this example, *Papaver somniferum* is the binomial (the basic unit of taxonomy and systematics). It is followed by a short abbreviation (in this case 'L.'), which indicates the botanist who provided the first scientific description of the species and who assigned the botanical name (in this example, 'L.' stands for Carl von Linnaeus (or Linné), a Swedish botanist (1707–1778) who developed the binomial.*
>
> **Species**: (*Papaver*) *somniferum,* here meaning 'sleep-producing'.
>
> **Genus**: *Papaver* (a group of species, in this case poppies, which are closely related).
>
> **Family**: Papaveraceae (a group of genera sharing certain traits, named after one of the genera).
>
> **Order**: Ranunculales.
>
> **Division** (=Phylum): Magnoliophyta (flowering plants with covered seeds).
>
> **Kingdom**: Plantae (the plants), one of three kingdoms, the others being the animals and fungi.
>
> In this textbook, we provide the full name of a plant species wherever possible, this includes the plant's binomial name (i.e. genus and species) as well as the abbreviated name of the person who described this taxon in a validated way. This is essential for exactly defining what species is used medicinally.

*In some cases, there is first a name in parentheses, followed by a second name not in parentheses. For example, in the case of the common aloe, *Aloe vera* (L.) Burm. f., the name in parentheses indicates the author (Linnaeus) who first described the species but assigned it to a different genus. The second name in this case, Burm. f., stands for the 18th century botanist Nicolaas Laurens Burman; f. stands for *filius* (son), since he is the son of another well-known botanist who provided numerous first descriptions of botanical species.

good characteristics of a species, others are more important from a botanical point of view.

Such characteristics include the form of the various parts of a flower; whether these parts are fused (joined) or separate (free); how many of each of these structures normally exist per flower; whether or not all flowers on a plant (or in a group of plants of the same species) are similar. Morphologically speaking, many parts of the flower are modified leaves, which during the development of higher plants have taken on specific functions for reproduction:
- The **calyx,** with individual sepals, generally serves as an outer protective cover during the budding stage of the flower. It is often greenish in colour, can be either fused or separate, and may sometimes drop off at the beginning of the flowering phase (e.g. *Chelidonium majus* L., greater celandine).
- The **corolla,** with individual petals, serves as an important element to attract the pollinator in animal-pollinated flowers. It is either fused or separate and may be very reduced, for example, in plants pollinated with the help of the wind. Most commonly, the number of petals is regarded as a key feature and can vary from a well-defined number (e.g. four, five or six) to a large number that is no longer counted (written as ∞). The colour of the petals is not a good characteristic generally, since it may vary within a genus or even within a species. All of these features—i.e. the number and form of the petals, whether they are fused or not and their size—are important pieces of information for identifying a plant.
- The **androecium,** with its individual **stamens** (also known as 'stamina') which produce the pollen, forms a ring around the innermost part of the flower. In some species, the anther is restricted to

only some of the flowers on a plant (whereas the others only have a gynaecium). In other species, androecium-bearing flowers are restricted to some plants, whereas the others bear flowers with only a gynaecium. Again, their number is important for identifying a plant.

- **Gynaecium** (pl. gynaecia; also called gynoecium) with individual carpels. This develops into the fruit (i.e. the seed covered by the pericarp) and includes the ovules (the part of the fruit bearing the reproductive organs which develop into the seeds).
- The **stigma** and **style**—together with the gynaecium—form the **pistil**. Their size and form are important differences between species.

Another essential aspect of the flower's morphology is the position of the gynaecium with respect to the position of the corolla on the pistil: i.e. epigynous (the corolla and other elements of the flower are attached to or near the summit of the ovary), or hypogynous (the corolla and other elements of the flower are attached at or below the bottom of the ovary).

Inflorescences

The way in which flowers are arranged to form an inflorescence is another useful feature for recognising (medicinal) plants, but this is beyond the scope of this introduction (Heywood, 1993).

Drugs

Although the flowers are of great botanical importance, they are only a minor source of drugs used in phytotherapy or pharmacy. A very important example is:

- Chamomile, *Matricaria recutita* L. (Matricariae flos).
  Other examples include
- Calendula, *Calendula officinalis* L. (Calendulae flos).
- Arnica, *Arnica montana* L. (Arnicae flos).
- Hops, *Humulus lupulus* L. (Humuli flos).

Fruit and Seed

The development of seeds occurred relatively late in the evolution of plants. The lower plants, such as algae, mosses and ferns, do not produce seeds. Gymnosperms such as the maidenhair tree (*Ginkgo biloba* L.) (see below) were the first group of organisms to produce seeds, from which the angiosperms or fruit-bearing plants evolved. The gymnosperms are characterised by seeds that are not covered by a secondary outer protective layer, but only by the testa—the seed's outer layer.

In the angiosperms, the ovule and later the seed are covered with a specialised organ (the carpels), which in turn develops into the pericarp (Fig. 3.2). This, the outer layer of the fruit, can either be hard as in nuts, all soft as in berries (dates, tomatoes), or hard and soft as in a drupe (cherry, olives). Drugs from the fruit thus have to be derived from an angiosperm species.

The morphology of a fruit provides important information as to the identity of a plant species or medicinal drug. Another distinction of fruits is based on the number of carpels and gynaecia per fruit, which may be:

- Simple (developed from a single carpel).
- Aggregate (several carpels of one gynaecium are united in one fruit, as in raspberries and strawberries).
- Multiple (gynaecia of more than one flower form the fruit).

Drugs

Fruits and seeds have yielded important phytotherapeutic products, including:
Fruit
- Caraway, *Carum carvi* L. (Carvi fructus).
- Fennel, *Foeniculum vulgare* Mill. (Foeniculi fructus).

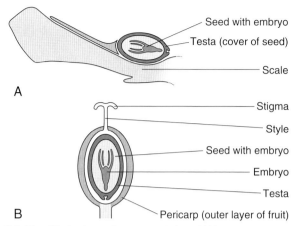

Fig. 3.2 Simplified schematic representation of (A) a gymnosperm seed sitting on a scale (as in a fir tree) and (B) an angiosperm fruit, covered by both the testa and the pericarp.

- Saw palmetto, *Serenoa repens* (Bartram) J.K. Small (Sabal fructus).
- Schizandra/schisandra, *Schisandra chinensis* (Turcz.) Bail. (Schisandrae fructus).

Seed
- (White) mustard, *Sinapis alba* L. (Sinapi semen).
- Horse chestnut seeds, *Aesculus hippocastanum* L. (Hippocastani semen).
- Ispaghula, *Plantago ovata* Forssk. and other *Plantago* spp. (Plantago ovatae semen), and psyllium, *Plantago afra* L. (syn *P. psyllium* L., Psylli semen).

Leaves

The leaves arise out of the stem; their key function is the assimilation of glucose and its derivative, starch, from water and carbon dioxide (photosynthesis) using energy provided by sunlight.

PHOTOSYNTHESIS: The net photosynthetic reaction is:

$$6CO_2 + 6H_2O \xrightarrow{hv} C_6H_{12}O_6 \text{ (glucose)} + 6O_2$$

This process is key not only to the survival of all plants but also in providing the energy and, ultimately, the basic building blocks for the secondary metabolites, which are used as pharmaceuticals.

The function of the leaves, as collectors of the sun's energy and its assimilation, results in their typical general anatomy with a petiole (stem) and a lamina (blade). In many cases, the petiole is reduced or may be missing completely. Plants have adapted to a multitude of environments and this adaptation is reflected in the anatomical and morphological features of the leaf. For example, adaptation to dry conditions gives rise to leaves that conserve moisture, which may be fleshy or possess a thick cuticle. These are termed xerophytic leaves, and include oleander (*Nerium oleander* L.).

The lower surface of the leaf is generally covered with stomata, pores that are surrounded by specialised cells and that are responsible for the gaseous exchange between the plant and its environment (uptake of CO_2 and emission of water vapour and O_2).

The nodes (or 'knots') are the parts of the stem where the leaves and lateral buds join; the intermediate area is called the internodium. A key characteristic of a species is the way in which the leaves are arranged on the stem. For example, they may be (Fig. 3.3):

- **Alternate**: the leaves form an alternate or helical pattern around the stem, also called spiral.

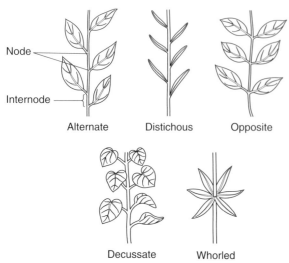

Fig. 3.3 Types of arrangements of leaves.

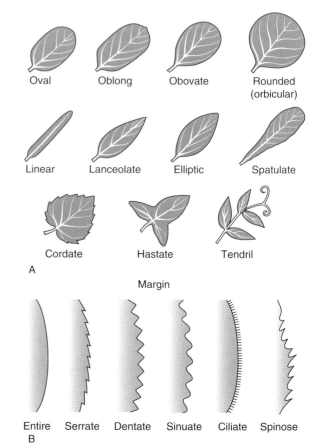

Fig. 3.4 (A) Characteristic shapes of leaves. (B) Characteristic margins of leaves.

- **Distichous**: there is a single leaf at each node, and the leaves of two neighbouring nodes are disposed in opposite positions.
- **Opposite**: the leaves occur in pairs, with each leaf opposing the other at the nodes.
- **Decussate**: this is a special case of opposite, where each successive pair of leaves is at a right angle to the previous pair (typical for the mint family).
- **Whorled**: three or more leaves are found at one node.

Another important characteristic is the form of the leaves. Typically, the main distinction is between simple and compound. Simple leaves have blades that are not divided into distinct morphologically separate leaflets, but form a single blade, which may be deeply lobed. In compound leaves, there are two or more leaflets, which often have their own small petioles (called petiolules). The form and size of leaves are essential characteristics (Fig. 3.4A). For example, leaves may be described as oval, oblong, rounded, linear, lanceolate, ovate, obovate, spatulate or cordate. The margin of the leaf is another characteristic feature. It can be entire (smooth), serrate (saw-toothed), dentate (toothed), sinuate (wavy) or ciliate (hairy) (Fig. 3.4B). Also, the base and the apex often have a very characteristic form.

Microscopic characteristics of leaves include the form and number of stomata, the inner structure of the leaves, specialised secretory tissues including trichomes or hairs, of two types: glandular and covering (very large, stiff, covering trichomes are often referred to as bristles), and the presence of calcium oxalate structures, which give a characteristic refractive pattern under polarised light.

The powdered leaves of several members of the nightshade family (Solanaceae), which yield some botanical drugs that are important for the industrial extraction of the alkaloid atropine, cannot be distinguished using normal chemical methods since they all contain similar alkaloids. On the other hand, they can easily be distinguished microscopically by the presence of different forms of crystals formed by the different species and deposited in the cells (Fig. 3.5).

Drugs

Numerous drugs contain leaf material as the main component. Some widely used ones include the following:
- (Lemon) balm, *Melissa officinalis* L. (Melissae folium).
- Deadly nightshade, *Atropa belladonna* L. (Belladonnae folium) (and other solanaceous species).

None of these are used in phytotherapy, but rather for the extraction of alkaloids, of which they have a high content.

- Ginkgo, *Ginkgo biloba* L. (Ginkgo folium).
- Green tea, *Camellia sinensis* (L.) Kuntze (Theae folium).
- Peppermint, *Mentha × piperita* L. (Menthae folium).
- (Red) bearberry, *Arctostaphylos uva-ursi* (L.) Spreng. (Uvae ursi folium).

Shoots (=Stem, Leaves and Reproductive Organs)

An essential differentiation needs to be made between herbaceous ('herbs') and woody plants (trees and shrubs). In both cases, the function of the stem is to provide the physical strength required for positioning the leaves/flowers and fruit in the most adaptive way. The stem is a cylindrical organ that, together with the root, forms the main axis of a plant. Herbaceous species are generally short-lived and often grow rapidly and the distinction between the outside and the inner stem can only be made by detailed examination. Woody species, on the other hand, show a clear distinction between the bark and the (inner) wood.

In the stem, the transport of water and inorganic nutrients (upward transport) is achieved in the **xylem**, which only occurs in the inner parts of the stem and forms an essential part of the wood. The **phloem**, on the other hand, is the plant part responsible for the transport of assimilates (sugars and polysaccharides), which generally occurs from the leaves downwards. Between the wood and the bark is the cambium, the tissue that gives rise to new cells, which then differentiate and form the outer (bark) and inner (wood) parts of a secondary stem. The fine structure of a bark or wood is an important diagnostic criterion for identifying a drug. The bark as an outer protective layer frequently accumulates biologically active substances; for example, several of the pharmaceutically important barks accumulate tannins.

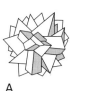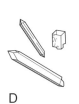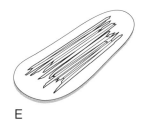

Fig. 3.5 Calcium oxalate crystals, main forms: (A) rosette (e.g. *Datura stramonium*, Solanaceae); (B) sand (e.g. *Atropa belladonna*, Solanaceae); (C) monoclinic prism (e.g. *Hyoscyamus niger*, Solanaceae); (D) needles (e.g. *Iris germanica*, Iridaceae); (E) raphides (e.g. *Urginea maritima*, Hyacinthaceae).

Drugs: Stem

Stem material is often part of those drugs that are derived from all above-ground parts (herb or herba). No stem-derived drug is currently of major importance. Some underground organs used as drugs (rhizome of tormentil) or food (potato) are in fact modified stems that have taken on specific new functions (storage, spreading of the plant) (as discussed in the following section).

Drugs: Bark

- Frangula, *Frangula alnus* Mill. (syn. *Rhamnus frangula* L.) (Frangulae cortex).
- Red cinchona, *Cinchona pubescens* Vahl (syn.: *C. succirubra* Pav. ex Klotzsch), *C. calisaya* Wedd. (The main cultivated species in southern Asia) and *Cinchona* spp. (Cinchonae cortex).
- Oak, *Quercus petraea* (Matt.) Liebl. and *Qu. robur* L. (Quercus cortex).
- Willow, *Salix alba* L. and *Salix* spp. (Salicis cortex).

Drugs: Aerial Parts (=Stem, Leaves Plus Flowers/Fruit)

- Ephedra, *Ephedra sinica* Stapf (Ephedra herba).
- Hawthorn, *Crataegus monogyna* Jacq. and *C. laevigata* (Poir.) DC. (syn. *C. oxycantha*) (Crataegi herba or Crataegi folium cum flore).
- Passion flower, *Passiflora incarnata* L. (Passiflora herba).
- Wormwood, *Artemisia absinthium* L. (Absinthii herba); in Africa and Asia, sweet or annual wormwood (*Artemisia annua* L.) is used in the treatment of malaria.

The substitution of leaves with aerial parts of the same species is a common problem with cheap phytopharmaceuticals used as 'health food supplements'. These adulterated drugs often contain fewer and/or other active constituents and this points to the need to define not only the species, but also the plant part to be used pharmaceutically.

Root

Three functions of a typical root are of particular importance to a plant:
- It provides an anchor in the ground or any other substrate and thus allows the development of the plant's above-ground organs (anchorage).
- It is the main organ for the uptake of water and inorganic nutrients (absorption and conduction).
- It often serves to store surplus energy, generally in the form of polysaccharides such as starch and inulin (storage).

The root is generally composed of an outer layer (the bark of the root including the hypodermis) and an inner cylinder, containing the xylem and the phloem. The two organs of the root are separated by the endodermis, an inner protective layer. Water and inorganic nutrients are transported upwards in the xylem; assimilates are transported in the phloem.

Very young plants have a primary root, which during development soon becomes thicker and adds layers of secondary tissue. It is the secondary roots—often roots or rootstocks with a special storage function—that are used in pharmacy.

Rootstock and Specialised Underground Organs

Some underground organs can be distinguished on botanical grounds from the root. Although they may have some functions similar to roots, botanically they are derived from other parts of the plants; they are therefore a separate group of plant organs and yield another group of botanical drugs. They include rhizomes and tubers (generally, both are morphologically a stem) and underground bulbs (morphologically derived from parts of the leaves).

Rhizome and Root (Radix) Drugs

Underground organs of only a few species have yielded pharmaceutically important drugs. Examples include the following:
- Devil's claw, *Harpagophytum procumbens* (Burch.) DC. ex Meisn. (Harpagophyti radix, thickened roots).
- Korean ginseng, *Panax ginseng* C.A. Mey. (Ginseng radix).
- Tormentill, *Potentilla erecta* (L.) Raeusch. (syn. *Potentilla tormentilla* Stokes, Potentillae radix).
- Echinacea, *Echinacea angustifolia* DC., *E. pallida* (Nutt.) Nutt. and *E. purpurea* (L.) Moench (Echinacea radix).
- Siberian ginseng, *Eleutherococcus senticosus* (Rupr. & Maxim.) Maxim. Maxim. (Eleutherococci radix).
- Kava-kava, *Macropiper methysticum* (G. Forst.) Miq. (better known under its synonym: *Piper methysticum* G. Forst.; Rhizoma Piperis Methystici, kava-kava rhizome).
- Chinese foxglove root, *Rehmannia glutinosa* (Gaertn.) DC. (Rehmannia radix).
- Rhubarb, *Rheum palmatum* L., and *Rh. officinale* Baill., as well as their hybrids (Rhei radix, thickened roots).
- Sarsaparilla, *Smilax ornata* Lem., *Smilax regelii* Killip & C.V. Morton, and *Smilax* spp. (Sarsaparillae radix).

Diverse and Unspecified Botanical Drugs

Some drugs are derived from the whole plant or from specialised organs (e.g. the bulbs in the case of garlic, *Allium sativum* L.). The exudates of *Aloe vera* (L.) Burm. f. (syn. *Aloe barbadensis* Mill.) leaves are used as a strong purgative.

REFERENCES

Heywood, V.H., 1993. Flowering Plants of the World. Batsford Ltd., London. (For further references, see Chapter 4).

4

Plant Families Yielding Important Medicines

Systematics has always been an important tool in pharmacognostical practice and research. Related families often contain similar types of compounds and, therefore, may have similar beneficial or toxic effects. Consequently, an understanding of the systematic position of a medicinal plant species allows some deductions to be made about the (biologically active) secondary natural products from the species. For example, many members of the mint family are known to contain essential oil.

In this chapter, the pharmaceutically most important families are highlighted, especially those that have yielded many, or very important, botanical drugs. Because a species may yield several botanical drugs (e.g. from the flowers and the leaves), these are not included in this chapter but can be found in Part B. Here, 20 families (out of a total of more than 200 recognised families) have been selected as being particularly important or interesting and are presented in alphabetical order within the groupings angiosperms and gymnosperms. The families are not classified further; more detailed information on the systematic position of these families can be found in relevant botanical textbooks.

ANGIOSPERMS (MAGNOLIOPHYTA)

These are the plants commonly known as 'fruit-bearing plants' (i.e. the seed is covered by closed carpels). The fruits are sometimes very large and yield many of the economically important botanical products used because of their nutritional properties. An important characteristic of these plants is double fertilisation, in which cells other than the egg unite during fertilisation to give a triploid endosperm. This then develops into the fruit, which may also include other parts of the flowers. The flowers are typically fertilised by animals (i.e. zoogamous; mostly insects, but also birds, bats and spiders). Many species of this huge group have secondarily lost this trait and are fertilised with the help of the wind (e.g. oak, birch). At least 240,000 species of angiosperm are known, making it the largest group of plants. However, many estimates are much higher.

The taxon was originally split into two large groups—the Dicotyledoneae and the Monocotyledoneae—distinguished, *inter alia*, by the different number of cotyledons (primary leaves), but modern systematic classifications reject this division into only two groups.

AMARYLLIDACEAE ('MONOCOTYLEDONEAE')

Allium is the only important genus of this family, which includes important food plants, such as the common onion (*Allium cepa* L.), wild leek (*Allium ampeloprasum* L.) and chives (*Allium schoenoprasum* L.), and the food and medicinal plant garlic (*Allium sativum* L.). The genus is often included in the Liliaceae (i.e. the broadly defined lily family).

Morphologic Characteristics of the Family

These perennial herbs have underground storage organs (onions), which are used for hibernation. Typically, the flowers are composed of a perianth of two whorls of three with the sepals and petals having identical shape (i.e. the calyx and corolla are indistinguishable), six stamens and three superior, fused gynaecia. This is, in fact, the typical composition of the flowers of many related families that were previously united with the Liliaceae. The leaves are simple, annual, spirally arranged, parallel veined and often of a round shape. The fruit is a capsule.

Distribution

The 700 species of this family are found in northern temperate to Mediterranean regions.

Chemical Characteristics of the Family

The genus *Allium* is particularly well known for its very simple sulfur-containing compounds, especially alliin and allicin (Fig. 4.1), which are thought to be involved in the reported pharmacologic activities of the plants as a bactericidal antibiotic, in the treatment of arterial hypertension and in the prevention of arteriosclerosis and stroke.

APIACEAE (ALSO CALLED UMBELLIFERAE)

Important Medicinal Plants in the Family

- *Carum carvi* L. (caraway), a carminative and also important as a spice.
- *Coriandrum sativum* L. (coriander), a carminative and also important as a spice.
- *Foeniculum vulgare* Mill. (fennel), a mild carminative.
- *Levisticum officinale* W.D.J. Koch (lovage), a carminative and antidyspeptic.
- *Pimpinella anisum* L. (anise fruit, wrongly called 'seed'), an expectorant, spasmolytic and carminative.

Morphologic Characteristics of the Family

This family of nearly exclusively herbaceous species is characterised by hermaphrodite flowers in a double umbel (Fig. 4.2); note that the closely related Araliaceae have a simple umbel. Typical for the family are the furrowed stems and hollow internodes, leaves with a sheathing base and generally a much-divided lamina. The flowers are relatively inconspicuous, with two pistils, an inferior gynaecium with two carpels, a small calyx and generally a white to greenish corolla, with free petals and sepals.

Distribution

Members of this family, which has approximately 3000 species, are mostly native to temperate regions of the northern hemisphere.

Chemical Characteristics of the Family

Unlike the Araliaceae, members of this family are often rich in essential oil, which is one of the main reasons for the pharmaceutical

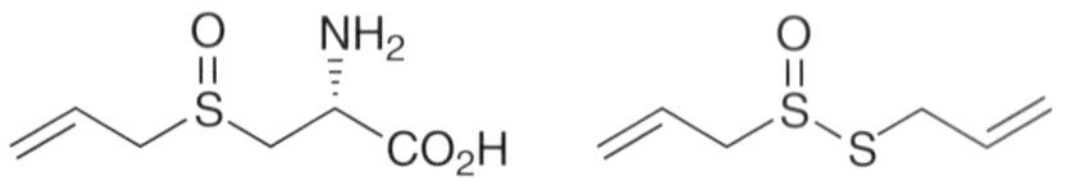

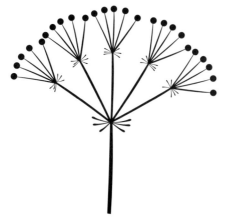

Fig. 4.1 Alliin *(left)*, allicin *(right)*.

Fig. 4.2 Double umbel.

importance of many of the apiaceous drugs (see earlier). Also common are 17-carbon skeleton polyacetylenes, which are sometimes poisonous, and (furano-)coumarins, which are responsible for phototoxic effects (e.g. in *Heracleum mantegazzianum* Sommier & Levier, hogweed). Some species accumulate alkaloids (e.g. the toxic coniine from hemlock, *Conium maculatum* L.).

ARALIACEAE

Important Medicinal Plants From the Family

- *Hedera helix* L. ((common) ivy), used as a cough remedy.
- *Panax ginseng* C.A. Mey. (ginseng), used as an adaptogen (a very ill-defined category) and to combat mental and physical stress (and sometimes replaced by *Eleutherococcus senticosus* (Rupr. & Maxim.) Maxim. (syn.: *Acanthopanax senticosus* (Rupr. & Maxim.) Harms) from the same family).

Morphologic Characteristics of the Family

This family consists mostly of woody species, characterised by hermaphrodite flowers in a simple umbel (see the closely related Apiaceae with a double umbel). The leaf lobes are hand shaped, and the flowers are relatively inconspicuous with two pistils, an inferior gynaecium, a small calyx and generally a white to greenish corolla, with free petals and sepals.

Distribution

This family of greater than 700 species is widely dispersed in tropical and subtropical Asia and in the Americas. *H. helix* is the only species native to Europe.

Chemical Characteristics of the Family

Of particular importance from a pharmacognostical perspective are the saponins, triterpenoids and some acetylenic compounds. The triterpenoids (ginsenosides) are implicated in the pharmacological effects of *P. ginseng*, while saponins (hederasaponins) are of relevance for the secretolytic effect of *H. helix*.

ASPHODELACEAE ('MONOCOTYLEDONEAE')

This family is often included in the Liliaceae (lily family).

Important Medicinal Plants From the Family

- *Aloe vera* (L.) Burman f. (syn. *Aloe barbadensis*, Barbardos aloe) and *Aloe ferox* Miller (Cape aloe), both strong purgatives

Morphologic Characteristics of the Family

Members of this family are generally perennials, and, in the case of *Aloe*, usually woody, with a basal rosette and the typical radial hermaphrodite flower structure of the Liliales. The petals and sepals are identical in form and colour and composed of 3+3 free or fused, 3+3 free stamens and three fused superior carpels.

Distribution

This family, with approximately 600 species, is widely distributed in South Africa (a characteristic element of the Cape flora); some species occur naturally in the Mediterranean (*Asphodelus*).

Chemical Characteristics of the Family

Typical for the genus *Aloe* are anthranoids and anthraglycosides (aloe-emodin), which are responsible for the species' laxative effects, as well as polysaccharides accumulating in the leaves. Contrary to other related families, the Asphodelaceae do not accumulate steroidal saponins.

ASTERACEAE—THE 'DAISY' FAMILY (ALSO KNOWN AS COMPOSITAE)

This large family has kept botanists busy for many centuries and still no universally accepted classification exists. All members of the family have a complex inflorescence (the capitula), which gave rise to the older name of the family: Compositae (= inflorescence composed of many flowers). In other features, the family is rather diverse, especially with respect to its chemistry.

Important Medicinal Plants From the Family

- *Arnica montana* L. (arnica), used topically, especially for bruises.
- *Artemisia absinthium* L. (wormwood or absinthium), used as a bitter tonic and choleretic.
- *Calendula officinalis* L. (marigold), used topically, especially for some skin afflictions.
- *Cnicus benedictus* L. (cnicus), used as a cholagogue (a bitter aromatic stimulant).
- *Cynara cardunculus var. scolymus* L. (artichoke), used in the treatment of liver and gallbladder complaints and several other conditions.
- *Echinacea angustifolia* DC., *E. pallida* (Nutt.) Nutt. and *E. purpurea* (L.) Moench (cone flower), now commonly used as an immunostimulant.
- *Matricaria recutita* L. (chamomille/camomille/chamomile; several botanical synonyms are also commonly used, including *Chamomilla recutita* and *Matricaria chamomilla*).
- *Tussilago farfara* L. (coltsfoot), a now little-used expectorant and demulcent.

Morphological Characteristics of the Family (Fig. 4.3)

The family is largely composed of herbaceous and shrubby species, but some very conspicuous trees are also known. The most important morphological trait is the complex flower head, a flower-like structure, which may in fact be composed of a few or many flowers (**capitulum** or **pseudanthium**). In some sections of the family (e.g. the subfamily Lactucoideae, which includes lettuce and dandelion), only ligulate (tongue-shaped) or disk (ray) florets are present in the dense heads. In the other major segment (subfamily Asteroideae), both ligulate and radiate/discoid flowers are present on the same flower head, the former generally forming an outer, showy ring with the inner often containing large amounts of pollen. The flowers are epigynous, bisexual or

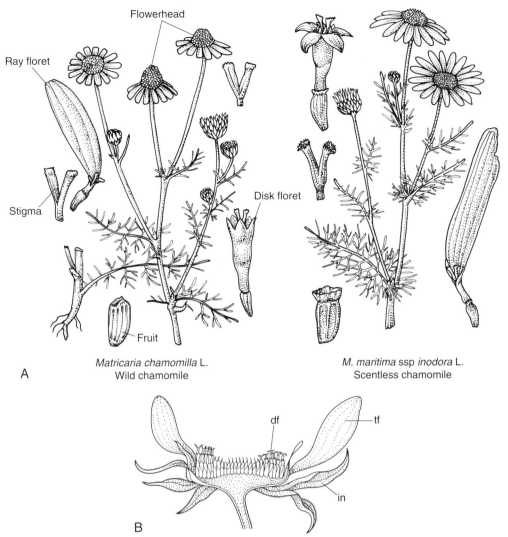

Fig. 4.3 (A) Two members of the genus *Matricaria*. (Left) *Matricaria chamomilla* L. is aromatic and used medicinally. (Right) *Matricaria maritima* L. subsp. *inodora* Schultz [=*Tripleurospermum perforatum* (Mérat) Wagenitz], also known as *Matricaria inodora*, is not aromatic and is not used medicinally. The illustration shows typical morphological differences in these two species, such as the form of the flower heads and the fruit, but it also shows how similar the two species are in many other characteristics. (B) Schematic of typical flower heads (a capitulum) of the Asteraceae (Compositae). *df*, Disk flowers; *in*, involucre; *tf*, tubular flowers. (A, From Fitch, 1924. B, From Brimble, 1942.)

sometimes female, sterile or functionally male. The (outer) calyx has five fused sepals and in many instances later develops into a pappus (feather-like in dandelions, in other instances more bristly), which is used as a means for dispersing the fruit; it is lacking in many other taxa. The fused petals (generally five) form a tubus or a ligula. The two gynaecia are epigynous and develop into tiny, nut-like fruits (achene or cypsela). The leaves are generally spirally arranged, simple, dissect or more or less compound.

Distribution

More than 21,000 species are known from practically all parts of the world, with the exception of Antarctica, and the family has found niches in a large variety of ecosystems. The family is particularly well represented in Central America and southern North America (Mexico).

Chemical Characteristics of the Family

A typical chemical trait of this family is the presence of polyfructanes (especially inulin) as storage carbohydrates (instead of polysaccharides)

in perennial taxa. Inulin-containing drugs are used for preparing malted coffee (e.g. from the rootstocks of *Cichorium intybus*, chicory). In many taxa, some segments of the family accumulate sesquiterpene lactones (typically with 15-carbon atoms, such as parthenolide; Fig. 4.4); these are important natural products responsible for the pharmacological effects of many botanical drugs, such as *Chrysanthemum parthenium* (feverfew) and *A. montana* (arnica). Polyacetylenic compounds (polyenes) and essential oil are also widely distributed. Some taxa accumulate pyrrolizidine alkaloids, which, for example, are present in *T. farfara* (coltsfoot) in very small amounts. Many of these alkaloids are known for their hepatotoxic effects. Other taxa accumulate unusual diterpenoids; for example, the diterpene glycoside stevioside (see Fig. 4.4) is of interest because of its intensely sweet taste.

CAESALPINIACEAE

This family was formerly part of the Leguminosae (or Fabaceae) and is closely related to two other families: the Fabaceae (see later) and the

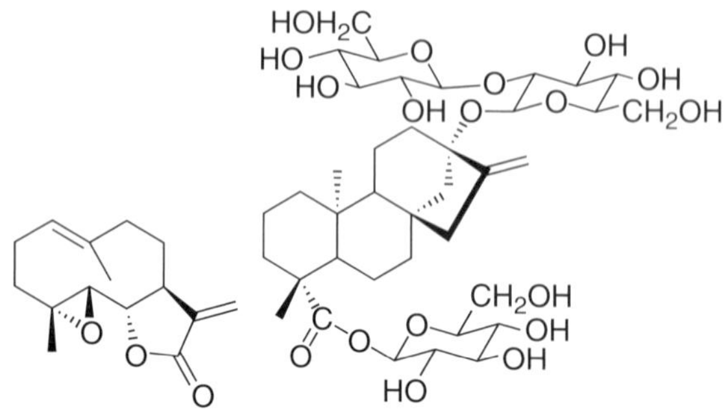

Fig. 4.4 Parthenolide *(left)*, stevioside *(right)*.

Mimosaceae (not discussed). Many contain nitrogen-fixing bacteria in root nodules. This symbiotic relationship is beneficial to both partners (for the plant, increased availability of physiologically useable nitrogen; for the bacterium, protection and optimal conditions for growth).

Important Medicinal Plants From the Family

- *Cassia senna* L. and other spp. (senna), used as a cathartic

Morphologic Characteristics of the Family (Fig. 4.5)

Nearly all of the taxa are shrubs and trees. Typically, the leaves are pinnate. The free or fused calyx is composed of five sepals, the corolla of five generally free petals and the androecium of 10 stamens, with many taxa showing a reduction in the number of stamens (five) or the development of staminodes instead of stamens. The flowers are zygomorphic and have a very characteristic shape if seen from above, resembling a shallow cup.

Distribution

The 2000 species of this family are mostly native to tropical and subtropical regions, with some species common in the Mediterranean region. The family includes the ornamental *Cercis siliquastrum* L. (the Judas tree), native to the western Mediterranean, which, according to (very doubtful) legend, was the tree on which Judas Iscariot hanged himself.

Chemical Characteristics of the Family

From a pharmaceutical perspective, the presence of anthranoids with strong laxative effects is of particular interest. Other taxa accumulate alkaloids, such as the diterpene alkaloids of the toxic *Erythrophleum*.

FABACEAE

This family is also classified together with the Mimosaceae and the Caesalpiniaceae as the Leguminosae (or Fabaceae, s.l.; see note under Caesalpiniaceae). One of its most well-known characteristics is that many of its taxa are able to bind atmospheric nitrogen.

Important Medicinal Plants From the Family

- *Cytisus scoparius* (L.) Link (common or Scotch broom), which yields sparteine (formerly used in cardiac arrhythmias, as an oxytocic, and in hypotonia to raise blood pressure).
- *Glycyrrhiza glabra* L. (liquorice), used as an expectorant and for many other purposes.
- *Melilotus officinalis* (L.) Pall. (melilot or sweet clover); the anticoagulant drug warfarin was developed from dicoumarol, first isolated from spoiled hay of sweet clover.
- *Physostigma venenosum* Balfour (Calabar bean), a traditional West African arrow poison, which contains the cholinesterase inhibitor

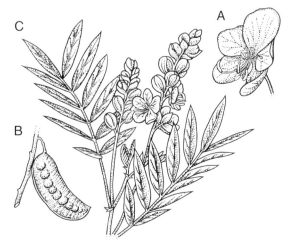

Fig. 4.5 *Cassia angustifolia*, a typical Caesalpiniaceae: (A) typical zygomorphic flower (yellow in its natural state); (B) fruit (one of the botanical drugs obtained from the species); (C) flowering branch showing leaves, composed of leaflets, and inflorescence. (Modified from Frohne & Jensen, 1998.)

physostigmine, used as a miotic in glaucoma, in postoperative paralysis of the intestine and to counteract atropine poisoning.

Morphological Characteristics of the Family

This family is characterised by a large number of derived traits. Most of the taxa of this family are herbaceous, sometimes shrubby and only very rarely trees. Typically, the leaves are pinnate, and sometimes the terminal one is modified to form a tendril, used for climbing. Bipinnate leaves are not found in this family. The five sepals are at least basally united. The corolla is formed of five petals and has a very characteristic butterfly-like shape (papilionaceous), with the two lower petals fused and forming a keel-shaped structure, the two lateral ones protruding on both sides of the flower and the largest petal protruding above the flower, being particularly showy. The androecium of 10 stamens generally forms a characteristic tubular structure with at least 9 out of 10 of the stamens forming a sheath. Normally, the fruit are pods containing beans (technically called legumes) with two sutures, which open during the drying of the fruit (Fig. 4.6).

Distribution

This is a cosmopolitan family with approximately 11,000 species and is one of the most important families. It includes many plants used as food, for example, numerous species of beans (*Phaseolus* and *Vigna* spp., *Vicia faba* L.), peas (*Pisum sativum* L.), soy (*Glycine max* (L.) Merrill), fodder plants (*Lupinus* spp.) and medicines (see earlier),

Chemical Characteristics of the Family

This large family is characterised by an impressive phytochemical diversity. Polyphenols (especially flavonoids and tannins) are common, but from a pharmaceutical perspective the various types of alkaloids are probably the most interesting and pharmaceutically relevant groups of compounds. In the genera *Genista* and *Cytisus* (both commonly called broom), as well as *Laburnum*, quinolizidine alkaloids, including cytisine and sparteine (Fig. 4.7), are common. The hepatotoxic pyrrolizidine alkaloids are found in this family (e.g. in members of the genus *Crotolaria*).

Other important groups of natural products are the isoflavonoids, known for their oestrogenic activity, and the coumarins used

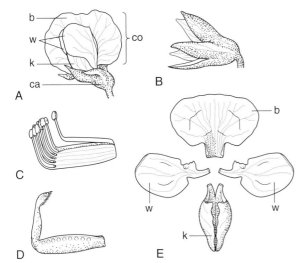

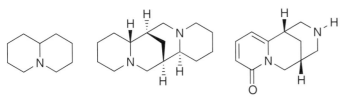

Fig. 4.6 Flower of *Pisum sativum* (common pea, Fabaceae, *sensu stricto*): (A) entire flower showing the various elements of the corolla (co): *b*, banner; *ca*, calyx; *k*, keel; *w*, wing (two); (B) calyx; (C) stamens (nine fused and one free); (D) gynaecium; (E) the four petals of the corolla. (Modified from Frohne & Jensen, 1998.)

Fig. 4.7 Quinolizidine *(left)*, sparteine *(middle)*, cytisine *(right)*.

as anticoagulants (see *Melilotus officinalis* above). *G. glabra* (licorice) is used because of its high content of the triterpenoid glycyrrhic acid, which, if joined to a sugar, is called glycyrrhizin (a saponin) and is used in confectionery as well as in the treatment of gastric ulcers (controversial). Last, but not least, the lectins must be mentioned. These large (MW 40,000 to 150,000), sugar-binding proteins agglutinate red blood cells and are a common element of the seeds of many species. Some are toxic to mammals; for example, phasins from the common bean (*Phaseolus* spp.) is the cause of the toxicity of uncooked beans.

HYPERICACEAE

This small family was formerly part of the Guttiferae and is of pharmaceutical importance because of St. John's wort, which in the last decade of the 20th century became one of the most important medicinal plants in Western medicine.

Important Medicinal Plant From the Family

• *Hypericum perforatum* L. (St. John's wort) has clinically well-established effects in mild forms of depression. It has also been used topically for inflammatory conditions of the skin.

Morphologic Characteristics of the Family

The leaves are opposite, often dotted with glands. A characteristic feature of this family is a secondary increase in the number of stamens (polyandrous flowers). The fruit are usually capsules, but berries may occur in some species.

Distribution

This family, with approximately 900 species, has its main area of distribution in the tropics and in temperate regions.

Chemical Characteristics of the Family

This small family was formerly part of the Guttiferae. St. John's wort is now one of the most important medicinal plants in Western medicine. For example, the hypericin glands, with a characteristic red colour, are present especially in the flowers and contain naphthodianthrones, including hypericin (Fig. 4.8) and pseudohypericin, which are characteristic for some sections of the genus. Typical of the family in general are also xanthones (found nearly exclusively in this family and in the Gentianaceae). The genus *Hypericum* is known to accumulate flavonoids and their glycosides (rutoside, hyperoside), as well as hyperforin (see Fig. 4.8) and its derivatives.

LAMIACEAE

The Lamiaceae is a family yielding a high number of medicinal taxa, especially due to their high content of essential oil.

Important Medicinal Plants From the Family

• *Lavandula angustifolia* Miller (lavender), a mild carminative and spasmolytic.
• *Melissa officinalis* L. (lemon balm), a mild sedative, carminative and spasmolytic.
• *Mentha arvensis* L. var. *piperascens* Malinvand (Japanese mint), yields a commonly used essential oil (e.g. for respiratory problems).
• *Mentha × piperita* L. (peppermint), a commonly used carminative and spasmolytic and a hybrid between *M. spicata* L. and *M. aquatica* L.
• *Mentha spicata* L. (spearmint), commonly used in toothpaste and chewing gum, with mild carminative effects.
• *Rosmarinus officinalis* L. (rosemary), a carminative and spasmolytic.
• *Salvia officinalis* L. (sage), used as a topical antiseptic (gargling) and orally as a carminative and spasmolytic.
• *Thymus vulgaris* L. (thyme), a carminative and spasmolytic.

Morphologic Characteristics of the Family (Fig. 4.9)

Most of the taxa in this family are herbs or small shrubs with the young stems often being four-angled. All of them have opposite simple or rarely pinnate leaves. The zygomorphic flowers, with very characteristic short-stalked epidermal glands, are very typical. They are bisexual, with five fused sepals, five generally zygomorphic petals, four or two stamens and two very characteristic fused gynaecia each divided into two partial units developing into a nut with a secondary division into nutlets.

Distribution

This important family with 5600 species is cosmopolitan and has a centre of distribution spanning from the Mediterranean to Central Asia.

Chemical Characteristics of the Family

Essential oil in the epidermal glands is very common. Some segments of the family are known to accumulate monoterpenoid glycosides (iridoids). Many species also accumulate rosmarinic acid and other derivatives of caffeic acid. Rosmarinic acid (Fig. 4.10) is of some pharmaceutical importance because of its nonspecific complement activation and inhibition of the biosynthesis of leukotrienes (leading to an antiinflammatory effect), as well as its antiviral activity.

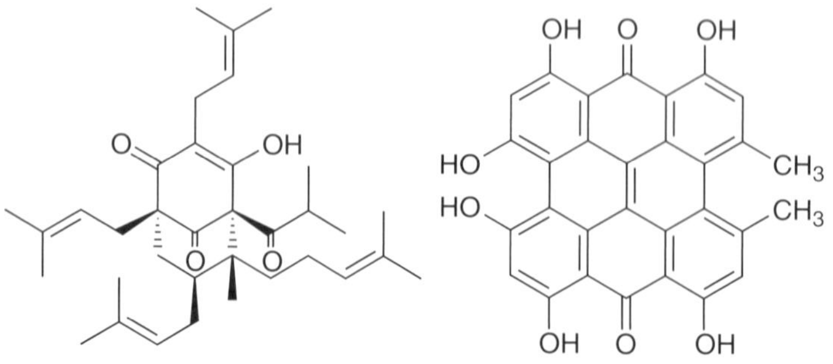

Fig. 4.8 Hyperforin *(left)*, hypericin *(right)*.

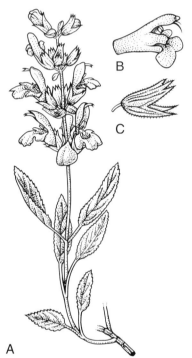

Fig. 4.9 *Salvia officinalis* (sage, Lamiaceae): (A) flowering branch showing typical leaves and the inflorescence; (B) corolla; (C) calyx. (Modified from Frohne & Jensen, 1998.)

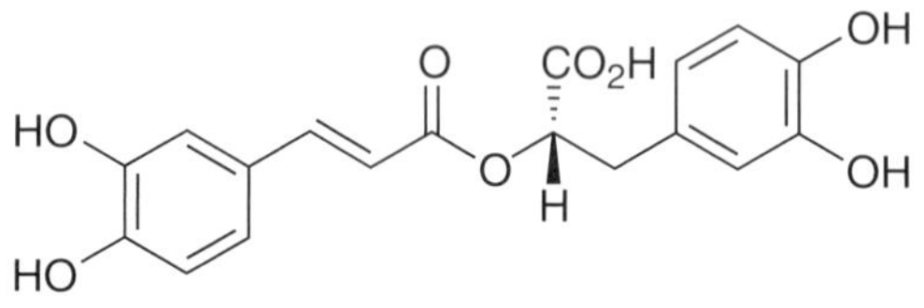

Fig. 4.10 Rosmarinic acid

Distribution

The family, with approximately 2700 exclusively evergreen woody species, is widely distributed in the tropics and subtropics.

Chemical Characteristics of the Family

The accumulation of polyphenols, some relatively simple alkaloids (especially pyridine derivatives) and steroidal saponins, as well as fatty acids (coconut (*Cocos nucifera* L.) and oil palm (*Elaeis guineensis* Jacq.)) is typical. However, the pharmaceutical use of *S. repens* seems to be due to the presence of relatively large amounts of the ubiquitous triterpenoid β-sitosterol.

PAPAVERACEAE

This rather small family has yielded a multitude of pharmaceutically or toxicologically important genera (e.g. *Chelidonium, Eschholzia, Glaucium, Papaver*), and natural products from two of its representatives are particularly widely used.

Important Medicinal Plants From the Family

- *Chelidonium majus* L. (greater celandine), which yields the alkaloid chelidonine, sometimes used as a cholagogue.
- *Papaver somniferum* L. ((opium) poppy), which yields a multitude of pharmacologically active alkaloids and is a well-known and dangerous narcotic.

Morphologic Characteristics of the Family (Fig. 4.11)

This family of (generally) herbs or subshrubs typically has spirally arranged leaves that are entire or lobed or dissected. The generally large flowers are bisexual, have an inferior gynaecium, a reduced number of sepals (two to occasionally four), often four petals and numerous stamens. The fruit is a capsule (e.g. *P. somniferum*, which is lanced to obtain opium), with valves or pores for seed dispersal.

Distribution

This small family with approximately 200 species is mostly confined to the northern temperate regions of the world.

PALMACEAE (ARECACEAE, PALMAE, 'MONOCOTYLEDONEAE')

The palms are particularly important because they include many species widely used as food, but in recent years at least one has become medically important.

Important Medicinal Plant From the Family

- *Serenoa repens* (Bartram) J.K. Small (saw palmetto, sabal), used for difficulty in micturition in benign prostate hyperplasia in the early stages.

Morphologic Characteristics of the Family

These are generally unbranched, mostly erect, trees with primary thickening of the stem and a crown of large, often branched, leaves. The flowers are generally unisexual and radial, consisting of two whorls with three perianth leaves and six stamens. The three-lobed carpels may be free or united and develop into a berry, drupe or nut.

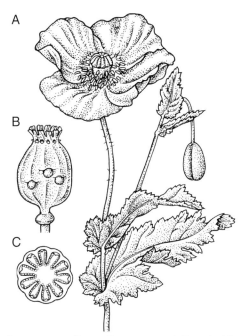

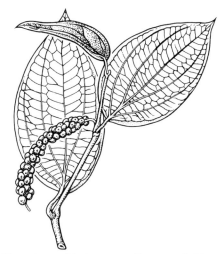

Fig. 4.13 *Piper nigram* (black pepper, Piperaceae). Line drawing of a fruiting shoot showing the typical leaves and the fruiting inflorescence. (Modified from Frohne & Jensen, 1998.)

Fig. 4.11 *Papaver somniferum* (Papaveraceae). Botanical line drawings showing (A) a flowering shoot; (B) the fruit (a capsule), with the latex shown at the lanced parts; (C) a cross-section of the fruit. (Modified from Frohne & Jensen, 1998.)

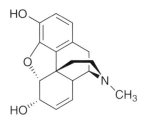

Fig. 4.12 Morphine.

Chemical Characteristics of the Family

The laticifers (or latex vessels) are rich in isoquinoline alkaloids, including morphine (Fig. 4.12), papaverine, codeine, thebaine and noscapine. Some of these alkaloids are typical benzylisoquinoline alkaloids (papaverine, noscapine); others are chemically modified and have two additional ring systems (morphinane-type skeleton).

PIPERACEAE

Important Medicinal Plants From the Family

- *Piper methysticum* Forster f. (kava-kava), traditionally used as a mild stimulant in Oceania and now used for conditions of nervous anxiety; reports of liver toxicity have resulted in withdrawal in many countries.
- *Piper nigrum* L. (black and white pepper), occasionally used in rubefacient preparations and as a spice.

Morphologic Characteristics of the Family (Fig. 4.13)

This family of shrubs and herbs or small trees generally has simple, spirally arranged leaves. The flowers are drastically reduced and sit in dense fleshy spikes.

Distribution

The family, with approximately 2000 species, is restricted to the tropics. The most important genera are *Piper* (including black pepper and kava-kava) and *Peperomia*. Some species are epiphytic (grow on other plants).

Chemical Characteristics of the Family

Pungent acidic amides, such as piperine, are known from several members of this family, and sometimes essential oil is present. The α-pyrone derivatives (e.g. kavain) from *P. methysticum* are another group of commonly found compounds known from species of *Piper*.

POACEAE ('MONOCOTYLEDONEAE')

The 'grass' family is not very important with respect to their bioactive contents, but many pharmaceuticals contain starches derived from corn, rice or wheat as excipients.

Important Medicinal Plants From the Family

- *Zea mays* L. (maize, corn) and other cereals, a common staple food; starches are also used in antidiarrhoeal preparations.

Morphologic Characteristics of the Family

Most are herbs, often with rhizomes, and sometimes perennial. The leaves are distichous (with a single leaf at each node and the leaves of two neighbouring nodes disposed in opposite positions), elongate with parallel main veins, often with a characteristic sheath at the base. A typical feature of the family is the wind-pollinated flowers, which form spike-like inflorescences (panicles).

Distribution

This cosmopolitan family has approximately 9000 species. Many of the economically important food staples are from this family and are grown all over the world.

Chemical Characteristics of the Family

Members of this family often accumulate silicates, and some members have fruits rich in polysaccharides (starch) and proteinaceous tissue, mostly in the endosperm.

RHAMNACEAE

Important Medicinal Plants From the Family

- *Rhamnus purshiana* DC. (American cascara) and *Rhamnus frangula* L. (syn. *Frangula alnus*, European alder buckthorn), both used as strong purgatives.

Morphological Characteristics of the Family

This family mostly consists of trees with simple leaves, which are arranged spirally or opposite. The flowers are small and unisexual with an epigynous gynaecium and four or five small petals. The fruit is a drupe (fleshy exocarp and mesocarp with a hard endocarp).

Distribution

A relatively small cosmopolitan family, mainly tropical and subtropical, with approximately 900 species.

Chemical Characteristics of the Family

The family is best known pharmaceutically because some taxa accumulate anthraquinones. In addition, alkaloids of the benzylisoquinoline type and the cyclopeptide type are known from many taxa.

RUBIACEAE

The family yields one of the most important stimulants, coffee (*Coffea arabica* L. and *Coffea canephora* Pierre ex Froehner) and one of the first and most important medicinal plants brought over from the 'New World', cinchona bark (see later).

Important Medicinal Plants From the Family

- *Cinchona succirubra* Weddell, *Cinchona calisaya* Weddell and *Cinchona* spp. (cinchona, Peruvian bark), used as a bitter tonic, febrifuge and against malaria.

Morphological Characteristics of the Family

This family consists mostly of trees or shrubs, with some lianas (climbing plants) and herbs. It has simple, entire and generally decussate leaves, which are nearly always opposed and which usually have connate stipules (sometimes as large as the leaves themselves, e.g. *Galium*). The usually bisexual and epigynous, insect-pollinated flowers have four to five petals and four to five sepals, and five (or four) stamens and two gynaecia. The type of fruit varies (berry, drupe, capsule).

Distribution

This is a large cosmopolitan family with more than 10,000 species, particularly prominent in the tropical and warmer regions of the world.

Chemical Characteristics of the Family

The family is known for a large diversity of classes of natural products, including iridoids (a group of monoterpenoids), alkaloids (including indole alkaloids, such as quinine from *Cinchona* spp.), methylxanthines, such as caffeine, theobromine and theophylline, and anthranoids in some taxa (e.g. the now obsolete medicinal plant *Rubia tinctorum*, which was withdrawn because of its genotoxic effect).

RUTACEAE

The family includes some of the most important fruit-bearing plants known: the genus *Citrus* with orange, lemon, lime, mandarin, grapefruit, etc.

Important Medicinal Plants From the Family

- *Pilocarpus jaborandi* Holmes and *Pilocarpus* spp. (pilocarpus), for the isolation of pilocarpine, which is used in ophthalmology.
- *Ruta graveolens* L. (rue), formerly widely used as an emmenagogue and spasmolytic, and which shows strong phototoxic side effects.

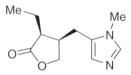

Fig. 4.14 Pilocarpine.

- Many species (especially of the genus *Citrus*) are aromatic and used as foods as well as in pharmacy and perfumery.

Morphological Characteristics of the Family

Most members of this family are trees or shrubs with spirally arranged, three pinnate or foliate (rarely simple) leaves. The bisexual flowers generally have five sepals and petals, 5+5 stamens and four or five hypogynous gynaecia.

Distribution

There are approximately 1700 species of this family distributed all over the world, but the tropics are particularly rich in them.

Chemical Characteristics of the Family

Essential oil is common in many taxa (*Citrus, Ruta*) and can be found in lysigenous secretory cavities in the parenchyma and pericarp. Alkaloids are also frequently found, especially benzyltetrahydroisoquinoline, acridone and imidazole types (pilocarpine; Fig. 4.14). The acridone alkaloids have so far only been reported from the Rutaceae. Other groups of natural products typically encountered are furanocoumarins and pyranocoumarins (e.g. bergapten from *Citrus aurantium* subsp. *bergamia*, used to flavour Earl Grey tea), as well as simple coumarins.

SOLANACEAE

This family contains the important food plants *Solanum tuberosum* L. (potato) and *Lycopersicon esculentum* Mill. (tomato), and many medicinal and toxic plants.

Important Medicinal Plants From the Family

- *Atropa belladonna* L. (deadly nightshade, belladonna)
- *Datura stramonium* L. (thorn apple, stramonium)
- *Hyoscyamus niger* L. (henbane)

These species contain tropane alkaloids with spasmolytic and anticholinergic properties such as hyoscine (scopolamine), and atropine, which is used in ophthalmology.

Morphologic Characteristics of the Family (Fig. 4.15)

The usually simple, lobed or pinnate/three-foliate leaves of these shrubs, herbs or trees are generally arranged spirally. The taxa have bisexual, radial flowers with five fused sepals, mostly five fused petals, five stamens and two gynaecia, which generally develop into a berry or a capsule.

Distribution

This family of approximately 2600 species is particularly well represented in South and Central America and is widely distributed in most parts of the world.

Chemical Characteristics of the Family

Typical for the family are alkaloids, especially of the tropane, nicotine and steroidal types (Fig. 4.16). Many taxa are characterised by oxalic acid, which often forms typical structures (e.g. sand-like in *A. belladonna*, irregular crystals in *D. stramonium*).

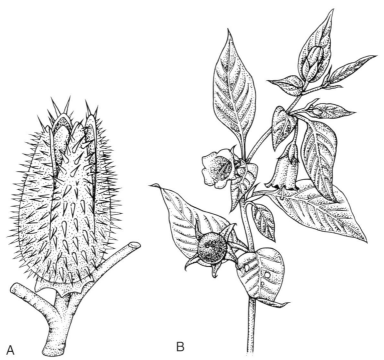

Fig. 4.15 (A) *Datura stramonium,* showing capsule enclosing the black seeds. (B) *Atropa belladonna,* showing a flowering and fruiting branch, with the violet-brown (outside) and dirty yellow (inside) flowers and the shiny black berries. (Modified from Frohne & Jensen, 1998.)

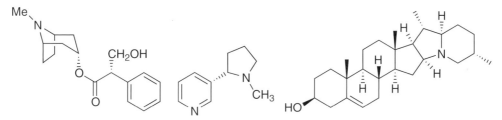

Fig. 4.16 Hyoscyamine *(left),* nicotine *(middle),* solanidine *(right).*

ZINGIBERACEAE ('MONOCOTYLEDONEAE')

In terms of pharmaceutical use, this family is the most important of the former class Monocotyledoneae (which includes the Liliaceae, Palmaceae and Poaceae). Many members of this family are native to the Indo-Malayan region and are thus particularly important in Asian medical systems.

Important Medicinal Plants From the Family

- *Curcuma zanthorrhiza* Roxburgh (Temu lawak, Javanese turmeric).
- *Curcuma longa* L. (syn. *C. domestica,* turmeric), a commonly used spice and popular remedy used, for example, for inflammatory and liver diseases, and in most Asian medical systems for a large variety of illnesses.
- *Elettaria cardamomum* (L.) Maton (cardamom), which is mostly used as a spice but also as a medicine.
- *Zingiber officinale* Roscoe (ginger), used for a large variety of illnesses, including travel sickness, respiratory and gastrointestinal disorders.

Morphological Characteristics of the Family

In general, the species of this family are aromatic herbs with very prominent thickened rhizomes. The latter are often rich in essential oil, stored in typical secretory cells. The leaves are arranged spirally or are distichous with a sheath around the stem (similar to the grasses). However, these sheaths are arranged in such a way that they form a stem-like structure, which supports the real, rather weak, stem. The zygomorphic and bisexual flowers are often very large and prominent and are pollinated by birds, bats or large (often nocturnal) insects.

Distribution

The family is distributed throughout the tropics, but many species are native to Asia (Indo-Malayan region).

Chemical Characteristics of the Family

This family is one of the few families of the former Monocotyledons, which is rich in essential oil with terpenes such as borneol, camphor and cineole (all oxygen-containing monoterpenes), camphene, pinene

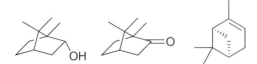

Fig. 4.17 Borneol *(left)*, camphor *(middle)*, α-pinene *(right).*

(monoterpenes) and zingiberene (a sesquiterpene), as well as phenylpropanoids (cinnamic acid derivatives) (Fig. 4.17). Typically, these compounds accumulate in oil cells, an important microscopical characteristic of the rhizomes of the Zingiberaceae.

GYMNOSPERMS

This much smaller group of seed-bearing plants differs from the angiosperms in not having the seeds enclosed in carpels (the seeds are naked) and in not having double fertilisation. The gymnosperms are generally fertilised with the help of the wind and are often characterised as having needles instead of broad leaves (the most important exception being *Ginkgo biloba*, the Chinese maidenhair tree). Only approximately 750 species are known, but some species are extremely important in the production of timber (European fir (*Abies* spp.), spruce (*Picea* spp.), Douglas fir (*Pseudotsuga menziesii* (Mirbel) Franco), all Pinaceae) and some yield medically important essential oil. The most important medicinal plant is *G. biloba*.

GINKGOACEAE

This is one of the most ancient families of the seedbearing plants and was widely distributed during the Mesozoic (180 million years ago). Only one species survives currently.

Important Medicinal Plant From the Family

- *G. biloba* L. (Chinese maidenhair tree), used for its memory-improving properties.

Morphological Characteristics of the Family (Fig. 4.18)

The characteristic fan-shaped leaves, which often have an indention at the apex, are well known. The tree does not bear fruit but has a pseudofruit, with the outer part of the seed (testa) developing into a fleshy cover, which has a strong unpleasant smell of butyric acid and a hard inner part. Fertilisation is not by pollen but by means of microspermatozoids, a characteristic of less well-advanced plants. Another typical aspect is the separation of the deposition of the microspermatozoids on the gametophytes and fertilisation (the unification of macrospermatozoid and microspermatozoid). Thus the seeds found on the ground during the autumn are not yet fertilised but will be during the winter.

Distribution

G. biloba is native to a small region in southeastern Asia and is now widely planted in many temperate regions of the world.

Chemical Characteristics of the Family

The most important, and unique, group of natural products are the ginkgolides (Fig. 4.19), which are unusual two-ringed diterpenoids with three lactone functions. Biflavonoids and glycosylated flavonoids are other groups of typical natural products.

PINACEAE

Important Medicinal Plants From the Family

- *Abies* spp. (fir).
- *Picea* spp. (spruce).

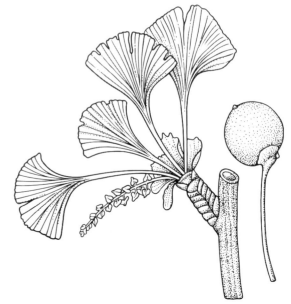

Fig. 4.18 *Ginkgo biloba* (Chinese maidenhair tree, Ginkgoaceae) showing the typical fan-shaped young leaves and a seed (sometimes wrongly called fruit). (Modified from Frohne & Jensen, 1998.)

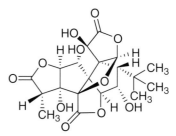

Fig. 4.19 Ginkgolide C.

Morphological Characteristics of the Family (Fig. 4.20)

The trees of this family (conifers) are evergreen and usually have opposed or whorled branches. Typically, the leaves of this family are needle shaped and linear ('pine needles'). The pollen- and gynoecium-producing flowers are separate but on one plant (monoecious). The pollen-producing cones are small and herbaceous. They produce large amounts of pollen, which is transported by the wind. The female cones are usually woody with spirally arranged scales, each usually with two ovules on the upper surface, and subtended by a more or less united bract. There are usually two winged, wind-distributed seeds per scale.

Distribution

This small family (approximately 200 species) is widely distributed in the north temperate regions of the world (including regions with long annual periods of extreme frost, such as high mountains (Alps), the northernmost parts of Western Europe and the Asian tundra) and extends into the warmer regions of the northern hemisphere. Many members of this family are accordingly very frost and drought resistant and form large tree- or shrub-dominated zones of vegetation.

Chemical Characteristics of the Family

The best-known pharmaceutical products from this family are essential oils and balsams, which are typically found in schizogenic excretion ducts of the leaves as well as in excretion pores of wood and bark. Both

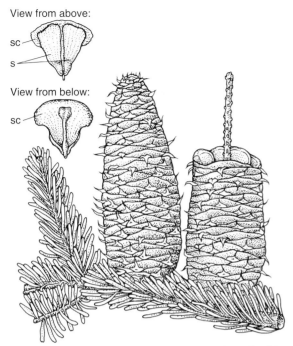

View from above:

View from below:

Fig. 4.20 *Abies alba* (fir tree, Pinaceae), showing a branch with cones, and a single scale viewed from above and below. *s*, Seed; *sc*, scale. (Modified from Frohne & Jensen, 1998.)

are rich in monoterpenoids, such as α-pinene and borneol. Mixtures of oil and resin from these species are called **turpentine**, while the resinous part is called **colophony** and is particularly rich in terpenoids (including diterpenoids such as abietic acid). Other widely reported groups of compounds from members of this family are flavonoids, condensed tannins and lignans (e.g. pinoresinol) (Fig. 4.21).

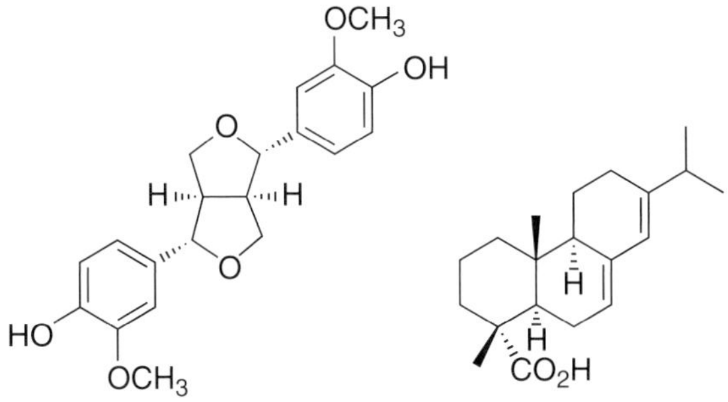

Fig. 4.21 Pinoresinol *(left)*, abietic acid *(right)*.

FURTHER READING

Angiosperm Phylogeny Group, 2016. An update of the Angiosperm Phylogeny Group classification for the orders and families of flowering plants: APG IV (PDF). Bot. J. Linn. Soc. 181 (1), 1–20.

Brimble, L.F.J., 1942. Intermediate Botany. Macmillan, London.

Evans, W.C., 2000. Trease and Evans' Pharmacognosy, fifteenth ed. WB Saunders, London.

Fitch, W.H., 1924. Illustrations of the British Flora. Reeve, London.

Frohne, D., Jensen, U., 1998. Systematik des Pflanzenreichs. 5 Aufl. Wissenschaftliche Verlagsgesellschaft, Stuttgart. http://www.wissenschaftliche-verlagsgesellschaft.de/service/widerrufsbelehrung.html.

Heywood, V.H., 1993. Flowering Plants of the World. Batsford, London.

Judd, W.S., Campbell, C.S., Kellogg, E.A., Stevens, P.F., Donoghue, M.J., 2002. Plant Systematics. A Phylogenetic Approach, second ed. Sinauer, Sunderland, MA.

Mabberly, D.J., 1990. The Plant Book. Cambridge University Press, Cambridge.

Raven, P.H., Evert, R.F., Eichhorn, S.E., 1999. Biology of Plants, sixth ed. WH Freeman, New York.

Robbers, J.E., Speedie, M.K., Tyler, V.E., 1996. Pharmacognosy and Pharmacobiotechnology. Williams & Williams, Baltimore.

Sitte, P., Ziegler, H., Ehrendorfer, F., Bresinsky, A., 1997. Lehrbuch der Botanik ('Strasburger'). 34 Aufl. Gustav Fischer Verlag, Stuttgart.

5

Ethnobotany and Ethnopharmacology

Many drugs that are commonly used today (e.g. aspirin, ephedrine, ergometrine, tubocurarine, digoxin, reserpine, atropine) came into use through the study of indigenous (including European) remedies—that is, through the scientific investigation of plants used by people throughout the world. Table 5.1 lists just a few of the many examples of drugs derived from plants. As can be seen, most plant-derived pharmaceuticals and phytomedicines currently in use were (and often still are) used by native people around the world. Accordingly, our information is derived from local knowledge as it was and is utilised throughout the world, although European and Mediterranean traditions have had a particular impact on these developments. The historical development of this knowledge is discussed in Chapter 2. This chapter is devoted to traditions as old as or older than the written records, but which have been passed on orally from one generation to the next. Some of this information, however, may have not been documented in codices or studied scientifically until very recently.

Today such 'traditional medicine' (TM) has become a priority for pharmaceutical and medical research in many countries. The World Health Organization (WHO) has developed a comprehensive strategy for developing it. The World Health Assembly resolution on TM (WHA62.13) has defined the following goals for all states:

harnessing the potential contribution of TM to health, wellness and people-centred health care;

promoting the safe and effective use of TM by regulating, researching and integrating TM products, practitioners and practice into health systems, where appropriate.

In 2018 the WHO highlighted the importance of a wide range of therapeutic approaches including TM in primary healthcare:

We support broadening and extending access to a range of health care services through the use of high-quality, safe, effective and affordable medicines, including, as appropriate, traditional medicines, vaccines, diagnostics and other technologies.
(https://www.who.int/teams/primary-health-care/conference/ declaration).

This declaration sets standards for primary healthcare at a global level (40 years after the first declaration—the Alma Ata Declaration) and it is intended to 'make bold political choices for health across all sectors'. Multisectoral approaches are endorsed, which incorporate health in all policies and prominently address the importance of the different forms of TMs, thus also setting a place for research in 'ethnopharmacology'.

Ethno*pharmacology* is an interdisciplinary field of research that looks specifically at such traditional medical systems and other empirical knowledge systems used throughout the world. Foods, toxins and other useful substances are often included in ethno*botanical* studies, which thus cover the whole range of local knowledge of and practice with useful plants. In the context of ethnopharmacology the potential

health benefits and (as with all drugs) the potential toxicological risks associated with such remedies are of particular importance. Empirical knowledge was sometimes recorded in herbals and other texts on *materia medica*. Written traditions are obviously better documented and easier to access, but both written and oral forms of indigenous phytotherapy are important factors influencing the use of medicinal plants in the Western world. Each year new plants become popular with some sections of the population (and often are as quickly forgotten again). Only a few are sufficiently well studied scientifically and can be recommended on the basis of bioscientific and/or clinical evidence.

ETHNOBOTANY

Shortly before the start of the 20th century (1896), the American botanist William Harshberger coined the term 'ethnobotany'—the study of plant use by humans.

> **Ethnobotany** studies the relationship between humans and plants in all its complexity and is generally based on a detailed observation and study of the use a society makes of plants, including all the beliefs and cultural practices associated with this use.

It is usual for ethnobotanists to live with indigenous people, to share the everyday life of their community and, of course, to respect the underlying cultures. Ethnobotanists have a responsibility both to the scientific community and to the indigenous cultures. According to the above definition, ethnobotany focuses not only on medicinal plants but also on other natural products derived from nature, such as
- Food.
- Plants used in rituals.
- Colouring agents.
- Fibre plants.
- Poisons.
- Fertilisers.
- Building materials for houses, household items, boats, etc.
- Ornamentals.
- Oil plants.

This broad definition is still used today, but modern ethnobotanists face a multitude of other tasks and challenges (as discussed in the following section). Medicinal plants have always been one of the main research interests of ethnobotany and the study of these resources has also made significant contributions to the theoretical development of the field; however, the more anthropologically oriented fields of research are beyond the scope of this introductory chapter.

ETHNOPHARMACOLOGY

Ethnopharmacology as a specifically designated field of research has had a relatively short history. The term was first used in 1967 in the title of a book on hallucinogens. The field is nowadays much more broadly defined.

TABLE 5.1   Botanical Drugs Used in Indigenous Medicine or of Importance in the Development of Modern Drugs

Botanical Name	English Name	Indigenous Use	Origin (Regional and Ethnic)	Medical Uses	Representative Active Constituents
Aesculus hippocastanum L. (Hippocastanaceae)[a]	Horse chestnut	Antiinflammatory	South-eastern Europe	Chronic inflammatory conditions, circulatory problems	Aescin (a saponin mixture)
Ammi visnaga (L.) Lam. (syn.: *Visnaga daucoides* Gaertn., Apiaceae)	Visnaga	Inflammatory and infectious conditions of the mouth, diuretic, 'palpitations of the aorta'	Northern Africa	Increase of cardiac activity	Khellin, and development of cromoglycate
Ananas comosus (L.) Merr. (Bromeliaceae)	Pineapple	Anthelmintic, expectorant, abortifacient	South America (today pantropical)	Antiinflammatory	Bromelain
Atropa belladonna L. (Solanaceae)	Deadly nightshade	Pain relief, asthma, inflammatory conditions	Europe, Middle East	Parkinsonism, antiemetic	(−)-Hyoscyamine
Camptotheca acuminata Decne. (Nyssaceae)	—	?	South and South-eastern Asia	Cancer chemotherapy (inhibitor of topoisomerase 1)	Camptothecin (under development)
Carapichea ipecacuanha (Brot.) L.Andersson (syn.: *Cephaelis ipecacuanha* (Brot.) Tussac, Rubiaceae)	Ipecacuanha	Amoebiasis, expectorant, emetic	Tropical regions of South America	Expectorant, emetic, amoebiasis	Emetine
Catharanthus roseus (L.) G. Don (Apocynaceae)	Madagascar periwinkle	Diabetes mellitus	Madagascar (today a pantropical garden plant)	Cancer chemotherapy	Vincristine, vinblastine
Chondrodendron tomentosum Ruiz & Pav. (Menispermaceae)	—	Arrow poison	Brazil, Peru	Muscular relaxation (during operations)	D-Tubocurarine (Fig. 5.1) (and derivatives)
Cinchona pubescens Vahl (syn.: *C. succirubra* Pav. ex Klotzsch) and spp. (Rubiaceae)	Jesuits' bark	No indigenous uses were recorded during the 16th and 17th centuries	Northern South America	Malaria, cardiac arrhythmia	Quinine
Colchicum autumnale L. (Colchicaceae)	Meadow saffron	Poison	Europe	Gout	Colchicine
Combretum caffrum (Eckl. & Zeyh.) Kuntze (Combretaceae)	Bushwillow tree	An ingredient of arrow poisons?	South Africa	Cancer chemotherapy	Combretastatin A-4
Cryptolepis sanguinolenta (Lindl.) Schltr. (Asclepiadaceae)	Cryptolepis/Ghana quinine	Various symptoms, which may possibly be associated with diabetes	West Africa (e.g. Ghana)	Diabetes	Cryptolepine
Curcuma xanthorrhiza Roxb. and spp. (Zingiberaceae)	Turmeric (curcuma)	Cholagogue, stomachic, carminative	India (?), today widely distributed in the tropics	Hepatic disorders	Curcumin, essential oil
Datura metel L./*D. innoxia* Mill. (Solanacaeae)	Thorn apple	Hallucinogen	Africa and Asia, Middle America	Travel sickness, preoperative medication	Scopolamine (hyoscine)
Digitalis spp. (Scrophulariaceae)	Foxglove	Dropsy	Europe	Cardiac arrhythmia, atrial fibrillation	Digitalis glycosides

TABLE 5.1 **Botanical Drugs Used in Indigenous Medicine or of Importance in the Development of Modern Drugs—cont'd**

Botanical Name	English Name	Indigenous Use	Origin (Regional and Ethnic)	Medical Uses	Representative Active Constituents
Drimia maritima (L.) Stearn (syn.: *Urginea maritima* (L.) Baker (Asparagaceae/ Hyacinthaceae)	Sea onion	Dropsy, emetic, diuretic	Mediterranean	Coronary insufficiency	C_{24}-steroidal cardiac glycosides
Echinacea angustifolia DC. and *E. purpurea* (L.) Moench (Asteraceae)[a]	Echinacea	Pain relief, antiinflammatory, wounds	North America	Immunostimulant	Combined effect of several groups of compounds
Ephedra sinica Stapf (Ephedraceae)	Ephedra	Chronic cough	China	Cough suppressant	Forskolin
Filipendula ulmaria (L.) Maxim. (Rosaceae)	Meadowsweet	Various uses, including as diuretic, kidney problems	Europe, northern Asia	Pain	Acetylsalicylic acid
Frangula purshiana (DC.) Cooper (syn.: *Rhamnus purshiana* DC.) and other *Frangula* and *Rhamnus* spp. (Rhamnaceae)[a]	Cascara sagrada	Widely used as a laxative	Western North America	Purgative	Anthraquinones
Galanthus nivalis L. and related spp. (Amaryllidaceae)	Snowdrop	According to Fuchs (1543), not used pharmaceutically (?)	Warmer regions of Europe	Dementia, including Alzheimer's disease	Galanthamine
Ginkgo biloba L. (Ginkgoaceae)[a]	Ginkgo	Asthma, anthelmintic (fruit)	Eastern China, today widely cultivated	Dementia, cerebral deficiencies, cerebral circulatory problems	Ginkgolides
Harpagophytum procumbens (Burch.) DC. ex Meisn. (Pedaliaceae)[a]	Devil's claw	Fever, unspecified illnesses of the blood, pain relief (especially after parturition), inflammatory conditions, as digestive	Southern Africa	Pain, especially rheumatism	Harpagoside (?), caffeic acid derivatives
Hyoscyamus niger L. (Solanaceae)	Henbane	Pain relief (topical as ointment and plaster), fever, respiratory illnesses	Europe	Anticholinergic	Hyoscyamine
Hypericum perforatum L. (Hypericaceae)[a]	St. John's wort	Very diverse uses including wounds, rheumatism, gout, menstrual problems	Europe	Mild forms of depression, topical for inflammatory conditions (oil)	Hyperforin, flavonoids, hypericin
Justicia adhatoda L. (syn.: *Adhatoda vasica* Nees, Acanthaceae)	Malabar nut	Antispasmodic, antiseptic, antiasthmatic, fish poison, insecticide	India, Sri Lanka	Antispasmodic, oxytocic, cough suppressant	Vasicin (model for expectorants bromhexine and ambroxol)
Macropiper methysticum (G. Forst.) Miq. (syn.: *Piper methysticum* G. Forst.; Piperaceae)[a]	Kava-kava	Ritual stimulant and tonic	Polynesia	Anxiolytic, mild stimulant	Kava pyrones and others
Papaver somniferum L. (Papaveraceae)	(Opium) poppy	Pain relief, tranquilliser, hallucinogen	Western Mediterranean	Pain (P), cough (C), antispasmodic (S)	Morphine (P), codeine (C), papaverine (S)

Continued

TABLE 5.1   Botanical Drugs Used in Indigenous Medicine or of Importance in the Development of Modern Drugs—cont'd

Botanical Name	English Name	Indigenous Use	Origin (Regional and Ethnic)	Medical Uses	Representative Active Constituents
Physostigma venenosum Balf. (Fabaceae *sensu stricto*)	Calabar bean	Poison ('ordeal' and arrow poison)	Tropical West Africa (Sierra Leone—Democratic Republic of the Congo)	Glaucoma	Physostigmine
Pilocarpus jaborandi Holmes (Rutaceae)	Jaborandi	Poison	Africa	Parasympathomimetic, glaucoma	Pilocarpine
Podophyllum peltatum L. (Berberidaceae)	May apple	Especially as laxative, also for skin infections	North-eastern North America	Cancer chemotherapy, warts	Podophyllotoxin (and other lignans)
Prunus africana (Hook. f.) Kalkman (Rosaceae)[a]	African plum	Laxative (veterinary) and diverse other uses	Tropical Africa	Prostate hyperplasia	Especially sitosterol
Psoralea corylifolia L. (syn.: *Cullen corylifolium* (L.) Medik., Fabaceae (*sensu stricto*))	Purple fleabane	Stomachic, various skin infections	Asia	Psoriasis	Psoralen
Rauvolfia spp.	Snake root	Emetic, cholera	Widely distributed in the tropics	Cardiac arrhythmia, high blood pressure	Ajmalin, reserpine
Salix spp. (Salicaceae)[a]	Willow	A variety of uses, especially for chronic and acute inflammatory conditions	Europe, Asia, North America	Various types of pain (lower back pain), chronic inflammatory conditions	Salicin and derivatives (model for aspirin)
Senna alexandrina Mill. (syn.: *Cassia senna* L.) and related spp. (Caesalpiniaceae)	Senna	Laxative	North-eastern Africa, Middle East	Laxative	Sennoside anthraquinones
Strophanthus gratus (Wall. & Hook.) Baill. and *Strophanthus* spp. (Apocynaceae)	—	Arrow poison	Tropical Africa	Coronary insufficiency	Strophantin, ouabain
Syzygium aromaticum (L.) Merr. & L.M. Perry (Myrtaceae)[a]	Clove	Stomachic, digestive, antidiarrhoea, oil for toothache and rheumatism	Molucca Islands (formerly Spice Islands)	Toothache	Eugenol
Taxus brevifolia Nutt. (Taxaceae)	Californian yew	Very diverse uses including for 'cancer' (Tsimshian)	Western USA	Cancer chemotherapy (induction of tubulin aggregation)	Paclitaxel

[a]Examples of plants commonly used in European phytotherapy. In general, the others are not used as an extract but as pure compounds, or served as a model for developing semisynthetic drugs or as standardised (normalised) extracts.

The observation, identification, description and experimental investigation of the ingredients and their effects, as well as the effects of such indigenous drugs, is a truly interdisciplinary field of research that is very important in the study of traditional medicine. **Ethnopharmacology** is here defined as 'the interdisciplinary scientific exploration of biologically active agents traditionally employed or observed by man' (Efron, see Further Reading).

This definition draws attention to the scientific study of indigenous drugs but does not explicitly address the issue of searching for new drugs. Medicinal plants are an important element of indigenous medical systems in many parts of the world, and these resources are usually regarded as part of the traditional knowledge of a culture. For many years, Europe has profited from the exchange of ideas with other continents, and many of the natural products and phytomedicines used today are derived from plants used in indigenous cultures. Examples of 18th century explorers who described indigenous plant use in detail are Richard Spruce (British), Hipolito Ruiz (Spanish) and Alexander von Humboldt (German), who codiscovered curare.

The Story of Curare

An interesting example of an early ethnopharmacological approach is provided by the study of the botanical origin of the arrow poison curare, its physiological effects and the compound responsible for

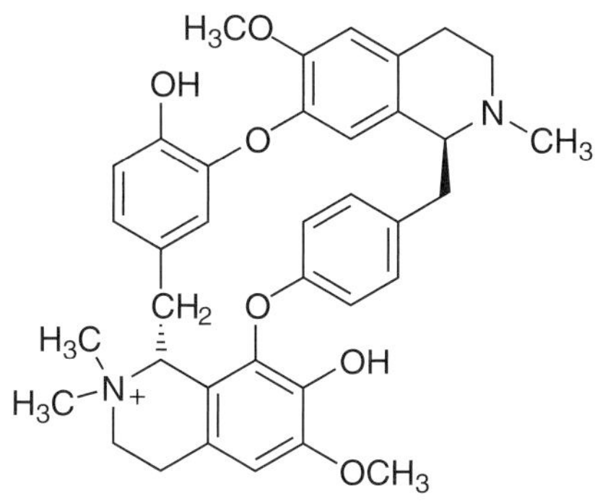

Fig. 5.1 Tubocurarine.

these effects. Curare was used by certain wild tribes in South America for poisoning their arrows and many early explorers documented this usage. The historical aspects of the scientific investigation of curare are outlined in Chapter 2, but the detailed descriptions made by Alexander von Humboldt in 1800, of the processes used to prepare poisoned arrows in Esmeralda on the Orinoco River, are equally interesting. Von Humboldt had met a group of native people who were celebrating their return from an expedition to gather the raw material for making the poison and he described the 'chemical laboratory' used to prepare the poison:

He [an old Indian] was the chemist of the community. With him we saw large boilers (Siedekessel) made out of clay, to be used for boiling the plant sap; plainer containers, which speed up the evaporation process because of their large surface; banana leaves, rolled to form a cone-shaped bag [and] used to filter the liquid which may contain varying amounts of fibres. This hut transformed into a laboratory was very tidy and clean.

The botanical source of curare was finally identified as the climbing vine *Chondrodendron tomentosum* Ruiz & Pavón. Other species of the Menispermaceae (*Curarea* spp. and *Abuta* spp.) and Loganiaceae (*Strychnos* spp.) are also used in the production of curares of varying types. Von Humboldt then eloquently described one of the classical problems of ethnopharmacology:

We are unable to make a botanical identification because this tree [which produces the raw material for the production of curare] only grows at quite some distance from Esmeralda and because [it] did not have flowers and fruit. I had mentioned this type of misfortune previously, that the most noteworthy plants cannot be examined by the traveller, while others whose chemical activities are not known [i.e. which are not used ethnobotanically] are found covered with thousands of flowers and fruit.

The Role of the Ethnobotanist

The role of the ethnobotanist in the search for new drugs was important until the second half of the 20th century, when other approaches became more 'fashionable'. Since the turn of the millennium, the study of ethnobotany has again received considerable interest in the media and in some segments of the scientific community. Also, the 'Western' use of such information has come under increasing scrutiny, and the national and indigenous rights to these resources have become acknowledged by most academic and industrial researchers. These developments result in a considerable challenge to (and increasing responsibilities for) ethnobotanists and ethnopharmacologists. Simultaneously, the need for basic scientific investigation of plants used in indigenous medical systems is becoming ever more relevant.

The public availability of research results is as essential for further developing and 'upgrading' indigenous and TM as it is for any other medical or pharmaceutical system.

ETHNOPHARMACOLOGY AND THE CONVENTION ON BIOLOGICAL DIVERSITY (CONVENTION OF RIO)

None of the studies discussed so far took the benefits for the providers (the states and their people) into account. Over the decades since the 1980s this has changed in multiple ways. Ethnopharmacological and related research using the biological resources of a country are today based on agreements and permits, which in turn are based on international and bilateral treaties. The most important of these is the Convention of Rio or the Convention on Biological Diversity (see https://www.cbd.int/convention/), which looks in particular at the rights and responsibilities associated with biodiversity on an international level:

The objectives of this Convention, to be pursued in accordance with its relevant provisions, are the conservation of biological diversity, the sustainable use of its components and the fair and equitable sharing of the benefits arising out of the utilization of genetic resources, including by appropriate access to genetic resources and by appropriate transfer of relevant technologies, taking into account all rights over those resources and to technologies, and by appropriate funding.

The basic principles of access are regulated in article 5:

States have, in accordance with the Charter of the United Nations and the principles of international law, the sovereign right to exploit their own resources pursuant to their own environmental policies, and the responsibility to ensure that activities within their jurisdiction or control do not cause damage to the environment of other States or of areas beyond the limits of national jurisdiction.

The rights of indigenous peoples and other keepers of local knowledge are addressed in article 8j:

Subject to its national legislation, respect, preserve and maintain knowledge, innovations and practices of indigenous and local communities embodying traditional lifestyles relevant for the conservation and sustainable use of biological diversity and promote their wider application with the approval and involvement of the holders of such knowledge, innovations and practices and encourage the equitable sharing of the benefits arising from the utilization of such knowledge, innovations and practices.

This and subsequent treaties significantly changed the basic conditions for ethnopharmacological research. Countries that provide the resources for natural product research and drug development now have well-defined rights. This specifically includes the sharing of any benefits that may accrue from the collaboration. Access to resources is addressed in article 15, which is crucial for an understanding of this and any other activity that may yield economically important products:

15.1. Recognizing the sovereign rights of States over their natural resources, the authority to determine access to genetic resources rests with the national governments and is subject to national legislation.

15.5. Access to genetic resources shall be subject to prior informed consent of the Contracting Party providing such resources, unless otherwise determined by that Party.

15.7. Each Contracting Party shall take legislative, administrative or policy measures…with the aim of sharing in a fair and equitable way the results of research and development and the benefits arising from the commercial and other utilization of genetic resources with the Contracting Party providing such resources. Such sharing shall be upon mutually agreed terms.

In the case of ethnopharmacological research, the needs and interests of the collaborating community become an essential part of the research and, in fact, there is an inextricable link between cultural and biological diversity. This principle was first formulated at the First International Congress on Ethnobiology held in Belem (Brazil) in 1988. No generally agreed upon standards have so far been accepted, but the importance of obtaining the 'prior informed consent' of the informants has been stressed by numerous authors.

After this first Convention the mutual obligations were developed further, including the Nagoya Protocol of 2010 (https://www.cbd.int/abs/about/), The protocol specifically calls for the promotion and safeguarding of 'the fair and equitable sharing of benefits arising from the utilisation of genetic resources' (Secretariat of the Convention on Biological Diversity 2011) with the expectation that commercial or noncommercial benefits result for the countries of origin. Each signatory country implements their own mechanisms to achieve this. Other relevant agreements include trade-related aspects of intellectual property rights (TRIPS) and World Trade Organization (WTO) agreements (cf. www.wto.org). While the implementation is complex and time consuming, in major academic circles it is the general consensus that their implementation is an essential foundation of any form of ethnopharmacological and related research.

BIOPROSPECTING AND ETHNOPHARMACOLOGY

Studies dealing with medicinal and other useful plants and their bioactive compounds have used many concepts and methodologies. These are interdisciplinary or multidisciplinary studies, combining such diverse fields as anthropology, pharmacology, pharmacognosy or pharmaceutical biology, natural product chemistry, toxicology, clinical research, plant physiology and others. In order to analyse their strengths and weaknesses, and especially the outcomes of research, two different but closely related approaches can be distinguished: **bioprospecting** and **ethnopharmacology** (Table 5.2).

Bioprospecting focuses on the development of new drugs for the huge markets of the northern hemisphere. Potentially highly profitable pharmaceutical products are developed, based on the biological and chemical diversity of the various ecosystems on Earth; this requires an enormous financial input. The research starts with the collection of biogenic samples (plants, fungi, other microorganisms and animals); progresses through analysis of the chemical, biological and pharmacological activities; and ends with the development of drug templates or new drugs. A key process in this search is high-throughput screening systems such as those that have been established by major international pharmaceutical companies. Huge libraries of compounds (and sometimes extracts) are screened for biological activity against specific targets. Active natural products are only one of the many sources of material for these batteries of tests but serve as a starting point for drug development. Currently, some companies envision screening 500,000 samples a week against a single target; thus, it becomes essential to have an enormous number of chemically diverse samples available.

The other approach may best be termed ethnopharmacological. Ethnobotanical studies generally result in the documentation of a rather limited set of well-documented useful plants, mostly medicinal, but also those known to be toxic or used in nutrition. In ethnopharmacology, an important goal is the development of improved preparations for use by local people. Thus, it is essential to obtain information on the bioactive compounds from these plants, their relative contribution to the effects of the extract (including, for example, synergistic or antagonistic effects), the toxicological profile of the extract and its constituents. By restricting ethnopharmacology to the bioscientific study of indigenous uses, attention is drawn to the need for improving indigenous phytomedical systems, especially in developing countries. This requires research strategies for studying indigenous medicinal plants and their uses.

The importance of conserving such nature-derived products in the healthcare of the original keepers of such knowledge must be the main goal of truly interdisciplinary research. Ethnopharmacology may contribute to the development of new pharmaceutical products for the markets of the northern hemisphere, but this is only one of several targets. Truly multidisciplinary research on medicinal plants requires the inclusion of other methodologies from such fields as medical or pharmaceutical anthropology or sociology. Not only do we need a detailed understanding, incorporating social scientific and bioscientific methods, but we also need to support all means available of making better use of these products. It has been pointed out that the two approaches—ethnopharmacology and biodiversity prospecting—are not mutually exclusive and the two concepts as they are outlined here are rarely realised in such extreme forms. Instead, any discussion should specifically draw attention to the particular strengths and roles of both approaches. In bioprospecting programmes, which are directed specifically towards infectious diseases, the use of 'ethnobotanical' information is very useful and promising. However, this is not necessarily the case in cancer chemotherapy, for example, where highly toxic plants are not used in TM because the dose cannot be controlled sufficiently well to ensure safety.

EXAMPLES OF MODERN ETHNOPHARMACOLOGICAL STUDIES

A project conducted by Hensel et al. (see Further Reading) focusing on the scientific study of indigenous uses of Ghanaian medicinal plants leading to the identification of some bioactive constituents in *Phyllanthus muellerianus* (Kuntze) Exell (Phyllanthaceae) is a good example. An ethnopharmacological field study in the Ashanti region of Ghana was initiated and the binational collaboration between Ghanaian and German researchers identified 104 plant species traditionally used for wound healing. In vitro studies of extracts from the most prominent candidates were conducted using primary human fibroblasts and human keratinocytes. A high degree of concordance with the traditional use was observed.

In case of the aqueous extract from the dried leaves of *P. muellerianus* a total tannin content of 14% was found. The ellagitannin geraniin (Fig. 5.2) with two isomers was identified as a major constituent. The compounds identified help to explain the rationale behind the indigenous uses. The tannins are known to have antibacterial activity, and antiinflammatory effects contribute to the therapeutic benefits (which, however, have not yet been studied clinically). Specifically, the stimulation of the epidermal keratinocyte barrier and the formation of extracellular matrix markers from the fibroblasts of typical skin cells were identified

TABLE 5.2	**Ethnopharmacology and Bioprospecting Compared**
Ethnopharmacology	**Bioprospecting**
Overall Goals	
(Herbal) drug development, especially for local uses	Drug discovery for the international market
Complex plant extracts (phytotherapy)	Pure natural products as drugs
Social importance of medicinal and other useful plants	—
Cultural meaning of resources and understanding of indigenous concepts about plant use and of the selection criteria for medicinal plants	—
Main Disciplines Involved	
Anthropology	—
Biology (ecology)	Biology including (very prominently) ecology
Pharmacology/molecular biology	Pharmacology and molecular biology
Pharmacognosy and phytochemistry	Phytochemistry
Number of Samples Collected	
Very few (up to several hundred)	As many as possible, preferably several thousand
Selected Characteristics	
Detailed information on a small segment of the local flora (and fauna)	Limited information about many taxa
Database on ethnopharmaceutical uses of plants	Database on many taxa (including ecology)
Development of autochthonous resources (especially local plant gardens, small-scale production of herbal preparations)	Inventory (expanded herbaria) economically sustainable alternative use to destructive exploitation (e.g. logging)
Pharmacological Study	
Preferably using low-throughput screening assays, which allow a detailed understanding of the local or indigenous uses	The assay is not selected on the basis of local usage, instead high-throughput screening systems are used
Key Problem	
Safety and efficacy of herbal preparations	Local agendas (rights) and compensation to access

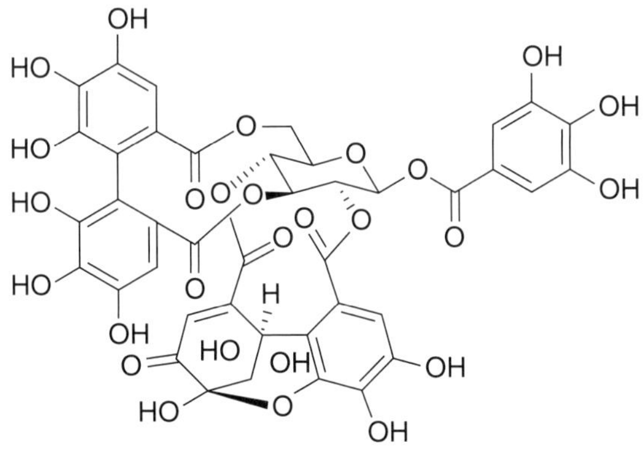

Fig. 5.2 Geraniin.

as key mechanisms. The extract also showed antiviral activity (in *Herpes simplex* virus 1—HSV-1). While this research is unlikely to result in new drug leads for a wider (global) commercial use as a licensed medicine, it offers a foundation for local uses of this species.

The second example is drawn from ethnobotanical fieldwork by Kufer et al. (unpublished) in Eastern Guatemala with a Mayan-speaking people, the Chorti. The Chorti use the fruit of *Ocimum micranthum* Willd. (Lamiaceae) in the treatment of infectious and inflammatory eye diseases. The fruits are approximately 1 mm in diameter and hard, and several of these are applied directly into the eye. At first glance, this seems an unlikely remedy for eye problems, but the rationale behind

it becomes evident when considering the morphological and chemical make-up of the fruits: they are covered with a mucilaginous layer containing complex polysaccharides, which form a soft layer around the fruit if it is put into water. This layer may well have a cleansing effect, and polysaccharides are known to be useful in the treatment of inflammatory conditions and bacterial or viral infections. Although there are no pharmacological data from experimental studies available to corroborate this use, information on the histochemical structure of the fruit makes it likely that the treatment has some scientific basis.

The previous two examples demonstrate the relevance of ethnopharmacology in relation to the scientific study of indigenous medical products. However, ethnopharmacology, as the science bridging the gap between natural sciences and anthropology, should also look at symbolic and cognitive aspects. People may select plants not only because of their specific pharmacological properties but also because of the symbolic power they may believe the plant to hold. Understanding these aspects requires cognitive and symbolic analysis of field data. Another example from field studies with the Mixe in Mexico can be used. At the end of a course of medical treatment, the patient is sometimes given a petal of *Argemone mexicana* L. (known to the Mixe as San Pedro Agats, Papaveraceae). This plant is known to contain a large number of biologically active alkaloids, including protopine. However, the yellow petals are presumably used, not because they exert a pharmacological effect (at this dose) but because they symbolise the bread of the Last Supper according to Christian mythology. Thus, they are a powerful symbol for the end of the healing process (for other examples of symbolic and empirical forms of plant use see Heinrich and other authors in Further Reading). This species, which has become (an often noxious) weed in many countries, has been studied in great detail for potential antimalarial effects. This is based on uses to treat the symptoms of malaria in Mali, and some clinical evidence has become available.

The role of ethnopharmacology can be extended beyond that defined previously. It looks not only at empirical aspects of indigenous and popular plant use but also at the cognitive foundations of this use. Only if these issues are to be included will it be a truly interdisciplinary field of research. The key tasks in this interdisciplinary process will be to:

- Study the pharmacological effects of the most widely used species (for selection criteria for the ethnopharmacologically most important taxa).
- Further develop local pharmacopoeias based on traditional use.
- Characterise the relevant constituents.
- Formulate improved (but relatively simple) galenical preparations (extracts).

This will result in a truly interdisciplinary approach to medicinal plants: the value of integrating ethnobotanical with phytochemical and pharmacological studies has been clearly demonstrated. While, for example, the likelihood of developing new therapeutic agents for use in biomedicine is relatively low (although it is certainly higher than with many other approaches), such studies confirm the therapeutic value and contribute to our knowledge of medicinal plants.

Another key development in recent decades has been the study of the use of herbal medicines and foods by migrants or in urban contexts. Such research is not primarily relevant for 'documenting and evaluating traditional knowledge' but often the focus is on understanding how people cope with the changes migration brings about and how such plant use helps to maintain and develop links with the country of origin. Importantly, it can contribute to improving primary health services for such populations, and as such, it has direct public health implications. This trend results in a merging of research in areas previously classified as 'phytotherapy research' or research in integrative medicines with ethnobotanical and ethnopharmacological research.

Some plants have many side effects or are highly toxic. In an example from the Highlands of Mexico, a species popularly used there contains hepatotoxic pyrrolizidine alkaloids, which pose potential health risks. The effects are cumulative and therefore delayed, and not immediately linked to consumption of the plant. Although this information is available to the scientific community, the general public may not be aware of these risks. Such data must be summarised appropriately and made available to local people. It is now essential to develop partnerships with institutions capable of translating these findings into an effective strategy.

CONCLUSION

With the increasing importance given to local and TMs, especially herbal medicines, and, for example, to the development of a global strategy on TMs, the study of indigenous, orally transmitted medical systems has become a priority in many countries, for example, in Asia, Africa and Southern America. It illustrates that the pharmaceutical sciences will profit in many ways by including such approaches. It is also important to further consolidate local knowledge. Ethnopharmacology in this context will provide patients in developing countries in Africa, South and Central America, Asia and South-East Asia with access to some evidence-based forms of their own 'traditional' medicine.

FURTHER READING

Bah, M., Bye, R., Pereda-Miranda, R., 1994. Hepatotoxic pyrrolizidine alkaloids in the Mexican medicinal plant *Packera candidissima* (Asteraceae: Senecioneae). J. Ethnopharmacol. 43, 19–30.

Berlin, B., 1992. Ethnobiological Classification: Principles of Categorization of Plants and Animals in Traditional Societies. Princeton University Press, Princeton, NJ.

Bernard, C., 1966. Physiologische untersuchungen über einige Amerikanische gifte. Das Curare. In: Bernard, C., Mani, N. (Eds.), Ausgewählte Physiologische Schriften. Huber Verlag, Bern, pp. 84–133. [orig. French 1864].

Bhamra, S.K., Slater, A., Howard, C., Johnson, M., Heinrich, M., 2017. The use of traditional herbal medicines amongst South Asian Diasporic Communities in the UK. Phytother. Res. 31, 1786–1794. https://doi.org/10.1002/ptr.5911.

Bisset, N.G., 1991. One man's poison, another man's medicine. J. Ethnopharmacol. 32, 71–81.

Bruhn, J.G., Holmstedt, B., 1981. Ethnopharmacology: objectives, principles and perspectives. In: Beal, J.L., Reinhard, E. (Eds.), Natural Products as Medicinal Agents. Hippokrates Verlag, Stuttgart, pp. 405–430.

Buenz, E.J., Verpoorte, R., Bauer, B.A., 2018. The ethnopharmacologic contribution to bioprospecting natural products. Annu. Rev. Pharmacol. Toxicol. 58, 509–530.

Dauncey, E.A., Howes, M.J., 2020. Plants That Cure. Kew Publishing/Royal Botanical Gardens, Kew London, UK.

Efron, D.H., Holmstedt, B., Kline, N.S., 1970. Ethnopharmacologic Search for Psychoactive Drugs. Public Health Service Publication no. 1645. Government Printing Office, Washington, DC (reprint, orig. 1967).

Graz, B., Willcox, M., Elisabetsky, E., 2015. Retrospective treatment-outcome as a method of collecting clinical data in ethnopharmacological surveys. In: Heinrich, M., Jaeger, A.K. (Eds.), Ethnopharmacology. ULLA Book Series. Wiley, Chichester, pp. 251–261.

Heinrich, M., 1992. Economic botany of American Labiatae. In: Harley, R.M., Reynolds, T. (Eds.), Advances in Labiatae Science. Royal Botanical Gardens, Kew, pp. 475–488.

Heinrich, M., 2013. Ethnopharmacology and drug discovery. In: Reedijk, J. (Ed.), Elsevier Reference Module in Chemistry, Molecular Sciences and Chemical Engineering. Elsevier, Waltham, MA.

Heinrich, M., Ankli, A., Frei, B., Weimann, C., Sticher, O., 1998. Medicinal plants in Mexico: Healers' consensus and cultural importance. Soc. Sci. Med. 47, 1859–1871.

Heinrich, M., Jaeger, A.K. (Eds.), 2015. Ethnopharmacology. ULLA Book Series. Wiley, Chichester.

Hensel, A., Kisseih, E., Agyare, C., Lechtenberg, M., Petereit, F., Asase, A., 2015. From ethnopharmacological field study to phytochemistry and preclinical research: the example of Ghanaian medicinal plants for improved wound healing. In: Heinrich, M., Jaeger, A.K. (Eds.), Ethnopharmacology. ULLA Book Series. Wiley, Chichester, pp. 179–197.

Lazarou, R., Heinrich, M., 2019. Herbal medicine: who cares? The changing views on medicinal plants and their roles in British Lifestyle. Phytother. Res. 33 (9), 2409–2420. https://doi.org/10.1002/ptr.6431.

Lewis, W., 2000. Ethnopharmacology and the search for new therapeutics. In: Minnis, P.E., Elisens, W.J. (Eds.), Biodiversity and Native America. University of Oklahoma Press, Norman, OK.

Posey, D.A., 2002. Kayapó ethnoecology and culture. In: Plenderleith, K. (Ed.), Studies in Environmental Anthropology, vol. 6. Routledge, London.

Schultes, R.E., Raffauf, R.F., 1990. The Healing Forest: Medicinal and Toxic Plants of the Northwest Amazonia. Discorides Press, Portland, OR.

Secretariat of the Convention on Biological Diversity, 2001. Handbook of the Convention on Biological Diversity. Earthscan, London.

Süntar, I., 2020. Importance of ethnopharmacological studies in drug discovery: role of medicinal plants. Phytochem. Rev. 19, 1199–1209. https://doi.org/10.1007/s11101-019-09629-9.

von Humboldt, A. (Ed.), 1997. Die Forschungsreise in Den Tropen Amerikas, Studienausgabe Bd 2, Teilband 3. Wissenschaftliche Buchgesellschaft, Darmstadt.

WHO, 2013. WHO Traditional Medicine Strategy: 2014–2023. World Health Organization, Geneva.

Natural Products: An Introduction

6

Natural Product Chemistry

This chapter looks briefly at the chemistry of natural products, the study of chemicals produced by the many diverse organisms of nature, including plants, microbes (fungi and bacteria), marine organisms and more exotic sources, such as frog skins and insects.

> **Natural products,** as included here, are organic compounds in the molecular weight range 100–2000. In a broader sense, the term natural products is applied to bulk substances from nature, such as crude plant material, foodstuffs, resins and exudates from plants (e.g. myrrh and frankincense) or extracts of plant material (water or alcoholic extracts). Here we will consider only **single chemical entities** or defined ranges of compounds.

Historically, natural products formed the basis of all medicines and, even now, many medicinally important compounds are derived from natural sources. It is highly likely that these chemicals are produced as part of a defence system to protect the organism from attack. Examples include the synthesis of antimicrobial compounds by plants infected by bacteria and fungi (compounds known as **phytoalexins**), and the synthesis of toxins in the skins of Central American frogs (to deter predation by other animals). Whatever the reasons for the presence of these compounds in nature, they are an invaluable and underexploited resource that can be used to find new drug molecules. They are produced as a result of primary or secondary pathways, as explained below.

PRIMARY AND SECONDARY PLANT METABOLISM

Primary metabolism is the set of metabolic pathways that synthesise compounds essential for the normal functioning of the plant cell. They include carbohydrates (sugars), lipids (fats), amino acids (proteins), nucleic acids (RNA, DNA) and vitamins. Each primary metabolite needs several steps, which constitutes a metabolic pathway, and each reaction is executed by one or several **enzymes**. Their expression is tightly controlled at the genetic level.

Secondary metabolites are not essential for the life of the plant, but give advantages for reproduction, evolutionary survival and ecological competition, and provide specific functions such as antimicrobial activity and as feeding deterrents to insects and animals. They are synthesised via complex metabolic pathways, starting from simple compounds, mostly sugars and amino acids.

The distinction between these two types of metabolites is a useful general classification and is commonly used in the scientific literature, but also has been criticised as no sharp distinction can be drawn between the two groups of pathways.

The plant (or microbe) may activate or repress one entire pathway (or even one of its enzymes only) depending on factors such as the life cycle, season, being under stress or attack. Furthermore, the biosynthesis of secondary metabolites is often under separate genetic control in each plant part. Thus, plant or other biomass harvested at the wrong time, or in the wrong way, may not yield the metabolites of interest.

Once a compound has been synthesised, it may accumulate as a stable end product, and stay intact if conditions do not change, or, in many cases, may be short lived as intermediates in the synthesis of others, and subject to rapid turnover. For example, **menthol** (see Fig. 6.26) has a half-life of just a few hours in the cells of mint (*Mentha × piperita*), whilst **pinene** (see Fig. 6.26), present in pine (*Pinus sylvestris*), can accumulate in the needles for almost 200 days.

The biosynthesis, storage and degradation of secondary metabolites is a dynamic process taking place simultaneously in different compartments within the cell. The energy involved in running the secondary metabolism is not to be underestimated, and every chemical metabolite shown in this chapter has been produced at a high energy cost to the cell and, ultimately, the plant.

There are many ways to classify the enormous chemical diversity of natural products. In this book we follow a mixed criterion to facilitate the task: all natural products, excluding alkaloids, are grouped by their biosynthetic origin, i.e. by end products of the same plant metabolic pathway. These may undergo further glycosylation, which results in significant changes in their solubility, reactivity, bioavailability and pharmacology, and thus glycosides will be considered separately.

CLASSES OF NATURAL PRODUCTS FROM DIFFERENT BIOSYNTHETIC PATHWAYS

Polyketides

These are a group of therapeutically important compounds comprising many antibiotics (macrolides and tetracyclines), fatty acids and aromatic compounds (anthrone purgative glycosides and anthracyclic antitumour agents).

Polyketides are mainly acetate (C_2)-derived metabolites and occur throughout all organisms (as fatty acids and glycerides), but it is the microbes, and predominantly the filamentous bacteria of the genus *Streptomyces*, that produce the structurally diverse polyketide antibiotics. The biosynthesis of these compounds begins (Fig. 6.1) with the condensation of one molecule of **malonyl-CoA** (CoA is short for coenzyme A) with one molecule of **acetyl-CoA** to form the simple polyketide acetoacetyl-CoA. In this reaction (Claisen reaction), one molecule of CO_2 and one molecule of HSCoA are generated. The reaction occurs because the carbon between both carbonyl groups of malonyl-CoA (the acidic carbon) is nucleophilic and can attack an electropositive (electron-deficient) centre (e.g. the carbon of a carbonyl group).

The curved arrows in Fig. 6.1 indicate the movement of a pair of electrons to form a bond. Further condensation reactions (between another molecule of malonyl-CoA and the growing polyketide) lead to chain elongation, in which every other carbon in the chain is a carbonyl group. These chains are known as **poly-β-keto esters** and are the reactive intermediates forming the polyketides. Using these esters, large chains such as fatty acids can be constructed and, in fact, reduction of the carbonyl groups and hydrolysis of the –SHCoA thioester leads to the fatty acid class of compounds. The expanding polyketide chain may be attached as a thioester to either CoA or to a protein called

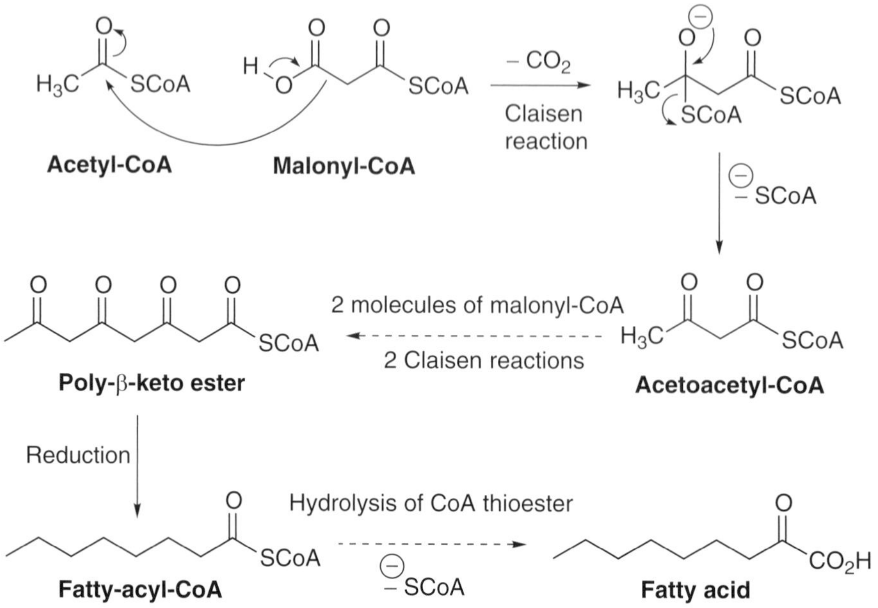

Fig. 6.1 Biosynthesis of polyketide antibiotics.

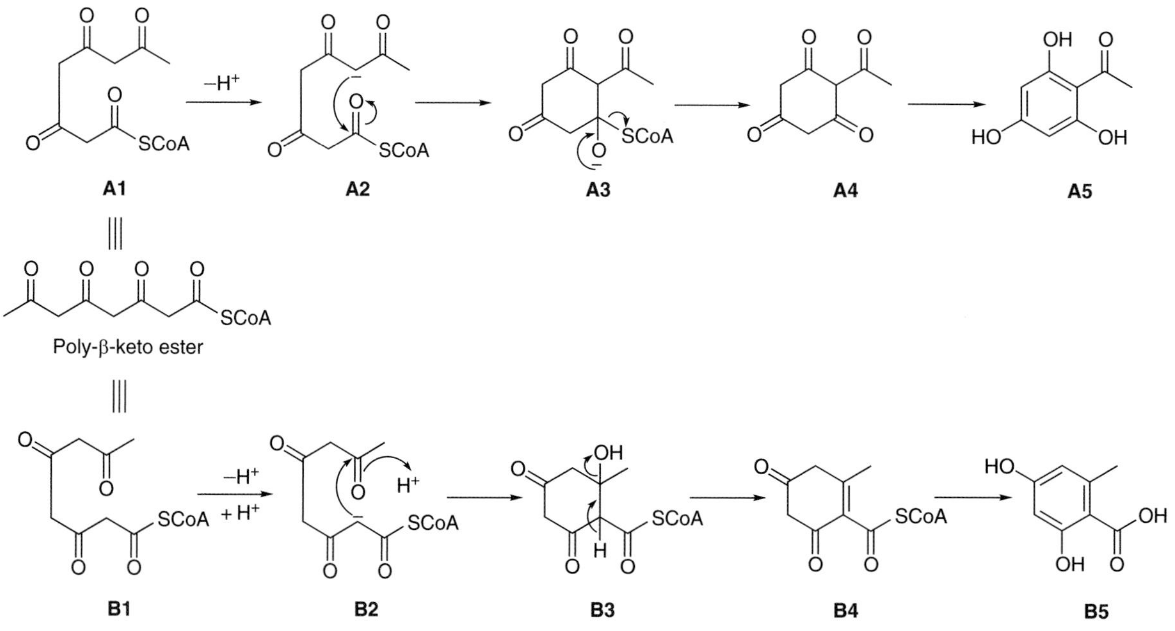

Fig. 6.2 Cyclisation of the poly-β-keto esters to form aromatic compounds.

an acyl-carrier protein. Multiple Claisen reactions with additional molecules of malonyl-CoA can generate long-chain fatty acids, such as stearic and myristic acids.

The poly-β-keto ester can also cyclise to form aromatic compounds, and the way in which the ester folds determines the type of structure generated (Fig. 6.2). If the poly-β-keto ester folds as **A1**, then loss of a proton, followed by an intramolecular Claisen reaction of intermediate **A2** (by attack of the acidic carbon on the carbonyl), would result in the formation of a cyclic polyketide enolate **A3**, which will rearrange to the keto compound with expulsion of the SCoA anion, resulting in the ketone **A4**. This ketone would readily undergo keto–enol tautomerism to the more favoured aromatic triphenol **A5** (**phloroacetophenone**).

Should the poly-β-keto ester fold as **B1**, then an aldol reaction on intermediate **B2** will occur by attack of the carbonyl by the acidic carbon, and, with the addition of a proton, an alcohol is formed, resulting in intermediate **B3**. This alcohol can then dehydrate to the

conjugated alkene **B4**, which can also tautomerise and, via hydrolysis of the thioester-SCoA, the aromatic phenolic acid **orsellinic acid (B5)** is formed.

The reactive nature of poly-β-keto esters gives rise to many useful pharmaceuticals and, because they are oxygen-rich starting precursors, the final natural products are generally rich in functional group chemistry. Ketone groups are often retained, but reduction to alcohols and the formation of ethers is common and many polyketides, particularly certain antibiotics and antitumour agents, also occur as glycosides.

Fatty Acids and Glycerides

These are widely distributed and part of the general biochemistry of all organisms, particularly as components of cell membranes. They are usually insoluble in water and soluble in organic solvents, such as hexane, diethyl ether and chloroform. They are sometimes referred to as fixed oils (liquid) or fats (solid), although both fixed oils and fats

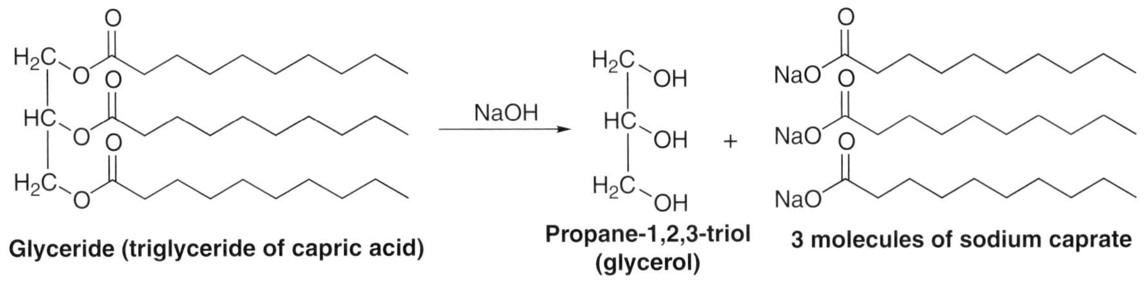

Fig. 6.3 Saponification of glycerides.

TABLE 6.1 Common Fatty Acids

Common Name	Formula	Oil and Source	Oil Use
Arachidic	$CH_3(CH_2)_{18}CO_2H$ (20:0)	Peanut oil, butter, *Arachis hypogaea* (Fabaceae)	Lubricant, food, emollient
Behenic	$CH_3(CH_2)_{20}CO_2H$ (22:0)	Carnauba wax, *Copernicia prunifera* (Arecaceae)	Polish for coated tablets
Butyric	$CH_3(CH_2)_2CO_2H$ (4:0)	Butter fat, cow, *Bos taurus*	Food oil
Caproic	$CH_3(CH_2)_4CO_2H$ (6:0)	Coconut oil, *Cocos nucifera* (Arecaceae)	Manufacture of flavours
Caprylic	$CH_3(CH_2)_6CO_2H$ (8:0)	Coconut oil, *C. nucifera* (Arecaceae)	Dietary supplement, perfumes
Capric	$CH_3(CH_2)_8CO_2H$ (10:0)	*Cuphea viscosissima, C. lanceolata* (Lythraceae)	Artificial flavours, perfumes
Docosahexaenoic	$CH_3CH_2(CH=CHCH_2)_6CH_2CO_2H$ (22:6) all *cis*	Cod liver oil and halibut liver oil	Dietary supplement
Eicosapentaenoic	$CH_3CH_2(CH=CHCH_2)_5(CH_2)_2CO_2H$ (20:5) all *cis*	Cod liver oil and halibut liver oil	Dietary supplement
Erucic	$CH_3(CH_2)_7CH=CH(CH_2)_{11}CO_2H$ (22:1) *cis*	Rapeseed oil, *Brassica napus* var. *oleifera* (Brassicaceae)	Food
Lauric	$CH_3(CH_2)_{10}CO_2H$ (12:0)	Coconut and palm kernel oil, *C. nucifera, Elaeis guineensis* (Arecaceae)	Food, soaps, shampoos
Linoleic	$CH_3(CH_2)_4(CH=CHCH_2)_2(CH_2)_6 CO_2H$ (18:2) all *cis*	Vegetable oils, soybean, corn, *Glycine max* (Fabaceae)	Essential fatty acid
α-Linolenic	$CH_3CH_2CH=CHCH_2CH=CHCH_2CH=CH(CH_2)_7CO_2H$	Linseed oil, *Linum usitatissimum* (Linaceae)	Liniments, paints, food
γ-Linolenic	$CH_3(CH_2)_4CH=CHCH_2CH=CHCH_2CH=CH(CH_2)_4CO_2H$	Evening primrose oil, *Oenothera biennis* (Onagraceae)	Dietary supplement
Myristic	$CH_3(CH_2)_{12}CO_2H$	Coconut and palm kernel oil, *C. nucifera, E. guineensis*	Food, soaps, shampoos
Nervonic	$CH_3(CH_2)_7CH=CH(CH_2)_{13}CO_2H$ (24:1) all *cis*	Honesty oil, *Lunaria annua* (Brassicaceae)	Supplement for patients with multiple sclerosis
Oleic	$CH_3(CH_2)_7CH=CH (CH_2)_7CO_2H$ (18:1) *cis*	Olive oil, *Olea europaea* (Oleaceae)	Food, emulsifying agent
Palmitic	$CH_3(CH_2)_{14}CO_2H$ (16:0)	Coconut and palm kernel oil, *C. nucifera, E. guineensis*	Food, soaps, candles
Ricinoleic	$CH_3(CH_2)_5CH(OH)CH_2CH=CH(CH_2)_7CO_2H$ (18:1) *cis*	Castor oil, *Ricinus communis* (Euphorbiaceae)	Soap manufacture
Stearic	$CH_3(CH_2)_{16}CO_2H$ (18:0)	Olive oil, *O. europaea* (Oleaceae)	Suppositories, tablet coatings

are mixtures of glycerides and free fatty acids and the state (i.e. liquid or solid) depends on the temperature as well as the composition. Glycerides are fatty acid esters of glycerol (propane-1,2,3-triol), and can be converted into soaps by a strong base (e.g. sodium hydroxide, NaOH). Saponification of fatty acids and glycerides with sodium hydroxide results in the formation of the sodium salts of the fatty acids (Fig. 6.3).

Glycerides are usually complicated mixtures as, unlike the example in Fig. 6.3, the substituents may be different from each other, and it is not uncommon for lipophilic plant extracts to contain many types of glycerides.

Fatty acids are very important as foods, and also as formulation agents and vehicles in and components of cosmetics and soaps. Table 6.1 lists the common names, chemical formulae, sources and uses of the more common fatty acids.

The saturated fats occur widely in nature. The most common are myristic, palmitic and stearic acids. The unsaturated fatty acids contain a varying number of double bonds. This, together with the length of the carbon chain, is indicated after the name of the fatty acid. For example, **oleic acid** (18:1), which is widespread in plant oils and is a

major metabolite in olive oil from *Olea europaea* (Oleaceae), has an 18-carbon chain and one double bond. α-**Linolenic acid** (18:3) is a metabolite in linseed oil from *Linum usitatissimum* (Linaceae), and the related compound, γ-**linolenic acid** (18:3), is found in evening primrose oil from *Oenothera biennis* (Onagraceae) and other widely used dietary supplements. **Ricinoleic acid** is a hydroxylated fatty acid and the main ingredient of castor oil (from the seeds of *Ricinus communis*, Euphorbiaceae), which was used as a purgative but is now used for the manufacture of soap and as a cosmetic base.

The **polyunsaturated** fatty acids contain three or more double bonds and are particularly beneficial as dietary components and in pharmaceuticals and cosmetics.

In humans, saturated fats are precursors for the biosynthesis of cholesterol, high serum levels of which are implicated in heart disease through the formation of atherosclerotic plaques in arteries.

Tetracyclines

These have four linear six-membered rings, from which the group was named and were discovered as part of a screening programme of filamentous bacteria (Actinomycetes), which are common components of

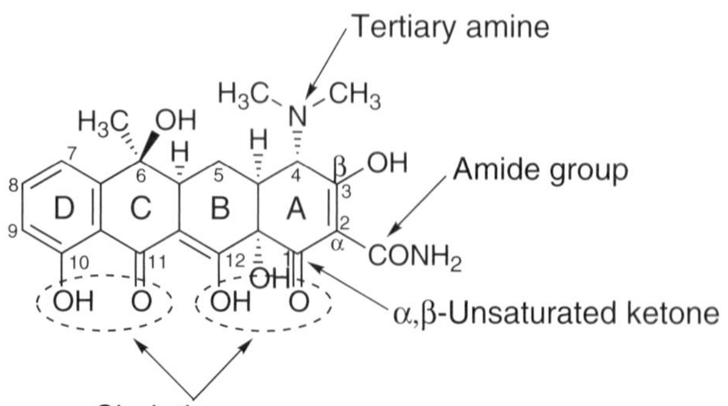

Fig. 6.4 Functional groups of tetracycline.

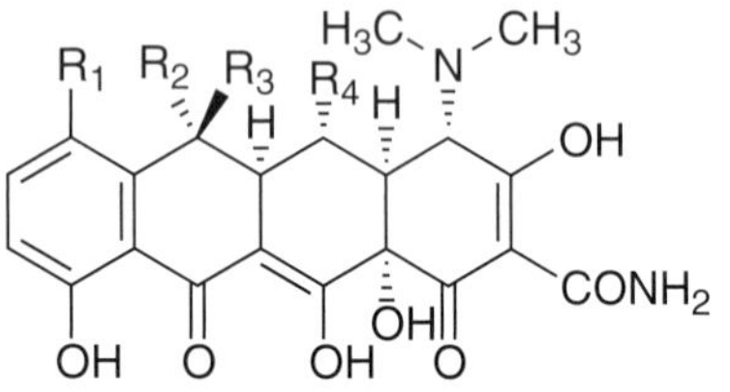

Tetracycline, $R_1 = H, R_2 = CH_3, R_3 = OH, R_4 = H$
Oxytetracycline, $R_1 = H, R_2 = CH_3, R_3 = OH, R_4 = OH$
Doxycycline, $R_1 = H, R_2 = H, R_3 = CH_3, R_4 = OH$
Minocycline, $R_1 = N(CH_3)_2, R_2 = H, R_3 = H, R_4 = H$

Fig. 6.5 Tetracycline and related compounds.

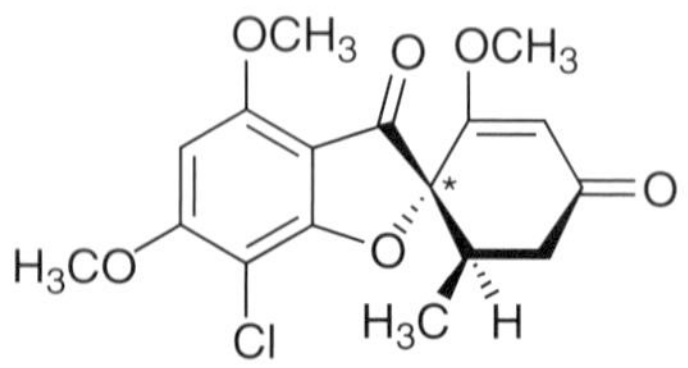

* denotes spiro carbon
Fig. 6.6 Griseofulvin.

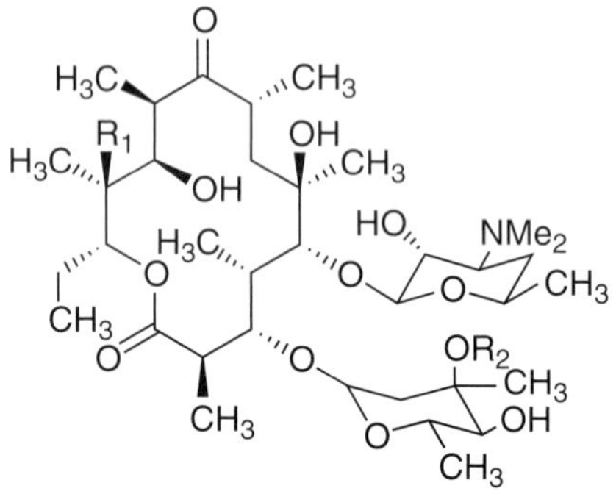

Erythromycin A, $R_1 = OH, R_2 = CH_3$
Erythromycin B, $R_1 = H, R_2 = CH_3$
Erythromycin C, $R_1 = OH, R_2 = H$

Fig. 6.7 Erythromycins.

soil. The most widely studied group is the genus *Streptomyces*, members of which produce many polyketide natural products, of which the antibiotic **tetracycline** (Fig. 6.4) and the **anthracyclic** antitumour agents are examples.

The key features of this class are shown in Fig. 6.4. Tetracycline has numerous functional groups, including a tertiary amine, hydroxyls, an amide, a phenolic hydroxy and keto group. The polyketide structure of tetracycline is still visible by looking at the lower portion of the molecule. C_{10}, C_{11}, C_{12} and C_1 are oxygenated, indicating that the precursor of this compound was a poly-β-keto ester. C_{10} and C_{11} and C_{12} and C_1 form part of a chelating system essential for antibiotic activity and may readily chelate metal ions, such as calcium, magnesium, iron and aluminium. This is one reason why tetracyclines are not administered with foods high in these (e.g. Ca^{2+} in milk), or with antacids (salts of Al^{3+}, Ca^{2+}, Mg^{2+}). These antibiotics have a very broad spectrum of activity against Gram-positive and Gram-negative bacteria, spirochetes, mycoplasma, rickettsiae and chlamydia. **Tetracycline** comes from mutants of *Streptomyces aureofaciens*, and the related **oxytetracycline** from *S. rimosus* (Fig. 6.5).

Minocycline and **doxycycline** are produced semisynthetically from natural tetracyclines. Minocycline has a very broad spectrum of activity and doxycycline is now used prophylactically against malaria in regions where there is a high incidence of drug resistance.

Griseofulvin

The polyketide antibiotic griseofulvin comes from the fungus (mould) *Penicillium griseofulvum* (Fig. 6.6). It is a **spiro** compound: it has two rings **fused** at one carbon. It is used to treat fungal infections, especially dermatophytic infections of the skin, hair, nails and feet caused by fungi belonging to the genera *Trichophyton*, *Epidermophyton* and *Microsporum*, and for the treatment of ringworm in animals.

Erythromycin A

Erythromycin A is a complex polyketide from *Saccharopolyspora erythraea* (Actinomycetes), which is a filamentous bacterium, originally classified in the genus *Streptomyces*. It is a member of the class of **macrolide** antibiotics; these can contain 12 or more carbons in the main ring system. The term macrolide is derived from the fact that erythromycin is a large ring structure (**macro**) and is also a cyclic ester referred to as an **olide** (a lactone). As can be seen from Fig. 6.7, erythromycin A has characteristic features of natural products, being highly chiral (possessing many stereochemical centres) and having many different functional groups, including a sugar, an amino sugar, lactone, ketone and hydroxyl groups.

The antibiotic medicinal product is a mixture containing predominantly erythromycin A with small amounts of erythromycins B and C. It is used to treat Legionnaire disease and for patients with respiratory tract infections who are allergic to penicillin. Semisynthetic analogues (including **clarithromycin** and **azithromycin**) are now widely used and there is interest in the genetic manipulation of *S. erythraea* to produce 'un-natural' natural products, which could potentially have antibiotic activity.

The Statins

The statins are named for their ability to lower (bring into stasis) the production of cholesterol, high levels of which are a major contributing factor to the development of heart disease. Statins are inhibitors of the enzyme hydroxymethylglutaryl-CoA (HMG-CoA) reductase, which catalyses the conversion of HMG-CoA (Fig. 6.8) to mevalonic acid, one of the key intermediates in the biosynthesis of cholesterol. HMG-CoA reductase was a target for the discovery of the natural product inhibitor **mevastatin**, which was initially isolated from cultures of the fungi *Penicillium citrinum* and *P. brevicompactum* (see Fig. 6.8).

Following this discovery, the methyl analogue **lovastatin** was isolated from *Monascus ruber* and *Aspergillus terreus*. It was found

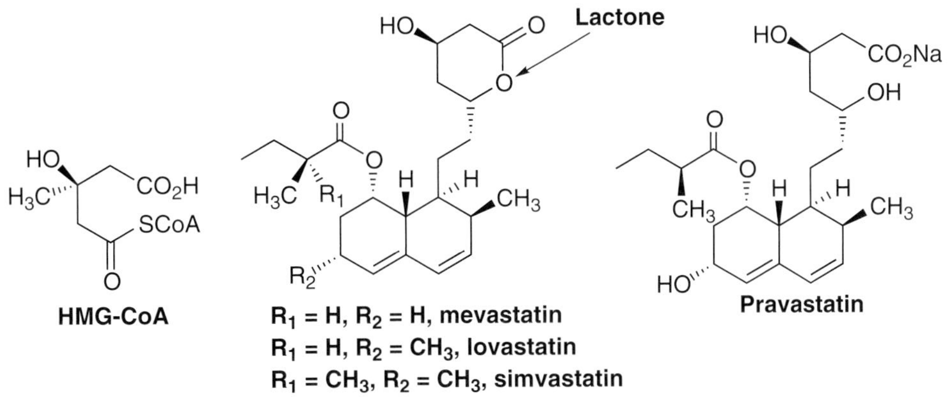

Fig. 6.8 Hydroxymethylglutaryl-coenzyme A (HMG-CoA) and statins.

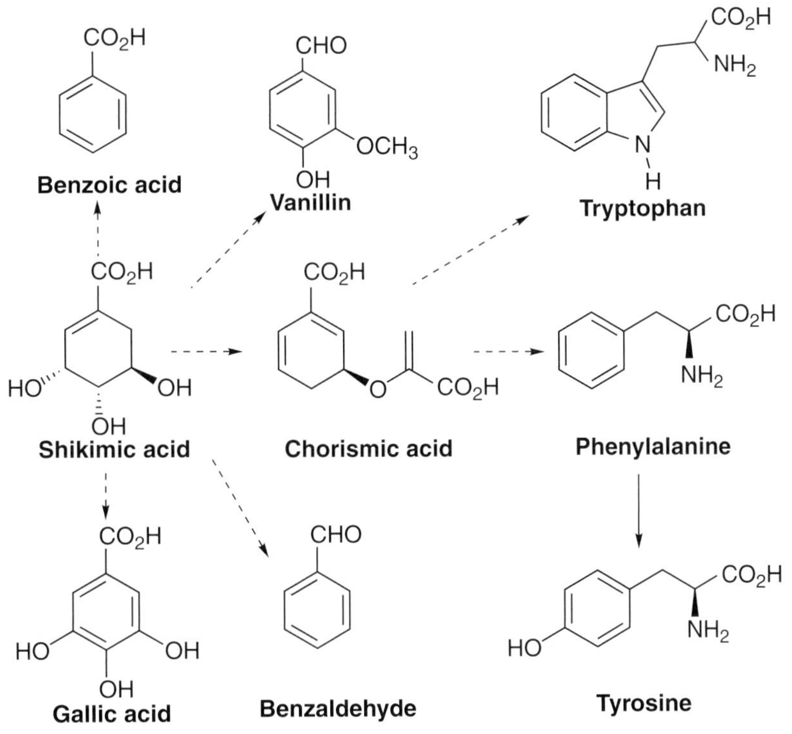

Fig. 6.9 Shikimic acid-derived natural products.

to also be an inhibitor of HMG-CoA reductase. **Simvastatin** is the dimethyl analogue of mevastatin and all three compounds are prodrugs, being activated by the hydrolysis (ring opening) of the lactone ring to β-hydroxy acids by liver enzymes. These acids are similar in structure to HMG-CoA and are inhibitors of HMG-CoA reductase. **Pravastatin** is semisynthetically produced by microbial hydroxylation of mevastatin by *Streptomyces carbophilus*. Unlike the previous examples, the lactone ring is opened to form the β-hydroxy acid, which is then converted into the sodium salt, increasing its hydrophilic water-soluble nature.

SHIKIMIC-ACID-DERIVED NATURAL PRODUCTS

Shikimic acid, sometimes referred to as shikimate, is a simple acid precursor for many natural products and aromatic amino acids, including phenylalanine, tyrosine, tryptophan, the simple aromatic acids that are common in nature (e.g. benzoic and gallic acids) and aromatic aldehydes, such as vanillin and benzaldehyde that contribute to the pungent smell of many plants (Fig. 6.9).

Several natural product groups are constructed from the amino acid phenylalanine, in particular the **phenylpropenes, lignans, coumarins** and **flavonoids**, all of which possess a common substructure based on an aromatic 6-carbon ring (C_6 unit) with a 3-carbon chain (C_3 unit) attached to the aromatic ring (Fig. 6.10). Many reactions can occur at this 9-carbon unit, including oxidation, reduction, methylation, cyclisation, glycosylation (addition of a sugar) and dimerisation, all of which contribute to the value of natural products as a resource for drug discovery by enhancing structural complexity with increased chirality and functionality.

Phenylpropenes

The phenylpropenes are the simplest of the shikimic-acid-derived natural products and consist purely of an aromatic ring with an unsaturated 3-carbon chain attached to the ring. They are biosynthesised by the oxidation of phenylalanine by the enzyme phenylalanine ammonia lyase, which through the loss of ammonia results in the formation of cinnamic acid. Cinnamic acid may then undergo **elaboration reactions** to generate many of the phenylpropenes. For example, in

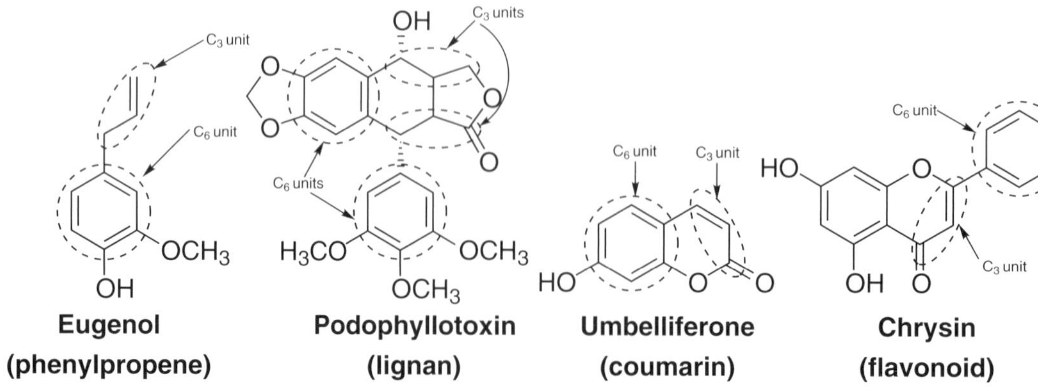

Eugenol
(phenylpropene)

Podophyllotoxin
(lignan)

Umbelliferone
(coumarin)

Chrysin
(flavonoid)

Fig. 6.10 Phenylpropene-derived natural products.

Phenylalanine   Cinnamic acid   Cinnamaldehyde

PAL = phenylalanine ammonia lyase

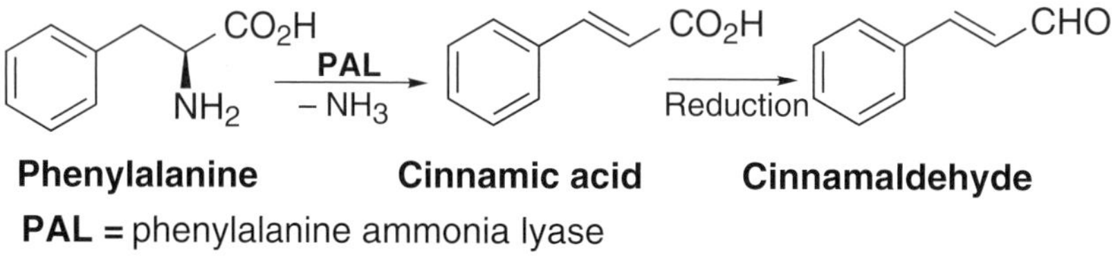

Fig. 6.11 Phenylalanine-derived natural products.

Eugenol   Myristicin   Safrole   Anethole

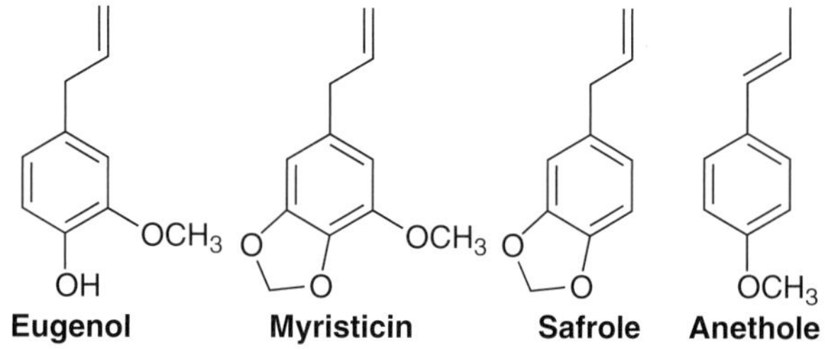

Fig. 6.12 Eugenol and related compounds.

Fig. 6.11, cinnamic acid is reduced to the corresponding aldehyde, **cinnamaldehyde**, which is the major metabolite in cinnamon oil derived from the bark of *Cinnamomum* species (Lauraceae) and used as a spice fragrance and flavouring, and for the treatment of fever and diarrhoea and other disorders.

Cinnamon leaf also contains **eugenol**, the major metabolite in oil of cloves derived from *Syzygium aromaticum* (L.) Merr. & L.M. Perry (Myrtaceae). Clove oil was used as a dental anaesthetic and antiseptic, both properties of which are due to eugenol, and the oil is still widely used as a short-term relief for dental pain. These phenylpropenes may have many different functional groups (e.g. OCH_3, $O–CH_2–O$, OH) and the double bond may be in a different position in the C_3 chain (e.g. eugenol versus **anethole**) (Fig. 6.12). They are common components of spices, have highly aromatic pungent aromas and many are broadly antimicrobial, with activities against yeasts and bacteria.

Myristicin is a metabolite in nutmeg (*Myristica fragrans* Houtt., Myristicaceae) and is psychoactive when ingested in large quantities. This phenylpropene is very lipophilic due to the presence of methylenedioxy and methyl ether substituent groups and it has been proposed that in vivo the double bond of this compound has an amino group added, resulting in the formation of a 3,4-methylenedioxymethamphetamine, MDMA, an illicit recreational drug. High doses of nutmeg can be fatal and the ingestion of large amounts should be avoided. Nutmeg also contains **safrole**, which is the toxic metabolite in sassafras (*Sassafras* spp., Lauraceae), and used as a precursor in the synthesis

of MDMA. ***Trans*-anethole** is the major metabolite of anise-flavoured essential oils from star anise (*Illicium verum* Hook. f., Illiciaceae), aniseed (*Pimpinella anisum* L., Apiaceae) and fennel (*Foeniculum vulgare* Mill. var. *vulgare*, Apiaceae). These oils are components of popular Mediterranean beverages such as anisette, ouzo and raki. When water is added to these drinks a cloudy white suspension results, which is attributable to a decrease in the solubility of these phenylpropenes as they are more soluble in ethanol than in water.

The phenylpropenes are generally extracted by **steam distillation** from plant material (e.g. cloves) to produce an essential oil, which is normally a complex mixture of phenylpropenes and other volatile natural products such as **hemiterpenes, monoterpenes** and **sesquiterpenes** (see later). The steam distillation procedure involves boiling the plant material with water and trapping the vapour in a distillation apparatus. The condensed liquid is transferred to a separating funnel and, as the oils are immiscible with water and form a less dense layer, they can be readily removed.

Lignans

Lignans are low-molecular-weight polymers formed by the coupling of two phenylpropene units through their C_3 side chains (Fig. 6.13) and between the aromatic ring and the C_3 chain. A common precursor of lignans is cinnamyl alcohol, which can readily form free radicals and enzymatically dimerise to form aryltetralin-type lignans of which the anticancer compounds **podophyllotoxin, 4-demethylpodophyllotoxin** and **α- and β-peltatin** (from *Podophyllum peltatum* L. and *P. hexandrum* Royle, Berberidaceae) are examples (Fig. 6.14). Lignans are common in the plant kingdom and are major metabolites in resinous exudates from roots and bark. The resin obtained from the roots of *P. peltatum* has long been used as a treatment for warts by North American Indians, and some preparations still contain 'podophyllin', an ethanolic extraction of the resin rich in podophyllotoxin, a lignan dimer of two 9-carbon ($C_6–C_3$) units with a 5-membered lactone ring or cyclic ester. Podophyllotoxin is highly toxic and not used clinically but was an important template on which to base the semisynthetic analogues **etoposide** and **teniposide**.

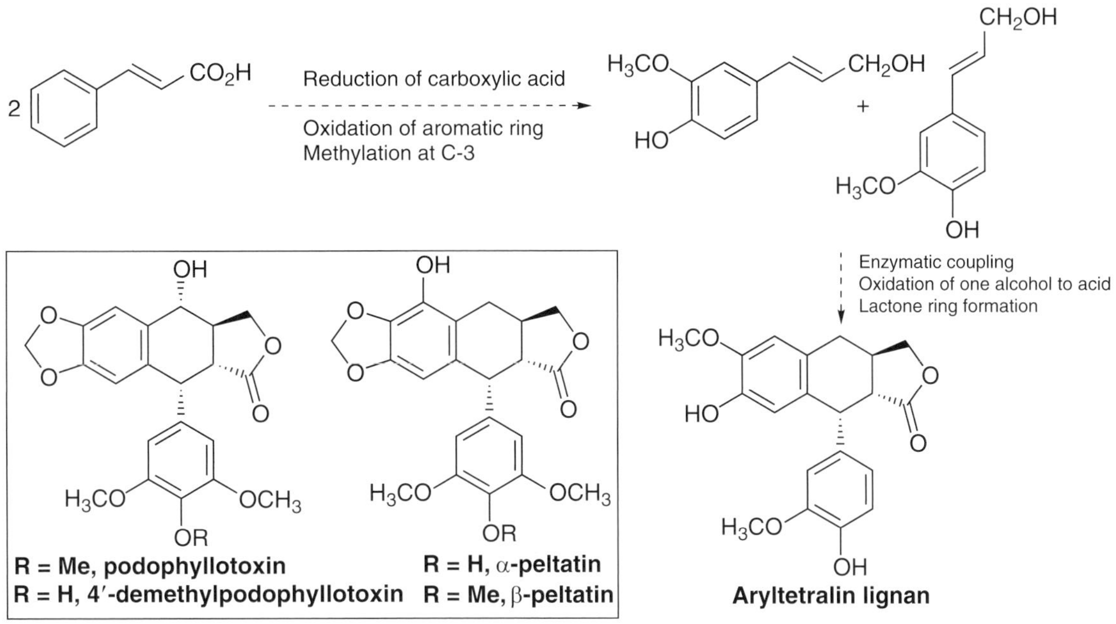

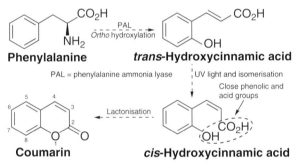

Fig. 6.13 Biosynthesis of lignans.

Coumarins

The coumarins are shikimate-derived metabolites formed when phenylalanine is deaminated and hydroxylated to *trans*-hydroxycinnamic acid (see Fig. 6.14). The double bond of this acid is readily converted to the *cis* form by light-catalysed isomerisation, resulting in the formation of a metabolite with phenolic and acidic groups in close proximity. These may then react **intramolecularly** to form a lactone and the basic coumarin nucleus, typified by the compound **coumarin** itself, which is recognisable as the scent of newly mown hay. Most coumarins are oxygenated at position C_7, resulting from *para* hydroxylation of cinnamic acid to give coumaric acid prior to further *ortho* hydroxylation, isomerisation and lactone formation.

Fig. 6.14 Biosynthesis of coumarins.

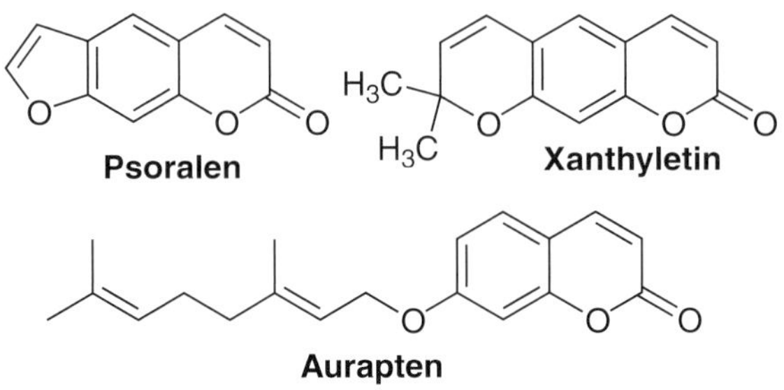

Fig. 6.15 Coumarin derivatives.

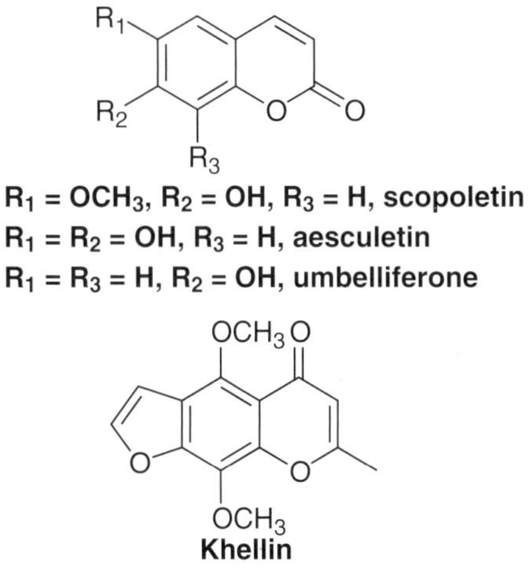

$R_1 = OCH_3$, $R_2 = OH$, $R_3 = H$, scopoletin
$R_1 = R_2 = OH$, $R_3 = H$, aesculetin
$R_1 = R_3 = H$, $R_2 = OH$, umbelliferone

Khellin

Fig. 6.16 Substituted coumarin derivatives.

Coumarins have a limited distribution in the plant kingdom and have been used to classify plants according to their presence (chemotaxonomy). They are commonly found in the families Apiaceae, Rutaceae, Asteraceae and Fabaceae and, as with all the natural products mentioned so far, undergo many elaboration reactions, including hydroxylation and methylation and, particularly, the addition of terpenoid-derived groups (C_2, C_5 and C_{10} units) (Fig. 6.15).

Some coumarins are **phytoalexins** and are synthesised de novo by the plant following infection by a bacterium or fungus. These phytoalexins are broadly antimicrobial; for example, **scopoletin** is synthesised by the potato (*Solanum tuberosum* L.) following fungal infection. **Aesculetin** occurs in the horse chestnut (*Aesculus hippocastanum* L.) and preparations of the seeds of this species are used to treat capillary fragility. *Hieracium pilosella* L. (now classed as *Pilosella officinarum* Vaill., Asteraceae), also known as mouse ear, contains **umbelliferone** and was used to treat infections; the antibacterial activity of this plant drug may in part be due to its presence (Fig. 6.16). **Khellin** is an **isocoumarin** (**chromone, furanochrome** and **furanocoumarin**) from *Ammi visnaga* (L.) Lam. (now classed as *Visnaga daucoides* Gaertn, Apiaceae) and has activity as a spasmolytic and vasodilator; it was the template for the development of drugs such as the antiallergic cromoglycate (see Chapter 21 Respiratory System), nifedipine (a calcium channel antagonist and vasodilator) used in heart disease, and amiodarone, a cardiac antiarrhythmic.

Coumarins are common in the Fabaceae, and it has long been known that animals fed with mouldy sweet clover, *Melilotus officinalis*, (L.) Pall. can die from haemorrhaging. The compound responsible was identified as the bishydroxycoumarin (hydroxylated coumarin dimer) **dicoumarol** (Fig. 6.17), produced by fungal spoilage of incompletely dried feeds or silage.

Dicoumarol has been used medicinally as an anticoagulant. Synthetic compounds based on the dicoumarol structure including salts of **warfarin** and **nicoumalone** are now more widely used. These agents interfere with vitamin K function in liver cells—necessary for the synthesis of 'normal' prothrombin—and a deficiency leads to abnormal prothrombin synthesis and a reduction in activity of the blood-clotting mechanism. Warfarin has also been used as rat poison.

The **psoralens** are coumarins with a furan ring and are sometimes known as **furocoumarins** or **furanocoumarins**. Examples are **psoralen, bergapten, xanthotoxin** and **isopimpinellin** (Fig. 6.18). Because of the extended chromophore of these compounds, they readily absorb light and fluoresce blue/yellow under long-wave ultraviolet light (UV-A, 320 to 380 nm). These compounds may be produced by the plant as a protection mechanism against high doses of sunlight: the psoralens are typical of the citrus (Rutaceae) and celery (Apiaceae) families. Some plants in these groups are known as 'blister bushes' as the psoralens they contain are known to cause phototoxicity or photosensitisation. The giant hogweed (*Heracleum mantegazzianum* Sommier & Levier), now a globally invasive species, but indigenous to Central Asia, is rich in psoralens and, in the presence of sunlight, can cause inflammation and blistering of the skin. Restrictions on the planting, breeding or otherwise encouraging the propagation of this species are legally enforceable in many countries. Other known phototoxic species include hogweed (*Heracleum sphondylium* L.), rue (*Ruta graveolens* L. and R. *chalepensis* L.) and some *Citrus* spp., particularly essential oils from bergamot (*Citrus* × *aurantium* subsp. *bergamia* (Risso & Poit.) Wight & Arn. ex Engl., Rutaceae, now included in *Citrus* × *limon* (L.) Osbeck) of which a major metabolite is **bergapten**. Many plants of the Apiaceae are of culinary importance, such as celery (*Apium graveolens* L.), parsley (*Petroselinum crispum* (Mill.) Fuss), parsnip (*Pastinaca sativa* L.) and angelica (*Angelica archangelica* L.), also contain furanocoumarins, and may be photosensitising in susceptible individuals.

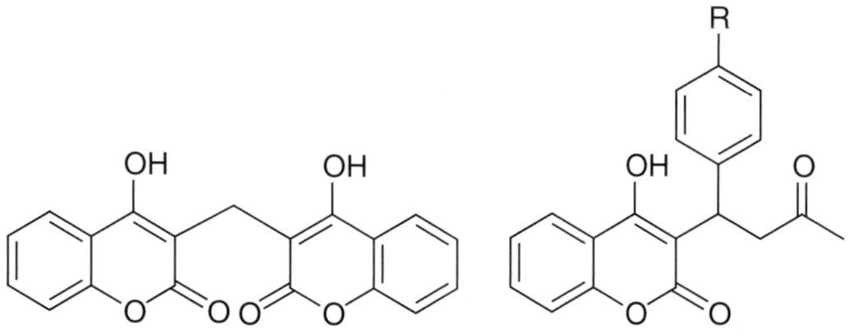

The psoralens are carcinogenic and mutagenic due to the formation of adducts with pyrimidine bases of DNA, such as thymine, via cycloaddition (Fig. 6.19). This reaction can occur with one (monoadduct) or two (di-adduct) pyrimidine bases and may result in cross-linking of DNA.

The ability of the psoralens to enhance the effects of UV light (photosensitisation) is exploited to promote skin pigmentation in the disease vitiligo, an autoimmune disease characterised by patches of skin that are deficient in the pigment melanin, and in severe psoriasis. Pure **xanthotoxin** (known as 8-methoxypsoralen, 8-MOP) is used to treat severe vitiligo and psoriasis and is given orally in combination with UV-A radiation. This results in coloration and pigmentation of non-pigmented skin areas and an improvement in the psoriatic skin by reducing cell proliferation. The treatment is referred to as PUVA (psoralen + UV-A) and is not without risks, requiring careful regulation to prevent skin cancer or cataract formation.

Flavonoids

The flavonoids are derived from a C_6–C_3 (phenylpropane) unit, which has as its source shikimic acid (via phenylalanine) and a further C_6 unit that is derived from the polyketide pathway. This polyketide fragment is generated by three molecules of malonyl-CoA, which combine with the C_6–C_3 unit (as a CoA thioester) to form a triketide starter unit (Fig. 6.20). Flavonoids are, therefore, of mixed biosynthesis, consisting of units derived from both shikimic acid and polyketide pathways.

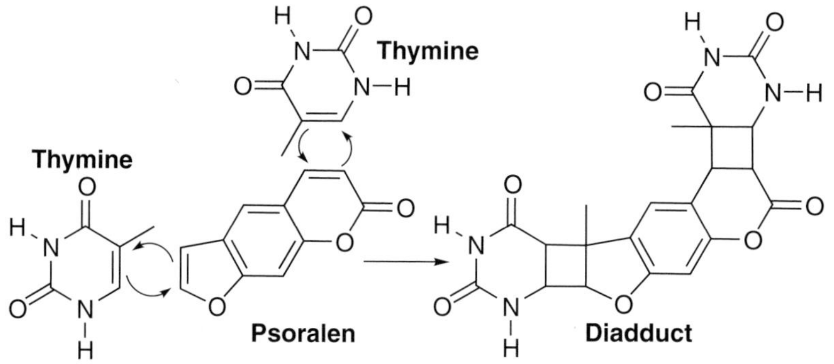

Dicoumarol

R = H, warfarin
R = NO₂, nicoumalone

Fig. 6.17 Dicoumarol and the synthetic anticoagulants warfarin and nicoumalone.

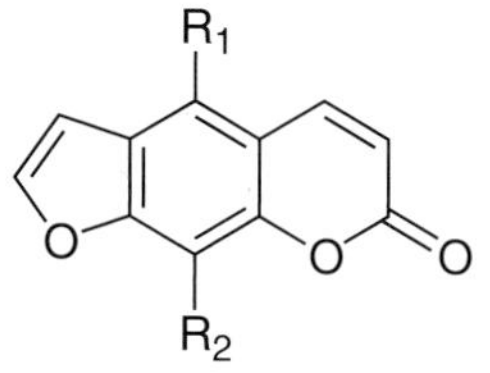

$R_1 = R_2 = H$,   psoralen
$R_1 = OCH_3$, $R_2 = H$, bergapten
$R_1 = H$, $R_2 = OCH_3$, xanthotoxin
$R_1 = R_2 = OCH_3$,   isopimpinellin

Fig. 6.18 Psoralens.

Fig. 6.19 Formation of a psoralen adduct with a pyrimidine base of DNA, thymine.

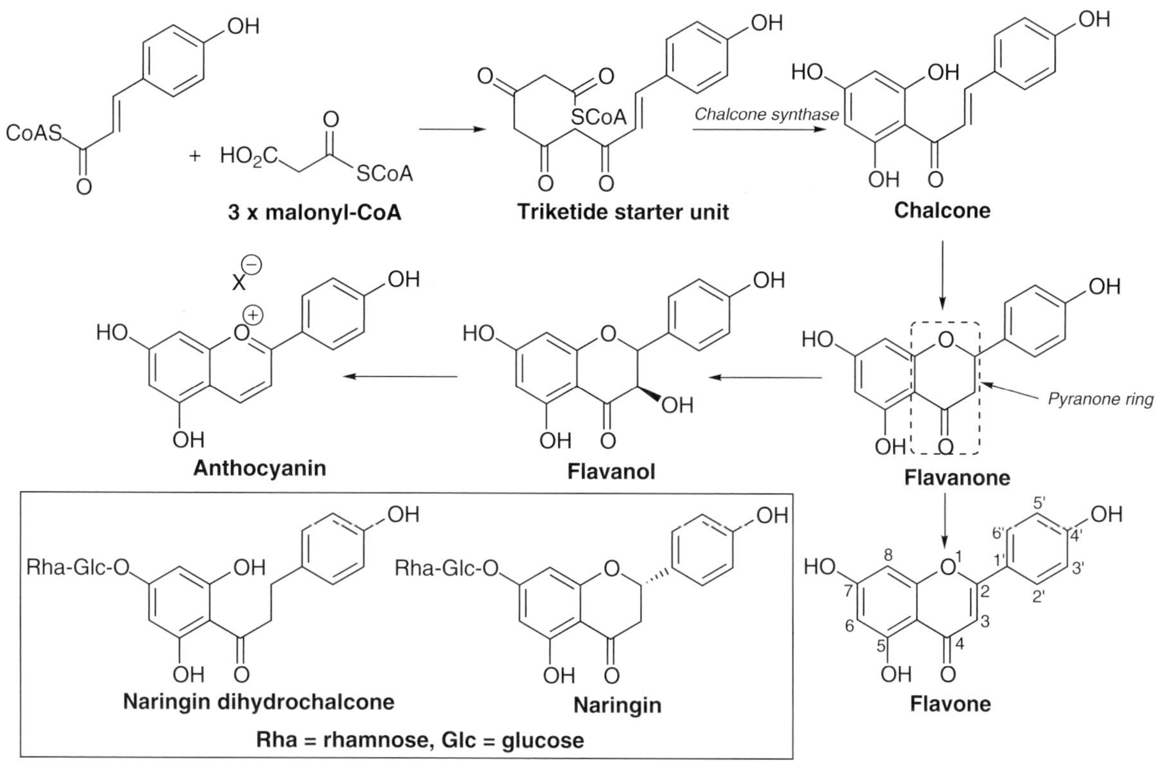

Fig. 6.20 Biosynthesis of flavonoids.

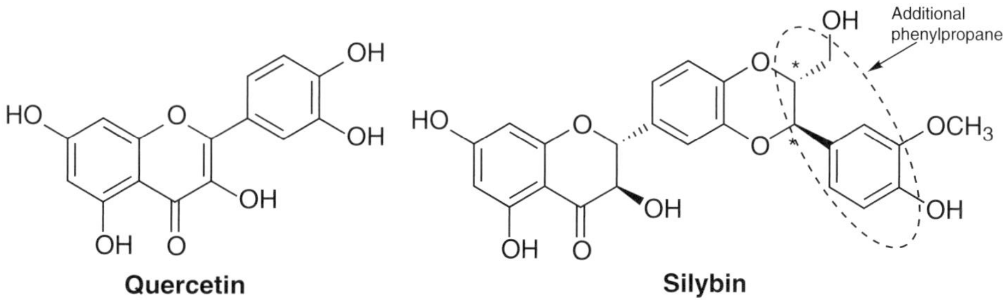

Fig. 6.21 Flavonols.

The triketide starter unit undergoes cyclisation by the enzyme chalcone synthase to generate the **chalcone** group of flavonoids. Cyclisation can then occur to give a pyranone ring-containing **flavanone** nucleus, which can either have the C_2–C_3 bond oxidised (unsaturated) to give the **flavones** or be hydroxylated at position C_3 of the pyranone ring to give the **flavanol** group of flavonoids. The flavanols may be further oxidised to yield the **anthocyanins**, which contribute to the brilliant blues of flowers and the dark colour of red wine. The flavonoids contribute to many of the other colours found in nature, particularly the yellow and orange of petals; even the colourless flavonoids absorb light in the UV spectrum (due to their extensive chromophores) and are visible to many insects. It is likely that these compounds have high ecological importance as colour attractants to insects and birds to aid plant pollination. Certain flavonoids also markedly affect the taste of foods; for example, some are very bitter and astringent such as the flavanone glycoside **naringin** (see Fig. 6.20), which occurs in the peel of grapefruit *Citrus × aurantium* L. (*Citrus × paradisi* Macfad.). Interestingly, the closely related **naringin dihydrochalcone** (see Fig. 6.20), which lacks the pyranone ring of naringin, is exceptionally sweet—some 1000 times sweeter than table sugar (sucrose).

Flavonoids are important dietary components because, being phenolic, they are strongly antioxidant. Many diseases are exacerbated by the presence of free radicals, such as superoxide and hydroxyl, and flavonoids scavenge and effectively 'mop up' these damaging oxidants.

Foods rich in flavonoids are important in preventing cancer and heart disease. **Quercetin** (Fig. 6.21), a flavonoid present in many foods, is a strong antioxidant and chemopreventant. Metabolites in milk thistle (*Silybum marianum* (L.) Gaertn.), in particular **silybin** (see Fig. 6.21), are antihepatotoxins; extracts of milk thistle are generally known as **silymarin** and are used to treat liver disease and reduce the effects of poisoning by fungi of the genus *Amanita*, which produce the deadly peptide toxins the amanitins. The mechanism of action is not entirely clear, but they may protect liver cells by reducing entry of the toxins through the cell membrane and scavenging the free radicals that can lead to hepatotoxicity. Silybin is a flavanol with an additional phenylpropane unit joined to it as a di-ether and it exists in the extract as a mixture of enantiomers at one of the positions where this additional unit is joined (* in Fig. 6.21).

The **stilbenes**, sometimes referred to as **bisbenzyls** or **stilbenoids**, are related to the flavonoids and have the basic structure C_6–C_2–C_6 (Fig. 6.22) arising from the loss of one carbon (as CO_2) from the triketide starter unit. The simplest member of this class is **stilbene**. **Resveratrol**, a component of red wine, has antioxidant and anti-inflammatory activity as well as alleged cancer-preventive effects. Together with other flavonoids and anthocyanins, it is associated with the low incidence of heart disease among the French population where there is also a high consumption of fats, a phenomenon known as 'the French paradox'. The **combretastatins**, such as **combretastatin A₁**,

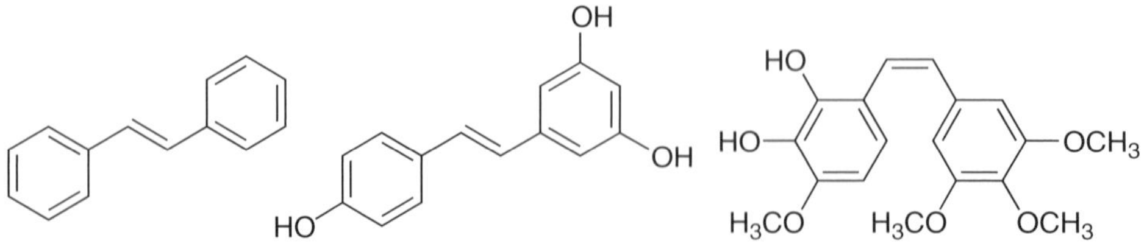

Stilbene   **Resveratrol**   **Combretastatin A₁**

Fig. 6.22 Stilbenes.

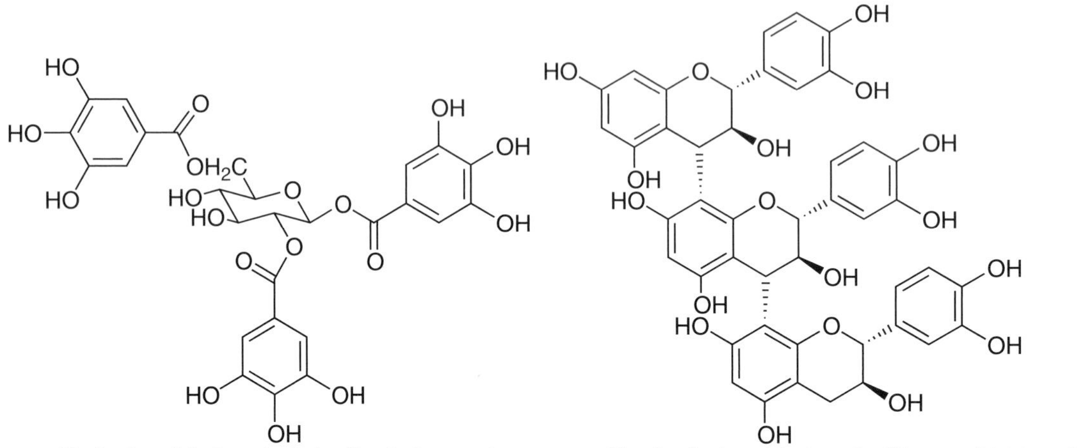

Hydrolysable tannin (trigalloyl glucose)   **Nonhydrolysable tannin (flavonoid trimer)**

Fig. 6.23 Hydrolysable and non-hydrolysable (condensed) tannins.

are cytotoxic stilbenoids that are inhibitors of microtubule assembly and exert their anticancer activity by targeting tumour vasculature. Combretastatin A₁ is derived from *Combretum caffrum* (Eckl. & Zeyh.) Kuntze (Combretaceae).

Tannins

Tannins are water-soluble polyphenolic compounds which may have a high molecular weight and are broadly divided into two groups: the **hydrolysable and nonhydrolysable** tannins. Hydrolysable tannins are formed by the esterification of sugars (e.g. glucose) with simple shikimate-derived, phenolic acids (e.g. gallic acid), and the **nonhydrolysable** (or **condensed**) tannins occur due to polymerisation (condensation) reactions between flavonoids (Fig. 6.23).

As their name suggests, the hydrolysable tannins may be hydrolysed with base to simple acids and sugars. A key feature of tannins is their ability to bind to proteins, and they have been used to tan leather, clarify beer and as astringent preparations in medicines and cosmetics. They have a very wide distribution in the plant kingdom and may be produced by a plant as a feeding deterrent, as their binding to proteins may reduce the dietary value of the plant as a food. They are currently attracting interest as animal feed additives for controlling nematode (worm) infections in grazing animals.

Tannic acid is a mixture of gallic acid esters of glucose and is obtained from nutgall, which is an abnormal growth of the tree *Quercus infectoria* G. Oliv. produced by insects. These growths (galls) are harvested and extracted with solvents (ether and water); the aqueous layer is collected and evaporated to yield tannic acid, which is further purified and used as a topical preparation for cold sores.

TERPENES

The terpenes are very widespread in nature and occur in most species, including humans. They are known as **isoprenes** because a common recurring motif in their structure (the branched repeating C_5 unit,

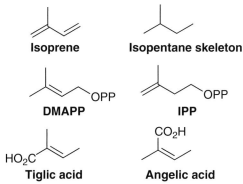

Isoprene   **Isopentane skeleton**

DMAPP   **IPP**

Tiglic acid   **Angelic acid**

Fig. 6.24 Biosynthesis of hemiterpenes.

the **isopentane** skeleton) is similar to isoprene (Fig. 6.24). Terpenes (**hemiterpenes, monoterpenes** and **sesquiterpenes**) contribute to many of the aromas associated with plants and range in complexity from simple C_5 units (**hemiterpenes**) up to the **polyisoprenes**, which include latex, leaf waxes and rubber. Terpenes are derived from a number of extensive reactions between two C_5 units (**dimethylallyl pyrophosphate (DMAPP)** and **isopentenyl pyrophosphate (IPP)**) (see Fig. 6.24); the products of these reactions will, therefore, have multiples of five carbons. DMAPP and IPP are biosynthesised from two sources (**mevalonic acid** or **deoxyxylulose phosphate**).

The terpenes are highly structurally diverse, and many are chiral and have extensive functional group chemistry. The simplest are the hemiterpenes (C_5) produced by modification reactions to either DMAPP or IPP and include simple acids such as the structural isomers **tiglic acid** and **angelic acid** (see Fig. 6.24), which form esters with many natural products. The monoterpenes (C_{10}), sesquiterpenes (C_{15}), **diterpenes** (C_{20}), **triterpenes** and **steroids** (C_{30}-derived) and the **tetraterpenes** (**carotenoids**, C_{40}) are all important medicinally and thus will be dealt with in more detail.

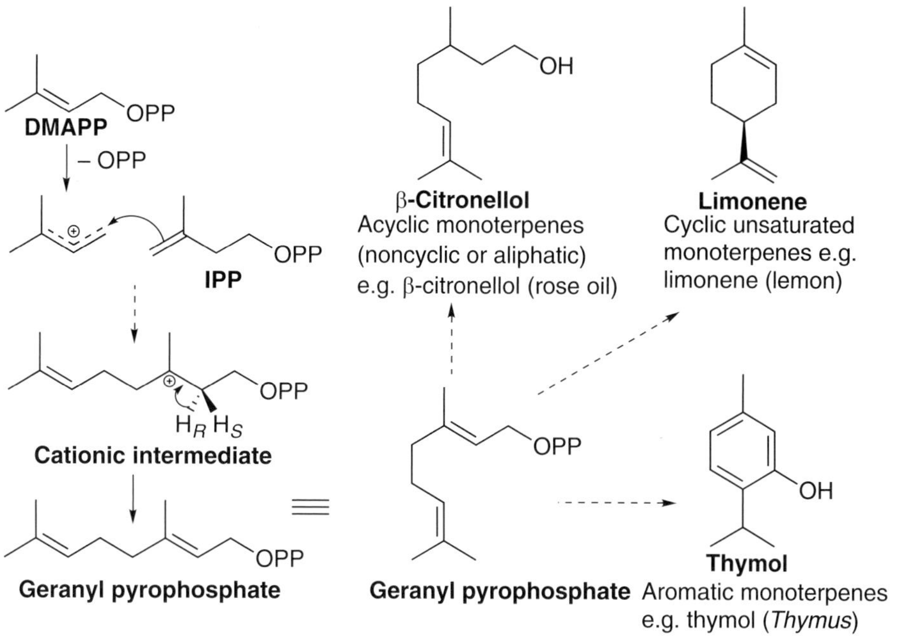

Fig. 6.25 Biosynthesis of monoterpenes.

Monoterpenes (C₁₀)

Together with the phenylpropenes, the **monoterpenes** are major constituents of the volatile (essential) oils that have highly characteristic odours and tastes and are used widely in the food and cosmetic industries in flavourings and perfumes. Monoterpenes are present in the leaf glands of plants and in the skin and peel of fruit (in particular *Citrus* spp.). The reasons for the presence of these compounds in the exterior organs of the plant are due to the complex interactions that plants have with other organisms: some monoterpenes are insect attractants (to aid pollination), others have a broad spectrum of antimicrobial activity to inhibit growth and invasion by bacteria and fungi (e.g. **thymol**). Volatile oils in plants are highly complex and their analysis can show the presence of hundreds of individual metabolites, many of which are monoterpenoid. These oils are highly prized in the perfume and food industry. Monoterpenes may be either aliphatic (**acyclic** or straight chain) or **cyclic** (saturated, partially unsaturated or fully aromatic) compounds. They usually possess functional groups such as ethers, hydroxyls, acids, aldehydes, esters or ketone moieties, and are generally highly volatile and fat-soluble (lipophilic).

Biosynthetically, the monoterpenes are produced by the reaction between DMAPP and IPP in the presence of the enzyme **prenyltransferase** (Fig. 6.25). The first step of this reaction is thought to be the ionisation of DMAPP to a cation (through the loss of pyrophosphate), which is then attacked by the double bond of IPP to generate a further cationic intermediate. Loss of a proton from the carbon neighbouring the cation (resulting in double bond formation) occurs in a stereospecific fashion (the R proton is lost) and this generates **geranyl pyrophosphate** (a C₁₀ unit).

Geranyl pyrophosphate can then undergo many reactions to generate the variety of monoterpenes observed, such as simple modification to give the acyclic monoterpene β-citronellol, which is a component of rose oil. Geranyl pyrophosphate can be cyclised to give cyclic monoterpenes, which may be fully saturated, partially unsaturated or fully aromatic products of which **menthol, piperitone** and **carvacrol** are examples, respectively (Fig. 6.26). The extensive structural diversity of this group is astounding considering that all of the monoterpenes are derived from just one C₁₀ unit, geranyl pyrophosphate.

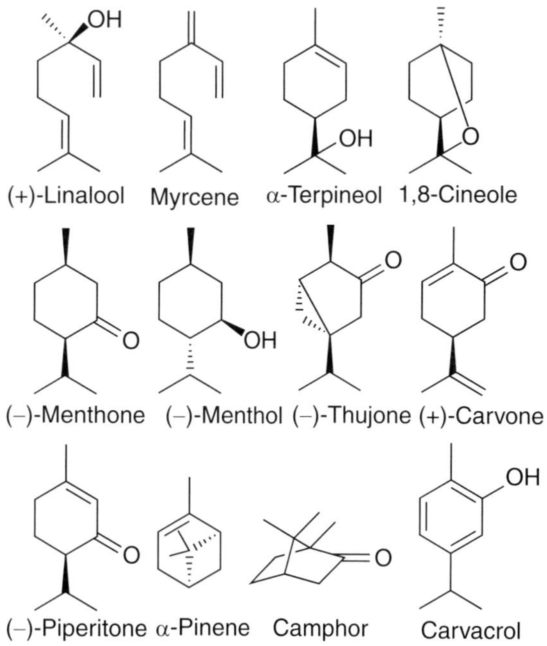

Fig. 6.26 Modified monoterpenes.

Linalool, a major constituent of coriander oil (*Coriandrum sativum* L.), is used as a flavouring and carminative. **Myrcene**, which is present in hop oil, is also used as a flavouring and currently some health benefits are being actively explored including anxiolytic, antioxidant, antiageing, antiinflammatory and analgesic properties (Surendran et al., 2021). Tea tree oil (from *Melaleuca alternifolia* (Maiden & Betche) Cheel) has been used by the Indigenous peoples of Australia as a treatment for skin infections. A main ingredient of this volatile oil is the tertiary hydroxylated monoterpene **α-terpineol**. **1,8-Cineole**, the structurally related ether, also has antibacterial properties and comes from species of *Eucalyptus* in the same family as *Melaleuca*, the Myrtaceae. **Menthol** and **menthone** are major metabolites in oils of plants belonging to the genus *Mentha* (Lamiaceae); in particular,

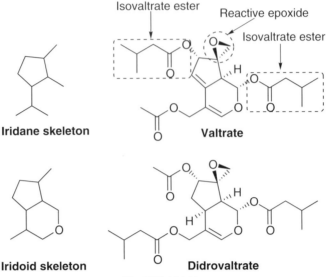

Fig. 6.27 Iridoids.

peppermint (*Mentha × piperita* L.) is used as a flavouring and carminative tea, and menthone is included in some pharmaceutical preparations as a nasal decongestant. **Thujone** has a cyclopropane ring as a functional group and is a metabolite in *Artemisia absinthium* L., an extract of which was used as an anthelmintic by the French army, hence the common name for this plant, wormwood. The liqueur absinthe was prepared by making an alcoholic extract of wormwood. **Carvone** is derived from dill (*Anethum graveolens* L.) and caraway oils (*Carum carvi* L.), which are used in carminative and digestive preparations. **α-Pinene**, which has a cyclobutane ring system, is the major metabolite in juniper oil (*Juniperus communis* L.), which is antiseptic and used in aromatherapy and as a flavouring. Essential oil from *Cinnamomum camphora* (L.) J. Presl (Lauraceae) is produced by steam distillation of the wood and is rich in **camphor**.

Natural oils have a very specific aroma, which accounts for the preference for these complex natural mixtures rather than cheaper synthetic alternatives. They are produced by **steam distillation** and, unless much is known about the stability of the oil components, care must be taken using this technique as some monoterpenes are **thermolabile** (i.e. they decompose on heating). The analysis of these complex mixtures is usually performed by gas chromatography (GC) or combined GC and mass spectrometry (GC–MS).

The **iridoids** are monoterpenes and oxidation products derived from geranyl pyrophosphate (Fig. 6.27). These normally esterified metabolites are common in the Lamiaceae, Gentianaceae and Caprifoliaceae. The ester element is often derived from hemiterpenes; for example, valeric acid is esterified to form **valtrate** and **didrovaltrate**. These compounds come from valerian (*Valeriana officinalis* L., Caprifoliaceae) and are often referred to as the **valepotriates**; they are highly functional, possessing isovalerate esters and an epoxide group that is possibly responsible for the in vitro cytotoxicity of valtrate and didrovaltrate.

Sesquiterpenes (C$_{15}$)

Sesquiterpenes have similar properties to the monoterpenes and are also metabolites in many volatile oils. They are broadly antimicrobial and antiinsecticidal, therefore contributing to the overall chemical defence of the producing organism. The starting unit for these compounds is **farnesyl pyrophosphate** (FPP), which is produced by the reaction of geranyl pyrophosphate (GPP) (the monoterpene precursor) with a molecule of IPP (Fig. 6.28). The reaction

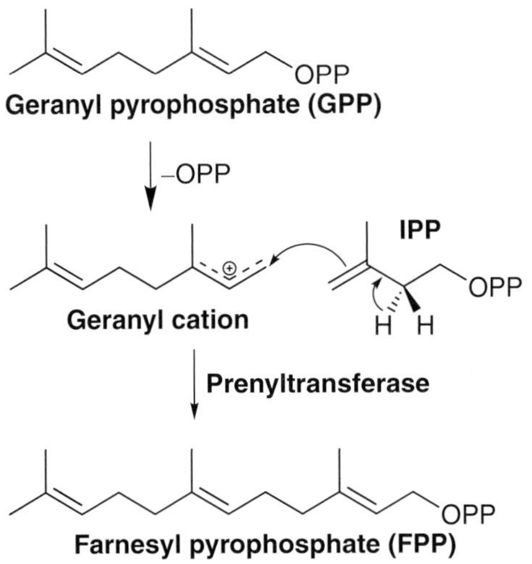

Fig. 6.28 Biosynthesis of farnesyl pyrophosphate and sesquiterpenes.

is analogous to the formation of the monoterpenes in which a cationic intermediate is formed that reacts with IPP with elimination of a hydrogen ion.

As with the monoterpenes, FPP can cyclise to form linear (acyclic) and cyclic sesquiterpenes. A key feature of these metabolites is their ability to undergo extensive elaboration chemistry, where they are highly functionalised, thus giving rise to the high structural diversity seen within this group of natural products. It is not always easy to see that these complex, functional, cyclic chiral compounds are derived from FPP due to these elaboration reactions. However, if the C$_{15}$ **skeleton** of FPP is compared to **arteannuin B**, it can be seen how even complex structures are constructed (Fig. 6.29).

The antimalarial **artemisinin** (Fig. 6.30) was isolated from sweet wormwood (...), used in China to treat fever (*Artemisia annua* L., Asteraceae). Artemisinin has a number of interesting features, including an ether, a lactone (cyclic ester) and an unusual peroxide functional group. The peroxide is essential for the antimalarial activity, and work has been carried out to enhance the solubility whilst retaining the biological activity. **Artemether**, the methyl ether of **dihydroartemisinin** (which possesses an acetal functional group), and **artesunic acid** (a succinic acid derivative) are very lipid-soluble.

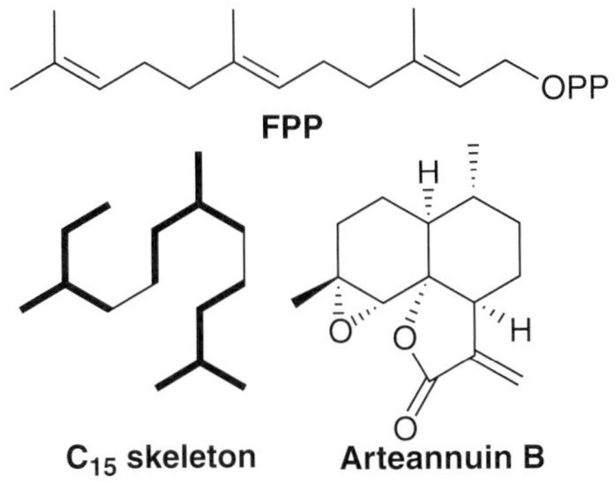

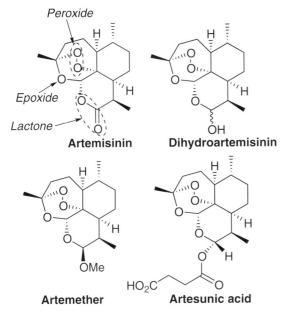

Fig. 6.29 Farnesyl pyrophosphate, the C15 skeleton and arteannuin B.

Fig. 6.30 Antimalarial sesquiterpene lactones.

Another Chinese medicinal plant used for treating malaria, *Artabotrys hexapetalus* (L.f.) Bhandari (*Annonaceae*), also contains a series of sesquiterpene peroxides (typically, **yingzhaosu A**; Fig. 6.31), which are responsible for the antimalarial activity.

Cottonseed oil (*Gossypium hirsutum* L.) has been shown to have contraceptive effects and restrict fertility in men and women when incorporated into the diet. In men, the oil has been shown to alter sperm maturation, motility and inhibit enzymes necessary for fertilisation. In women, inhibition of implantation has been observed. The active metabolite is the **bis-sesquiterpene** (**sesquiterpene dimer**) (−)-**gossypol**, which exists in the plant with the (+)-isomer. These compounds are optically active due to restricted rotation around the bond that joins the two naphthalene ring systems.

Diterpenes

Diterpenes are formed by the reaction of FPP, a C_{15} unit, with IPP, the C_5 unit that is the common building block for all of the terpenes. The first step of this reaction is the formation of a **farnesyl allylic cation** (analogous to the other examples of terpenes seen), which then reacts with IPP with stereospecific loss of a proton, resulting in the formation of **geranylgeranyl pyrophosphate** (GGPP). Depending on how GGPP folds and cyclises, a very large number of products may result (Fig. 6.32).

Loss of a proton from an allylic methyl (* in Fig. 6.32) and migration of bonds to form a bicyclic structure results in the formation of **labdadienyl pyrophosphate** (LDPP), which is a member of the **labdane** class of diterpenes of which **sclareol** from the clary sage (*Salvia sclarea*, Lamiaceae) is widely used in the perfumery industry. Sclareol is generated by hydrolysis of LDPP. If the *exo*methylene of LDPP reacts with a proton to form a cationic intermediate, this may undergo a series of **Wagner–Meerwein** hydride and methyl shifts (Fig. 6.33).

These reactions are sometimes referred to as **1,2-shifts** (indicating a movement of a group from a position to a neighbouring carbon) or **NIH shifts** (after the National Institutes of Health, where this reaction was studied). The hydride on C_9 migrates to C_8, the methyl on C_{10} migrates to C_9, the hydride on C_5 migrates to C_{10}, the β-methyl on C_4 migrates to C_5 and, finally, a proton is lost at C_3 resulting in the formation of a C_3–C_4 double bond. This series of migrations yields **clerodadienyl pyrophosphate** (CDPP; a **clerodane** diterpene) with many members of this class (for example, **hardwickiic acid,** which possesses a furan ring (produced by oxidation and cyclisation of the six-carbon side chain at C_9) and a carboxylic acid (produced by oxidation of C_{20})). An important facet of these Wagner–Meerwein shifts is the inversion of stereochemistry at the chiral centres where migration has occurred. For example, in LDPP, the methyl at C_{10} is β (coming up out of the plane of the page), whereas the corresponding group in CDPP is an α hydrogen (going down into the plane of the page). GGPP can cyclise to give an extraordinarily wide range of diterpene groups, some of which are shown in Fig. 6.34. Once a simple skeleton has been produced, a wide array of further elaboration reactions can occur. Plants producing diterpenes containing a nitrogen atom (**diterpene alkaloids**), such as *Aconitum* spp. and *Delphinium* spp., have historically been used medicinally. However, these compounds (e.g. **aconitine**) are highly toxic and are no longer used except in Chinese medicine, where they are specially processed, but still cause toxic reactions, including fatalities.

The antitumour diterpene paclitaxel (Fig. 6.35) was discovered in 1971. It belongs to a small class of taxanes with a four-membered ether (also called an oxirane) and a complex nitrogen-containing ester side chain; both of these functional groups are essential for antitumour activity. The solution to the problem of low concentration of the drug came from the knowledge that related compounds, such as **baccatin III** and **10-deacetylbaccatin III** (see Fig. 6.35), were present in greater concentrations than paclitaxel and could be converted to paclitaxel by simple reactions. Most importantly, 10-deacetylbaccatin III is also present in the needles (leaves) of the faster growing English yew (*Taxus*

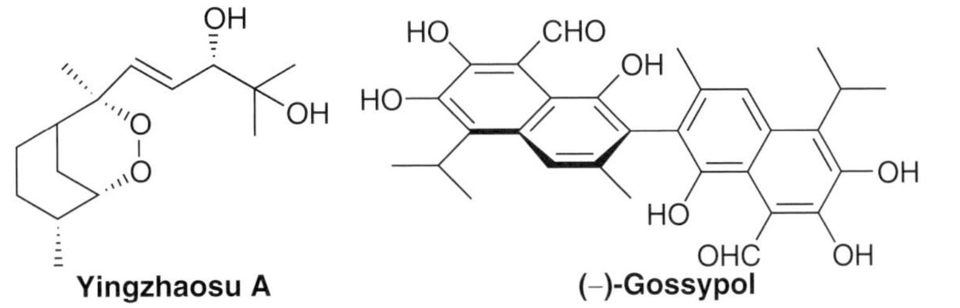

Fig. 6.31 Sesquiterpene derivatives.

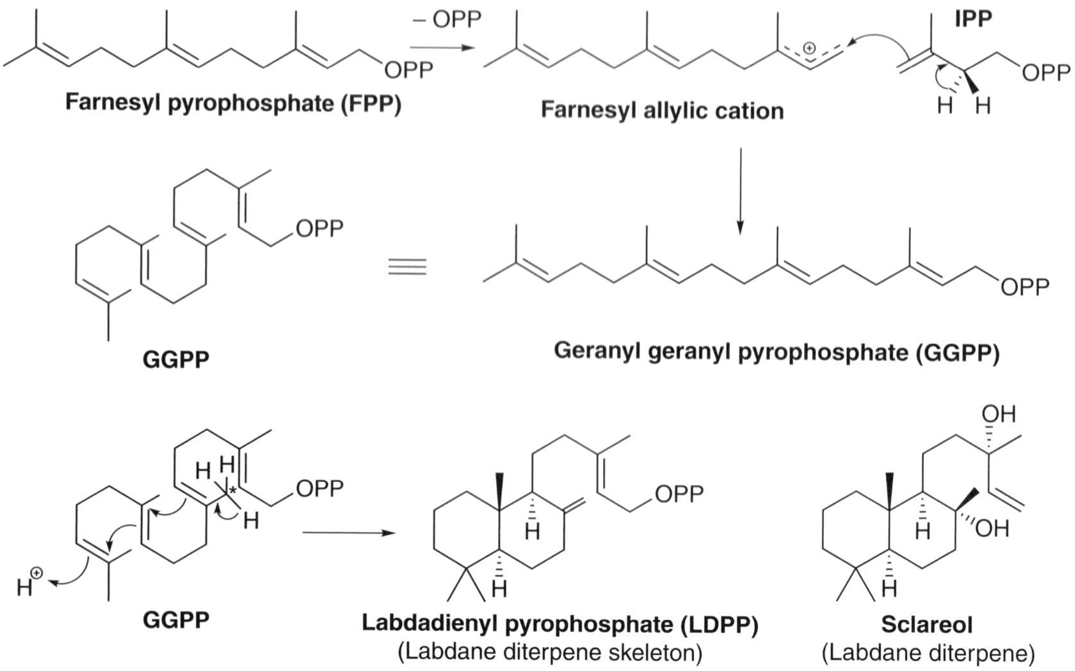

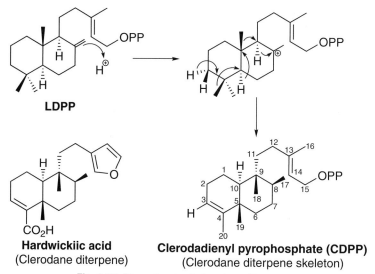

Fig. 6.32 Biosynthesis of labdane diterpenes from geranyl geranyl pyrophosphate (GGPP).

LDPP

Hardwickiic acid
(Clerodane diterpene)

Clerodadienyl pyrophosphate (CDPP)
(Clerodane diterpene skeleton)

Fig. 6.33 Biosynthesis of clerodane diterpenes.

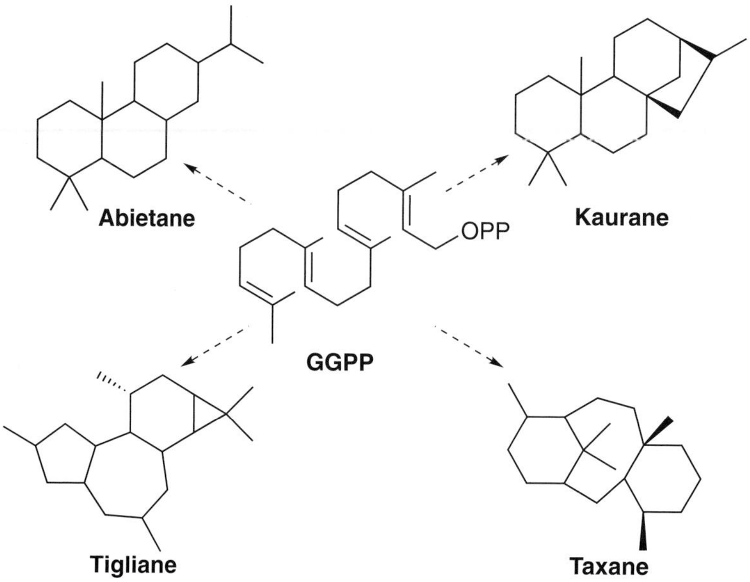

Abietane

Kaurane

GGPP

Tigliane

Taxane

Fig. 6.34 Terpene skeletons derived from geranyl geranyl pyrophosphate (GGPP).

baccata L.) at a higher concentration (0.1%) and, unlike the bark, the needles can be harvested without destroying the tree. Renewable resources are important in natural product chemistry: if a biologically active compound is developed into a drug, then large-scale production is always necessary. This is not problematic if a compound from a plant can be synthesised (semi- or fully synthesised) or produced by cell culture, and in the case of paclitaxel, a mixture of taxanes is extracted and treated with enzymes that specifically cleave ester groups from the taxane nucleus, resulting in a higher concentration of 10-deacetylbaccatin.

A fungus living in close association with the yew tree (*Taxomyces andreanae* Strobel, A. Stierle, D. Stierle & W. M. Hess) produces small concentrations of paclitaxel in fermentation culture. It is possible that the fungus has inherited the gene from the tree (or vice versa), which allows the organism to produce paclitaxel. Another fungus, isolated from the Himalayan yew tree (*Taxus wallichiana* Zucc.), is *Pestalotiopsis microspora* (Speg.) G. C. Zhao & N. Li, which produces higher concentrations of paclitaxel than *T. andreanae*. Paclitaxel is now produced by large-scale plant cell culture fermentation. **Docetaxel** (see Fig. 6.35), a related semi-synthetically produced taxane with a modified side chain to that of paclitaxel, is also used in the treatment of ovarian and other cancers.

Triterpenes

The triterpenes are C_{30}-derived terpenoids with an exceptionally wide distribution, including in humans, animals, plants, fungi, bacteria, soft corals and amphibia. The triterpenes include some very important

molecules, such as the **steroids** (e.g. **testosterone**), which are degraded triterpenes with many important functions in mammals, notably as sex hormones. Other types include the **sterols** (e.g. **β-sitosterol**), which are common tetracyclic steroidal alcohols with ubiquitous distribution in plants, the **pentacyclic triterpenes** such as **glycyrrhetic acid** found in liquorice and the **limonoids** (e.g. **limonin**), which are highly oxidised bitter principles present in the *Citrus* family (Rutaceae) (Fig. 6.36).

Triterpenes are also components of **resins** and resinous exudates from plants (e.g. frankincense and myrrh); myrrh is derived from the Arabic word for bitter, a characteristic which many triterpenes display. These resins are common from trees belonging to the family Burseraceae (which includes the myrrh-producing *Commiphora* sp.) and are produced following damage to the tree as a physical barrier to attack by fungi and bacteria. Many of the terpenoid components of these resins have high antimicrobial activity, killing potentially invasive microbes and slowing their growth until the tree has repaired the damage.

Their biosynthesis starts with the reaction between two molecules of FPP to form the true precursor of all triterpenes, **squalene** (Fig. 6.37). Squalene is then enzymatically epoxidised to **squalene epoxide** which, when folded in a particular conformation such as the 'chair-boat-chair-boat' conformation, can cyclise to give **sterol intermediate 1**, which is the precursor of the steroids and sterols (Fig. 6.38). This intermediate can undergo a series of Wagner–Meerwein shifts to give **lanosterol**, a common metabolite in plants and of wool fat.

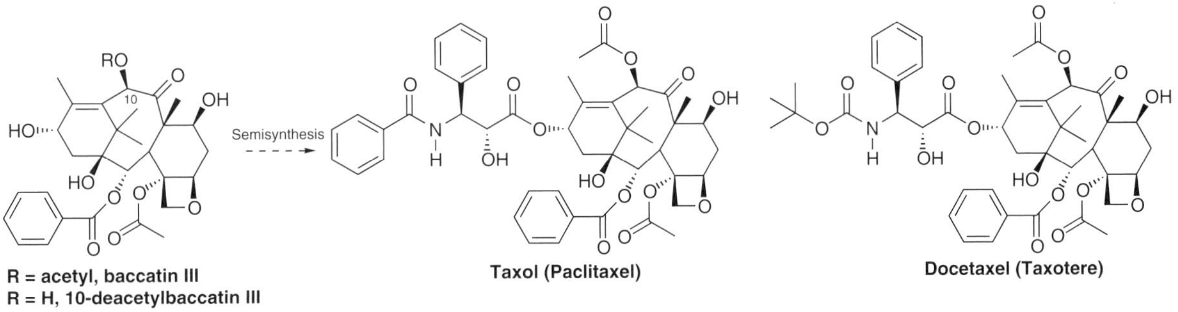

R = acetyl, baccatin III
R = H, 10-deacetylbaccatin III

Taxol (Paclitaxel)

Docetaxel (Taxotere)

Fig. 6.35 Taxane diterpenes.

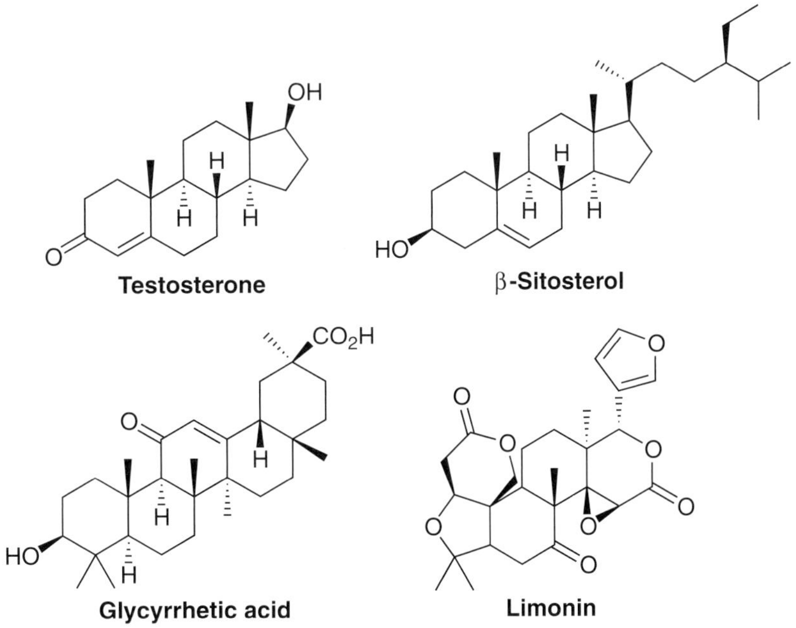

Testosterone

β-Sitosterol

Glycyrrhetic acid

Limonin

Fig. 6.36 Triterpenes.

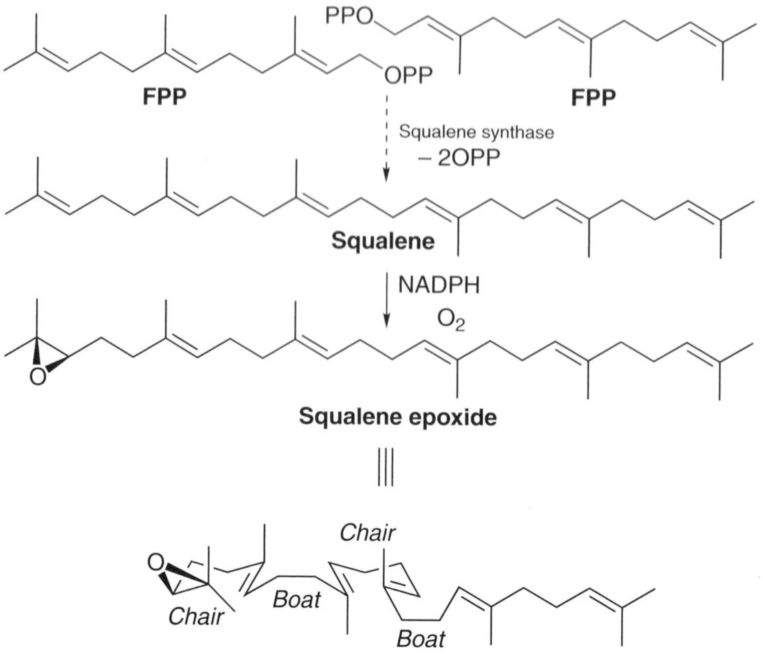

Squalene epoxide (chair-boat-chair-boat conformation)

Fig. 6.37 Biosynthesis of the sterol precursor, squalene epoxide.

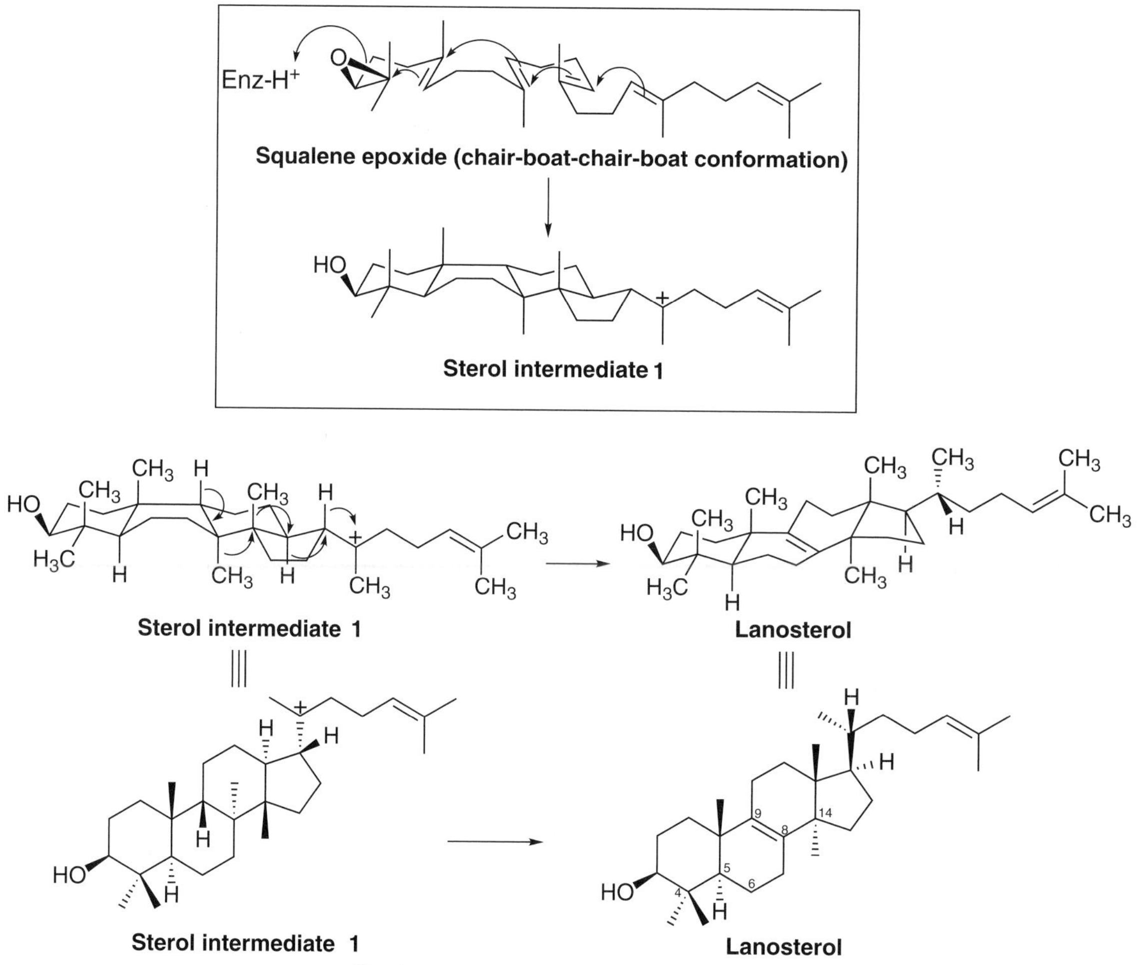

Fig. 6.38 Biosynthesis of the sterol skeleton.

Oxidation and loss of methyls at positions C_4 and C_{14}, introduction of a C_5–C_6 double bond (oxidation) and loss of two double bonds (one at C_8–C_9 and one in the side chain) results in the formation of **cholesterol**. Cholesterol is the main animal sterol, a component of cell membranes, and control of the levels of this sterol is important in the management of heart disease. The basic steroid nucleus and numbering of the ring system depicting the A, B, C and D rings are given for cholesterol (Fig. 6.39).

Other common sterols include the **phytosterols** (plant sterols) β-**sitosterol** and **stigmasterol** (which differs from β-sitosterol only by the presence of a double bond at position C_{22}–C_{23}), which are widespread in plants, and **ergosterol**, which is ubiquitous in fungi as a cell-wall component (see Fig. 6.39).

There is a great need for steroids in the pharmaceutical industry and this is met by using the plant sterol **diosgenin** from the wild yam (*Dioscorea* spp.). Diosgenin also occurs naturally as a glycoside (a sugar is attached at the hydroxyl position) and without the sugar the compound is referred to as a **genin**. Unlike the other plant sterols mentioned, the side chain normally present at position C_{17} has been transformed into a two-ring structure. Diosgenin can be converted into **progesterone** via a chemical process known as the marker degradation, which gives access to many important steroids such as **testosterone** (a male sex hormone) and **oestradiol** (a female sex hormone), which has had the A ring aromatised, resulting in the loss of a methyl group from C_{10} (Fig. 6.40).

Another semisynthetic compound lacking this methyl is the oral contraceptive **norethisterone**, which has an unusual acetylene group at position C_{17}. One of the most widely used steroids in pharmaceutical preparations is the antiinflammatory drug **hydrocortisone** (cortisol). This compound has a hydroxyl group at C_{11} that is introduced into

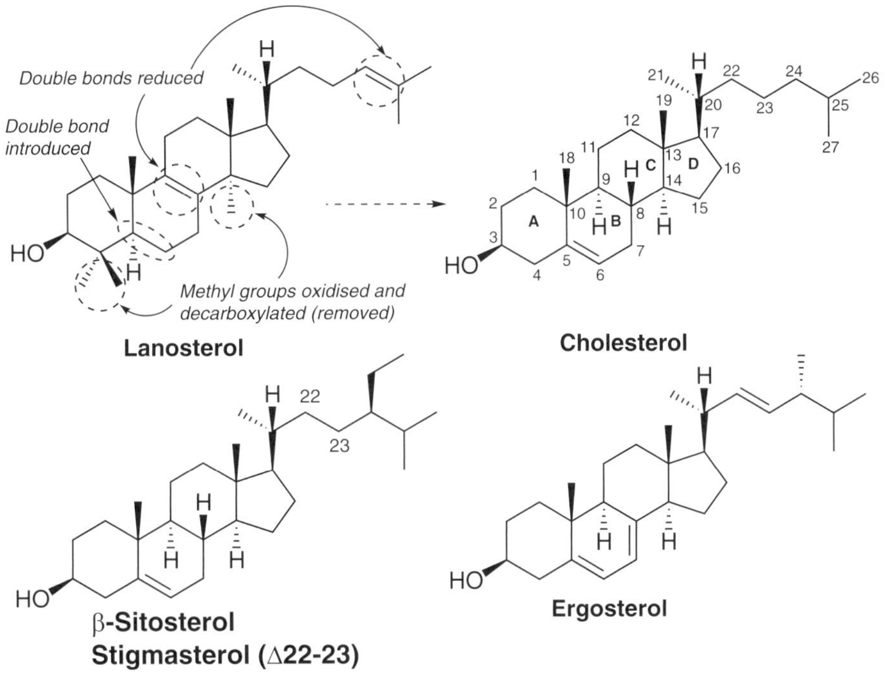

Fig. 6.39 Sterols.

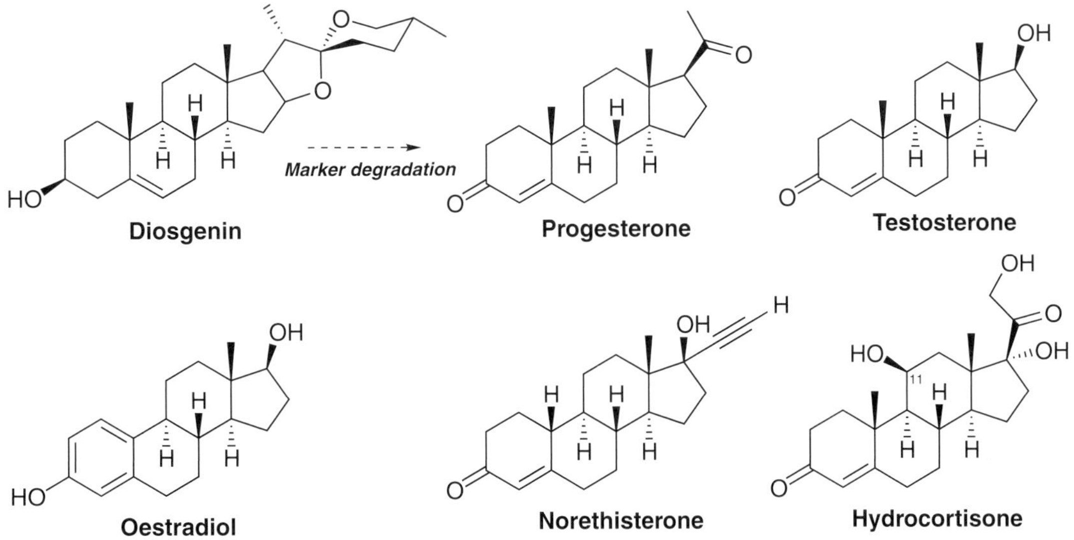

Fig. 6.40 Steroids derived from the sterol diosgenin.

the molecule in a stereospecific manner in fermentation culture using fungi of the genus *Rhizopus*.

If squalene is folded in a different conformation (chair-chair-chair-boat), then cyclisation mediated by a cyclase enzyme results in the formation of a different intermediate, **sterol intermediate II**, which is the precursor of the pentacyclic triterpenes (Fig. 6.41).

Migration of the C_{16}–C_{17} bond to satisfy the positive charge results in the formation of **sterol intermediate III**. This may undergo several rearrangements to give different triterpene skeletons. Pathway 1 involves formation of a bond between C_{18} and C_X, resulting in a positive charge on C_Y (through removal of one pair of electrons from the double bond to form the C_{18}–C_X bond). This may be satisfied by a series of Wagner–Meerwein methyl and hydride shifts with loss of a proton from C_{12} resulting in a C_{12} double bond. This pathway gives us the **ursane**-type triterpenes of which α-**amyrin** is an example, possessing a double bond in position C_{12} (referred to as a Δ^{12}-ursene) (see Fig. 6.41).

Pathway 2 occurs through the formation of a C_{18}–C_Y bond, which leaves a positive charge on C_X which is stabilised by the two methyls attached to it. This intermediate may then lose a hydrogen ion from one of these methyls to form a neutral double bond and the **lupane** skeleton (pathway a), or the bond between C_Y and C_Z may migrate to C_X, giving a carbocation at C_Y. Wagner–Meerwein migrations and loss of a hydrogen ion from C_{12} forming a double bond give the **oleanane** triterpene skeleton, of which β-**amyrin** is typical, again possessing a double bond at C_{12}. This compound may be referred to as a Δ^{12}-oleanene.

Pentacyclic triterpenes are common in plants and herbal remedies such as horse chestnut (*A. hippocastanum* L.) and liquorice (*Glycyrrhiza glabra* L.). The examples **protoaescigenin, baringtogenol** (both from horse chestnut) and **glycyrrhetic acid** (from liquorice) (Fig. 6.42) have a high degree of functionality and chirality, and usually occur in the plant material in the form of glycosides.

Liquorice has a long history of use as an antiinflammatory (anti-ulcer) agent. **Carbenoxolone sodium,** a semisynthetic derivative of glycyrrhetic acid, was formerly used to treat gastric ulcers, but has now been superseded by anti-*Helicobacter* therapy with proton pump inhibitors and antibiotics.

Tetraterpenes (C_{40})

The **tetraterpenes** are C_{40} natural products derived from the reaction of two molecules of GGPP (C_{20}). This class is sometimes referred to as the **carotenoids** because of their occurrence in the vegetable. The tetraterpenes are highly pigmented and are responsible for the colours of certain plants, in particular, the orange of carrots (β-**carotene**) and the red colour of tomatoes and chilli peppers, which is due to **lycopene** and **capsanthin**, respectively (Fig. 6.43). These highly conjugated compounds are strongly UV light absorbing and involved in photosynthesis; they are widely distributed in plants and may act as a protection against UV light damage.

The tetraterpenes are strong antioxidants, being preferentially oxidised over biological molecules such as nucleic acids and proteins. Their presence in the diet is linked to many health benefits, including cancer chemoprevention.

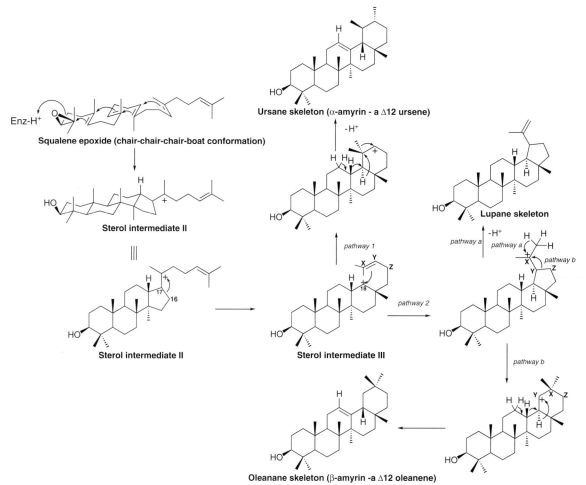

Fig. 6.41 Biosynthesis of pentacyclic triterpenes from squalene epoxide.

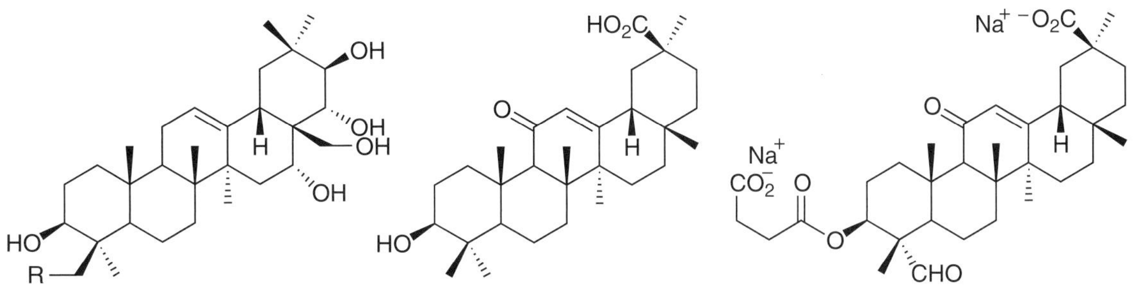

R = OH, protoaescigenin
R = H, barringtogenol

Glycyrrhetic acid

Carbenoxolone sodium

Fig. 6.42 Pentacyclic triterpenes.

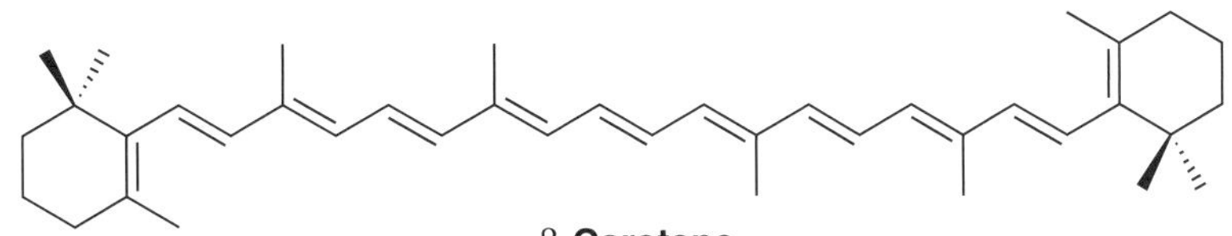

β-Carotene

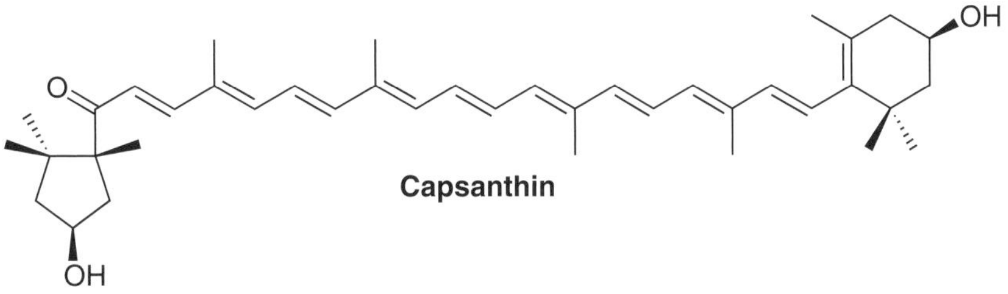

Capsanthin

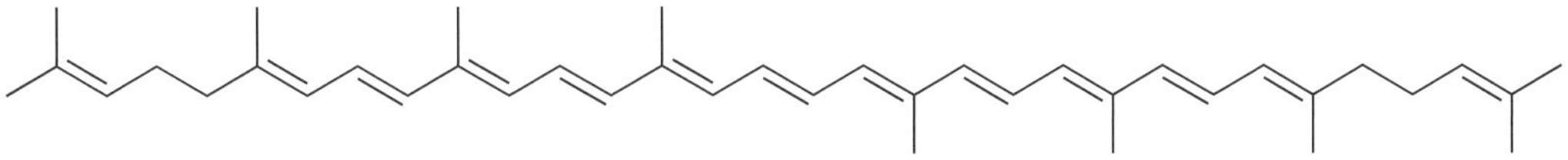

Lycopene

Fig. 6.43 Tetraterpenes (carotenoids).

The tetraterpenes are precursors of **vitamin A₁** (**retinol**), a deficiency in which results in reduced eyesight through changes to the cornea and conjunctiva. Vitamin A₁ occurs naturally in fish liver oils, carrots, green and yellow vegetables, and dairy products. It is biosynthesised by the oxidative cleavage of β-carotene to **retinal**, which is then reduced to **retinol** (**vitamin A₁**) (Fig. 6.44). Vitamin A acid (retinoic acid) and derivatives are used as treatments for acne.

THE GLYCOSIDES

The glycosides are discussed separately here because they enhance the structural diversity of other natural product classes. The term glycoside is a generic term for a natural product chemically bound to a sugar. Thus, the glycoside is composed of two parts: the **sugar(s)** and the **aglycone**. The aglycone may be a terpene, a flavonoid, a coumarin or practically any other compound. If the aglycone is a triterpene, it is sometimes referred to as a **genin** (e.g. protoaescigenin; see Fig. 6.42). Glycosides are very common in nature and provide extra chemical diversity and structural complexity.

There are two basic classes of glycosides: the **C-glycosides**, in which the sugar is attached to the aglycone through a carbon–carbon bond, and the **O-glycosides** in which the sugar is connected to the aglycone through an oxygen–carbon bond (Fig. 6.45). Glycosides are usually more polar than the aglycone, and glycoside formation generally increases water solubility. This may allow the producing organism to transport and store the glycoside more effectively.

Cyanogenetic Glycosides

Some glycosides are undoubtedly used by plants as a chemical defence and this is certainly so with the cyanogenetic (cyanide-generating) glycosides. These compounds, in the presence of enzymes, such as β-glucosidase, lose their sugar portion to form a **cyanohydrin,** which, in the presence of water, can undergo hydrolysis to give **benzaldehyde** and the highly toxic **hydrogen cyanide** (HCN) (Fig. 6.46).

Cyanogenetic glycosides such as **amygdalin** (see Fig. 6.50) are present in many species of the genus *Prunus*, which includes commercially important fruit, such as peaches, cherries, plums and apricots. Fortunately, the enzymes that convert these compounds to the cyanohydrins are localised in different parts of the plant or are absent. In the case of sweet almonds (*Prunus amygdalus* Batsch var. *dulcis* (Mill.) Koehne Deut.), the enzymes are present but not cyanogenetic glycosides.

Cassava (*Manihot esculenta* Crantz) is consumed widely as a food, and both the enzymes and cyanide glycosides are present. Extensive boiling of cassava removes toxic HCN.

Glucosinolates

The Brassicaceae includes cabbages, sprouts and the mustards and produces a group of glycosides known as **glucosinolates**. These are sulphur- and nitrogen-containing glycosides previously referred to

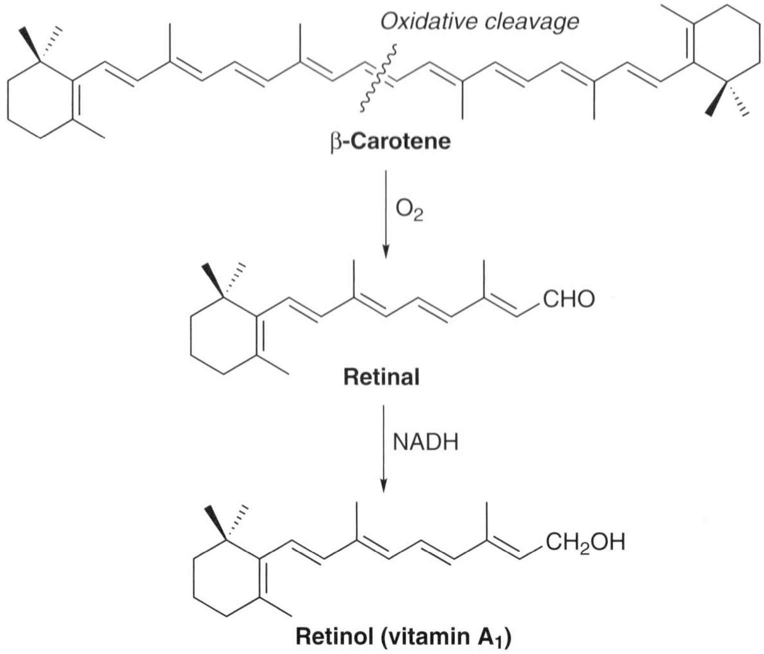

β-Carotene

Oxidative cleavage

O_2

Retinal

CHO

NADH

CH_2OH

Retinol (vitamin A₁)

Fig. 6.44 Biosynthesis of retinol.

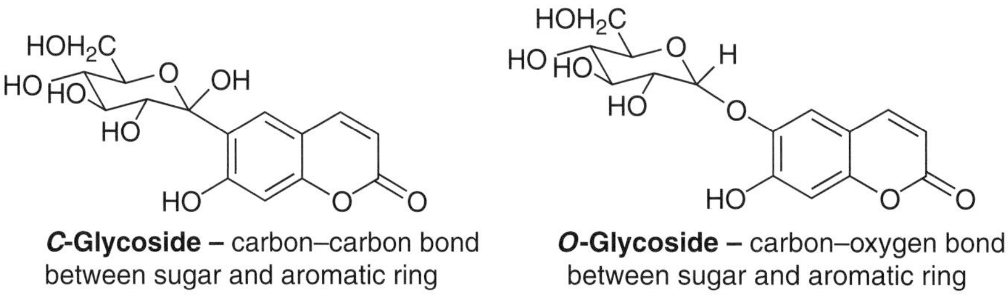

C-Glycoside – carbon–carbon bond between sugar and aromatic ring

O-Glycoside – carbon–oxygen bond between sugar and aromatic ring

Fig. 6.45 *C*-glycoside and *O*-glycosides.

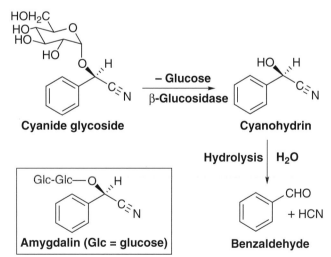

Cyanide glycoside

– Glucose
β-Glucosidase

Cyanohydrid

Hydrolysis | H_2O

CHO

+ HCN

Glc-Glc—O

Amygdalin (Glc = glucose)

Benzaldehyde

Fig. 6.46 Cyanogenetic glycosides.

as nitrogen mustards. An example is **sinalbin** from white mustard (*Sinapis alba* L.), which in the presence of the enzyme **myrosinase** is converted into a **thiohydroximate**, which rearranges with the loss of a hydrogen sulphate salt to the **isothiocyanate, acrinylisothiocyanate** (Fig. 6.47).

These isothiocyanates are exceptionally pungent and impart a strong aroma to mustards, and hot taste. In black mustard (*Brassica*

nigra W.D.J. Koch), the simple glucosinolate **sinigrin** is converted in the same fashion to **allyl isothiocyanate** (see Fig. 6.51), which is an oil and far more volatile than acrinylisothiocyanate. The oils derived from mustards are rich in these isothiocyanates and are mildly irritant; they have been used medicinally, externally applied, for muscular pain.

Cardiac Glycosides

Many plants contain **cardioactive** or **cardiac glycosides**, which have a profound effect on heart rhythm. They are commonly found in the genera *Convallaria, Nerium, Helleborus* and *Digitalis*. The aglycone portion is steroidal in nature and is sometimes referred to as a **cardenolide**, being **card**ioactive and possessing an alkene and an **olide** (a cyclic ester) (Fig. 6.48). The aglycone (genin) portion may have a wide variety of sugars attached. The foxglove (*Digitalis purpurea* L., Scrophulariaceae) was used as long ago as the 18th century for the treatment of heart failure and oedema described as 'dropsy'. The basis of this use was well founded, as it contains **digoxin** and **digitoxin** (see Fig. 6.48). Digoxin has been widely used in congestive heart failure and is now produced from the related species *Digitalis lanata*. Related cardiac glycosides no longer used include **lanatoside C** and **deacetyl-lanatoside C**.

Triterpene glycosides have widespread distribution in plants and are sometimes referred to as **saponins** as they have soap-like properties and readily form foams. Medicinally important examples include **glycyrrhizic acid** from liquorice (*G. glabra* L.) (Fig. 6.49), a popular confectionery ingredient, formerly used as a treatment for

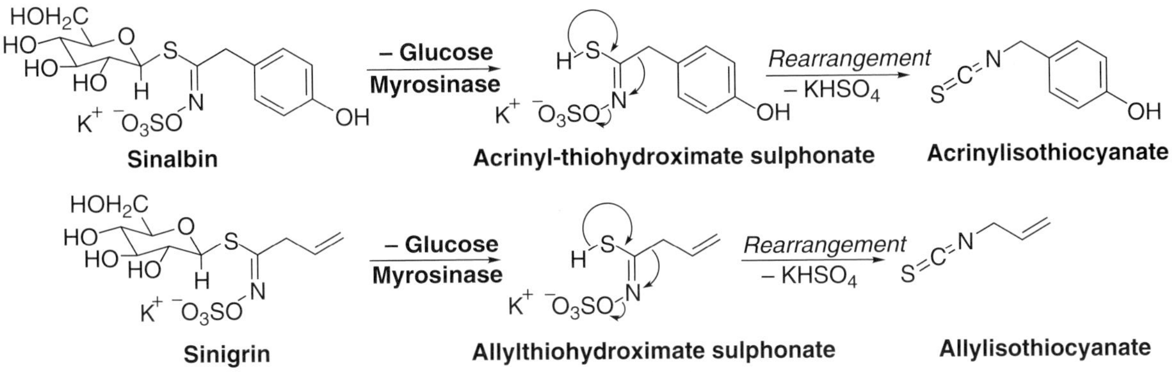

Fig. 6.47 Glucosinolates and isothiocyanates.

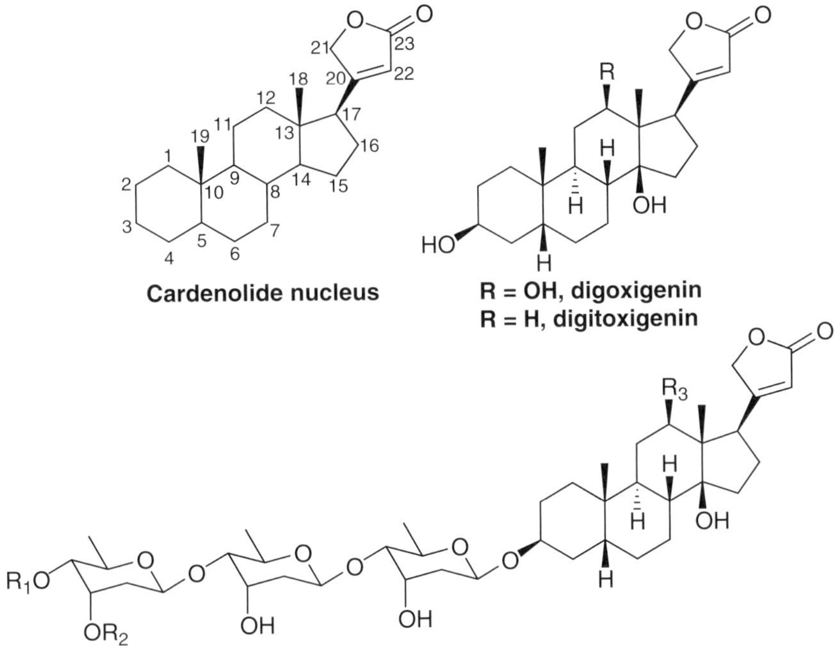

Cardenolide nucleus

R = OH, digoxigenin
R = H, digitoxigenin

$R_1 = R_2 = H$, $R_3 = OH$, digoxin
$R_1 = R_2 = R_3 = H$, digitoxin
$R_1 = glucose$, $R_2 = acetyl$, $R_3 = OH$, lanatoside C
$R_1 = glucose$, $R_2 = H$, $R_3 = OH$, deacetyl-lanatoside C

Fig. 6.48 Cardiac glycosides (cardenolides).

stomach ulcers, the salts of which are intensely sweet. The sugars in Fig. 6.49 are of the **glucuronic acid** type and are shown as their Fischer projections.

Anthraquinone Glycosides

Plants that contain **anthraquinone** or **anthrone glycosides** (Fig. 6.50) have long been known for their laxative properties. They include **cascara**, **senna** and **aloe**. Aloe is used as a laxative (as well as a treatment for minor burns). Aloe is the drained exudate from the cut leaves; it contains a mixture of anthraquinone glycosides of which **barbaloin** is the major metabolite and is a mixture of 10R and 10S isomers; the purified metabolites are referred to as **aloin A** and **B**.

Cascara bark (from *Frangula purshiana* (DC.) A.Gray ex J.G. Cooper) was in use in the late 19th century as a laxative; the main active principle is the diglucoside **cascaroside**, which, in common with barbaloin, exists as a mixture of epimers at position C10 as **cascaroside A** (10S) and **B** (10R).

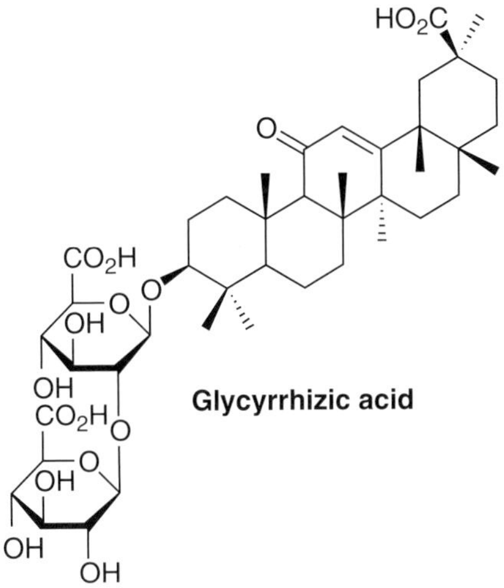

Glycyrrhizic acid

Fig. 6.49 Glycyrrhizic acid (remove embedded duplicate).

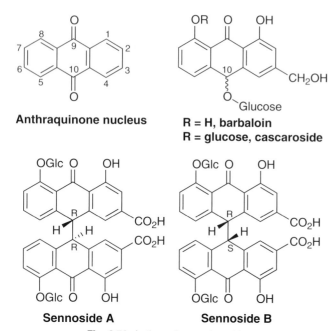

Fig. 6.50 Anthraquinone glycosides.

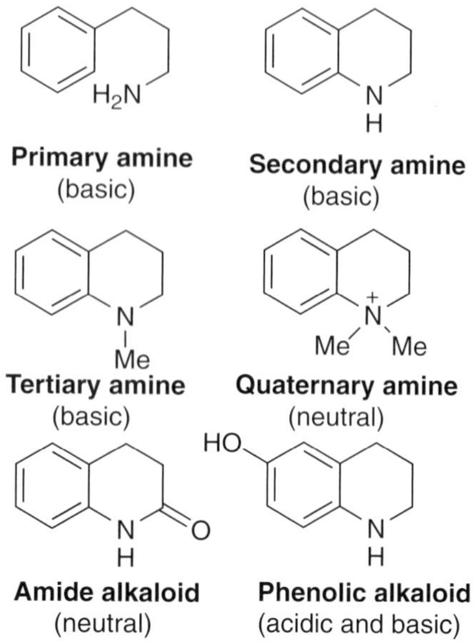

Fig. 6.51 Alkaloid types.

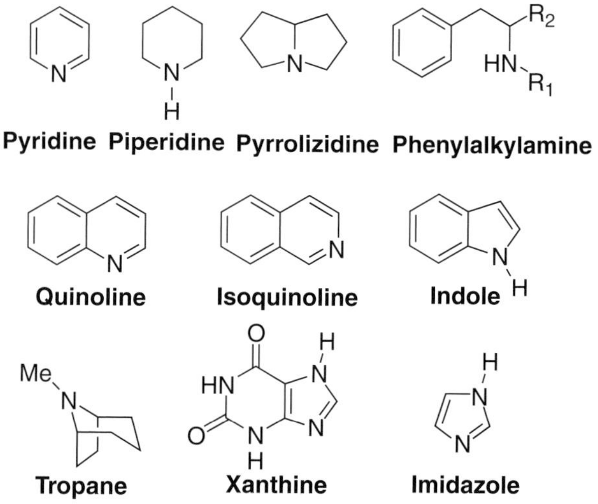

There is little difference in the chemistry of the two senna species. The active metabolites are **sennosides A** and **B** (see Fig. 6.50), which are **dianthrones** (dimers) of the **anthrone** skeleton. Fresh leaves of senna contain glycosides with additional sugar groups present and these are naturally hydrolysed to sennosides A and B. In vivo, the sennosides are hydrolysed to the dianthrones (lacking the sugars). Senna is a widely used stimulant laxative, suitable for occasional use.

ALKALOIDS

As a group, the alkaloids display an exceptionally wide array of biological activities and have an equally wide distribution, being present in plants, fungi, bacteria, amphibia, insects, animals and humans. Plants and fungi rich in alkaloids were used by early humans to relieve pain and treat other illnesses, as recreational psychoactive drugs, in religious ceremonies, and to poison people. The German pharmacist Carl Friedrich Wilhelm Meissner (1792–1853) first coined the term 'alkaloid' in 1818, to describe substances with alkaline properties. Many alkaloids are, indeed, alkaline in nature (Fig. 6.51) as they possess either a **primary, secondary** or **tertiary amine** functional group and the alkaline (basic) properties of these groups are used to aid their extraction and purification. However, some alkaloids exist as quaternary amine salts in which a lone pair of electrons from the nitrogen atom is used to form a bond with another group (e.g. methyl) and, therefore, a positive charge resides on the nitrogen making this group essentially neutral (neither basic nor acidic). Care must, therefore, be taken with the alkali or base definition of alkaloids as some are neutral, especially the amides (see Fig. 6.51), and some alkaloids possess phenolic groups, which confer acidic properties to the molecule, as in the ability to form salts. They are heterocyclic compounds containing nitrogen, but this class usually includes compounds containing nitrogen in an aliphatic chain (e.g. the **phenyl-alkylamines**; see later). Biosynthetically, alkaloids are produced from different amino acids, giving rise to diverse fundamental structures (Fig. 6.52).

Pyridine, Piperidine and Pyrrolizidine Alkaloids

Nicotine is the stimulant alkaloid of tobacco (*Nicotiana tabacum* L., Solanaceae) (Fig. 6.53). The compound has a pyrrole ring attached to

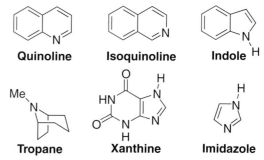

Fig. 6.52 Alkaloid skeletons.

the pyridine ring. It has no medical use except in the alleviation of the withdrawal symptoms of nicotine itself, as an aid to cessation of smoking where it is formulated as transdermal (skin patches) and oral delivery (chewing gums etc.) systems.

Hemlock (*Conium maculatum* L., Apiaceae) produces the highly poisonous piperidine alkaloid **coniine**, which has an alkyl (C_3) side chain at the 2-position of the piperidine ring. This plant is famous as a poison: the Greek philosopher Socrates, when found guilty of treason, was forced to drink a preparation of hemlock.

In many Asian countries, betel nuts (*Areca catechu* L., Arecaceae) are consumed for their stimulant and relaxing properties and to alleviate fatigue. The nuts are red (due to the presence of tannins), which causes staining of the teeth. The active compound is the piperidine alkaloid **arecoline**. Like nicotine, arecoline binds to the nicotinic receptors and has a stimulant effect on the CNS.

Lobeline is found in the leaves and tops of *Lobelia inflata* L. (Campanulaceae), traditionally known as wild tobacco or pukeweed. It has similar effects to those of nicotine and arecoline and has been used as a tobacco substitute and smoking deterrent.

Castanospermine, from *Castanospermum australe* A. Cunn. ex Mudie (Fabaceae), is an inhibitor of α-glucosidase, an enzyme involved in glycoprotein processing, which is important in the formation of viral coating, abnormalities of which stop infection of white blood cells. Castanospermine is a **polyhydroxylated alkaloid** (PHA) and is in fact a sugar analogue (compare with glucose in Fig. 6.53), explaining its activity against glucosidase enzymes in the formation of glycoproteins. It is sometimes classified as an indolizidine alkaloid, but also has a piperidine ring system.

Senecionine is a pyrrolizidine alkaloid, which like similar compounds has hepatotoxic properties. These compounds possess a reactive carbon (* in Fig. 6.53) that is readily alkylated by reactive thiol groups present in many enzymes found in the liver. Herbal medicines containing these compounds are banned from sale in many countries. Pyrrolizidine alkaloid are sometimes found as contaminants in herbal teas and medicines and European and other agencies have defined maximum amounts of pyrrolizidine alkaloid permissible in

certain herbal preparations as well as additional testing protocols for regulated medicines. These compounds are, however, also found in some foods including honey (due to bees collecting pollen and nectar from plants containing pyrrolizidine alkaloids) and spices. (EMA 2016, Schrenk et al., 2022). Senecionine occurs in ragwort (*Jacobaea vulgaris* Gaertn., better known under its synonym, *Senecio jacobaea* L.) and other *Senecio* spp. (Asteraceae), and has caused poisoning of livestock that have ingested the plants in feeds, mainly during times of drought.

Phenylalkylamine Alkaloids

These do not have a cyclic nitrogen atom but either a free amine or an alkyl-substituted amine. In Chinese medicine, Ma Huang (*Ephedra sinica* Stapf, Ephedraceae) has a long tradition of use as a treatment for colds, asthma and other bronchial conditions. The active metabolite is **ephedrine** (Fig. 6.54), which possesses CNS stimulatory, vasoconstrictive and bronchodilatory properties, and is used in respiratory

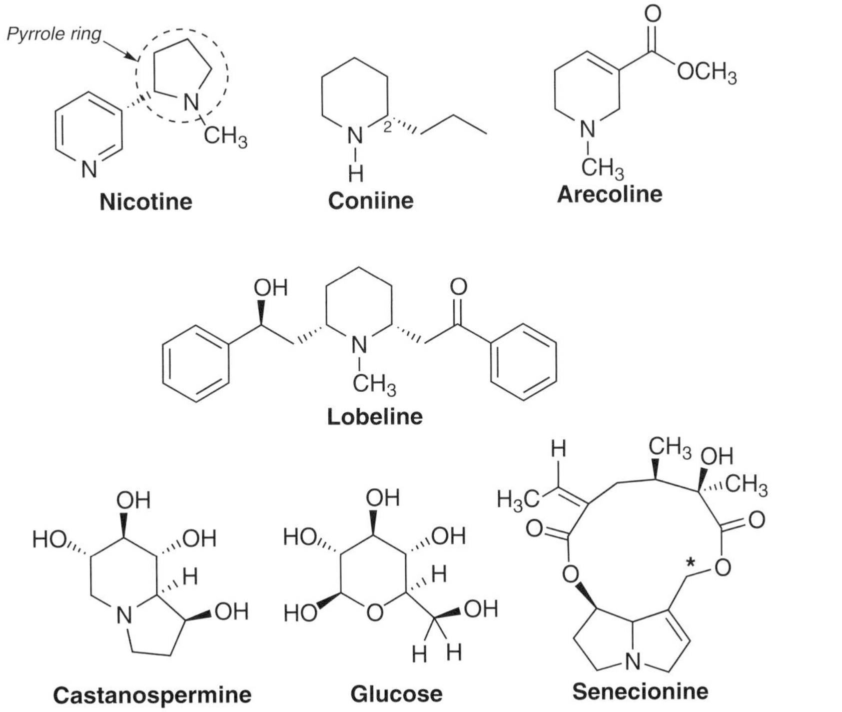

Fig. 6.53 Pyridine, piperidine and pyrrolizidine alkaloids.

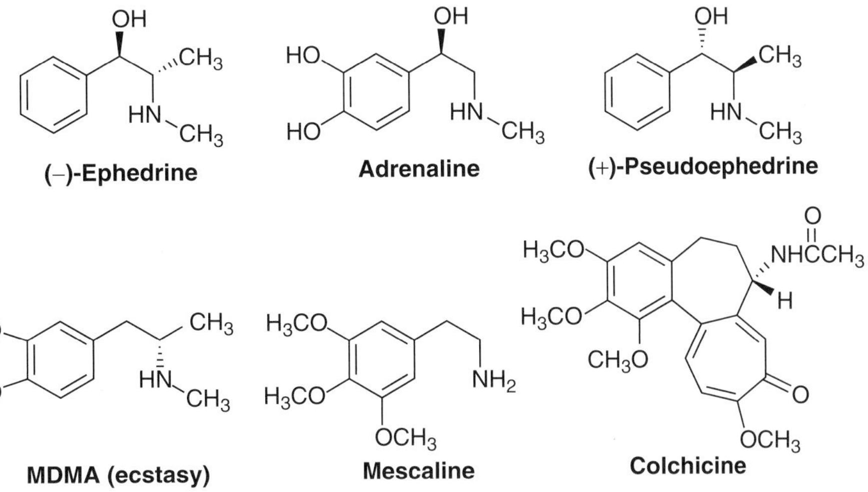

Fig. 6.54 Phenylalkylamine alkaloids.

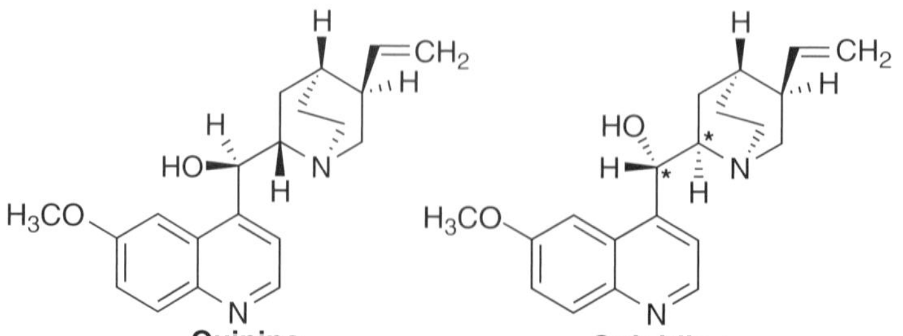

Fig. 6.55 Quinoline alkaloids.

disorders. They have properties in common with the natural hormone **adrenaline** (**epinephrine**), which is structurally similar (see Fig. 6.54). Ephedrine has two stereogenic (chiral) centres and, therefore, has four possible isomers. An isomer of ephedrine, (+)-**pseudoephedrine**, is used in decongestant preparations. Herba Ephedra has some notoriety as 'herbal ecstasy', but these preparations are dangerous and should be avoided.

Indigenous peoples of central and north Mexico and the southwestern United States have ingested the dried heads ('buttons') of the **peyote** or mescal cactus (*Lophophora williamsii* (Lem.) J.M. Coult, Cactaceae) as part of their religious ceremonies. It induces vivid dreams and hallucinations, due to the presence of **mescaline**, a trimethoxylated phenylethylamine.

Colchicine is an alkaloidal amine from the autumn crocus (*Colchicum autumnale* L., Colchicaceae). It is highly cytotoxic and antimitotic, being an inhibitor of microtubule formation. It is used to treat gout, and more recently as an adjunctive treatment for severe inflammatory pulmonary and cardiovascular inflammation in patients with COVID-19.

Quinoline Alkaloids

The Spanish conquistadors who invaded Peru in the latter part of the 16th century discovered that the indigenous Incas of this area used a preparation of the bark of a rain-forest tree to treat fevers, especially malaria. The Jesuit priests accompanying the invading force collected large amounts of this bark and used it to prevent and treat malaria. The bark was shipped back to Europe where it became known as **Jesuit bark** or Peruvian bark and gained great fame as a treatment for malaria. The trees responsible for this are of the genus *Cinchona* (Rubiaceae), and produce the quinoline alkaloid **quinine**, first isolated in 1820 by the French pharmacists Pelletier and Caventou (Fig. 6.55). The structure of this compound was not known until 1908 and total synthesis was only achieved in the mid-1940s. It has been used extensively as an antimalarial and as a template for the development of synthetic antimalarials such as **chloroquine** and **mefloquine**.

Quinine is an ingredient of Indian tonic water, to which gin was added to mask the taste. It gives a brilliant fluorescence under UV light. It was formerly used as a treatment for night cramps in older people, but its cardioactive effects make this unsuitable. **Quinidine** is an isomer of quinine with a different configuration at the positions marked * in Fig. 6.55. Quinidine was formerly used to treat type I cardiac arrhythmias but has been superseded by safer drugs.

Isoquinoline Alkaloids

The isoquinolines have had a profound effect on human society, as medicinal agents and as drugs of abuse. **Opium**, which is rich in **morphinane**-type isoquinoline alkaloids, has been used for millennia in the treatment of pain and as a narcotic substance. Opium is the latex exuded from the unripe capsules of the opium poppy (*Papaver somniferum* L., Papaveraceae). It contains more than 30 alkaloids, of which

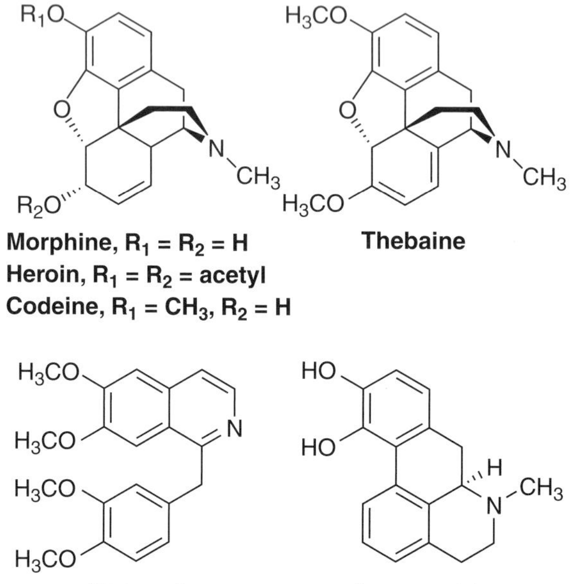

Morphine, R₁ = R₂ = H
Heroin, R₁ = R₂ = acetyl
Codeine, R₁ = CH₃, R₂ = H

Thebaine

Papaverine   **Apomorphine**

Fig. 6.56 Isoquinoline alkaloids.

the major metabolites are **morphine, codeine, thebaine, papaverine** and **noscapine** (Fig. 6.56).

Morphine, derived from the name for the Greek god of sleep *Morpheus*, possesses both a basic tertiary amine and an acidic phenol functional group. These groups allow morphine to be readily purified by acids and bases. Morphine is readily converted into **diamorphine** (**heroin**) by acetylation of both hydroxyl groups using acetic anhydride. The mechanisms of the analgesic effects of morphine were a mystery until the discovery of the **endorphins**, natural **end**ogenous morphine-like substances, which act at the same receptor sites as morphine. **Codeine** is the phenolic methyl ether of morphine and is widely used as an analgesic and cough suppressant. Both are important for the management of moderate to severe pain. Semisynthetic derivatives have been produced (cough suppressants including **pholcodine** and analgesics such as **dihydrocodeine**), and morphine was used as a template for the development of **pethidine** and other synthetic opiates. Other alkaloids, such as **thebaine,** are the starting point for the synthesis of codeine and veterinary sedatives such as **etorphine.**

Papaverine is an antispasmodic and was formerly used as a treatment for male impotence before the introduction of vastly superior drugs. Its activity as a Ca^{2+} channel blocker led to the development of **verapamil. Apomorphine** is prepared by heating morphine with concentrated hydrochloric acid. It is a dopamine agonist and used in the treatment of Parkinson disease. **Papaveretum** is a total alkaloid extract of opium from which the minor alkaloid **noscapine** was removed as it is genotoxic. Papaveretum was formerly used as a premedication

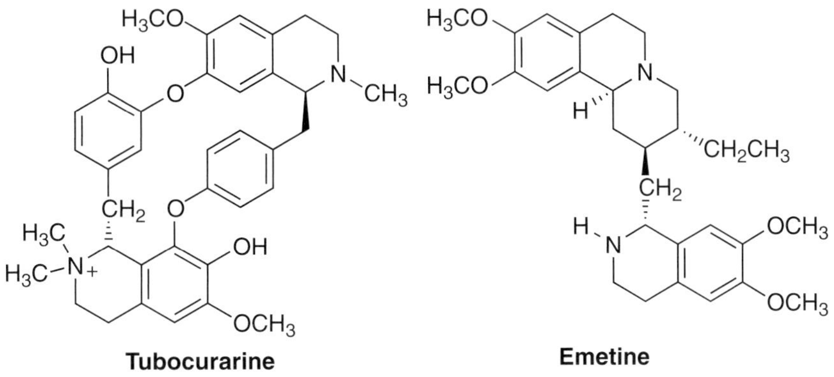

Fig. 6.57 Dimeric isoquinoline alkaloids.

and for postoperative pain relief, but more effective opioid drugs and improved formulations are now available.

Indigenous peoples of South America use a variety of arrow poisons for hunting purposes, of which **curare** is one type, and acts as a strong muscle relaxant. Curare is prepared from species of the family Menispermaceae, notably *Chondrodendron tomentosum* Ruiz & Pavón, which kills by paralysis of the muscles required to breathe. The major active metabolite in curare is the isoquinoline alkaloid **tubocurarine**, so named because the poison was carried in bamboo 'tubes' prior to use (Fig. 6.57). Tubocurarine is a quaternary salt and, as the chloride, was used as a muscle relaxant in surgical procedures. The compound was also a template for the development of other muscle relaxants of which **atracurium** is an important example.

Ipecacuanha or **Ipecac** (*Carapichea ipecacuanha* (Brot.) L. Andersson, Rubiaceae) is a shrub indigenous to Brazil and produces rhizomes (underground stems) used by the Indigenous peoples to treat diarrhoea. The main alkaloids are **emetine, psychotrine** and **cephaeline**. Ipecac was used to treat amoebic dysentery, but the side effects (vomiting, nausea and severe gastrointestinal disturbance) stopped its use, including as an emetic after poisoning or drug overdose. Emetine (see Fig. 6.57) is an expectorant and is 'ipecac' added to many cough medicines.

Indole Alkaloids

The indole alkaloids are a rich source of bioactive compounds. Snake root (*Rauvolfia serpentina* (L.) Benth. ex Kurz, Apocynaceae) is a shrub common to the Indian subcontinent; it is used in the Ayurvedic system of medicine, with uses described for the treatment of snakebite and madness. **Reserpine**, the major alkaloid, was used to treat psychotic illness and as an antihypertensive agent, but due to its side effects (neurotoxicity, cytotoxicity and depression) it is rarely used (Fig. 6.58). Reserpine is now used as a probe in mechanistic studies of multidrug resistance, as it inhibits P-glycoprotein and hence drug efflux.

In the Calabar coast area of West Africa (Nigeria and Cameroon) 'trial by ordeal' was allegedly conducted using the Calabar or 'Ordeal' bean (*Physostigma venenosum* Balf., Fabaceae). When an individual was accused of a crime, they were forced to consume an extract of the bean. Should the individual live, then they were deemed innocent of the crime, but death indicated guilt and summary justice served. The margin between 'innocence' and 'guilt' was probably a result of the degree of alkaloid extraction from the plant, but if vomiting could be induced quickly, survival was also possible. The toxic alkaloid is **physostigmine** (see Fig. 6.58), which is a potent inhibitor of acetylcholinesterase. Derivatives such as rivastigmine are used in the treatment of Alzheimer disease, which shows reduced levels of acetylcholine in the brain. **Neostigmine** and **pyridostigmine** are used to treat myasthenia gravis, a rare disease characterised by severe muscle weakness

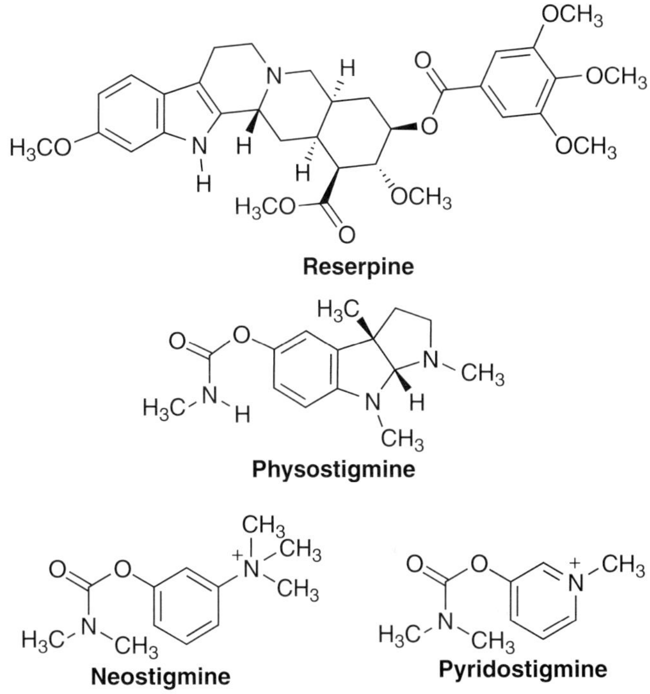

Fig. 6.58 Indole alkaloids.

caused by destruction of acetylcholine receptors at the neuromuscular junction and failed nerve transmission.

Poisoning through contamination of rye grain by fungi, particularly *Claviceps purpurea* (Fr.) Tul., has been described since the Middle Ages. Infected cereal grains produce dark-coloured structures (sclerotia) called **ergot**; these are rich in indole alkaloids. Poisoning from ingestion of bread made from contaminated grain gave rise to epidemics characterised by burning, 'fire-like' sensations throughout the extremities, blackened limbs and gangrene, vivid hallucinations and a high incidence of abortion. This condition became known as St Anthony's fire after the saint who spent much of his life meditating in the fire-like heat of the Sinai desert but is now known as ergotism. These epidemics were also considered the work of witchcraft. Bread was the staple diet in the Middle Ages, so this condition could be widespread, especially during wet weather. As bread made from infected flour was rather unpleasant, such epidemics were much more common among the poor who had little choice in the matter.

The ergot alkaloids are responsible for all these effects. Ergot was used in the 1500s to shorten labour during childbirth as it causes contraction of the womb, which explains the abortifacient effect in

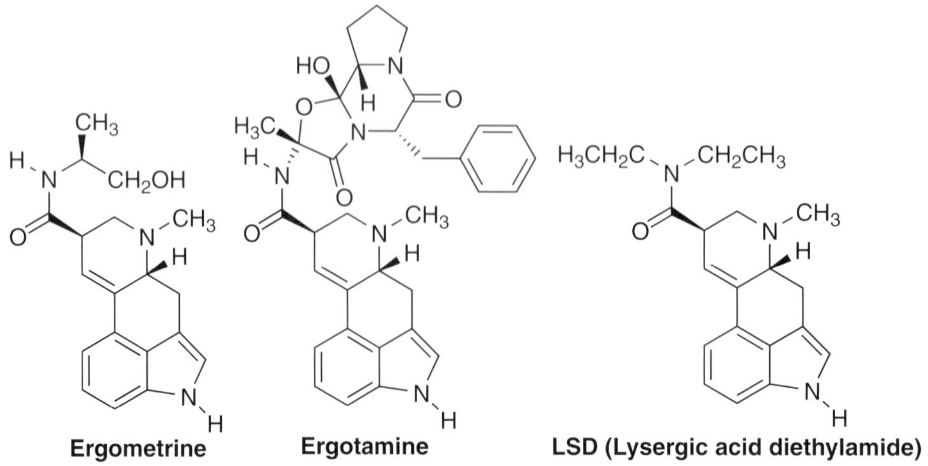

Fig. 6.59 Ergot alkaloids.

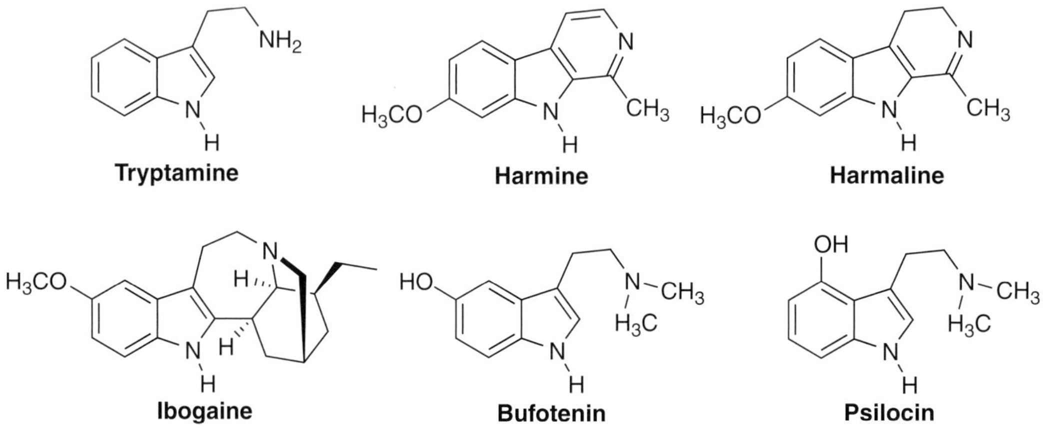

Fig. 6.60 Psychoactive indole alkaloids.

ergotism. It contains several groups of indole alkaloids such as the **ergometrine** type, which have simple amide side chains, and the **ergotamine** group, which possess complex amino-acid-derived side chains (Fig. 6.59).

Ergometrine is an oxytocic used to expel the placenta after childbirth, or to increase contractions. It acts on the pituitary as well as on the uterine muscles. **Ergotamine** is a vasoconstrictor introduced in the 1920s for the relief of migraine, and occasionally used today. Ergot derivatives (ergolines) have such diverse pharmacological effects they have been used as a template for the semisynthesis of **bromocriptine, pergolide** and **cabergoline**. Ergolines interact with dopamine, serotonin and adrenergic receptors, and are used in neurological disorders such as Parkinson disease and pituitary disorders. Ergot causes hallucinations, and the hallucinogen **LSD (lysergic acid diethylamide)** is structurally related to these compounds (see Fig. 6.59).

Many psychoactive compounds (including LSD) are structurally related to **tryptamine**, as are the **harmine** and **harmaline** alkaloids from *Peganum harmala* L. (Syrian Rue, Nitrariaceae) and the yahé or ayahuasca preparations (*Banisteriopsis caapi* (Spruce ex Griseb.) Morton (syn.: *B. inebrians* (C.V. Morton) J.F. Macbr, Malpighiaceae), which are prepared by Amazonian shaman. Ayahuasca is used as part of the community rituals of some Peruvian groups to preserve their traditional ways and to promote bonding and the establishment of social order. **Ibogaine**, from iboga (*Tabernanthe iboga* Baill., Apocynaceae), is hallucinogenic and anticonvulsant, and has recently been studied as a treatment for heroin addiction. Psychoactive indole derivatives are

even found in amphibia, notably in the skin of species of the genus *Bufo*, which produce **bufotenin** (Fig. 6.60).

Mushrooms of the genera *Psilocybe, Panaeolus, Conocybe* and *Stropharia* are known to produce psychoactive substances, such as **psilocybin**, which is a phosphate salt in the fungi and is converted into **psilocin** in vivo (see Fig. 6.60). The Aztecs of Mexico revered certain fungi (*Psilocybe mexicana* Heim, Hymenogastraceae) as the 'flesh of the Gods' and gave it the name Teonanacatl. The reverence for these mushrooms is attributed to the profound hallucinogenic effects they exert, and, in Europe, many related species, such as the liberty cap (*Psilocybe semilanceata* (Fr.) P. Kumm.), are collected for recreational abuse. These fungi are colloquially referred to as 'magic mushrooms', but as fungal taxonomy is highly complex there are risks of collecting poisonous species and the outcome may not be 'magic' at all.

The anticancer agents **vincristine** and **vinblastine** from the Madagascar periwinkle (*Catharanthus roseus* (L.) G. Don, Apocynaceae) are complex **bisindole** (dimeric indole) natural products present in small quantities in the plant material. They are used for the treatment of Hodgkin lymphoma, acute leukaemia and some solid tumours (Fig. 6.61).

Strychnine and **brucine** (Fig. 6.62) are intensely bitter indoles from the seeds of nux-vomica or 'vomiting nut' (*Strychnos nux-vomica* L., Loganiaceae), which is a tree indigenous to India. Preparations of nux-vomica were used as a stimulant tonic until the middle of the 20th century. However, these compounds are highly poisonous (strychnine is used as a rodenticide) and of historical interest only in medicine.

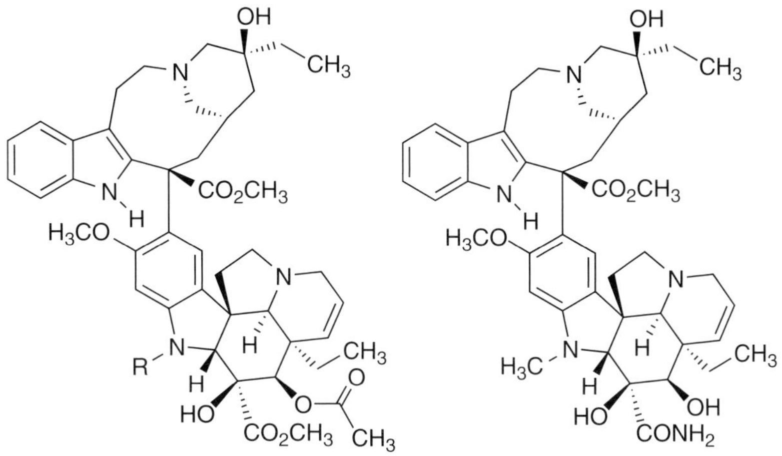

Vincristine, R = CHO
Vinblastine, R = CH$_3$

Vindesine

Fig. 6.61 Bisindole *Vinca* alkaloids.

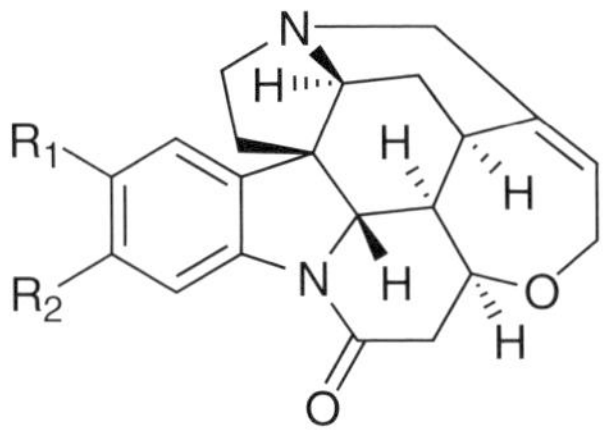

Strychnine, R$_1$ = R$_2$ = H
Brucine, R$_1$ = R$_2$ = CH$_3$O

Fig. 6.62 *Strychnos* alkaloids.

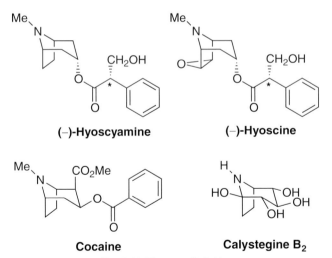

(–)-Hyoscyamine

(–)-Hyoscine

Cocaine

Calystegine B$_2$

Fig. 6.63 Tropane alkaloids.

Tropane Alkaloids

The European plant deadly nightshade (*Atropa belladonna* L., Solanaceae) produces **hyoscyamine** (Fig. 6.63), which occurs in the plant as a racemic mixture [(+) and (−) isomers, sometimes denoted (±)] at the chiral centre denoted * in Fig. 6.63. This mixture is referred to as **atropine**. The generic name of the plant refers to Atropos, the ancient Greek Fate who, in mythology, cut the thread of life. Belladonna, the species name, means 'beautiful lady' in Italian and refers to the use of the juice of the berries of this plant by ladies in the 16th century to dilate the pupils of their eyes, which was considered an attractive feature. Atropine is anticholinergic and has been used to treat acute arrhythmias and to dilate the pupil of the eye (a mydriatic) for ophthalmic examinations. Semisynthetic short-acting derivatives are also used (such as **tropicamide**). Hyoscyamine also occurs in other species of Solanaceae, notably henbane (*Hyoscyamus niger* L.) and thornapple (*Datura stramonium* L.), together with **hyoscine**, also known as **scopolamine**, which is the epoxide derivative of hyoscyamine. Hyoscine is widely used as a premedication prior to operations to dry up secretions produced by inhalant anaesthetics and reduce nausea caused by opiates. It is also a component of many travel (motion) sickness preparations.

Cocaine comes from the South American plants *Erythroxylum coca* Lam. and *E. novogranatense* var. *truxillense* (Rusby) Plowman (syn.: *E. truxillense* Rusby, Erythroxylaceae), which grow at high altitudes in the Andes in Colombia, Peru and Bolivia. It is a highly addictive CNS stimulant and its illicit use with huge public health (and crime) consequences is well known. Medicinally, cocaine has limited use, but drugs developed using cocaine as a template, such as lidocaine, are widely used as local anaesthetics for dental and dermatological conditions. Cocaine can cause cardiac arrhythmias, leading to heart attacks in large doses, but lidocaine is an antiarrhythmic and used to treat ventricular tachycardia.

The calystegines, typically **calystegine B$_2$**, are *nor*-tropane alkaloids ('nor' meaning lacking a carbon), which lack the N-methyl group of the tropanes. These compounds are widely distributed in the plant kingdom, particularly in the Solanaceae and Convolvulaceae, and are found in trace amounts in some fruits and vegetables (e.g. aubergines and tomatoes). The calystegines are inhibitors of glycosidase enzymes and may have potential toxicity, but the evidence base is insufficient including potential uses in foods.

Xanthine Alkaloids

The xanthines are very widely known (and consumed), being constituents of tea (*Camellia sinensis* (L.) Kuntze, Theaceae) and coffee (*Coffea arabica* L., Rubiaceae). Both contain the **xanthine** (or **purine**) alkaloid **caffeine.** Caffeine is a CNS stimulant and taken to counter fatigue and drowsiness. It is also a diuretic and is used in combination with analgesics for pain relief.

Theophylline and **theobromine** (Fig. 6.64) are minor metabolites in tea; theobromine also occurs in cocoa (*Theobroma cacao* L., Malvaceae). They differ only in the number and position of methyl

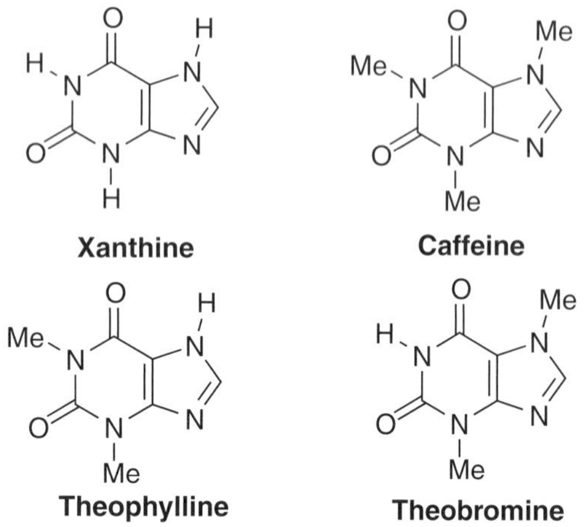

Fig. 6.64 Xanthine (purine) alkaloids.

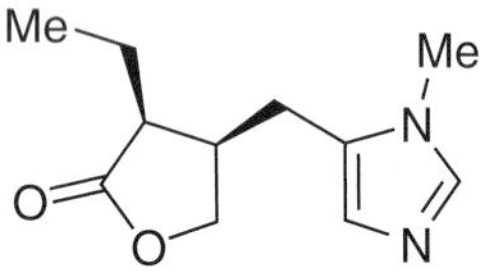

Fig. 6.65 Pilocarpine (remove embedded duplicate).

substituents around the xanthine ring system. Theophylline is used to treat chronic respiratory disease by relaxing the smooth muscle of the bronchi.

Imidazole Alkaloids

Pilocarpine comes from jaborandi (*Pilocarpus jaborandi* Holmes, Rutaceae), a tree common to South America (Fig. 6.65). Pilocarpine is a cholinergic agent and is in eye drops to stimulate muscarinic receptors of the eye in the treatment of glaucoma. It causes pupillary constriction (miosis) and relieves eye pressure by facilitating ocular drainage. Its cholinergic effects are used to enhance lacrimation and saliva production in dry eye and xerostomia after head and neck irradiation, and Sjögren syndrome.

In summary, natural products have led to the development of many valuable drugs; new methods of investigating targets and genomics, and modifying their synthesis, will ensure that they continue to do so for many years. These new approaches are outside our scope, but important review references are listed in the Further reading section.

FURTHER READING

Chopra, B., Dhingara, A.K., 2021. Natural products: a lead for drug discovery and development. Phytother. Res. 35 (9), 4460–4702.

Cragg, G.M., Kingston, D.G.I., Newman, D.J. (Eds.), 2005. Anticancer Agents from Natural Products, first ed. CRC Press, Boca Raton, USA.

Dewick, P.M., 2009. Medicinal Natural Products: A Biosynthetic Approach, third ed. John Wiley and Sons, Chichester, UK.

EMA, European Medicines Agency, 2016. Public Statement on Contamination of Herbal Medicinal Products/Traditional Herbal Medicinal Products with Pyrrolizidine Alkaloids. EMA/HMPC/328782/2016. Committee on Herbal Medicinal Products (HMPC).

Harvey, A.L., Edrada-Ebel, R., Quinn, R.J., 2015. The re-emergence of natural products for drug discovery in the genomics era. Nat. Rev. Drug Discovery 14 (2), 111–129.

Kinghorn, A.D., Falk, H., Gibbons, S. (Eds.), 2017. Progress in the Chemistry of Organic Natural Products, first ed. Springer, Switzerland.

Newman, D.J., Cragg, G.M., 2020. Natural products as sources of new drugs over the nearly four decades from 01/1981 to 09/2019. J. Nat. Prod. 83 (3), 770–803.

Rodrigues, T., Reker, D., Schneider, P., Schneider, G., 2016. Counting on natural products for drug design. Nat. Chem. 8 (6), 531–541.

Schrenk, D., Fahrer, J., Allemang, A., Fu, P., Lin, G., Mahony, C., et al., 2022. Novel insights into pyrrolizidine alkaloid toxicity and implications for risk assessment: occurrence, genotoxicity, toxicokinetics, risk assessment—A workshop report. Planta Med. 88 (2), 98–117. https://doi.org/10.1055/a-1646-3618.

Surendran, S., Qassadi, F., Surendran, G., Lilley, D., Heinrich, M., 2021. Myrcene-what are the potential health benefits of this flavouring and aroma agent? Front. Nutr. 8, 699666. https://doi.org/10.3389/fnut.2021.699666.

Wright, G.D., 2019. Unlocking the potential of natural products in drug discovery. Microb. Biotechnol. 12 (1), 55–57.

7

Analytical Methods for Natural Products

There are different approaches to extracting natural compounds from the biomass, but with all, there is a need to initially extract as many as possible of the constituents. If the plant has not been previously chemically investigated, this ('crude' or total) extract can be screened to identify classes of compounds. Usually, thin-layer chromatography (TLC) is the first step, sometimes using similar visualisation reagents which have been used for well over a century (e.g. Dragendorff's reagent for alkaloids).

Natural product chemistry has mainly focused on plants; consequently, much more is known about their chemistry than that of other living organisms. A plant may have related species that have been previously investigated, giving an indication of chemical composition, thus streamlining the process while acknowledging that new, potentially useful, structural classes of chemicals may be isolated also.

Whether samples are plants, algae, fungi, microbes (including fermented), marine organisms (corals, sea slugs, tunicates) or insects, the raw material is referred to as the **biomass**. Marine, fungal and bacterial organisms have yielded many important drugs, especially in anticancer (Chapter 9), antimicrobial (Chapter 10) and immunosuppressant therapies. Their collection, extraction and purification may be very different, and outside the scope of this book.

PREPARATION AND LIQUID EXTRACTION

In the case of plants, samples may be collected from the aerial parts (leaves, stem and stem bark), the trunk bark and roots or, in the case of large trees, the timber or the heartwood. Samples are then gently air-dried, although better control is achieved with drying cabinets or lyophilisers (freeze-driers). The biomass must be dried quickly to avoid degradation or spoilage (see Chapter 12). Care must be taken with lyophilisers as the high vacuum can remove volatile components that may be of interest.

Once dried, the biomass is chopped or ground (comminuted). This process determines the effective extraction: large particles will be poorly extracted, whereas small particles provide an overall higher surface area and, therefore, will be extracted more efficiently. However, a fine powder may not be optimal—it may not be necessary—and the comminution process may contribute to degradation (by heating, and loss of highly volatile constituents). Fine powders make the filtration process more time-consuming, and some, such as milled flours, are highly flammable.

The nature of the solvent determines the composition of extract. Traditional herbal medicines are mainly used as aqueous infusions, decoctions and hydroalcoholic tinctures (see Chapter 12); for these plants, it is usual to start with water and ethanol combinations. If a plant has a particular method of preparation used by Indigenous people or healers, the extraction should follow the traditional use method as far as possible to confirm activity. Most researchers take a more systematic approach by using multiple, sequential extraction steps to ensure all compounds of interest have been collected. (The −80°C freezers in phytochemistry laboratories are full of obscure green extracts, some decades old, which no-one dares discard!). Traditionally, plant material was extracted sequentially with solvents of increasing polarity: typically,

hexane (or petroleum ether), followed by dichloromethane, ethyl acetate, acetone, ethanol and, finally, water, at room temperature, limiting degradation. Cold extraction allows most compounds to be extracted, although some may have limited solubility at room temperature. In hot percolation, the biomass and solvent are heated gently under reflux. The concern over environmental pollution, carcinogenicity and hepatotoxicity of chlorinated solvents has resulted in the banning of the worst (e.g. carbon tetrachloride), and a general reduction in use of all organic solvents where possible, replacing them with more environmentally friendly methods such as aqueous and supercritical fluid methods of extraction, as explained below. Modern approaches aim to produce extracts with a broad range of metabolites, which can then be fractioned (usually into microwell plates) for *in vitro* testing and simultaneous chemical analysis (e.g. with LC-MS/MS), enabling the dereplication of known compounds.

Typically, plant material is macerated (stewed) in the solvent, often ethanol or aqueous ethanol mixtures. Both polar and (relatively) nonpolar compounds are extracted. Heating the extracts for long periods may degrade labile compounds and remove volatiles; preliminary studies may need to be conducted to see if any biological activity has been lost during extraction. Extraction is never truly total; for example, some highly lipophilic natural products (oils, fats) are insoluble in polar solvents.

Supercritical fluid extraction exploits the property of some gases to behave as liquids when under pressure, and these have solvating properties. Supercritical carbon dioxide can be used to extract biomass and has the advantage that, once the pressure has been removed, the gas evaporates, can be recycled and leaves behind a clean extract. Carbon dioxide is nonpolar, but its polarity as a supercritical extraction solvent may be increased by adding a modifying agent, usually another solvent.

The most widely used classical method for extraction of plant natural products is **Soxhlet extraction** (Fig. 7.1). This technique can produce continuous extraction by solvents of increasing polarity. The biomass is placed in a Soxhlet thimble constructed of filter paper, through which solvent is continuously refluxed. The apparatus empties its contents into a round-bottomed flask once the solvent reaches a certain level. As fresh solvent enters the apparatus at each cycle, via a reflux condenser, extraction is very efficient. This method is suitable for the recovery of large quantities of extract but suffers from the same drawbacks as other hot extraction methods—the possible degradation of products during the long boiling process.

Regardless of the process used, extracts can broadly be classified into two main types: **lipophilic** (fat-soluble), yielded by nonpolar solvents (e.g. petroleum, ethyl acetate, dichloromethane), and **hydrophilic** (water-soluble), yielded by polar solvents (e.g. acetone, methanol, water). The variable solubility of individual constituents in different solvents is the basis of the fractionation process. Certain classes of compounds have high solubility in a particular solvent (e.g. the monoterpenes in hexane), which can be exploited to simplify their purification. Others show a broad spectrum of solubilities and are more challenging to analyse.

Extracts are concentrated under vacuum using rotary evaporators (or under nitrogen for small volumes), and removal of solvent should be carried out immediately to minimise degradation and the

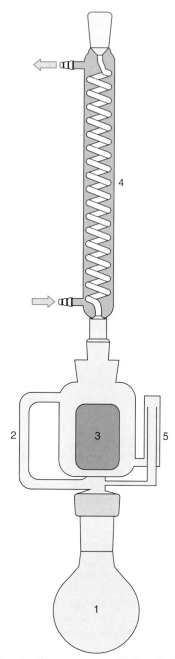

Fig. 7.1 Soxhlet extraction apparatus. *(1)* The flask containing the extractive solvent is heated up and the solvent vapours are directed through *(2)* into the extraction chamber, which contains the plant material in a thimble *(3)*. The solvent vapours condense in *(4)* and drop over the plant material producing a liquid extract. When this reaches a certain level, it is syphoned through *(5)* down into the flask *(1)* and the cycle repeats. (© José M. Prieto-Garcia.)

loss of volatile components. Aqueous extracts are generally lyophilised (freeze-dried). Dried extracts should be stored at (at least) −20°C to reduce decomposition.

If acidic or basic compounds are present, they can be extracted using a more tailored protocol. The most common group extracted this way is the alkaloids. These are basic, nitrogen-containing compounds, which are usually present in the plant as salts: many have potent biological activities and are used as medicines in their purified form. Their extraction typically follows these steps:

1. **Basification:** this converts the alkaloid salt (ionic) to the free base (nonionic) form by dispersing the extract in aqueous ammonia, rendering it alkaline. The alkaloids, as bases, are no longer ionic, less polar and much more soluble in organic solvents.
2. This allows **partitioning** of the free bases into an immiscible solvent such as ethyl acetate. This is carried out in a funnel in which the two layers can easily be separated, simply by turning a tap. The 'unwanted' layer can be discarded (but most researchers do not, learning from past mistakes). The organic layer can be either the top or bottom layer, depending on relative density. It is important to know which one.
3. **Acidification** converts the alkaloids from the free basic form in the organic layer back to the salt (ionic) form. If the extraction is carried out with dilute (2 M) hydrochloric acid, for example, the alkaloids transfer from the organic phase to the aqueous phase as the hydrochlorides.
4. **Rebasification** reverses this process, converting the alkaloids back to their free form, where they may even precipitate, but are more usually extracted back into an organic solvent, which can easily be evaporated and concentrated.

This acid/base duplication process appears repetitive, but in fact is a useful way of 'cleaning up' an extract, ensuring selective transfer of the alkaloids, leaving behind many very polar, nonbasic, lipophilic or other constituents. As illustrated in Fig. 7.2, it generates a mixture of alkaloids that are essentially free of neutral or acidic plant components and it is specific for compounds that can form free bases. However, the acids and bases used in the process may destroy active compounds that have functional groups susceptible to degradation (e.g. glycosides, epoxides and esters), and stereochemistry may be affected by their presence. The most important factor to consider is whether the biological activity has been retained following the extraction protocol.

Steam Distillation

Essential (volatile) oils are extracted from aromatic plants. A typical essential oil may contain over a hundred compounds, mainly terpenes and phenylpropenes (see Chapter 6). These volatile compounds are usually extracted by steam distillation and recovered via a water-cooled condenser. The plant material can be fresh (e.g. peppermint oil), which reduces loss of volatiles on drying, or dried (e.g. cloves and other spices); dried material is either submersed in water and boiled, or steam is passed through it, to directly vaporise the volatile compounds. The condensed liquid contains two immiscible phases: the essential oil and the hydrosol, which is water containing some of the more polar volatiles. Essential oils are usually less dense than water and therefore present as the upper phase of the distillate, but a few are denser and form the lower phase. Exceptions to the use of steam distillation are for the peels of *Citrus* sp. fruits (lemon, orange, grapefruit, lime), which are mechanically pressed in cold conditions to retain the more delicate labile constituents.

ANALYTICAL TECHNIQUES IN NATURAL PRODUCTS CHEMISTRY

The following techniques are used both in the quality assessment of herbal medicines, as in pharmacopoeial monographs, where they are complemented by other tests and assays (see Chapter 12), and as analytical methods for investigating the identity of novel compounds.

Phytochemical Screening

Classical (noninstrumental) qualitative or quantitative methods, such as precipitation, extraction and/or distillation, and colour changes induced by specific reagents, can be used to identify the presence of related compounds sharing similar functionality. These tests are simple, quick and cheap, and many form part of the 'General tests' in a pharmacopoeial monograph (see Chapter 12). They are most suited to testing bulk samples, and in forensic science to detect drugs of abuse, many of which are natural products, before more sophisticated (expensive) instrumental techniques are used. Table 7.1 shows some examples. If the sample has been monitored from cultivation to extraction, these initial methods are superfluous, and analysis can move directly to full assay and control of impurities.

Highly specific colour reactions can differentiate between subclasses of compounds: for example, as alkaloids, the tropanes (such as atropine or hyoscine, see Fig. 6.63) will test positive in the Dragendorff's test, but they will also form a purple colour when treated with fuming nitric acid followed by a solution of dimethylformamide and a few drops of concentrated tetraethylammonium hydroxide, whereas other alkaloids (without the tropane ring) do not.

CHROMATOGRAPHIC TECHNIQUES

Chromatography, first developed in the mid-20th century as a pharmacognostical tool, made it possible to separate small amounts of

complex mixtures of chemicals, such as those found in plant extracts, allowing for the identification of single compounds. It is a physico-chemical method of separation in which components are distributed between two phases, one of which is the **stationary phase** (usually solid, or a liquid chemically attached to a solid—known as 'reverse phase', RP), while the **mobile phase** (usually liquid) moves over it, progressively separating the 'solutes' according to their affinity for each phase. The solute is subjected to two opposing forces: the impelling force provided by the mobile phase (solvent flow) and the solubility of each solute in it, and the retarding forces of interaction with the stationary phase, such as adsorption (by hydrogen bonding etc.) or partition. Each interaction of the solute with the stationary phase will impede it to some extent, depending on the functional groups in the solute, and its stereochemistry, and influence the retention time/elution speed, as shown in Fig. 7.3.

Stationary phases have been developed to offer different chemical selectivity. Initially, chromatography was based on natural materials, such as cellulose, kieselguhr and aluminium oxide, and although not

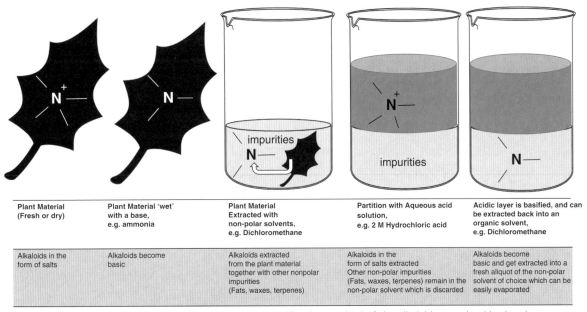

Plant Material (Fresh or dry)	Plant Material 'wet' with a base, e.g. ammonia	Plant Material Extracted with non-polar solvents, e.g. Dichloromethane	Partition with Aqueous acid solution, e.g. 2 M Hydrochloric acid	Acidic layer is basified, and can be extracted back into an organic solvent, e.g. Dichloromethane
Alkaloids in the form of salts	Alkaloids become basic	Alkaloids extracted from the plant material together with other nonpolar impurities (Fats, waxes, terpenes)	Alkaloids in the form of salts extracted Other non-polar impurities (Fats, waxes, terpenes) remain in the non-polar solvent which is discarded	Alkaloids become basic and get extracted into a fresh aliquot of the non-polar solvent of choice which can be easily evaporated

Fig. 7.2 Classical scheme of the extraction and purification method of the alkaloids contained in dry plant materials using **Liquid-liquid** partition.

TABLE 7.1 General Tests Used in Phytochemical Screening

Alkaloids	**Extracts dissolved in dilute hydrochloric acid and filtered**	**Positive result**
Dragendorff's test	Filtrate treated with potassium bismuth iodide	Red precipitate
Anthranol glycosides	**Extract hydrolysed in dilute hydrochloric acid and filtered**	
Modified Borntrager's test	Filtrate treated with ferric chloride solution, immersed in boiling water for 5 min, cooled and extracted with chloroform; chloroform layer treated with ammonia	Rose-pink colour in the ammoniacal layer
Flavonoids	**Plant material extracted with distilled water and filtered**	
Alkaline reagent test	Filtrate treated with a few drops of sodium hydroxide solution	Intense yellow colour, becomes colourless on addition of dilute acid
Phenols	**Plant material extracted with distilled water and filtered**	
Ferric chloride test	Filtrate treated with 3–4 drops of ferric chloride solution	Positive result: formation of bluish-black colour
Phytosterols	**Plant material extracted with dichloromethane and filtered**	
Liebermann Burchard's test	Filtrate treated with a few drops of acetic anhydride, boiled and cooled. Then conc. sulfuric acid added	Positive result: formation of a brown ring at the water–chloroform interphase
Saponins	**Extract diluted with distilled water and filtered**	
Foam test	Filtrate shaken with 2 mL of water	Positive result: foam produced persists for 10 min
Tannins	**Plant materials are extracted with distilled water and filtered**	
Gelatin test	Filtrates are treated with 1% gelatin solution containing sodium chloride	Positive result: formation of white precipitate

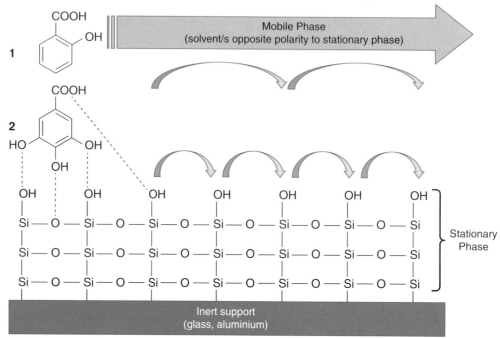

Fig. 7.3 Physicochemical mechanisms underlying chromatography. Different degrees of interaction between the phytochemicals salicylic acid *(1)* and gallic acid *(2)*, stationary phase (silica gel, acting as a polar adsorbent) and mobile phase (a less polar solvent, providing partition) result in one molecule *(1)* eluting faster than the other *(2)*.

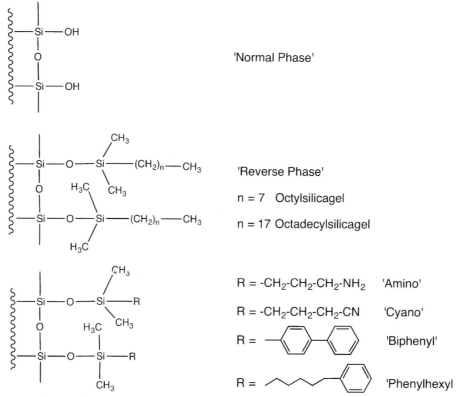

Fig. 7.4 Common stationary phases used in adsorption/partition chromatography.

entirely phased out, silica gel and its bonded derivatives, such as cyano, diol, amide and RP, are preferred due to their superior resolution, reproducibility and versatility (Fig. 7.4). These stationary phases are based on adsorption/partition fundamental interactions; others use different principles, such as size exclusion and ion-chromatography.

The detection of individual solutes can be achieved by chemical or physical means. The latter mostly comprise spectroscopic and spectrometric analysis by detectors at the exit of the chromatograph and provide information on each separated solute to aid its identification. Multiple detectors can be linked—as many as is technically feasible given the size of the sample and capacity of the chromatograph—and these are termed 'hyphenated' techniques and provide much more information than a single detector system. When an eluate passes through several detectors sequentially, it is referred to as 'linear hyphenation'. When using a linear system, all nondestructive methods (e.g. ultraviolet UV), (nuclear magnetic resonance NMR) must (obviously) be used before terminating the analysis with a destructive one (such as mass spectrometry (MS)).

If the eluate is split before analysis, a parallel detection system can be used. The main limitation here is the availability of sufficient eluate, and the sensitivity of the detectors, but a great advantage is that each solute is detected *as it is present in the original eluate*, and not after passage through systems (UV, NMR etc.) which may have altered the chemistry. Examples of parallel coupling in liquid chromatography (LC) include ultraviolet-mass spectrometry and light scattering, whilst a gas chromatograph eluate may be split to both combustion and MS detectors.

Thin-Layer Chromatography Including High-Performance Thin-Layer Chromatography

TLC is a widely used and simple analytical method for the fingerprint and/or quality control of crude extracts. High-performance TLC (HPTLC) is a more sensitive, highly controlled and usually automated technique, giving high resolution, and is preferred where available. TLC uses plastic, aluminium or glass plates, precoated with sorbent (e.g. silica gel) of varying thickness dependent on the amount of material to be loaded, but generally of 0.2 mm. The mixture (extract) is loaded at 1–2 cm from the bottom edge of the plate as a spot or, more usually, a small band. The plate is then lowered into a tank containing the solvent system and, as the band migrates along the plate by capillarity, components will separate according to their affinity for each phase (mainly polarity). Samples of medicinal plant extracts (e.g. *Ginkgo biloba*) or drugs of abuse (e.g. cannabis resin) may be compared with reference substances (bilobalide and tetrahydrocannabinol, respectively) for quick identification.

TLC allows micrograms of material to be separated and, although still used, it is being replaced by more accurate HPTLC, in which all steps that introduce variables—mainly human factors—are controlled by automatisation, greatly increasing reproducibility. Accurate volumes of samples are loaded onto high-resolution plates and developed within tanks under controlled temperature, humidity and solvent saturation conditions. Development of the plates is by immersion in the reagent and drying on hot plates at controlled temperature is usually carried out robotically.

The Stationary Phase

Typically, these consist of ultrapure silica with spherical particles of 7 μm, significantly lower than the 10–12 μm particle size in classical TLC. They produce very compact bands with high resolution. This reproducibility of HPTLC (unlike TLC) allows for quantitation of solutes if the plates are scanned under UV or visible light followed by densitometric computer analysis. HPTLC is used routinely for quality control in the pharmaceutical industry and is the method of choice for herbal identification and quality assurance process in pharmacopeial monographs (see Chapter 12).

Choice of Sorbent and Solvent

Many stationary phases are commercially available, but silica gel 60 is still the most popular; it can achieve many types of separation if used with a suitable mobile phase. Several solvent systems are already optimised for good resolution for different classes and subclasses of natural compounds. In pharmacopoeial monographs, systems are, where possible, harmonised. This means that the same protocol can be used for related species and/or compound analysis, such as flavonoids, saponins, essential oils and alkaloids. Using a harmonised (e.g. pharmacopoeial) HPTLC system has the following advantages:

1. Herbal extracts can be more easily compared
2. The systems have been checked many times for validity and reproducibility
3. Safer methods are introduced as soon as they are available
4. Systems can be set up in advance for immediate use when needed
5. There is no need to keep a wide range of solvents in stock—with their associated problems of environmental disposal, storage, hazard to staff, and cost.

Regardless of system, (HP) TLC, with a carefully constituted mobile phase, can give excellent results, and even differentiation of derivatives of the same compounds. For example, a solvent system of ethyl acetate–formic acid–acetic acid–water in the proportions 100:11:11:27 gives an excellent separation of flavonoid *glycosides* only. Under these conditions, the less polar (nonglycosylated) aglycones, such as quercetin, elute near the solvent front, whilst the more polar glycosides, such as rutin, and the polyphenolic chlorogenic acid, are somewhat retained and show as well-resolved bands in the middle zone of the plate (Fig. 7.5).

Sorbent-coated plates often incorporate a fluorescence indicator (F_{254}) so that compounds absorbing short-wave UV light (e.g. 254 nm) will appear as black bands on a bright green background. Under long-wave UV light (e.g. 365 nm), certain compounds may emit a brilliant fluorescence on a dark background (see Fig. 7.5). Both properties may be used to monitor separations, without harm to the solutes, which is useful when running a plate more than once. TLC plates are finally visualised using chemical reagents. They are either quickly immersed or lightly sprayed with specific development reagents and may need heating. These reagents may be specific for a certain class of natural products, or general in that they will show almost any organic compound (such as concentrated sulfuric acid with heating, which carbonises everything, used only as a last resort). Examples of some common TLC developing reagents are shown in Table 7.2.

For each band, the retention factor (R_f) is calculated; this is the ratio between the distance travelled along the plate by the solute and that travelled by the leading edge of the mobile phase, measured from the point of application. Reference substances (standards) applied to the same plate can thus be compared to aid identification: these are usually pure compounds, but as herbal medicines are complex mixtures, extracts from herbal drugs of pharmacopoeial quality may be supplied as standards. 'Type chromatograms', which are examples of profiles of extracts are available on Pharmacopoeia websites; these are for references only. A similar R_f is not enough for identification: a band must show the same R_f and colour reaction as the reference standard in *at least three different systems* before it can be considered to be the same compound; even then, structure elucidation must be used for confirmation.

Resolution of very similar compounds may be improved with bidimensional TLC. Here, a single sample is applied (as a spot, not a band) close to a corner of the TLC plate, which is developed in a suitable mobile phase. The plate is then dried, turned 90 degrees and developed again in a second solvent system.

(HP) TLC has several advantages in the analysis and isolation of natural products:

- Cost-effective compared with instrumental methods and usually more robust
- Requiring less expertise and training of personnel
- Easy scale-up to preparative mode—from milligram to gram yields
- Flexibility in choice of mobile and stationary phases

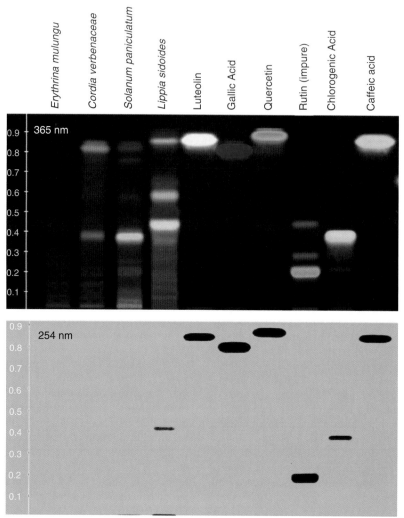

Fig. 7.5 Thin-layer chromatography plate under UV light at 365 nm after derivatisation with Natural Products Reagent. Phenolic substances appear as bands of varying colours on a dark background *(upper image)*. Viewed under 254 nm, all compounds show as black bands on a green fluorescent background (quenching) using an indicator (F_{254}) embedded into the stationary phase *(lower image)*.

TABLE 7.2 Common Developing Reagents Used in Thin-Layer Chromatography Visualisation

Reagent	Test Procedure	Positive Result, Compounds Detected
p-Anisaldehyde—H_2SO_4	Spray with a solution of freshly prepared 0.5 mL p-anisaldehyde in 50 mL glacial acetic acid and 1 mL 97% sulfuric acid. Heat to 105°C until maximum visualisation of spots	Phenols, terpenes, sugars, and steroids turn violet, blue, red, grey or green
Ninhydrin	Spray with a solution of 0.2 g ninhydrin in 100 mL ethanol and heat to 110°C until spots appear	Reddish spots appear. For detection of amines (alkaloids) but also amino acids, amino sugars
Natural substance—polyethylene glycol reagent (NST/PEG)	Spray a 1% methanol solution of natural substance reagent A (diphenylboric acid β-aminoethyl ester) and a 5% ethanol PEG 4000 solution, one after the other onto the TLC plate (approx. 10 and 8 mL). Adding PEG will lead to an increase in detection sensitivity	Intensive fluorescent colours will appear immediately or after 15 min in UV 365 nm. For detection of flavonoids
Vanillin—H_3PO_4	Spray plate with 1 g vanillin in 100 mL 50% aqueous H_3PO_4 Heat for 5–30 min at 110°C	Chars all natural products resulting in brown, grey or black spots. Coloured or fluorescent spots (at 254 and 360 nm) may be seen

TLC, Thin-layer chromatography.

- Separations may be optimised to 'zero in' on one or more components
- Most separations can be achieved with suitable mobile and stationary phases
- Many samples can be analysed simultaneously and comparisons are more easily made.

The major disadvantages of (HP)TLC are that:
- Loading and speed are poor compared with high-performance liquid chromatography (HPLC)
- Less efficient detection and control of elution compared with HPLC.

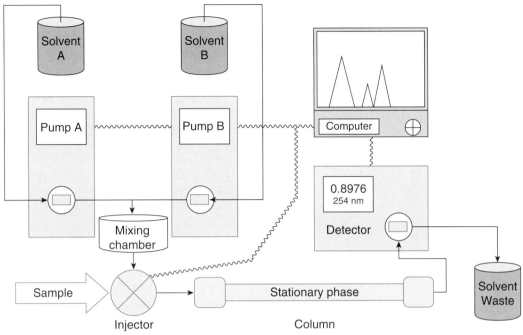

Fig. 7.6 HPLC instrument. (© José M. Prieto-Garcia.)

High-Performance Liquid Chromatography

HPLC is widely used for the analysis and isolation of natural products. It is based on the same principles—adsorption and partitioning—previously discussed. Similar stationary and mobile systems are used, although these are not directly transferable. The sensitivity of the HPLC, particularly when coupled with UV/VIS detection, enables the acquisition of spectra of eluting peaks ranging from 190 to 800 nm. Solvent flowrates are typically 0.5–2.0 mL/min and sample loading in the analytical mode allows the rapid detection and separation of submicrogram amounts of material; the system can easily be scaled up for preparative work.

HPLC systems pump solvents at high pressures (up to 15,000 psi in modern ultra-HPLC machines) through stainless steel columns densely packed with the stationary phase, thus maximising interaction with solutes. Modern HPLC systems are computer-driven and not only run samples but can be programmed to process data and print out chromatograms and spectra automatically. A scheme of an HPLC instrument is shown in Fig. 7.6.

Standard sorbents, such as normal phase silica and reverse-phase (RP-C_{18} and C_8) systems, and more specialised stationary phases, such as phenyl, cyano, C_4 and chiral phases, provide an array of adsorption/partition chromatography methods tailored to separate most types of natural product. Other techniques, such as ion exchangers (for highly polar/ionic compounds) and gel size-exclusion (for large molecules such as proteins), can be incorporated.

The use of such stationary phases has made HPLC a highly versatile method of separation, and the most versatile of all is still C_{18} (RP), which generally employs water/acetonitrile or water/alcohol mixtures as the mobile phase—and avoiding chlorinated and other toxic solvents. Despite the presence of water, it can be used for most natural products that are soluble in organic solvents. These mobile phases may be run in **isocratic elution** mode, in which a constant composition (e.g. 70% acetonitrile in water) is maintained throughout the separation, or in **gradient elution** mode, in which the concentration of a solvent is gradually increased during the run-time, starting, for example, with 100% water and increasing to 100% acetonitrile over 30 minutes. Gradient elution is achieved with computer-controlled pumps,

accurately mixing solvents over time, resulting in improved resolution and shorter run times.

HPLC detectors use either a UV/VIS detector, which records at one wavelength, or a photo-diode array (PDA) detector, which can monitor and record all wavelengths at the same time. This is very useful as plant extracts contain compounds with very diverse UV/VIS properties. Despite the analytical power packed in a HPLC-UV/VIS-PDA system, phytochemical separations pose such a challenge—in terms of polarities and UV spectra—that not all the components of an extract may be fully resolved.

Fig. 7.7 shows a typical HPLC-UV/VIS chromatogram (at 254.4 nm) of a plant extract together with the UV/VIS spectra of each major peak. Not all peaks represent a pure compound but a group of compounds with very similar polarities eluting together (such as 1, 2 and 5). Other peaks in the chromatogram are single compounds, well resolved from each other. Their identification must be carried out by matching both the retention time (t_R) and UV/VIS spectra with those of pure standards under the same conditions. Co-injection of the sample and reference substance should result in a perfect overlap producing a single larger peak—a procedure known as 'spiking'.

Compounds with poor UV characteristics cannot be detected by PDA UV/VIS detection. This is especially true of natural products, such as terpenoids or polyketides, which may have no unsaturation or chromophores that give rise to a characteristic UV signature. In these cases, a **refractometry index** (RI) detector has been the classical alternative. However, they are 100–1000 times less sensitive than UV detectors and can be used with isocratic conditions only. To overcome these limitations **evaporative light scattering** (ELS) detectors were developed. Three processes occur within the ELS detector: (1) the eluate is nebulised, (2) the mobile phase is evaporated and (3) the light scattered by the solute particles is detected. This detector works better with volatile mobile phases; its response is related to the quantity of the solute (mass not concentration) and its molecular mass. The ELS detector is suitable for the analysis of high molecular weight, UV/VIS transparent compounds, such as polysaccharides.

Fluorescence detectors contain an excitation light, axial to the detector cell, to produce fluorescence in susceptible compounds. Its

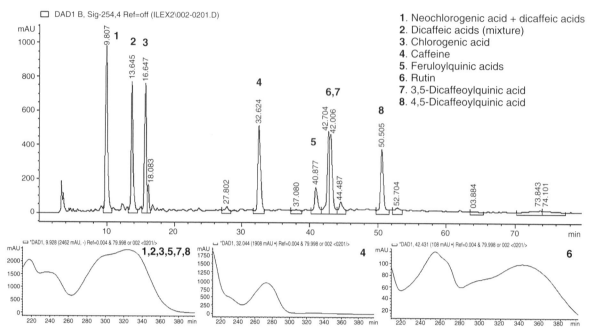

Fig. 7.7 Typical HPLC-UV-VIS-PDA chromatogram of a plant extract (in this case at 254.4 nm, up) and the UV spectra of every major peak (down). *HPLC,* High-performance liquid chromatography; *PDA,* photo-diode array; *UV,* ultraviolet, *VIS,* visible light. (© José M. Prieto-Garcia.)

sensitivity is up to 1000 times higher than UV/VIS. Unfortunately, not all molecules are endowed with this property and in some cases a derivatisation reagent is added pre- or post-column to form a fluorescent derivative that can be detected.

The most important addition to the detection power in HPLC systems is MS. As with gas chromatography-mass spectrometry (GC-MS) (see later), HPLC-MS becomes even more powerful when coupled to an electronic library capable of searching and comparing compounds with known UV/VIS spectra and MS ionisation patterns and is now considered to be the gold standard in terms of versatility and sensitivity for most analyses.

FINGERPRINTING EXTRACTS

These are depictions of the overall chemical composition of herbal extracts *without necessarily identifying them.* The degree of similarity between profiles (fingerprints) generated from UV/VIS-MS spectra, or patterns of chromatographic peaks, can be compared as an aid to identification. In order to be of any use, the conditions under which the fingerprint was taken must be disclosed: all analytical parameters, processing and extraction protocols, brand of equipment, columns and solvents, and every other detail of the program and settings, to provide reproducibility. In many pharmacopoeias, fingerprints, known as 'type-chromatograms', are included, not as official standards, but as useful visual guidance.

Using multivariate analysis and chemometrics, fingerprints can be used to check consistency across batches of the same herbal product, and rule out adulterations, which may otherwise be missed by focusing on one phytochemical marker only. Fig. 7.8 shows the overlapped fingerprint analysis of 19 samples of *Ginkgo biloba.* The chemometric analysis (scatter plot) reveals that samples 1, 2 and 4 stand out from the others because peak 8 is too predominant (as seen in the single chromatograms on the right). These samples were adulterated by addition of the inexpensive flavonoid rutin, thus artificially increasing their total flavonoid content.

Gas Chromatography

GC, also known as vapour-phase or gas-liquid chromatography (GLC), is a partition technique in which the mobile phase is an inert gas (usually helium or nitrogen), referred to as the **carrier gas,** which flows through a column containing the stationary phase, a liquid, coated on the interior of the narrow capillary column as a thin film. This provides a mechanism for partition between the gas and liquid phases. Former GC systems used larger columns, packed with particles of adsorbent or RP materials. These are rarely used now, as they give poor resolution and are easily degraded.

The mixture to be analysed is heated until vaporised immediately after injection into the system, and carried by the gas flowing through the column, which is enclosed in a temperature-controlled oven. Components become separated according to their affinity between the gas and stationary phase, as in other forms of chromatography. The choice of gas is mainly dictated by the detector system used. Optimal elution of the components is achieved by a balance of the pressure of the gaseous mobile phase and the temperature of the column. Carrier gas flow rates are typically between 1 and 10 mL/min and the temperature from 50 to 300°C. Electronic pressure control allows the instrument to compensate for changes in gas pressure as the oven temperature rises. Fig. 7.9 shows the scheme of a GC chromatograph; it can be run in fully automated mode, and with carousel autosamplers it is possible to analyse tens to hundreds of samples per 'run'.

Detection in GC has been classically based on **combustion detectors,** particularly flame ionisation detection (FID). Combustion detectors require the addition of a 'fuel gas' (usually hydrogen) and an 'oxidising gas' (usually dry air). Noncombustion detectors, such as **electrochemical detectors** (ECDs), do not require any added gas but may use argon or methane gas to increase detector sensitivity. ECDs are able to detect down to 10^{-13} g (one tenth of a picogram!) of solute.

The analytical power of GC is greatly increased by the addition of MS detectors, which can provide the molecular weight of a compound: once a molecular ion has been identified, it is possible to measure it accurately to ascertain the exact number of hydrogens, carbons,

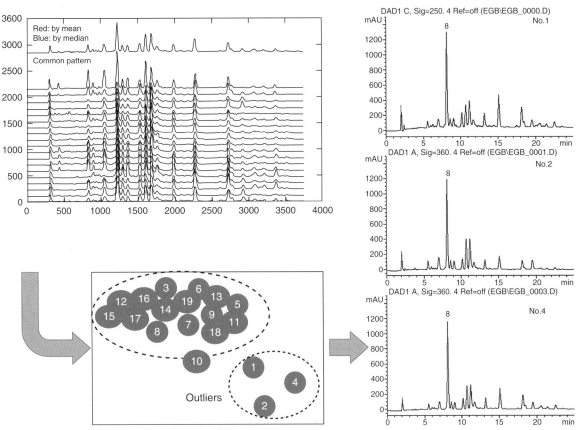

Fig. 7.8 (A–C) High-performance liquid chromatography fingerprints of 19 commercial samples of *Ginkgo biloba* L. extracts analysed by computer-aided-similarity-evaluation software help to pinpoint adulterated products. (Adapted from Xie, P., Chen, S., Liang, Y.-z., Wang, X., Tian, R., Upton, R., 2006. Chromatographic fingerprint analysis—a rational approach for quality assessment of traditional Chinese herbal medicine. J. Chromatog. A 1112 (1–2), 171–180.)

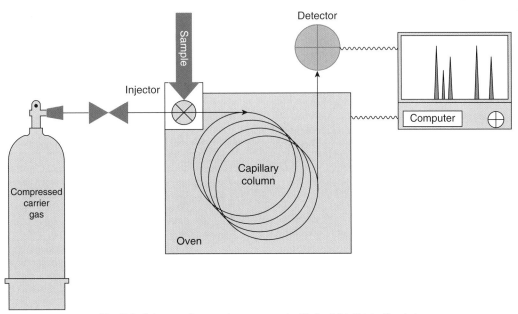

Fig. 7.9 Scheme of a gas chromatograph. (© José M. Prieto-Garcia.)

oxygens and other atoms in the molecule and, thus, the molecular formula. Several ionisation techniques are available in MS; **electron impact** gives good fragmentation patterns and is useful for assigning functional groups present in the molecule.

Molecular ions are not always present. Softer techniques such as **chemical ionisation** (CI), **electrospray ionisation** (ESI) and **fast atom bombardment** (FAB) MS can ionise the molecule with less energy; consequently, molecular ions are more likely to be generated, although

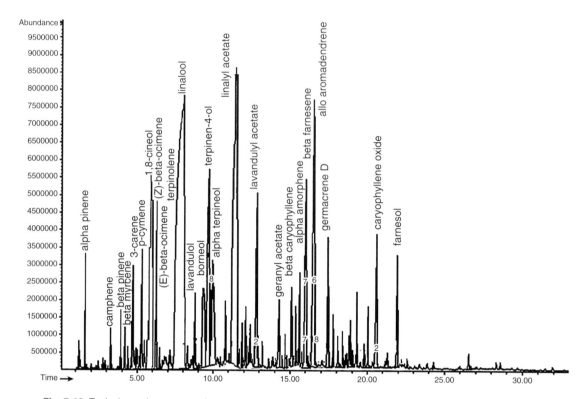

Fig. 7.10 Typical gas chromatography–mass spectrometry chromatogram of *Lavandula angustifolia* essential oil showing the separation of chemical components.

less fragmentation means less information for structure elucidation purposes.

GC-FID-MS or GC-ECD-MS, coupled to an electronic library enables early identification of known compounds, or the comparison of novel compounds with known MS spectra. GC is only suitable for relatively volatile compounds that are not degraded by heat. It is the method of choice for some essential oils, which are by definition mixtures of volatile compounds. It provides fast resolution and identification of typically 80–99% of the components, which is unmatched by any other instrumental technique. Fig. 7.10 shows the GC chromatogram of lavender essential oil.

Less volatile/more polar compounds can be chemically modified to improve volatility, usually by silylation of their hydroxyl and carboxylic acid groups, using trimethylchlorosilane in pyridine; however, this technique is rarely used now, as HPLC can produce better separations of polar compounds, without the losses induced by derivatisation and/or the use of highly reactive and toxic reagents.

CURRENT TRENDS IN NATURAL PRODUCTS CHEMICAL ANALYSIS

Phytochemical analysis benefits from developments in the wider field of analytical chemistry and the application of computation and statistical analyses (see Further Reading). The next frontier making separation an unnecessary step—the direct analysis of a natural substance in a mixture by purely spectroscopic techniques, such as near-infrared (NIR), MS or NMR spectroscopy. This vastly reduces processing times and generation of artefacts but requires high sensitivity and computational power. NIR is useful for the direct characterisation of herbal medicinal and food products and can ascertain whether they contain synthetic or natural adulterants. It is a powerful technique—enough that tablets can sometimes be analysed without even taking them out of their blister packets—thus allowing for continuous quality control during the manufacturing process.

FURTHER READING

Booker, A., Frommenwiler, D., Johnston, D., et al., 2014. Chemical variability along the value chains of turmeric (*Curcuma longa*): a comparison of nuclear magnetic resonance spectroscopy and high-performance thin layer chromatography. J. Ethnopharmacol. 152, 292–301.

Cozzolino, D., 2009. Near infrared spectroscopy in natural product analysis. Planta Med. 75 (7), 746–756.

Cozzolino, D., 2022. An overview of the successful application of vibrational spectroscopy techniques to quantify nutraceutical in fruits and plants. Foods 11 (3), 315.

European Pharmacopoeia. https://pheur.edqm.eu/home; British Pharmacopoeia https://www.pharmacopoeia.com.

Fanali, S., Haddad, P.R., Poole, C., 2017. Liquid Chromatography: Applications, second ed. Elsevier.

Fanali, S., Haddad, P.R., Poole, C., 2017. Liquid Chromatography: Fundamentals and Instrumentation, second ed. Elsevier, Amsterdam.

Kowalska, T., Sherma, J., Cazes, J., 2020. Preparative Layer Chromatography. Taylor and Francis, Boca Raton, FL.

McNair, H.M., Miller, J.M., Snow, N.H., 2019. Basic Gas Chromatography, third ed. Wiley, Hoboken, NJ.

Politi, M., Zloh, M., Pintado, M.E., et al., 2009. Direct metabolic fingerprinting of commercial herbal tinctures by nuclear magnetic resonance spectroscopy and mass spectrometry. Phytochem. Anal. 20, 328–334.

Poole, C., 2021. Gas Chromatography. Elsevier, Amsterdam.

Poole, C., Reich, E., 2023. Instrumental Thin-Layer Chromatography, 2nd Edition. Elsevier, Amsterdam.

Prieto, J.M., Mellinas-Gomez, M., Zloh, M., 2016. Application of diffusion-edited and solvent suppression ¹H-NMR to the direct analysis of markers in valerian-hop liquid herbal products. Phytochem. Anal. 27, 100–106.

Reich, E., Schibli, A., 2011. High-performance Thin-Layer Chromatography for the Analysis of Medicinal Plants. Thieme, New York.

Sarker, S.D., Nahari, L., 2012. Hyphenated techniques and their applications in natural products analysis. Methods Mol. Biol. 864, 301–340.

Schmidt-Traub, H., Schulte, M., Seidel-Morgenstern, A., 2020. Preparative Chromatography, third ed. Wiley, Weinheim.

Sherma, J., Vander Heyden, Y., Komsta, L., 2018. Chemometrics in Chromatography. CRC Press, Boca Raton, FL.

Sultanbawa, Y., Smyth, H.E., Truong, K., Chapman, J., Cozzolino, D., 2021. Insights on the of chemometrics and vibrational spectroscopy in fruit metabolite analysis. Food Chem. 3, 100033.

Wagner, H., Bauer, R., Melchart, D., Xiao, P.G., Staudinger, A., 2016. Chromatographic Fingerprint Analysis of Herbal Medicines: Thin-Layer and High-Performance Liquid Chromatography of Chinese Drugs. Vol 1 (2nd ed), 2011; Vol 2 (2nd ed), 2011; Vol 3, 2014; Vol 4. Springer, Cham, Switzerland.

Wagner, H.., Barghouti, T., Melchart, D., Pühls, S., Staudinger, A. (Eds.). 2018. Chromatographic Fingerprint Analysis of Herbal Medicines: Thin-Layer and High Performance Liquid Chromatography of Chinese Drugs, Vol 5. Springer, Cham, Switzerland.

8

Natural Product Isolation and Structure Elucidation

Public interest in natural product drugs (and particularly in miracle drugs from tropical rainforests) remains high, but investment in their discovery by industry or in academic research is generally low and cyclical due to the development of alternative ways of finding new leads (e.g. combinatorial chemistry). However, synthetic chemistry cannot yet mimic the ability of living organisms to produce such complex and diverse structures, and novel techniques in natural product chemistry ensure they will continue to provide new molecules for years to come.

A natural product-derived drug may be:

- Isolated directly from the producing organism, such as the β-lactamase inhibitor **clavulanic acid**, from the bacterium *Streptomyces clavuligerus*.
- A semisynthetic compound, i.e. one that has undergone a minor chemical modification, such as **aspirin**, which is derived from **salicylic acid** and occurs which occurs as esters and glycosides in willow bark (*Salix* spp.) and other plants.
- A synthetic compound, based on a natural product possessing biological activity (e.g. **pethidine**, which was based on **morphine** from the opium poppy, *Papaver somniferum* L.). These compounds are used as templates to 'design' molecules posing the important skeletal structure and functional groups needed for specific pharmacological effects and, as such, it is sometimes difficult to see how the fully synthetic compound was modelled on the natural product (Fig. 8.1).

Drug leads are compounds that may be developed into medicines. Examples include the anticancer drugs **paclitaxel** (Fig. 8.2), irinotecan, etoposide and others (see Chapter 9). Paclitaxel shows the qualities which make natural products ideal as drug leads, having many functional groups and chiral centres (11), giving rise to distinctive shapes and biological activities.

There are several approaches used to identify potential new drug leads:

Ethnobotanical approaches use the knowledge of the use of a particular plant by an indigenous people to direct a search for a drug lead in a specific therapeutic area, such as infection, pain relief or digestive disorders (see Chapter 5).

Chemotaxonomic approaches rely on the relationships between plants and their chemistry; taxonomically related plants often contain structurally similar compounds.

Random approaches ignore existing knowledge of plant chemistry or biological activity. They take advantage of the availability of plants and include most screening processes. Random selection is purely serendipitous; there is a chance it will find compounds with bioactivity, but it may however identify useful properties in a plant that are unrelated to the traditional use, as with the discovery of the anticancer *Vinca* alkaloids (see Chapter 9).

Information-driven approaches use a combination of these, linked in a database used to prioritise candidates to be screened. This approach is necessary when screening thousands of samples to avoid the repeated discovery of known compounds, a process, known as **dereplication**, which is crucial when investment costs are so high.

The steps involved in drug discovery are shown in Fig. 8.3. Many further preclinical, pharmacological and toxicological assessments must be conducted prior to a drug being subjected to clinical trials, and it may take 10–20 years before it is marketed as a medicine. Regardless of the scale involved, the biomass is collected, (usually) dried, extracted into a suitable organic solvent and screened in a bioassay. In **low-throughput screening** (LTS), small numbers of extracts are tested; this is usually the case in academic research. In **high-throughput screening** (HTS), thousands of extracts are screened, an approach more suitable to the pharmaceutical industry, which may have hundreds of thousands of samples (both natural and synthetic) available for evaluation.

Active extracts are further fractionated using bioassay-guided isolation, with chromatographic techniques used to separate the extract (eventually) into individual component(s), designated as lead compounds, to be further assessed in a process of cross-screening. This gives information on the selectivity of the compound: is it active in many assays or does it exhibit activity only in a particular type of assay? Specificity is an important criterion during selection of a compound for further development.

Whilst biological evaluation is ongoing, structure elucidation methods are conducted to identify the active molecule(s) at each stage, to establish whether a compound appears to be novel, the chemical class it belongs to, and if that type of compound has previously been reported to possess biological activity.

If these criteria are satisfied, larger amounts of the lead compound are extracted and investigations are conducted to establish its potency, mechanism of action and toxicity, as well as whether chemical modification is needed to enhance activity. It will undergo extensive preclinical and in vivo studies before clinical trials can even be considered, and during this extensive evaluation, many drug candidates fail through toxicity or lack of efficacy in humans. Given the complexity, it is not surprising that many natural product drug leads fail to make their way onto the market.

Bioassay-guided isolation is the process used to isolate active compounds by monitoring their biological effects—and potency—during each stage of their fractionation and purification.

INITIAL FRACTIONATION METHODS

Once an extract has been produced using a suitable protocol (see Chapter 7) and activity is demonstrated in a bioassay, different separation methods, usually in combination, can be used to isolate a biologically active pure compound. Partitioning, a simple technique widely used as an initial 'clean up' step, separates lipophilic from polar

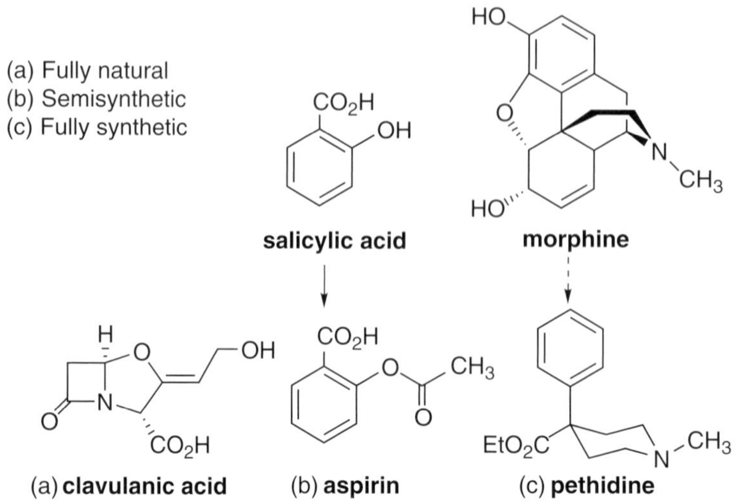

(a) Fully natural
(b) Semisynthetic
(c) Fully synthetic

salicylic acid   **morphine**

(a) **clavulanic acid**   (b) **aspirin**   (c) **pethidine**

Fig. 8.1 Medicinal agents from natural sources.

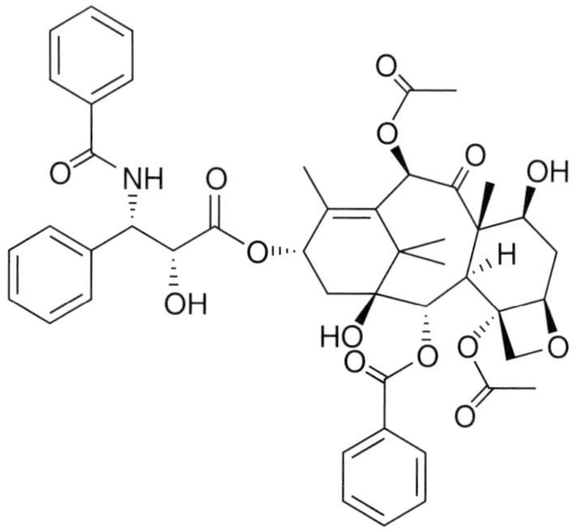

Fig. 8.2 Paclitaxel (Taxol).

compounds. It requires two immiscible solvents, to which the extract is added in a separating funnel: depending on their solubility, different components will migrate to either aqueous or organic layer, and can be easily separated. This is usually repeated sequentially using immiscible organic solvents of increasing polarity; typically, starting with water/light petroleum ether (hexane) to generate a nonpolar fraction in the organic layer; followed by water/dichloromethane or water/chloroform or water/ethyl acetate to give a medium-polar fraction in the organic layer. The remaining aqueous layer will contain polar water-soluble natural products. This separation method relies on the solubility of natural products and not a physical interaction with another medium (as in chromatography, see Chapter 7). Partitioning gives excellent separations of compounds that differ greatly in solubility; for example, monoterpenes are easily separated from phenolics such as tannins. The next steps involve sequential chromatographic separations.

Gel Chromatography

A widely used initial clean-up technique is **gel chromatography**, also known as **size-exclusion chromatography**. This technique employs a cross-linked dextran (sugar polymer) that, when added to a suitable solvent (e.g. chloroform or ethyl acetate), swells to form a gel matrix. The gel contains pores of a finite size that allow small molecules (<500 Da) to be retained in the matrix; larger molecules (>500 Da) are excluded and move quickly through the gel. This gel is loaded into a column and the extract is added on top. Large molecules are the first to

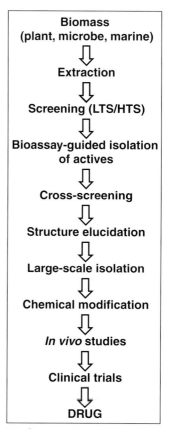

Biomass
(plant, microbe, marine)
⇓
Extraction
⇓
Screening (LTS/HTS)
⇓
Bioassay-guided isolation of actives
⇓
Cross-screening
⇓
Structure elucidation
⇓
Large-scale isolation
⇓
Chemical modification
⇓
In vivo studies
⇓
Clinical trials
⇓
DRUG

Fig. 8.3 Steps involved in Drug Discovery.

elute, followed by molecules of a smaller size. This is a useful method for separating out chlorophylls, fatty acids, glycerides and other large molecules that may interfere with the biological assay. Different gels are available, to be used in organic solvents (e.g. LH-20) or aqueous preparations such as salts and buffers (e.g. G-25). Both nonpolar and polar compounds can thus be fractionated. The dextran from which the gel is made contains hydroxyl groups which further facilitate separation according to polarity.

This nondestructive method has a high recovery rate (compounds are rarely strongly adsorbed) and large quantities of extract (hundreds of milligrams to grams) may be separated. Different gels are available with a variety of pore sizes that can separate compounds from 500 to 250,000 Da. This is the method of choice for large molecules, in particular proteins, polypeptides, carbohydrates, tannins and glycosides, saponins and triterpene glycosides.

Ion-Exchange Chromatography

The separation of small, polar, ionic compounds is often problematic. It is possible to separate these from larger molecules (using gels), but they are generally very strongly adsorbed on sorbents such as silica or alumina, and even when using polar solvents and pH modifiers, efficient separations may not be achievable. These compounds are not retained in reverse-phase systems such as C_{18} or C_8. However, their functional groups (including CO_2H, –OH, –NH_2) contribute to the polarity of the molecule, which is exploited in **ion-exchange chromatography**. The technique is limited to compounds that can carry a charge on a functional group. The stationary phase has charged groups and mobile counter ions, and as the mobile phase moves through the column, separation is achieved by differences in affinity between the ionic solutes and the stationary phase. Ion-exchange sorbents or resins may be **cation** exchangers, which have acidic groups (CO_2H, –SO_3H) and exchange their protons with cations of the solute, and **anion** exchangers, which have basic groups (–N^+R_3) incorporated into the resin, and exchange anions with the solute. Ion-exchange resins may be used in open-columns, and in closed-column systems such as high-performance liquid chromatography (HPLC).

Flash Chromatography

Flash chromatography uses prepacked solvent-resistant plastic cartridges (Fig. 8.4), which contain the sorbent (silica, alumina, C_{18}, HP-20 or ion-exchange resin). These cartridges are introduced into a **radial compression module** (see the metal cylinder in Fig. 8.4), which pressurises the cartridge and sorbent radially. This results in a very homogeneous packed sorbent, reducing solvent channelling when the system is running and minimising void spaces on the column head.

The extract is dissolved in solvent and loaded onto the column directly; solvent is then pumped through the column and fractions are collected. With flash chromatography, larger amounts of extract can be fractionated rapidly (typically 30 minutes) using a step gradient solvent system, and high resolution achieved. This speed minimises contact with reactive and/or hazardous sorbents such as silica, which are contained within the cartridges. These are re-used, reducing the cost.

Fractions and compounds eluting from the column may be detected by further chromatographic methods such as thin-layer chromatography (TLC) or passing the eluent through a UV detector. Running several flash columns simultaneously enables sufficient extract to be generated for further purification.

Preparative Thin-Layer Chromatography

Preparative TLC is widely used for purifying a small number of components, typically following a flash separation. As with TLC, this method employs glass or aluminium plates precoated with sorbent of varying thickness, dependent on the amount of material to be loaded onto the plates. The coating of preparative plates may be 1–2 mm thick, up to 10 times thicker than analytical plates, but the principles are the same. The higher loading can produce enough purified material for biological assays and structure elucidation; it is rapid and cheap, and the method of choice for separating lipophilic compounds. Preparative plates can be modified to offer greater flexibility by incorporation of modifying agents into the sorbents (e.g. silver nitrate for separation of olefinic compounds), use of other sorbents (ion exchange, polyamide, cellulose) and the addition of indicators and binders.

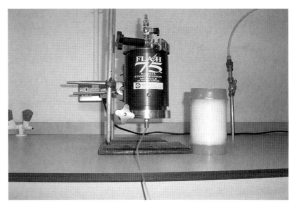

Fig. 8.4 Biotage flash chromatograph. Fast separations are achieved with good resolution.

The scale-up from analytical to preparative mode may change the separation of the components. Normally, the method developed on the analytical scale needs to be modified, generally by reducing solvent polarity. Preparative TLC is mostly used as a simple, final clean-up procedure to separate 2–4 compounds. An edge of the plate is sprayed with the reagent (taking care that the rest of the plate is covered) and separated compounds are visualised as coloured bands. The bands containing purified compounds are scraped off the plate and desorption carried out in a sintered glass funnel, by eluting with a suitable solvent. The eluate is collected, concentrated and assessed for purity by analytical TLC.

Preparative High-Performance Liquid Chromatography

The scaling up of an analytical HPLC method allows for the separation of up to gram quantities of samples. Coupled with intelligent fraction collectors that can 'peak collect' compounds as they elute, by receiving input from the ultraviolet–visible (UV–Vis), Evaporative Light Scattering (ELS) or mass spectrometry (MS) detectors, they are highly efficient, and also expensive in terms of instrumentation, consumables as well as environmental and disposal costs.

Isolation Strategies

A typical isolation protocol starting with extraction of the biomass using a Soxhlet apparatus, cold or hot percolation, or supercritical fluid extraction, is shown in Fig. 8.5.

Hydrophilic extracts may initially undergo ion-exchange chromatography with bioassay of generated fractions. Further isolation of active fractions eventually yields pure compounds, which can be submitted for structure elucidation. Lipophilic extracts may initially be partitioned to generate a further, more hydrophilic fraction, which is subjected to the same procedures.

Lipophilic extracts may undergo initial gel chromatography (to remove or separate large components, e.g. chlorophylls, fatty acids or glycerides), or be subjected directly to flash chromatography to generate a series of fractions for bioassay.

Active fractions can then be further purified by using either HPLC or TLC to give pure compounds for structure elucidation. This is only a general outline; there is no tailored protocol, and the isolation of chemicals from nature can be difficult and intellectually challenging. Most extracts is highly complex, and the active component(s) may be present at very low concentrations or be unstable. It is also possible that activity may diminish during the separation process; this could be due to a synergistic effect of components working in concert in the bioassay. It is likely that the efficacy of certain herbal medicines (which contain tens to hundreds, or even thousands, of constituents) is due to several active compounds; thus, the bioassay-guided isolation approach may not be appropriate for their study.

STRUCTURE ELUCIDATION

Ideally, separation methods should afford a pure natural compound of at least 5 mg in weight. Current structure elucidation techniques are available that can determine the structures of micrograms of material, although larger quantities are needed for further biological assays. Normally, large quantities of biomass are extracted, in case of a potentially lengthy bioassay-guided isolation process and to ensure sufficient quantities of compounds are produced for pharmacological investigation, without having to source and duplicate the extraction.

The structure elucidation of chemical entities generally employs classical spectroscopic techniques, especially **mass spectrometry** (MS) and **nuclear magnetic resonance** (NMR) **spectroscopy**. The first steps, however, should be the recording of infrared (IR) and UV–Vis spectra to determine the presence of certain functional groups and conjugation in the molecule.

Rather than a theoretical approach, a real case can be used to illustrate the steps involved in purification, with an explanation of the spectra produced by each technique, and how these are used in tandem. In a project to isolate and characterise antimicrobials from plants, *Thymus vulgaris* L. (thyme, Lamiaceae), was extracted with hexane and ethyl acetate to yield a lipophilic, and a more polar (but not aqueous) extract, following the scheme shown in Fig. 8.5. Both extracts were highly active in a methicillin-resistant *Staphylococcus aureus* (MRSA) assay, and when analysed by TLC, were found to be chemically very similar and therefore bulked. Flash chromatography, followed by preparative HPLC, led to the isolation of a pure active natural product, compound X, which was a pale-yellow volatile oil with a pungent aroma. The UV spectrum showed a maximum at 277 nm, indicative of the presence of an aromatic ring. The IR spectrum showed absorptions attributable to aromatic and aliphatic C–H groups and a broad peak at 3600 nm indicative of a hydroxyl functional group.

Compound X was submitted to fast atom bombardment mass spectrometry (FAB-MS); the spectrum is shown in Fig. 8.6. The scale on the x-axis is the mass (m) to charge (z) ratio (m/z). As compound X readily forms single ions, m/z is in effect m/1 and therefore directly related to the weight of fragments and, in the case of the molecular ion, the molecular weight of the compound.

A molecular ion (M+) is seen at m/z 150. This is supported by additional peaks where the molecule picks up a hydrogen ion at m/z 151

[M+H]+ and loses a hydrogen ion at m/z 149 [M–H]+. The spectrum was run using FAB ionisation and little fragmentation is evident. There are some useful fragments, however, in particular at m/z 135, which is 15 mass units less than the molecular ion and almost certainly corresponds to [M–Me]+, indicating that this molecule contains a methyl group (15 mass units), which is readily lost in the mass spectrometer.

Accurate mass measurement of the molecular ion at m/z 150 gave a figure of 150.104700. If a computer program is used to calculate the number of carbon, hydrogen and oxygen atoms that would be required to give this weight, a formula of $C_{10}H_{14}O$ is produced. The theoretical mass of this formula is 150.104465, which is very close to the measured accurate mass. The theoretical mass takes into account the accurate masses of carbon, hydrogen and oxygen, and the nearest 'fit' to the measured mass gives the $C_{10}H_{14}O$ formula. Interestingly, compound X has 10 carbon atoms and, as it is a volatile oil, it is likely to be a monoterpene.

At this stage, it would be possible to perform a database search on this molecular formula and the producing organism (*T. vulgaris*) from reference sources. However, there are many natural products with this formula and therefore further structure elucidation is required.

NMR Spectroscopy
¹H NMR Spectroscopy

The next step in this process is the recording of an ¹H NMR spectrum (Fig. 8.7). This will indicate the number of hydrogen atoms associated with a particular group (**integration**) and how **shielded** or **deshielded** that group is. Shielding and deshielding occur due to the presence of groups that are either electron withdrawing (deshielding) or electron donating (shielding).

Inspection of the ¹H NMR spectrum of compound X recorded in the solvent deuterated chloroform $CDCl_3$, which has a peak at 7.27 ppm (**Z** in the spectrum), shows three deshielded peaks (**A**, **B** and **C**), each integrating for one proton (the figures under the x-axis are the integration and indicate how many protons are associated with each peak). These protons occur in the aromatic region (6.00–8.00 ppm) and have a particular coupling pattern. Additional signals include a broad peak (**D**), indicating that it is exchangeable and possibly a hydroxyl group, a multiplet at 2.84 ppm (**E**) integrating for one proton and a singlet at 2.23 ppm (peak **F**) integrating for three protons, which is due to a methyl group. The last peak in the spectrum (**G**) is a doublet (two lines) integrating for six protons. This is due to two methyl groups occurring in the same position of the spectrum as they are equivalent. This equivalence occurs because they are in the same 'environment'. This signal appears as a doublet because these methyl

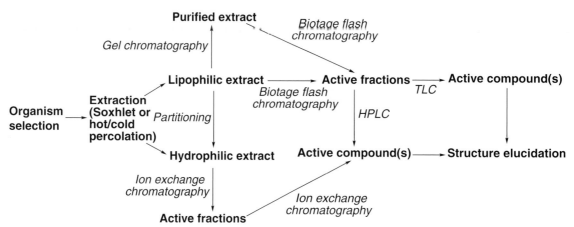

Fig. 8.5 General isolation strategy for purification of bioactive natural products. *HPLC,* High-performance liquid chromatography; *TLC,* thin-layer chromatography.

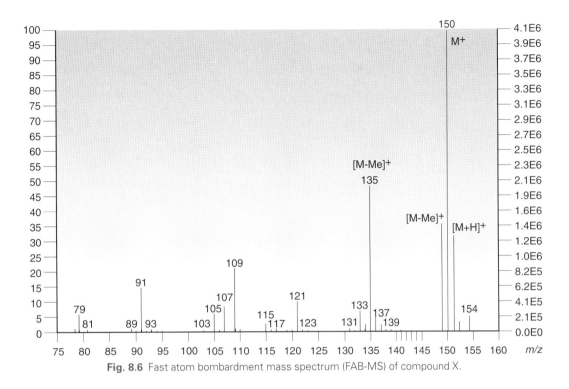

Fig. 8.6 Fast atom bombardment mass spectrum (FAB-MS) of compound X.

groups are coupled to one proton (multiplicity = *n* + 1, where *n* is the number of nearest neighbouring protons), and the most likely candidate for this single proton is the multiplet at 2.84 ppm. This proton is a complex multiplet because it couples to all six of the protons of the two coincident methyl groups. This coupling system indicates that these two groups form an isopropyl group [(CH₃)₂CH–]. The one-proton multiplet at 2.84 ppm (peak **E**) and methyl group at 2.23 ppm (**F**) are slightly deshielded (higher ppm) with respect to the methyl groups at 1.23 ppm (**G**), indicating that they are attached to a group that causes electron withdrawal (possibly an aromatic ring, which is inferred by the presence of the aromatic protons).

Expansion of the aromatic region 6.6–7.1 ppm (Fig. 8.8) shows the coupling pattern of the aromatic ring. Inspection of this area allows measurement of coupling constants, referred to as *J* values. Taking peak **A**, which is a doublet (two lines), as an example, this is done by subtracting the lower ppm value for this peak from the higher ppm value and multiplying the difference by the field strength at which this experiment was measured (400 MHz in this case). This gives: (7.066 – 7.046 ppm) × 400 = 8 Hz.

The size of this coupling constant indicates that peak A is coupled to another proton that is *ortho* to itself (*ortho*-coupling constants are of the order of 6–9 Hz). Peak **B** is a double doublet (and has four lines) with two couplings (8 and 1.6 Hz), indicating that this is the proton that is *ortho* to peak **A** (it has the same coupling constant of 8 Hz) and the smaller coupling constant (1.6 Hz) is indicative of a *meta* coupling to another proton (*meta*-coupling constants are typically 1–2 Hz). Peak **C** at 6.67 ppm is a doublet (1.6 Hz) that has the same coupling constant as one of those for peak **B**, indicating that this is the proton that is *meta* to **B**. This part of the spectrum therefore tells us that we have an aromatic ring with three protons attached to it in the 1, 2 and 4 positions (see Fig. 8.7).

Taking all of the fragments from the ¹H spectrum into consideration, there are three aromatic protons, a broad exchangeable peak, a multiplet, a methyl singlet and a six-proton doublet corresponding to two coincident methyl groups. This total of 14 protons is identical to the number found in the molecular formula using MS.

¹³C NMR Spectroscopy

The proton spectrum has revealed much about the number of protons present and their chemical environments, i.e. whether they are shielded or deshielded by electron-donating or electron-withdrawing groups, respectively. The next step is the acquisition of a ¹³C NMR spectrum, which will give further information regarding the environment of the different groups and the number of carbons present. Two ¹³C NMR spectra of compound X are shown in Fig. 8.9.

The top spectrum is the **broadband decoupled** spectrum that shows all of the carbons present; the carbons appear as singlets due to proton decoupling. The top spectrum of compound X was recorded in CDCl₃, which occurs as three lines at 77.0 ppm. There are only nine carbons evident, which might be confusing as we know from the mass spectrum that compound X should contain 10 carbons. However, as the ¹H spectrum has two coincident methyl groups, it is possible that there are two carbons associated with the peak at 24 ppm. If both methyl groups were in the same environment (as they are in an isopropyl group), then they would occur at the same position in the spectrum. As with the proton spectrum, the carbon signals occur over a large range, which is again determined by whether the carbons are deshielded (high ppm value) or shielded (low ppm value). The lower ¹³C spectrum has been produced by a special experiment called **DEPT-135**, which lacks the solvents' signals, but, more importantly, it only shows carbons that have protons attached to them (CH, CH₂ and CH₃). As compound X does not have any CH₂ groups (there are no groups in the ¹H spectrum that integrate for two protons), only CH and CH₃ carbons are shown. This allows quaternary carbons (carbons with no protons attached) to be identified, and there are three additional aromatic quaternaries in the top spectrum, at 153.6, 148.5 and 120.8 ppm. The range for aromatic carbons is 110–160 ppm. The carbon at 153.6 is highly deshielded and it is possible that this carbon is attached to an oxygen atom (from the OH group in compound X). The three peaks at 130.8, 118.8 and 113.0 are all carbons bearing one proton (CH or methine carbons); these correspond to proton peaks **A**, **B** and **C** in the ¹H spectrum (see Fig. 8.7). The remaining peaks at 33.7, 24.0 and 15.3 are carbons associated

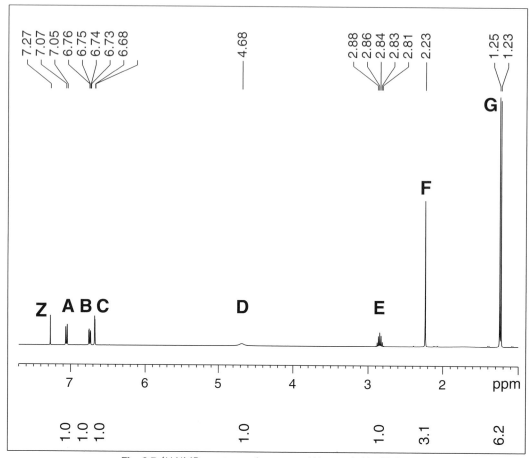

Fig. 8.7 ^{1}H NMR spectrum of compound X recorded in CDCl$_3$.

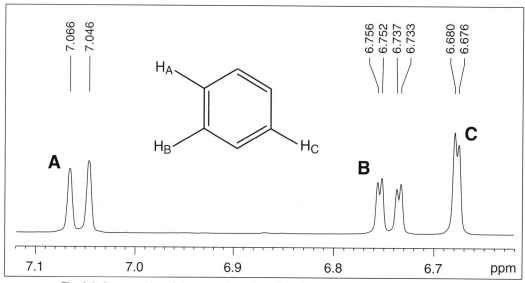

Fig. 8.8 An expansion of the aromatic region of the ^{1}H NMR spectrum of compound X.

with the multiplet (peak **E**), two coincident methyl groups (peak **G**) and a methyl singlet (peak **F**).

Homonuclear Correlation Spectroscopy

COrrelation SpectroscopY (COSY) reveals couplings between protons that are close (two, three or four bonds distant from each other). It is referred to as a **homonuclear** (same nuclei, both of which are ^{1}H) two-dimensional technique because the data are displayed in a

matrix format with two one-dimensional experiments (^{1}H spectra) displayed on the x- and y-axes (Fig. 8.10). A diagonal series of peaks correspond to the ^{1}H spectrum signals. Peaks that are away from the diagonal (referred to as **cross-peaks**) indicate coupling between signals.

Fig. 8.10 shows a cross-peak between the signal at 1.23 ppm (coincident methyl groups, **G**) and the multiplet signal at 2.84 ppm (group **E**), confirming that they are coupled to each other (implied

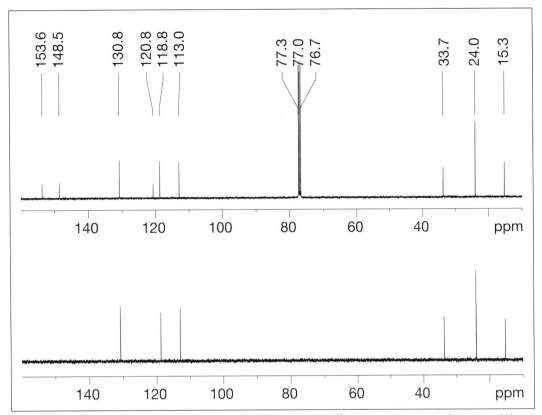

Fig. 8.9 Broadband decoupled ^{13}C spectrum *(top)* and DEPT-135 ^{13}C spectrum *(bottom)* of compound X.

by the couplings in the ^{1}H spectrum) and that together **E** and **G** are an isopropyl group. Additionally, group **F** (a methyl singlet at 2.23 ppm) shows a coupling to proton **A**, indicating that the methyl group is *ortho* to this proton (see Fig. 8.10).

Expansion of the aromatic region (Fig. 8.11) provides further support for the coupling pattern suggested by the ^{1}H spectrum. H_A has an *ortho* coupling to H_B and, in addition to coupling to H_A, H_B has a *meta* coupling to H_C and appears as a double doublet (four lines). This coupling pattern is indicative of a 1,2,4-protonated aromatic ring and confirms the data from the ^{1}H spectrum.

The related technique of **Nuclear Overhauser Effect SpectroscopY** (NOESY) shows through-space correlations and through-bond coupling between protons. Once the through-bond correlations are determined by a COSY spectrum, the through-space correlations can be seen. This allows the measurement of how close one proton is to another, which is very useful in assigning the stereochemistry of a compound.

Heteronuclear Correlation Spectroscopy

Homonuclear spectra, such as COSY, detect only one type of nucleus (^{1}H), but it is also possible to detect the interactions between two different nuclei, such as ^{1}H and ^{13}C. This is known as **heteronuclear correlation spectroscopy**, and includes **Heteronuclear Single Quantum Coherence** (HSQC) and **Heteronuclear MultiBond Coherence** (HMBC).

HSQC shows which protons are attached to which carbons. Fig. 8.12 shows an HSQC spectrum for compound X from which clear correlations can be seen for protons **A–C** and **E–G** with the carbons to which they are attached. Proton **D** is attached to oxygen (a hydroxyl group), so there is no carbon to correlate to (and therefore no signal). The aromatic protons all correlate to carbons at higher ppm; the aliphatic protons correlate to lower ppm carbons.

HMBC shows correlations between protons and the carbon atoms that are two and three bonds distant; these couplings are referred to as ^2J and ^3J, respectively. The experiment is set to show correlations that occur where the coupling constant between protons and carbons is of the order of 7 Hz. Two-bond correlations are not always present in the spectrum as the coupling constant for ^2J correlations may be less or greater than 7 Hz. Fig. 8.13 shows the HMBC spectrum for compound X. HMBC spectra allow partial structure fragments to be identified, which may enable the full elucidation of the structure of a compound. The correlations for each proton group of compound X are shown schematically in Fig. 8.14 and described below.

The HSQC spectrum has shown which protons are attached to which carbons, and the HMBC spectrum allows the final structure of compound X to be pieced together. For peak **A** (1 H aromatic doublet proton at 7.05 ppm) there are three correlations: one to the carbon associated with peak **F** and two to quaternary carbons.

Peak **B** (1 H aromatic double doublet proton at 6.74 ppm) correlates to the carbon to which peak **E** is attached; this fixes the isopropyl group next to peak **B** on the aromatic ring (peak **E** is part of the isopropyl system with peak **G**). Further correlations for peak **B** include couplings to carbons that are directly attached to peak **C** and to a quaternary carbon.

Peak **C** (1 H aromatic doublet proton at 6.68 ppm) also couples to the carbon bearing the proton associated with peak **E**; this confirms the position of the isopropyl side chain between protons **B** and **C**. Proton **C** also couples to the same quaternary carbon as **B** and to the carbon attached to proton **B**. There is also a small coupling to the most downfield carbon at 153.6 ppm.

Peak **D** (hydroxyl group, 4.68 ppm) is broad, and long-range correlations to carbons are absent. Peak **E** (1 H multiplet proton at 2.84 ppm) shows correlations to the carbons attached to peak **G** (these are

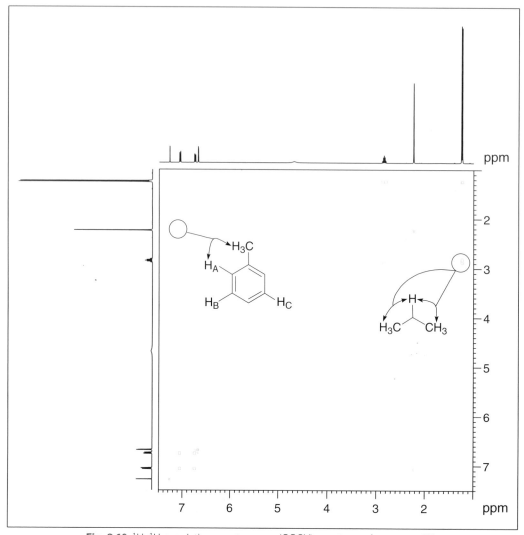

Fig. 8.10 ¹H–¹H correlation spectroscopy (COSY) spectrum of compound X.

the coincident methyl groups), to both carbons attached to peaks **B** and **C** and to a quaternary carbon, which is the carbon to which the isopropyl group is directly attached.

For peak **F** (3 H singlet protons at 2.23 ppm) there are two correlations that appear equidistant at 15.3 ppm in the carbon domain and are an artefact of the HMBC spectrum (they are in fact the unsuppressed direct correlation between the protons of peak **F** and the carbon to which they are directly attached; compare with the HSQC spectrum in Fig. 8.12). There are three couplings for peak **F**: to the carbon attached to proton A, and to two quaternary carbons, one of which is the most downfield carbon (153.6 ppm).

Finally, peak **G** (6 H doublet at 1.23 ppm) shows a correlation to the neighbouring methyl carbon of the isopropyl group (and an unsuppressed one-bond signal equidistant to the peak **G** signal), a correlation to the carbon directly attached to peak **E** and to an aromatic quaternary carbon.

Fig. 8.14 shows all correlations for each peak. The position of the hydroxyl group has yet to be assigned, but, as there is only one position available on the aromatic ring, the hydroxyl must be placed *ortho* to the methyl group. This is supported by the fact that the carbon to which this hydroxyl group is attached is the most downfield aromatic quaternary carbon (153.6 ppm), and heteroatoms such as oxygen are known to deshield carbon nuclei (compare the ppm value

of this quaternary carbon with other quaternary aromatic carbons in compound X).

A database search indicates that compound X is **carvacrol** (see Fig. 8.14), which is a common component of volatile oils, especially those from plants in the mint family (Lamiaceae).

X-ray Structural Analysis

Carvacrol is a simple example, but the same techniques are also widely used for complex natural products such as cardiac glycosides and polyketides. However, the most comprehensive way to determine the three-dimensional structure of a molecule is to use x-ray structural analysis. This technique requires the compound to be in the form of a crystal, as pure as possible, which is then placed in the path of an x-ray source. The atoms of the crystal diffract the x-rays in a pattern that is characteristic of the arrangement and type of atoms present. The pattern can then be interpreted by computer programs to give a three-dimensional structure of the compound. Unfortunately, natural products do not always form crystals (for example, carvacrol is an oil); moreover, the yield of compounds by some organisms may be small and can make the production of crystals challenging. However, x-ray structural analysis can provide information on the stereochemistry of a molecule and the structure can be solved in a matter of hours.

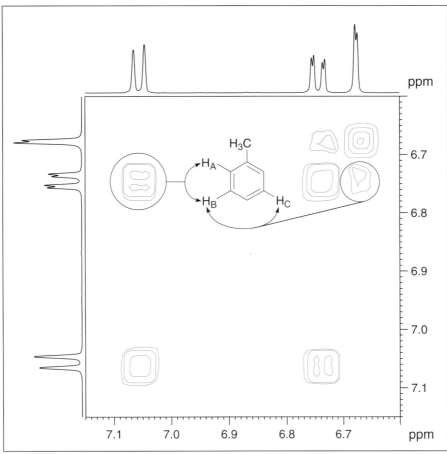

Fig. 8.11 An expansion of the aromatic region of the correlation spectroscopy (COSY) spectrum of compound X.

APPROACHES TO DRUG LEAD DISCOVERY

Companies involved in natural product drug discovery use a highly organised approach to reduce the time taken to find a biologically active compound and put it into drug development. All researchers use similar approaches, albeit on different scales.

Choice of Biological Target

The first decision is to choose a target relevant to the disease state for which a drug is sought. In the pharmaceutical industry, this decision is necessarily economic, and results in a focus on conditions in (richer) Western countries with enormous potential markets and an emphasis on anticancer or antiarthritis drugs. Drugs for tropical and diseases of poverty, such as malaria, amoebic dysentery and tuberculosis, for which there is an enormous need, are often neglected, or only investigated by government or charitable organisations.

Assay Selection and Development

Clearly, assays should show a good correlation with, and reflect, the disease state under investigation, and both cellular and molecular mechanisms are investigated using several assays. Specificity for the target, ease and speed of performing the assay, sensitivity to common natural products and the ability to perform assays in an automated system—large numbers of samples are involved—determine selection of a bioassay.

Assay arrays form the first part of specific drug discovery programmes, such as for **antiinfectives** (assays for antibacterial, antifungal and antiviral agents), **immune-inflammation** (assays for arthritis, eczema, asthma, psoriasis, etc.) and **anticancer agents** (assays for cytotoxic agents and resistance reversing agents).

Dereplication

After a screening process (the assay), a series of fractions may be active, so it is important to establish that no replicates (i.e. extracts with the same chemistry) are present, or that no compounds are present that are already known to be active in the assay. This is done by the process of **dereplication**, to avoid known compounds or common molecules that interfere with assays (e.g. tannins which may bind in a nonspecific manner to many proteins, including enzymes). The main reason for dereplication is cost in time and money; it can take weeks, sometimes months, to isolate active components, so it is important that they are novel and/or are not already known to be active in an assay. It is possible to avoid some known compounds by literature searching relevant databases, usually more than one, as none is perfect. Most dereplication methods conduct chemical analysis on extracts before the bioassay, particularly automated **HPLC-MS**. which can provide information on retention times of peaks, their UV spectra (with photo-diode array) and molecular weight (and fragment) information, which is acquired as peaks elute from the UV detector into the mass spectrometer. These data can be built into a spectral library to allow searching of peaks with characteristic retention times, UV and mass spectra with those already acquired.

For compounds that are lipophilic and volatile, a combination of **gas chromatography and mass spectrometry (GC-MS)** can be used to separate components to give retention times and eluting peaks that

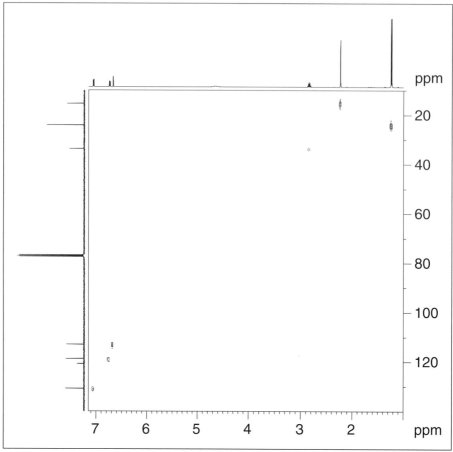

Fig. 8.12 Heteronuclear single quantum coherence (HSQC) spectrum for compound X showing correlations between protons and the carbon atoms to which they are directly attached.

can be fed into a mass spectrometer to acquire characteristic molecular weight and fragmentation information. This technique can be applied to polar water-soluble components such as the calystegines and other polyhydroxylated alkaloids if they are first derivatised with a suitable agent (e.g. trimethylsilyl chloride) to increase their volatility, but is now rarely used.

Positively or negatively charged compounds may be further analysed using **capillary electrophoresis–mass spectrometry (CE–MS)**. Extracts are separated in a capillary filled with buffer, which has a potential difference (voltage) applied. Compounds of varying charge can be separated and, when coupled to a UV detector and mass spectrometer, easily identified.

Natural Product Libraries

Traditionally, drug-lead discovery has used HTS of extracts in large numbers to identify active extracts, which are then produced in large amounts to enable compound isolation and further bioassay. This process is highly productive, and there are many examples of drugs that have been discovered in this way. It is, however, expensive, time-consuming and may not lead to a drug candidate if it turns out to be a known compound with an uninteresting broad spectrum of activities.

Combinatorial chemistry 'libraries' contain large numbers of sample compounds that are available for screening for bioactivity. Natural product chemistry has taken a similar approach, and several companies and organisations now compile natural product libraries (NPLs). NPLs are banks of microtitre plates containing pure natural products in individual wells at a known concentration and, in effect, the chemistry has already been done.

There are several benefits to this procedure over conventional HTS and synthetic libraries:

- The isolation chemistry in HTS has always been the bottleneck. The process is faster in NPL generation, which enables decisions about active compounds to be made rapidly.
- Compounds in the NPL have a defined concentration and so the potency of the compound in the assay can be determined immediately; this is not true with extract screening. 'Active' extracts may contain high concentrations of a component with weak activity or, even worse, a weakly active extract may contain a low concentration of a very potent compound, which may therefore be overlooked.
- Screening a pure compound gives a more accurate assay response, as single components have a cleaner interaction with the biological target and there are no interfering components which may mask the presence of an active compound in the extract.
- The dereplication process is more successful with pure compounds and a large amount of data can be acquired.
- Chemical characterisation of the active compound before screening gives useful information on structure–activity relationships with other screened compounds.
- The cost is less than HTS as the time for discovery of a natural lead is reduced.

The Culture and Fermentation of Fungi and Other Microbes

Many fungi and bacteria do not produce natural products when fermented in isolation, and require an external stimulus from another organism, such as other microbes or molecules secreted into their environment by another organism. Additionally, only 5% of microbes

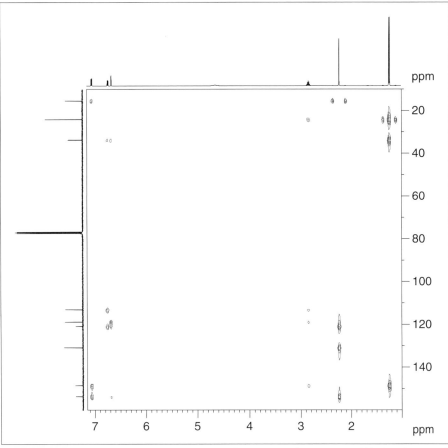

Fig. 8.13 Heteronuclear multibond coherence (HMBC) spectrum for compound X showing correlations between protons that are two and three bonds distant from carbon atoms.

may be culturable and fermentable and there is, therefore, great potential to discover new therapeutic agents if new ways—possibly genetic—are found to tap into their chemical diversity.

The procedure of combinatorial biosynthesis is one in which DNA is taken from uncultivable organisms, or from soil, and used to build a library of characterised DNA fragments. It is then possible to insert this DNA into a host, such as *Escherichia coli* or a yeast, which is readily fermentable, based on the assumption that the host may use this DNA in the biosynthesis of new molecules. The host is then fermented and screened for bioactivity; this process may also be used to generate compounds for NPLs. Unfortunately, the host may not utilise the foreign DNA, or it is possible that the DNA inserted may not code for the proteins that make new natural products.

The Importance of Biodiversity and Its Associated Ethics

A high range of biological diversity gives rise to a high degree of chemical diversity (i.e. a wide array of structurally unrelated molecules). This applies not only to plants, but also to fungi, filamentous bacteria, corals, sea animals and amphibia. The tropics hold a vast repository of numbers of such species, and therefore enormous potential to discover new bioactive entities, which is now being exploited. In Costa Rica, for example, the Instituto Nacional de Biodiversidad (INBio) has been conducting a national inventory of plants, insects, microbes and animals, and has so far assessed almost 500,000 species. This incredible genetic resource could generate many new chemical structures to be assessed for biological activity. Individual species are adept at producing not only different classes of natural products (e.g. flavonoids and monoterpenes simultaneously), but also analogues in the same natural product class (Fig. 8.15).

The **Convention on Biological Diversity** is a treaty between 182 countries that recognises the authority that countries/states have over their genetic resources (see also Chapter 5), whether plant, microbial or animal. It is not possible to acquire biological specimens from an area without 'prior informed consent' on 'mutually agreed terms' and, should any commercial benefit arise from collection of organisms (e.g. in the discovery of a new drug), then 'equitable sharing of benefits' should occur. This is an important concept for profit sharing and one that can be illustrated by the example of **prostratin** (Fig. 8.16) from *Homolanthus nutans* (G. Forst.) Guill. (Euphorbiaceae). The ethnobotanist Paul Cox, while working in Samoa, became intrigued by the local use of the inner bark of *H. nutans* to treat jaundice, a symptom of viral hepatitis. He collected samples and sent them for testing at the National Cancer Institute (NCI) for assessment of antiviral activity in anti-AIDS assays. The active component, **prostratin**, was isolated and its structure determined as a diterpene of the phorbol ester group. It has been shown to flush latent HIV from infected cells, but research is slow due to low yields of the natural compound. Whilst prostratin is still in development, the authorities of the village from which the discovery originated have negotiated an agreement, signed by the prime minister of Samoa, whereby 20% of any commercial profits generated from prostratin will go back to Samoa. Revenues will go back to the village and to the families of the healers who provided the initial information on the traditional use of *H. nutans*. This example highlights the principles that it is not only important that financial recompense is made to the originators, but also that this traditional knowledge, and the maintenance of biodiversity, have immense value that must be preserved.

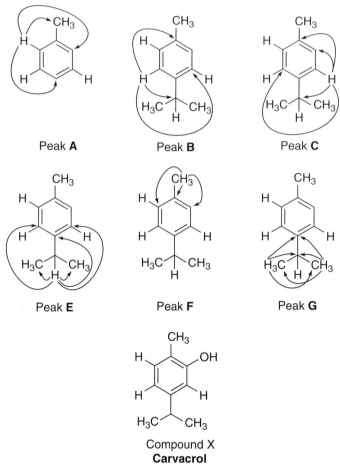

Peak **A**   Peak **B**   Peak **C**

Peak **E**   Peak **F**   Peak **G**

Compound X
Carvacrol

Fig. 8.14 Heteronuclear single quantum coherence (HSQC) and heteronuclear multibond coherence (HMBC) correlations confirming the structure and identity of compound X.

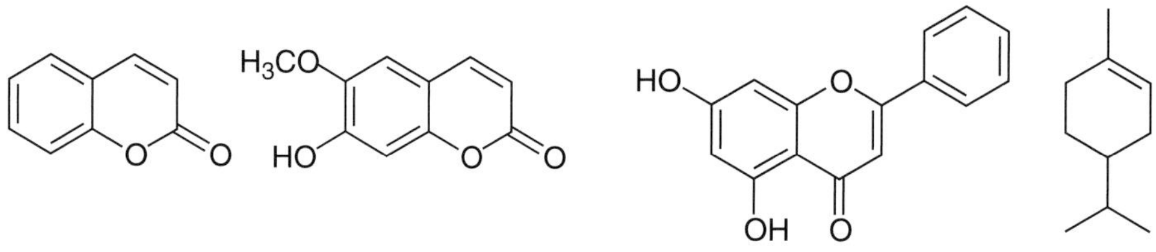

Fig. 8.15 Analogues *(left)* and different classes *(right)*.

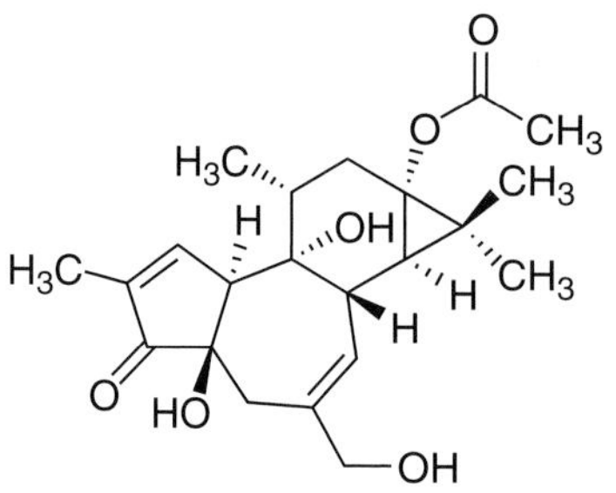

Fig. 8.16 Prostratin.

FURTHER READING

Balick, M.J., Cox, P.A., 2020. Plants, People and Culture: The Science of Ethnobotany, second ed. Garland Science, New York.

Brown, P.D., Lawrence, A.L., 2017. The importance of asking 'how and why' in natural product structure elucidation. Nat. Prod. Rep. 34 (10), 1193–1202.

Crews, P., Rodriguez, J., Jaspars, M., 2009. Organic Structure Analysis, second ed. Oxford University Press, Oxford.

Hanson, J.R., 2017. A hundred years in the structure elucidation of natural products. Sci. Prog. 100 (1), 63–79.

Hostettmann, K., Hostettmann, M., Marston, A., 2014. Preparative Chromatography Techniques: Applications in Natural Product Isolation. Springer, Berlin.

Klika, K.D., 2020. A critique of formulaic description of in natural product structure elucidations. Chem. Biodiversity. 17 (1), e1900607.

Sarker, S.D., Nahar, L. (Eds.), 2012. Natural Products Isolation: Methods and Protocols, third ed. Springer, New Jersey.

Fleming, I., Williams, D.H., 2019. Spectroscopic Methods in Organic Chemistry, seventh ed. Springer, Cham, Switzerland.

9

Natural Products With Anticancer and Chemopreventive Effects

Anticancer agents from natural products, including from plants, cover a spectrum of activity ranging from preventing carcinogenesis and inhibiting tumour development (chemoprevention) and invasion to those that treat cancer once it has developed. The former are termed chemoprevention agents, and the latter are anticancer or cytotoxic drugs. The mechanisms of cancer initiation and progression are diverse, interconnected and apply to all aspects of carcinogenesis. In contrast, chemopreventive agents may have properties that affect both healthy and cancer cells, the anticancer drugs target cancer cells specifically, although their effects on normal cells confer substantial toxicity and adverse effects.

Considering the processes and pathways involved in cancer evolution and progression is necessary to understand how these different phytochemicals work. Cancer chemotherapy typically uses a multitarget approach, recognising the value of using drugs with complementary mechanisms to increase efficacy of the treatment and reducing resistance to a particular drug. Therapeutic options can encompass chemopreventive approaches, such as inhibiting pathways and enzymes involved in cancer progression. Many natural compounds also inhibit the metabolic enzymes involved in activation of carcinogens, and those that are involved in drug resistance.

CANCER CHEMOPREVENTION

Common tumours in adults, such as cancers of the breast, cervix, colon, lung, ovary and prostate, develop over many years via the accumulation of mutations in the cancer-cell genome and changes in the cellular environment, including the immune system. This development can be divided into the initiation, promotion, conversion, progression, invasion and metastasis stages. This generally slow evolution from normal through increasingly aggressive neoplastic stages presents an opportunity to intervene with chemopreventive agents.

Cancer chemoprevention includes the inhibition, suppression or reversal of the initiation of carcinogenesis or the progression of neoplastic cells to invasive cancer. The molecular mechanisms that drive this are not necessarily unique to one organ site, and chemopreventive agents usually work by more than one mechanism.

An overview of the progression to invasive cancer is shown in Fig. 9.1 with the site(s) of action of some chemopreventive phytochemicals. Many of these also protect against other inflammatory disorders (e.g. atherosclerosis, arthritis, diabetes): inflammatory responses contribute to these diseases, as well as to cancer progression in many ways, and the use of antiinflammatory drugs such as ibuprofen is correlated with a reduced incidence of oesophagus, stomach, colon and rectal cancer.

Antiinflammatory Targets

Tumour-associated macrophages and tumour-infiltrating lymphocytes produce a range of proinflammatory cytokines, in particular tumour necrosis factor (TNF), chemokines, including interleukins 1, 6, 8 (IL-1, IL-6, IL-8), growth factors, and signal transducers and activators of transcription (STATs), which can be targeted by phytochemicals. These inflammatory mediators promote cancer growth, invasion and metastasis by inducing DNA damage by reactive oxygen species/reactive nitrogen species (ROS/RNS) and inhibiting DNA repair mechanisms, inactivating tumour suppressor genes (mainly p53), induction of vascular permeability by activation of matrix metalloproteinases, modulation of cell adhesion and stimulating of angiogenesis by induction of growth factors such as vascular endothelial growth factor (VEGF), basic fibroblast growth factor (bFGF) and IL-8.

The number of potential targets for chemoprevention is vast; they are interdependent and may differ according to cancer type. Common mechanisms for reducing inflammation-induced carcinogenesis include cyclooxygenase-2 (COX-2) inhibition and modulation of the transcription factor nuclear factor kappa B (NF-κB), which is involved in the inflammatory response to many stimuli, including bacterial endotoxins, free radicals and ultraviolet irradiation. Intracellular signalling cascades are triggered, which act independently, or in combination to regulate the expression of target genes. These transcription factors mediate cellular transformation and tumour promotion by transactivating genes that have inflammatory, immunoregulatory, antiapoptotic and cell cycle regulatory functions. Although outside the scope of this introduction, these complex cascades offer opportunities for targeting steps that may reduce carcinogenesis, and details can be found in Further Reading.

Nuclear Factor Kappa B

This transcription factor regulates the expression of genes, including COX-2, matrix metalloproteinase 9 (MMP-9) and inducible nitric oxide synthase (iNOS). Carcinogens, proinflammatory agents and tumour promoters have been shown to activate NF-κB. NF-κB binds to the inhibitory κB kinase, forming a complex that is activated during inflammation, and if this is prevented, translocation of NF-κB to the nucleus is inhibited. This presents a target for antiinflammatory drugs and many phytochemicals with identified effects on NF-κB: some are shown in Table 9.1. However, after initial optimism, the view on NF-κB as a potential therapeutic target is much more sceptical since this transcription factor interferes with many cellular processes, pointing to a lack of *specific* and therapeutically relevant anticancer effects.

It is notable that many of the compounds listed in Fig. 9.1 are used for therapeutic purposes other than cancer, reflecting their actions on protein synthesis and basic cell metabolism; these compounds include andrographolide, berberine, emodin and isothiocyanates, which have significant antimicrobial properties and are discussed in Chapter 10 (Antimicrobial Natural Products).

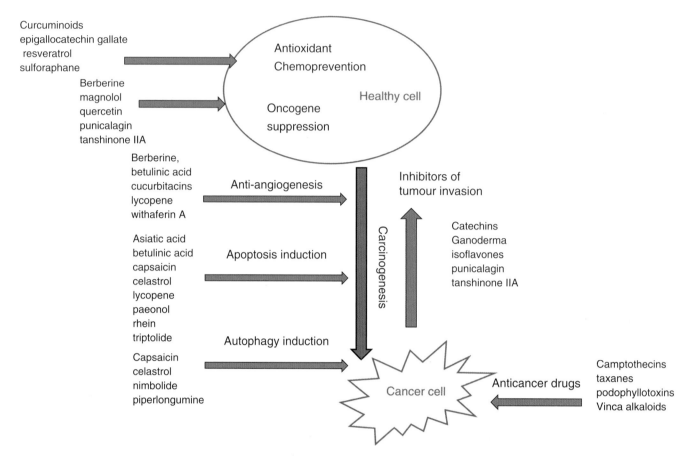

Fig. 9.1 Cancer progression and phytochemical interactions.

Cyclooxygenase-2

COX exists in two isoforms: COX-1 and COX-2. COX-1 is normally present in tissues, while COX-2 is expressed in response to inflammatory stimuli, such as bacterial endotoxins and cytokines. It is closely associated with mechanisms of carcinogenesis: COX-2 overexpression is correlated with increased cell proliferation and reduced apoptosis, and COX-2 may promote carcinogenesis at most stages of progression (shown in Fig. 9.1) and by several pathways (Fig. 9.2).

COX-2 inhibition is common among plant compounds, with various stages of the pathway targeted by phytochemicals. Some of these are shown in Table 9.2. Compounds known to interact with the NF-κB pathway (see Table 9.1) also affect COX-2 expression. Many of these phytochemicals have demonstrated health benefits in addition to their chemopreventive effects and are described in Part B and Chapter 6 as important plant secondary metabolites. If so, their structures in other chapters are marked in Table 9.2.

Dietary Chemopreventive Compounds

As shown in Box 9.1, these are widely found in fruits, vegetables, herbs and spices. Many are included in Fig. 9.1 and Tables 9.1 and 9.2.

Evidence for chemopreventive effects is largely epidemiological and mechanism-based: clinical trials in this area are very difficult to carry out, but there is no doubt of the public health benefits of plant-based compounds in the prevention and treatment of cancer and other degenerative and inflammatory conditions.

Chemoprevention targets the same pathways as do anticancer drugs, as shown in Fig. 9.1 at similar phases of the cell cycle (Fig. 9.3), although chemopreventive agents must be nontoxic as they are taken over long periods and often in high doses. Anticancer drugs, however, are expected to be toxic: they can paradoxically promote some cancers,

reduce the activity of the immune system and have many unpleasant and distressing side effects. They are, therefore, only used for treatment over as short a time as possible.

The phases of the cell cycle that anticancer compounds target correspond to the cellular processes occurring at each: i.e. interfering with microtubule assembly and spindle formation at the M (mitosis) phase, with the inhibition of DNA synthesis at the S phase, and so on, as shown in Fig. 9.4. The sites of action of some natural-product derived anticancer drugs on DNA and protein synthesis are shown in Fig. 9.5.

ANTICANCER NATURAL PRODUCT DRUGS

Natural products have made an enormous impact on the discovery of compounds that kill cancer cells; in fact, possibly 60% of all cancer drugs that are used clinically are either natural products or owe their origin to a natural source. The National Cancer Institute (NCI), in particular, the M. E. Wall and M. Wani groups, were involved in many discoveries in the characterisation of natural cytotoxic products, screening and evaluating them in preclinical and clinical studies. The story of the NCI and later initiatives is fascinating but outside our scope and is documented in reviews in Further Reading.

Natural anticancer drugs from microbial sources (antibiotics) are well known, and marine organisms (molluscs, sea squirts) show great future potential. Unfortunately, there is a tendency to use incorrect terminology when reporting on the activities of natural drugs in cancer research, and as a result, we have hundreds of scientific papers on false 'anticancer' natural products. Where a compound is active at the in vitro level only, the correct adjective is **cytotoxic** or **antiproliferative,** and only where it is also active in vivo animal models can it be described as having **antitumour** properties. Only when the

TABLE 9.1 Phytochemicals Interacting With the NF-κB Pathway

Compound	Effects on the NF-κB Pathway
Andrographolide	Forms a covalent adduct with p50, blocks the binding of NF-κB to nuclear proteins
Baicalein	Blocks IκB-α degradation
Berberine	Inhibits FAK, IKK, NF-κB, MMP-2, MMP-9
Capsaicin	Inhibits NF-κB activation
Curcumin	Blocks IκB-α degradation, downregulates NF-κB, inhibits IκB kinase, COX-1 and -2, suppresses COX-2 and iNOS gene expression
Emodin	Inhibits NF-κB activation
(–)-Epigallocatechin-3-gallate	Blocks IκB-α degradation and induction of nitric oxide synthase by downregulating NF-κB, inhibits TNF-α and IκB kinase
Gingerols	Block IκB-α degradation
Grapeseed procyanidins	Decrease nuclear translocation of NF-κB, inhibit NO and PGE2 production, suppress iNOS expression
Guggulsterone	Suppresses NF-κB DNA-binding activity
Isothiocyanates	Decrease nuclear translocation of NF-κB and inhibit activation
Lupeol	Inhibits the PI3K-AKT pathway
Lycopene	Directly suppresses p65 nuclear translocation
Parthenolide	Inhibits IκB kinase and activation of the NF-κB pathway, thus inhibiting interleukin 1- and TNF-α
Resveratrol	Suppresses reactive oxygen species, blocks degradation of IκB-α, inhibits nuclear translocation of NF-κB

COX, Cyclooxygenase; *FAK,* focal adhesion kinase; *IKK,* I kappa B kinase; *iNOS,* inducible nitric oxide synthase; *IκB,* nuclear factor of kappa light polypeptide gene enhancer in B-cells inhibitor; *MMP,* matrix metalloproteinase; *NF-κB,* nuclear factor kappa B; *NO,* nitric oxide; *PGE2,* prostaglandin E2; *PI3K-AKT,* phosphoinositide-3-kinase-protein kinase B; *TNF,* tumour necrosis factor.

drug proves to be of therapeutic value in clinical trials (i.e. involving human patients) can we talk about an **anticancer** effect.

An overview of the progression from cell mutation to tumour is shown in Fig. 9.4. Signalling pathways control cell growth and division, cell death, and cell motility, and when disturbed, drive cancer progression. Mutations that convert proto-oncogenes to oncogenes cause activation of these signalling pathways.

A full review of antitumour agents is beyond the scope of this text, but three primary sources of anticancer agents (plants, marine organisms and microbes) will be outlined, with selected examples.

Plant Anticancer Agents

The track record of plant anticancer agents is excellent, and since about 1960, several major chemotherapy drugs have been developed, such as **alkaloids** from *Vinca* species (**vinblastine, vincristine, vindesine** and **vinorelbine**), the **camptothecin**-derived cytotoxics (**topotecan** and **irinotecan**), **homoharringtonine** from *Cephalotaxus* shrubs and trees, **lignans** based on the **podophyllotoxins** (**etoposide** and **teniposide**), **terpenes** such as **betulin**, the **taxanes** (**paclitaxel** and **taxotere**) and **ingenol mebutate** and others.

Alkaloids

Alkaloids are highly bioactive natural products due to the presence of the amine functional group. Many alkaloids are endowed with an exquisite selectivity for their targets, allowing them to exert their effects at very low concentrations. They are easily extracted and purified with simple partition and precipitation methods, so they were isolated in high purity early in the history of drug discovery.

Camptothecin (Fig. 9.6) is found in *Camptotheca acuminata* Decne. (Nyssaceae). It has a unique structure, possessing an α-hydroxylactone and being a highly unsaturated alkaloid (nitrogen-containing) natural product of the quinoline alkaloid group. Camptothecin was shown to be extremely active in life-prolongation assays in mice, but clinical trials in the United States did not show good responses, and there were toxic side effects. Larger clinical trials in China involving 1000 patients gave better results against head, neck, gastric, intestinal and bladder carcinomas. This may be because the US patients had already been treated with other cytotoxic drugs, and their tumours may have become multidrug-resistant. Wall and Wani continued to isolate and evaluate *Camptotheca* metabolites and found that **10-hydroxycamptothecin** (see Fig. 9.6) was more active than camptothecin. Interest in this compound and its analogues was initially low until it was discovered many years later, in 1985, that camptothecin works by inhibiting topoisomerase I and inhibits tumour growth. The derivatives **irinotecan** and **topotecan** (Fig. 9.7) are less toxic than camptothecin and have much greater water solubility than camptothecin.

Vinca Alkaloids

Catharanthus roseus (L.) G. Don (Apocynaceae), the Madagascar periwinkle (syn. *Vinca rosea* L.), has been widely cultivated for hundreds of years and can now be found growing wild in most countries, including the UK. The natural wild plants are pale pink with a purple eye in the centre, but many colours have been developed by horticulturalists, ranging from white to pink and purple. The plant has had a long history of treating a wide assortment of diseases and was used as a folk remedy for diabetes in Europe for centuries. In China, the plant has been used for its astringent and diuretic properties and as a cough remedy. In the Caribbean, it is used to treat eye infections and diabetes. Historically, the periwinkle has had a reputation as a magical plant: Europeans thought it could ward off evil spirits, and the French referred to it as 'the violet of the sorcerers'. Jamaicans reportedly used a tea from *C. roseus* to treat diabetes.

Over 150 alkaloids have been characterised, mainly **indole alkaloids**, including **dimeric** or **bis-indole alkaloids**.

The discovery of the vinca alkaloids from the Madagascan periwinkle is a classic example of serendipitous drug discovery in that, although the plant had a reputation for being useful in the treatment of diabetes, routine screening found that extracts inhibited the growth of certain types of cancer cells, and led to the discovery of **vincristine** and **vinblastine** (Fig. 9.8).

These dimeric indole alkaloids can be synthesised but are very costly to produce in this way, and the natural yield of the drugs in the plant is exceptionally low (0.0002% for vincristine), which makes them very expensive antitumour agents. They inhibit mitosis by binding to tubulin, thus preventing the cell from making the spindles it needs for cell division. Vinblastine is useful for treating Hodgkin disease, lymphomas, and advanced testicular and breast cancers. Vincristine treats acute leukaemia, Hodgkin disease and other lymphomas. Semisynthetic vinca alkaloids of note include **vindesine**, used to treat leukaemia and lung cancers, and **vinorelbine**, used for ovarian cancer. Vinorelbine has a wider range of antitumour activity than the other vinca alkaloids and is used, in combination with cisplatin, in treating patients with non-small-cell lung cancers.

Homoharringtonine

Homoharringtonine (= omacetaxine) is a naturally occurring alkaloid in *Cephalotaxus fortunei* Hook. (Taxaceae) and related species. Isolated in China, it is used as a mepesuccinate ester for treating chronic myeloid leukaemia (CML) in cases resistant to other therapies. The development of homoharringtonine is possibly the longest

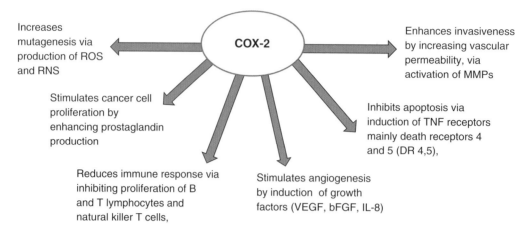

Fig. 9.2 Proinflammatory effects of cyclooxygenase-2 (COX-2) and its role in carcinogenesis. *bFGF*, Basic fibroblast growth factor; *IL-8*, interleukin-8; *MMPs*, matrix metalloproteinases; *RNS*, reactive nitrogen species; *ROS*, reactive oxygen species; *TNF*, tumour necrosis factor; *VEGF*, vascular endothelial growth factor.

TABLE 9.2   Phytochemicals Interacting With COX-2 Expression and Activity

Compound	Type	Effects on COX-2 Expression in Experimental Modes
Astaxanthin	Xanthophyll	Inhibits expression of COX-2 and NF-κB; inhibits COX-2 stimulation of apoptosis
β-Carotene	Carotene Fig. 6.43	Decreases expression of COX-2 but not COX-1; decreases ROS production via the peroxidase function of COX
Lutein	Xanthophyll	Free radical scavenger; decreases COX-2 and NF-κB expression
Lycopene	Carotene Fig. 6.43	Inhibits NF-κB and COX-2 expression; induces apoptosis and modulates cytokine expression
Curcumin	Curcuminoid Fig. 23.2	Downregulates COX-2 expression inhibits COX-1 and -2 activity; blocks nuclear translocation of NF-κB and inhibits DNA binding; prevents degradation of IκB
Chrysin	Flavonoid Fig. 10.4	Inhibits NF-IL-6 DNA binding activity
Quercetin	Flavonoid Fig. 6.22	Downregulates COX-1 and COX-2 expression; attenuates TNF-α-induced NF-κB activation
(–)-Epigallocatechin-3-gallate	Polyphenolic flavan-3-ol Fig. 10.5	Inhibits NF-κB DNA binding; decreases protein and mRNA expression levels of COX-2 and the inflammatory cytokines TNF-α, IFN-γ, IL-6, IL-12 and IL-18
Genistein	Isoflavone Fig. 24.1	Suppresses COX-2 expression; prevents IκB degradation via inhibition of IκB kinase; inhibits hepatocellular carcinoma cell migration
Ferulic acid	Polyphenolic phenylpropanoid	Inhibits COX-1 and COX-2; inhibits NF-κB activation and migration via IκBα degradation; reduces iNOS-2 gene expression and serum TNF-α and IL-6
α-Linolenic acid	Omega-3-fatty acid	Inhibits COX-2, inducing 15 prostaglandin dehydrogenase, leading to apoptosis
Resveratrol	Stilbene Fig. 6.22	Downregulates COX-2 expression through the inhibition of NF-κB DNA binding; inhibits COX-1 and -2 activity
Aurapten	Prenylated coumarin Fig. 6.15	Suppresses COX-2 expression; inhibits the production of PGE2
Osthole	O-Methylated coumarin	Inhibits TNF-α, NO and COX-2 expression through suppression of the NF-κB and MAPK signalling pathways
Sulforaphane	Isothiocyanate	Inhibits NF-κB DNA binding
Schisandrins	Lignan Fig. 26.3 and Chapter 26	Inhibition of IκB degradation; inhibition of LPS-induced phosphorylation of JNK and p38 MAPK

COX, Cyclooxygenase; *IL,* interleukin; *iNOS,* inducible nitric oxide synthase; *IκB,* nuclear factor of kappa light polypeptide gene enhancer in B-cells inhibitor; *JNK,* Jun N-terminal kinase; *LPS,* lipopolysaccharide; *NF-IL-6,* nuclear factor interleukin 6; *NF-κB,* nuclear factor kappa B; *NO,* nitric oxide; *p38 MAPK,* p38 mitogen-activated protein kinase; *PGE2,* prostaglandin E2; *ROS,* reactive oxygen species; *TNF,* tumour necrosis factor.

in the history of anticancer research due to several factors, including difficult production and unreliable source supply, the toxicity profile of the original dose schedules, and the initial success of other synthetic drugs in CML.

Cephalotaxus trees grow in humid valleys or forests in Japan, India and China. Crude extracts from Chinese *Cephalotaxus* trees showed promising antitumour activity in early screenings. Further research revealed that alkaloids from any part of the trees (bark, roots, leaves,

dried stems) had similar activity. One of the alkaloids, **cephalotaxine** (Fig. 9.9), was biologically inactive, indicating that the antitumour activity was due to one or more of the remaining alkaloids. After much effort, the structures of the remaining alkaloids were elucidated as the cephalotaxine esters **harringtonine, homoharringtonine, isoharringtonine** and **deoxyharringtonine** (see Fig. 9.9). Homoharringtonine emerged as the better overall drug lead, but further clinical studies were hampered by the large quantities of *Cephalotaxus* trees required to maintain a

- *Anthocyanins:* cyanidin, pelargonidin: in bilberry, blackberry and many other berries
- *Carotenoids:* lycopene, in tomatoes, many fruits and vegetables
- *Catechins:* epigallocatechin: in green tea, chocolate
- *Curcuminoids:* curcumin, from turmeric
- *Flavonoids:* quercetin, luteolin, in apples, onions, citrus fruits, parsley, celery
- *Glucosinolates, isothiocyanates:* sulforaphane in *Brassica* spp., broccoli, sprouts, mustards, watercress.
- *Hydroxycinnamic acids:* rosmarinic, caffeic, etc., in fruit and culinary herbs
- *Phenolic acids:* ellagic, gallic, in tea, berries, nuts
- *Stilbenoids:* resveratrol, in many herbs
- *Tannins:* condensed or hydrolysable polymers of polyphenols in wine, tea, pomegranate and berries
- *Triterpenes:* lupeol, in many fruits and vegetables including cucumber, figs, olives, peppers and strawberries

steady supply of the drug. These species are rare in China and cannot be grown easily. Although homoharringtonine is present in low concentrations, cephalotaxine is abundant in all parts of *Cephalotaxus* species, and methods of semisynthesis by addition of acyl moieties to the cephalotaxine ring were developed to ensure a sustainable supply of semisynthetic homoharringtonine, which is known as omacetaxine and is structurally identical to its natural counterpart.

Homoharringtonine and its analogues are inhibitors of protein synthesis, although direct effects at the DNA level cannot be ruled out. Interestingly, they do not interfere with protein synthesis when this has already started, and in vivo studies show the recovery of protein synthesis within 24 hours of injection. This implies that continuous drug exposure is required to achieve a maximal antitumour effect, with its associated adverse effects, which include cardiotoxicity and hyperglycaemia. To reduce patient exposure to homoharringtonine, combinations with other cytotoxic agents were investigated, and a significant synergistic effect was found with cytarabine. This combination showed a better therapeutic outcome in vivo, characterised by a dramatic increase in the cure rates (up to 40%) with fewer adverse effects. Furthermore, the reduced doses could be administered by subcutaneous injections, making self-administration by patients possible.

By the time homoharringtonine was ready for regulatory approval as an anticancer drug, a synthetic tyrosine kinase inhibitor (imatinib) took the clinical world by storm and temporarily outclassed all other drugs. It took the increased clinical experience to appreciate that homoharringtonine has a therapeutic edge in a subset of patients suffering CML and T315I mutations; the failure of several tyrosine kinase inhibitors to increase survival in these cases led to the approval of omacetaxine for CML in chronic or accelerated phases post-failure of two or more tyrosine kinase inhibitors.

Terpenes

Terpenes made their entry in the anticancer therapy arena later than other natural products due to difficulties in their isolation and characterisation. These properties are inherent to their chemistry: they do not precipitate or form crystals easily, and they have very low polarity making separation of the very complex mixtures of naturally occurring terpenes a challenge. Triterpene and phytosteroid structures mimic those of many physiologically relevant animal metabolites, such as hormones. This is less obvious for the diterpenes; however, after the discovery of the taxanes and ingenol esters, this class is becoming a promising source of therapeutic approaches for the future.

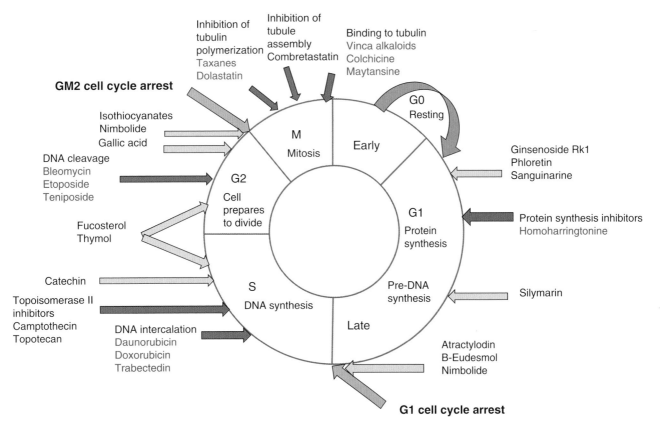

Fig. 9.3 Cell cycle phases and anticancer targets.

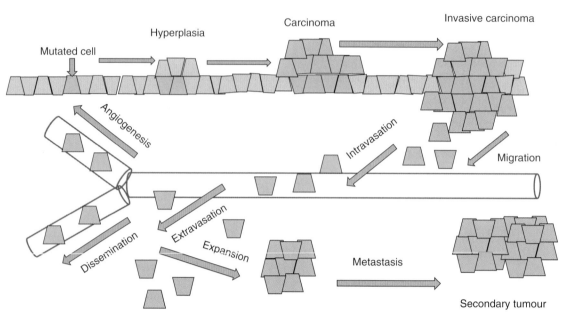

Fig. 9.4 Overview of cancer progression.

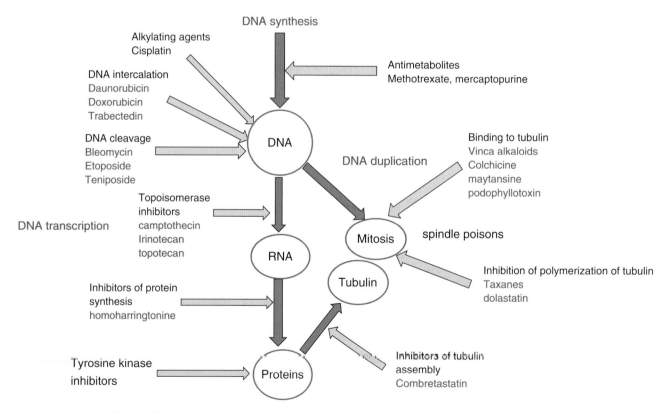

Fig. 9.5 Sites of action of natural-product derived anticancer drugs on DNA and protein synthesis.

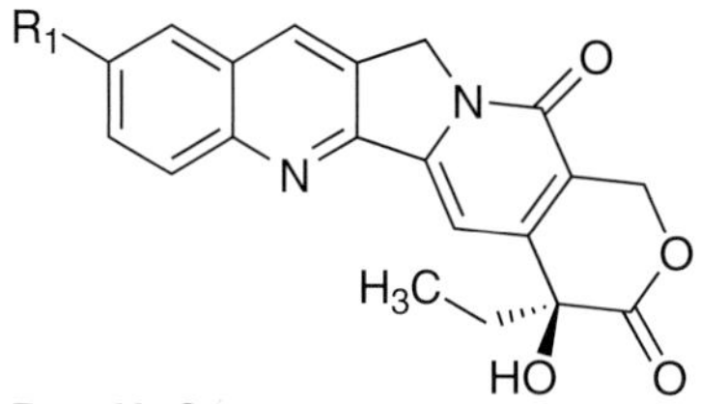

R₁ = H, **Camptothecin**
R₁ = OH, **10-Hydroxycamptothecin**

Fig. 9.6 Camptothecin and 10-hydroxycamptothecin.

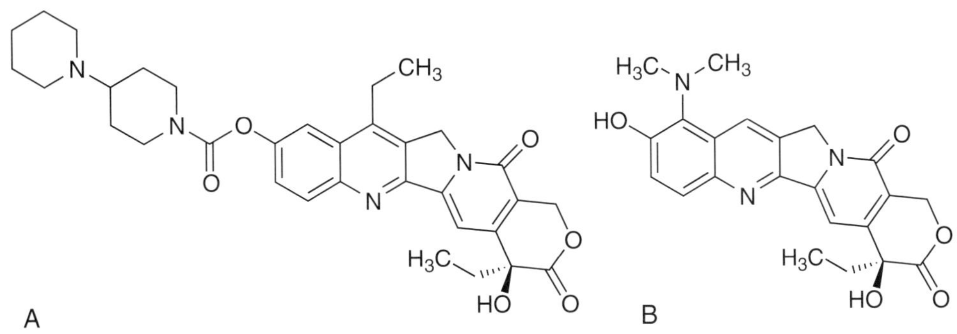

Fig. 9.7 A) Irinotecan and B) Topotecan.

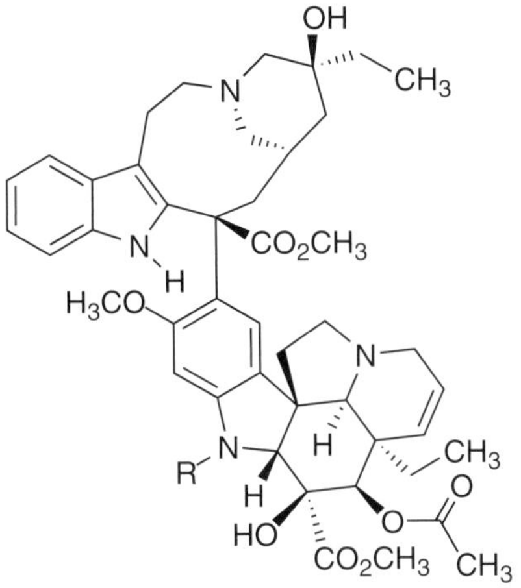

Vincristine, R = CHO
Vinblastine, R = CH₃

Fig. 9.8 Vincristine and vinblastine.

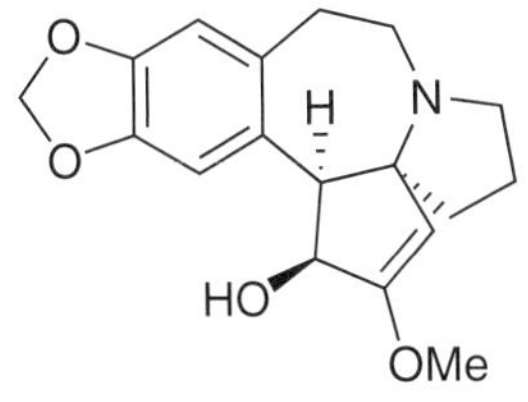

Cephalotaxine

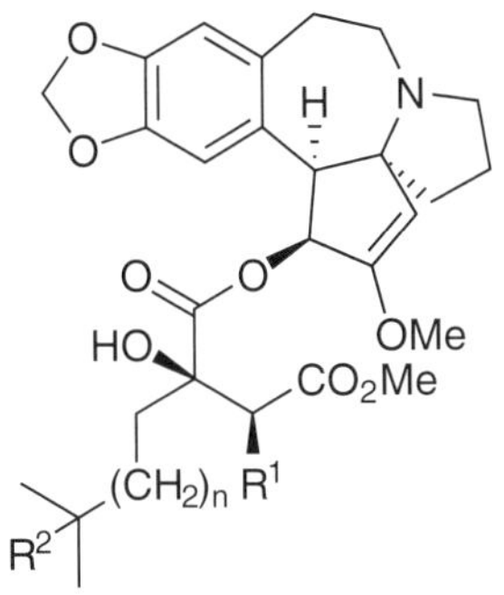

Harringtonine: R¹ = H, R² = OH, n = 1
Isoharringtonine: R¹ = OH, R² = H, n = 1
Homoharringtonine: R¹ = H, R² = OH, n = 2
Deoxyharringtonine: R¹ = H, R² = H, n = 1

Fig. 9.9 Cephalotaxine, harringtonine, homoharringtonine etc.

Taxanes

In the early 1960s, as part of the NCI-supported programme, extracts of *Taxus brevifolia*. Nutt. (Taxaceae), commonly known as the Pacific yew, were investigated. The Pacific yew is a slow-growing tree common to the western coast of the United States. The isolation of paclitaxel (marketed initially as Taxol, Fig. 9.10) required a highly extensive partitioning procedure utilising many steps between aqueous and organic solvents, and an exceptionally low yield (0.004%) was obtained. Structure elucidation was not a trivial process in the 1960s (it can still be difficult today!), and the elucidation of paclitaxel is an example of a masterful piece of natural product research (see Further Reading). This was the first report of a taxane diterpene with cytotoxic activity. Paclitaxel is a highly functional molecule possessing esters, epoxides, hydroxyls, amides, ketone groups and unsaturation. It has a large number of chiral centres (11) and is very difficult to synthesise; this was achieved in 1994 after 26 steps and is not a feasible option for production on a large scale. Work on paclitaxel ended in 1971 as it was thought that the concentration in the plant was too low, the extraction and isolation too difficult, and the tree supply too limited. However, two developments reignited interest in this paclitaxel: its activity in a melanoma cell line and the discovery of its unique mode of action. Initial work suggested that paclitaxel had similar activity to other agents that were 'spindle poisons', such as vincristine and colchicine, but Susan Horowitz's group demonstrated that whilst paclitaxel inhibited mitosis, it actually stabilised microtubules and inhibited their depolymerisation back to tubulin. This is the exact opposite of other agents that bind to soluble tubulin and inhibit the polymerisation of tubulin into microtubules.

Since paclitaxel worked by a new mechanism and is a highly unusual and novel structure, this encouraged further research, resulting in the development of analogues such as docetaxol (Taxotere, see Fig. 9.10). The supply issues concerning paclitaxel were overcome with its semisynthesis by the conversion of metabolites present in larger amounts (e.g. 10-deacetylbaccatin III; see Fig. 9.10) in the needles of the related English yew (*Taxus baccata*), which is common in churchyards in the UK. As needles are a renewable resource, there is no need to destroy trees by the removal of bark. Taxanes are now commercially produced by plant cell culture by large-scale fermentation of the plant cells and are widely used for the treatment of many forms of cancer. Docetaxel, like paclitaxel, prevents the mitotic spindle from being broken down by stabilising microtubule bundles and is slightly more water-soluble than paclitaxel. Both are administered intravenously.

Stilbenoids

Combretastatins (see Chapter 6, Fig. 6.22) have been isolated from the Cape Bushwillow tree *Combretum caffrum* (Eckl. & Zeyh.) Kuntze (Caffraceae). Combretastatin A4-phosphate is undergoing clinical

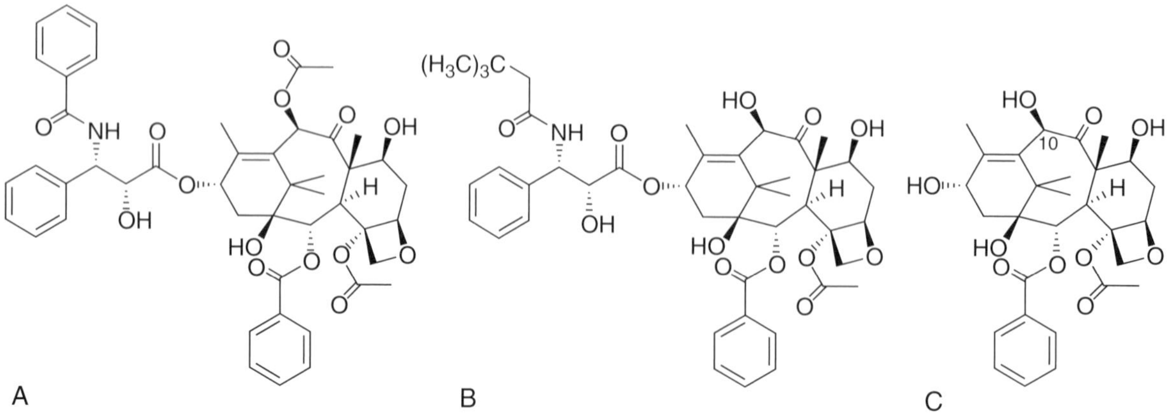

Fig. 9.10 A) Paclitaxel B) Docetaxel C) 10-Deacetylbaccatin III.

trials for hepatic cancers, but no derivatives have as yet been registered as anticancer drugs.

Ingenol Esters

The spurges (a group of *Euphorbia* species) have been known since ancient times for their topical proinflammatory activity and drastic laxative effects when taken internally. Their characteristic milky latex, when applied to warts, removes them very effectively, although usually accompanied by painful oedema. Chronic application of diterpenes in the latex of spurges, notably phorbol esters, is known to induce cancerous changes in normal cells and differentiation in cancer cells for the topical treatment of actinic keratosis.

The development of **ingenol mebutate** (Fig. 9.11) originates in the use of *Euphorbia peplus* L. in Australian folk medicine for the treatment of actinic keratoses and skin cancer. Actinic keratosis is a precancerous condition that, if untreated, usually leads to melanoma.

The diterpene ingenol was first isolated in 1968 during a search for the skin irritant and tumour-promoting compounds in *Euphorbia ingens* E. Mey. ex Boiss. At the same time, relatively nonirritant ingenane esters were also isolated. These were 90% less irritant than TPA (tetradecanoylphorbol acetate, also known as PMA, phorbol 12-myristate 13-acetate), a naturally occurring protein kinase C activator diterpene in *Croton* spp., which is classified as a Category 2 carcinogenic chemical hazard.

Work carried out during the 1990s showed that ingenol is endowed with both antitumor and in vitro anti-HIV activities. Mechanistic studies of its effects on actinic keratosis unveiled a dual mechanism of action, including rapid necrosis of the affected skin cells and a specific neutrophil-mediated, antibody-dependent cellular cytotoxicity. Destruction of actinic keratosis lesions was accomplished in 2 or 3 days, and the subsequent immune-mediated response prevented the development of residual dysplastic epidermal cells. Post-marketing studies reported adverse effects are mild to moderate in intensity (i.e. erythema, flaking/scaling and crusting) and resolve quickly. However, in 2020, safety concerns were raised about the product causing squamous cell skin carcinoma, and the medication was withdrawn from the market, illustrating the fine line between cytotoxicity and tumour promotion and the inherent difficulties in developing anticancer drugs.

Triterpenes

Triterpenoids are widely occurring in plants (see Chapter 6 and Fig. 6.41) and are currently under scrutiny for their potential as anticancer agents. Several pentacyclic lupane-, oleanane-, ursane-, cucurbitane- and dammarane-type tetracyclic triterpenes, including ginsenosides dichapetalins, have been identified as anticancer leads.

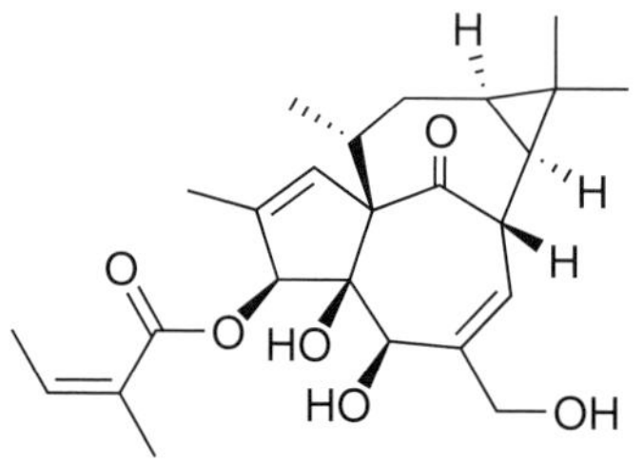

Fig. 9.11 Ingenol mebutate.

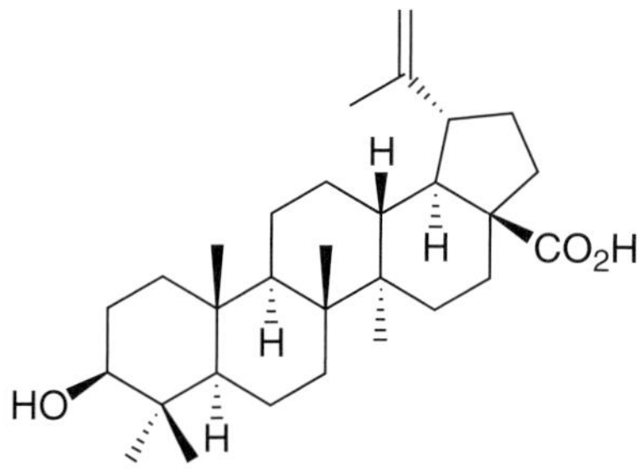

Fig. 9.12 Betulinic acid.

Betulinic acid (Fig. 9.12) is a lupane triterpene occurring in several plants, and the closely related **betulin** is a product found in abundance in the outer bark of white birch trees *Betula pubescens* Ehrh. (Betulaceae), formerly known as *Betula alba* L.

Betulinic acid selectively kills human melanoma cells, leaving healthy cells alive. The incidence of melanoma has been increasing at a higher rate than any other type of cancer, and therefore, there is a need for new anticancer agents that selectively target melanoma. Betulinic acid has been shown to be an inducer of apoptosis with a high degree of specificity for melanoma cells. This is unusual when compared with other cytotoxic agents, such as camptothecin or paclitaxel, which exhibit a far broader spectrum of activity, and the relative lack of toxicity makes triterpenes an attractive therapeutic option.

The oleanane triterpenoid (+)-oleanolic acid interacts with multiple molecular targets, showing cytotoxic and antimetastatic activities by decreasing the expression of the angiogenic VEGF and the development of melanoma-induced lung metastasis. It inhibits the proliferation of human gallbladder cancer cells through the mitochondrial apoptosis pathway, and further effects and mechanisms are under investigation.

Glycyrrhizin (glycyrrhizic acid, Fig. 18.6) is the major active constituent of liquorice, *Glycyrrhiza* species. Studies suggest an antitumor potential for glycyrrhizin based on its cytotoxicity toward hepatocellular carcinoma cells. *Glycyrrhiza uralensis* Fisch. ex DC. is a component of the licensed medicine PHY906, a traditional four-herb formula used in Chinese medicine to improve the efficacy and reduce adverse effects of standard anticancer drugs.

Lignans

Lignans are polymers of phenylpropene units providing a wide array of different arrangements. They are discussed in Chapter 6.

Podophyllotoxins

Podophyllum peltatum L. (Berberidaceae), also known as the mayapple, Devil's apple and American mandrake, is a perennial found in the woodlands of Canada and eastern United States. The rhizomes are known to be poisonous, containing high concentrations of **podophyllotoxin** (Fig. 9.13) and α- and β-**peltatin**, all of which are cytotoxic. The closely related species, *P. emodi* (syn. *P. hexandrum*), or Indian podophyllum, contains these at lower concentrations. Podophyllotoxin and related lignans are also found in the rhizomes of *P. pleianthum*, which in Japan and China is used to make a preparation to treat snakebites and genital tumours.

The rhizomes of *P. peltatum* have a long history of medical uses among indigenous North Americans, who use them as a laxative or to treat intestinal worms. The powdered rhizome was also used as a poultice to treat warts and skin growths.

Ethanolic extracts of the rhizomes, known as **podophyllin**, are included in many pharmacopoeias for the topical treatment of warts and condylomata acuminata, which are benign tumours. Podophyllin resin is highly irritant and toxic and cannot be used systemically. It contains many components in podophyllin, the most important of which are the lignans.

The hypothesis that podophyllin resin may contain anticancer lignan glycosides that are more water-soluble and less toxic than podophyllotoxin led to the isolation of several lignan derivatives which did, indeed, possess greater water solubility but unfortunately had less antitumour activity. In an entirely serendipitous event, a crude fraction of podophyllin was treated with benzaldehyde, resulting in a mixture of products that were mainly benzyl derivatives of lignan glycosides. This crude reaction mixture was highly cytotoxic and active in the mouse life-prolongation assay and against a leukaemia cell line. The components of this mixture were isolated but were not as active as the whole mixture. Crucially, the crude mixture worked by a different mechanism from the purified products by inhibiting tumour cells from undergoing mitosis. The most abundant component of this mixture was **podophyllotoxin benzylidene glucoside** (**1**), with lesser amounts of **4′-demethylepipodophyllotoxin benzylidene glucoside** (**2**), which was more active (see Fig. 9.13). Synthetic work to develop analogues that retain the same structural features of **4′-demethylepipodophyllotoxin benzylidene glucoside** (**2**), which is epimeric at position 1 and lacking a methyl at position 4 with respect to **podophyllotoxin benzylidene glucoside** (**1**), produced **etoposide** and **teniposide** (Fig. 9.14), which have much more potency than the parent compound. Etoposide is indicated for small-cell lung cancer, testicular cancer and lymphomas; teniposide is also used in the treatment of brain tumours.

Podophyllotoxin binds to tubulin and is a 'spindle poison' that functions by preventing microtubule formation, whereas etoposide and teniposide work via a different mechanism, inhibiting the enzyme topoisomerase II, preventing DNA synthesis and replication. The difference in mechanism is attributable to the small adjustment in structure with etoposide and teniposide being 4′-demethyl compounds and having different stereochemistry at position C_1.

Macrolides

Macrolides are traditionally a class of microbial secondary metabolites contributing to the defence against other organisms. Many have powerful antibiotic and cytotoxic properties towards other microbes and mammal cells, respectively. Macrolides have been found in plant extracts and were initially considered 'exotic' plant polyketides. In fact these 'plant-derived' compounds are biosynthesised by endophytic microorganisms. However, they can only be obtained from plant biomass and are included here on that basis. They also form a link with cytotoxic antibiotics, which are also isolated from soil bacteria in the rhizosphere.

Maytansine

Maytansine (Fig. 9.15) was originally isolated from *Gymnosporia buchananii* Loes. (Celastraceae), formerly *Maytenus ovatus* L., after crude extracts of the fruit, root and stems showed significant inhibitory activity in vitro and in vivo against animal tumour models. Bioassay-led fractionation of the acetylated extract yielded a derivative with the structure and configuration of a novel ansamycin macrolide, **maytansine**, which showed significant antileukaemic activity. It has since been shown that maytansine is instead synthesised by bacteria in the rhizosphere (the narrow soil zone around the root) and not by the plant. Maytansine exerts its cytotoxic activity by interacting with tubulin, in a similar manner to that of the vinca alkaloids and the dolastatins (see the section on marine drugs later). Poor results from early clinical studies showed that selective, targeted delivery of maytansine was necessary for efficacy, and a maytansine–Herceptin-linked monoclonal antibody has been approved to treat HER2-positive breast cancer that has spread to other parts of the body (metastatic breast cancer) after prior treatment with Herceptin (trastuzumab) and a taxane.

Microbial Anticancer Agents

Like plants, microbes are a rich source of bioactive natural products; anticancer drugs being good examples, with important classes such as the **anthracyclines, bleomycins** and **actinomycin**s represented. The streptomycetes, a large family of G gram-positive, filamentous bacteria, in particular have produced, and continue to provide, anticancer antibiotics. These bacteria occur predominantly in soil and decaying vegetation, in the rhizosphere of many plant species: the exchange of bioactive compounds from plant to the soil to bacteria, and in reverse, constitutes a unique environment that contributes to the diversity of antibiotics produced.

Anthracyclines

This family of antibiotics is structurally and biosynthetically related to the tetracyclines (Chapter 6), and is derived from the polyketide pathway. One of the first agents described was **daunorubicin** from *Streptomyces peucetius* and *S. coeruleorubidus* (Fig. 9.16). A widely used, related antitumour agent is **doxorubicin** from *S. peucetius* var. *caesius*, discovered in the late 1960s. Semisynthetic analogues have been produced, of which **idarubicin** has enhanced antitumour potency and is less cardiotoxic than doxorubicin. These agents bind to DNA and inhibit DNA and RNA synthesis, with the main antitumour activity mediated via the inhibition of topoisomerase II.

Bleomycins

This group of closely related glycopeptide antibiotics from the filamentous bacterium *Streptomyces verticillus* was discovered in 1966. It

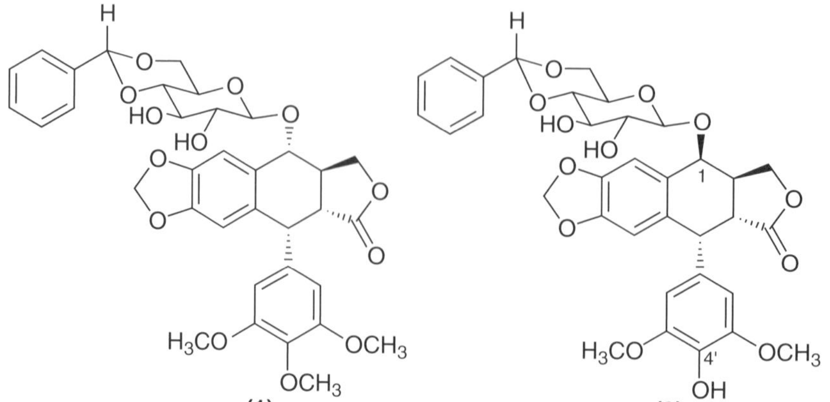

Fig. 9.13 Podophyllotoxin.

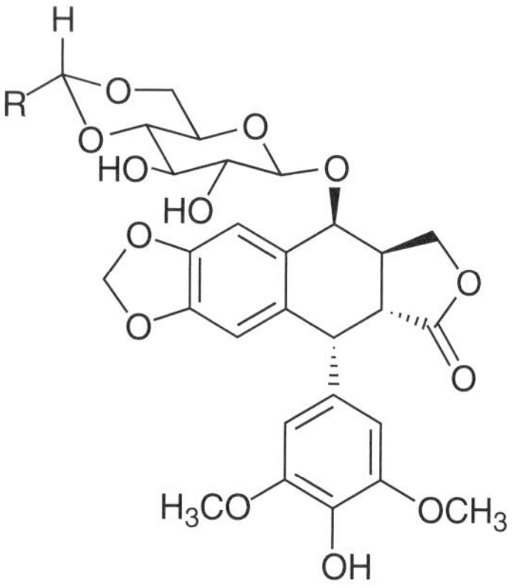

R = CH$_3$, **Etoposide**

R = ⟨thiophene⟩ **Teniposide**

Fig. 9.14 Etoposide and teniposide.

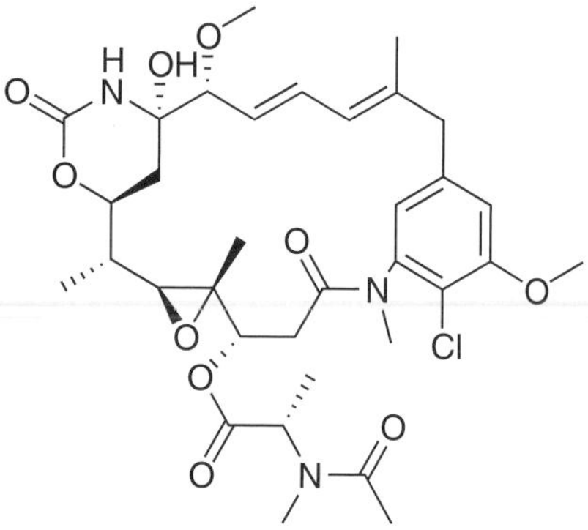

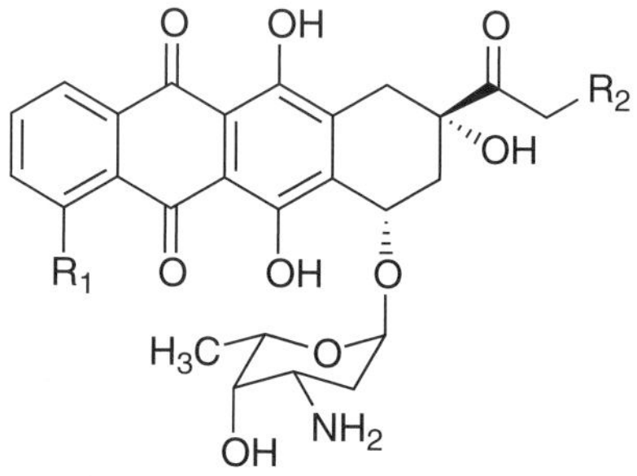

R$_1$ = OCH$_3$, R$_2$ = H, Daunorubicin
R$_1$ = OCH$_3$, R$_2$ = OH, Doxorubicin
R$_1$ = H, R$_2$ = H, Idarubicin

Fig. 9.16 Daunorubicin, doxorubicin and idarubicin.

Actinomycins

Actinomycin D (**dactinomycin**), from *Streptomyces parvulus* first isolated in 1940, structurally consists of a planar phenoxazinone dicarboxylic acid attached to two identical pentapeptides (Fig. 9.18). A number of analogues of different peptide compositions are known.

The planar group of this agent intercalates with double-stranded DNA, inhibits topoisomerase II and RNA synthesis, and can also cause single-strand DNA breaks. The principal use of this group is in paediatric tumours, including kidney (Wilms) tumours, but the use is limited due to its high incidence of toxic side effects.

MARINE ANTICANCER NATURAL PRODUCTS

Marine natural product research is comparatively new, but increasing interest and closely related to phytochemistry, with similar isolation, bioassay, structure elucidation and pharmacological methods used to identify active constituents and to assess their bioactivity. Marine organisms have limited history of medicinal use, but the oceans cover 70% of the Earth's surface and suggest a vast reserve for the discovery of new natural product drugs. Collection of biomass is usually carried out by divers, and in some cases, submersibles can give access to organisms that occur in deeper sites, but it is generally more challenging than plant collecting!

Important marine compounds with potential and demonstrated antitumour properties are described below.

Bryostatin-1 is a novel macrocyclic lactone derived from the marine bryozoan, *Bugula neritina*. This compound modulates protein kinase C activity, and phase I studies have demonstrated activity

Fig. 9.15 Maytansine.

consists of a mixture of **bleomycin A$_2$** (55%–70%) and **bleomycin B$_2$** (30%) (Fig. 9.17) and occurs naturally as blue copper chelates.

The bleomycins are DNA-cleaving drugs and cause single- and double-strand breaks in DNA. The dithiazole groups are essential for activity and are believed to be important in binding the bleomycins to DNA. They are used in the treatment of lymphomas, head and neck tumours, and testicular cancer.

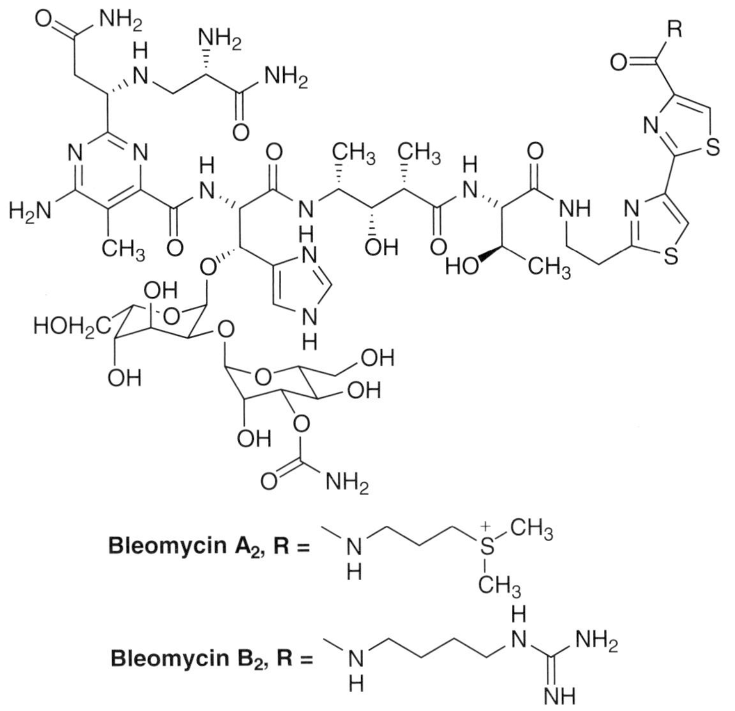

Fig. 9.17 Bleomycins.

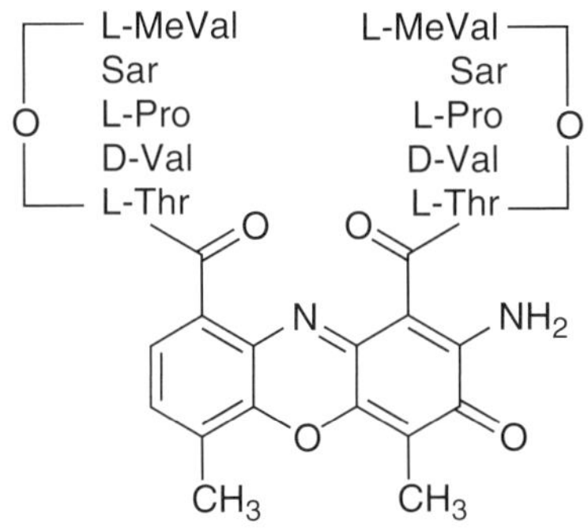

Fig. 9.18 Actinomycin D.

R = Lac-Pro-*N*-Me-L-Leu; DidemninB

against several tumour types. It has been investigated in phase II clinical trials as a single agent, and data suggest that it may have potential in combination with other cytotoxic agents.

Tunicates, or **sea squirts**, are organisms that attach themselves to submerged objects and feed by removing microscopic organisms from the water that is drawn through them. **Didemnin B** (Fig. 9.19) (*Trididemnum solidum*) has recently been shown to induce apoptosis (programmed cell death) in a wide range of cell lines. **Aplidine** (see Fig. 9.19) is a marine **depsipeptide** obtained from *Aplidium albicans*, originally found in the Mediterranean. Depsipeptides are cyclic peptides that also possess a cyclic ester functional group. Aplidine blocks the cell division cycle in human tumour cell lines and prevents the onset of DNA synthesis. Like didemnin B, it has also been shown to be an inducer of apoptosis in many cell models, and in the mouse xenograft assay, aplidine demonstrated considerable activity against bladder, colon, lung, lymphatic, prostate, skin and stomach tumours.

The first anticancer drug to be developed from marine organisms was **ecteinascidin-743** (= trabectedin) (Fig. 9.20), from *Ecteinascidia turbinata*, a tunicate found in the Caribbean and Mediterranean.

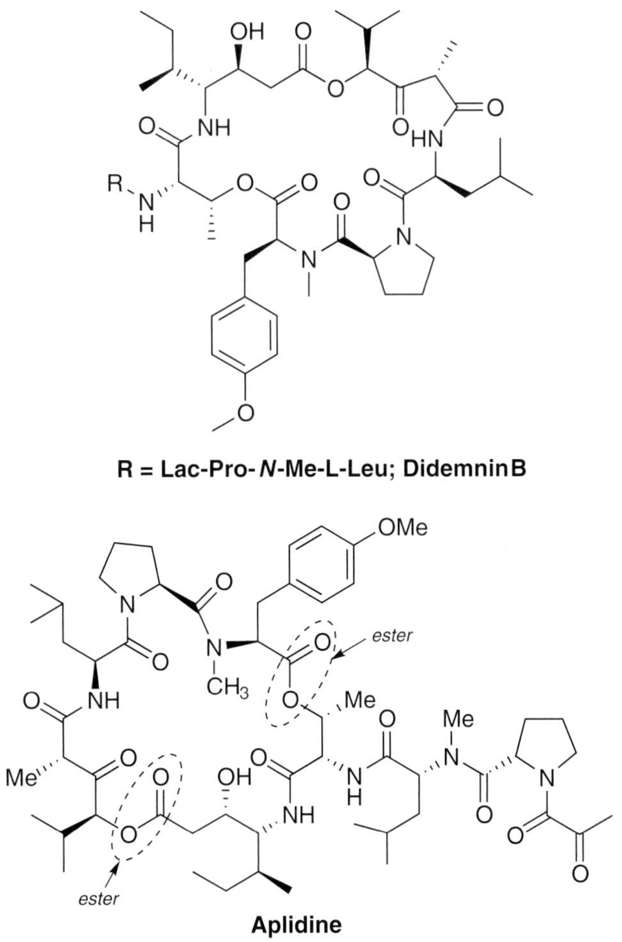

Aplidine

Fig. 9.19 Didemnin B and Aplidine.

Ecteinascidin-743 has very potent activity against a broad spectrum of tumour types in animal models; it binds to the minor groove of the DNA double helix and inhibits cell proliferation, leading to the apoptosis of cancer cells. This binding to the minor groove of DNA allows an alkylation reaction to occur between a guanine residue of the DNA and an electron-deficient carbon on the molecule (* in Fig. 9.20).

Ecteinascidin-743–DNA adducts are recognised by the nucleotide excision repair system, which is inherent to each cell and is present to protect the cell from the accumulation of mutations and DNA damage. When this repair system encounters the adduct, rather than repairing the cell, apoptosis occurs. Ecteinascidin-743 cytotoxicity only occurs during the active transcription of genes; this has obvious potential in cancer cells, which rely on increased transcription and translation. Ecteinascidin-743 also inhibits the induction of the gene *MDR1*, which encodes a membrane pump responsible for multidrug resistance, and this can drastically affect the potency of antitumour agents. These properties make ecteinascidin-743 unique, and it has been approved as an anticancer drug in combination with doxorubicin, particularly for the treatment of relapsed ovarian cancer.

The sea hare (*Dolabella auricularia*), a herbivorous (feeding on plants) mollusc from the Indian Ocean, produces cytotoxic linear peptides, such as **dolastatin-10** (Fig. 9.21), an inhibitor of microtubule assembly.

While there has been no breakthrough yet based on marine natural products, the structural diversity of the metabolites found in biologically very diverse organisms offers important opportunities for drug development. The contribution of natural products to the treatment of cancers has been one of the most important public health benefits of pharmacognosy and research on the world's biodiversity.

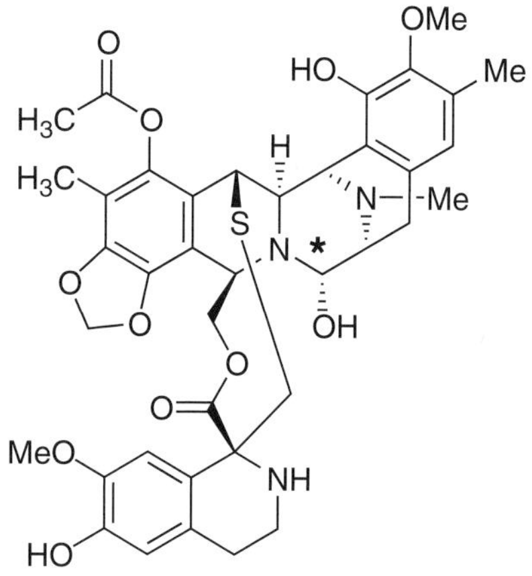

Fig. 9.20 Ecteinascidin-743.

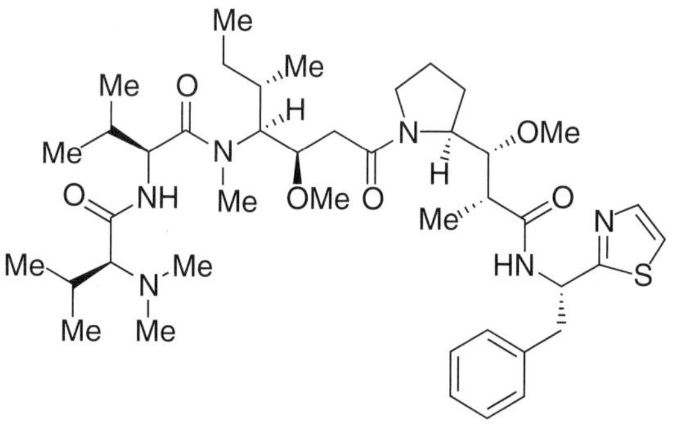

Fig. 9.21 Dolastatin-10.

FURTHER READING

Cerella, C., Sobolewski, C., Dicato, M., Diederich, M., 2010. Targeting COX-2 expression by natural compounds: a promising alternative strategy to synthetic COX-2 inhibitors for cancer chemoprevention and therapy. Biochem. Pharmacol. 80, 1801–1815.

Cragg, G.M., Pezzuto, J.M., 2016. Natural products as a vital source for the discovery of cancer chemotherapeutic and chemopreventive agents. Med. Princ. Pract. 25 (Suppl. 2), 41–59. https://doi.org/10.1159/000443404.

Cui, Q., Yang, D.-H., Chen, Z.-S., 2018. Special issue: natural products: anticancer and beyond. Molecules 23 (6), 1246. https://doi.org/10.3390/molecules23061246.

Desai, S.J., Prickril, B., Rasooly, A., 2018. Mechanisms of phytonutrient modulation of cyclooxygenase-2 (COX-2) and inflammation related to cancer. Nutr. Cancer 70 (3), 350–375. https://doi.org/10.1080/01635581.2018.1446091.

Ernst, M., Grace, O.M., Saslis-Lagoudakis, C.H., Nilsson, N., Simonsen, H.T., Rønsted, N., 2015. Global medicinal uses of *Euphorbia* L. (Euphorbiaceae). J. Ethnopharmacol. 176, 90–101.

Goodman, J., Walsh, V., 2001. The Story of Taxol. Cambridge University Press, Cambridge.

Grever, M.R., Schepartz, S.A., Chabner, B.A., 1992. The National Cancer Institute: cancer drug discovery and development program. Semin. Oncol. 19, 622–638.

Guerra, A.R., Duarte, M.F., Duarte, I.F., 2018. Targeting tumor metabolism with plant-derived natural products: emerging trends in cancer therapy. J. Agric. Food Chem. 66, 10663–10685.

Kim, C., Kim, B., 2018. Anti-cancer natural products and their bioactive compounds inducing ER stress-mediated apoptosis: a review. Nutrients 10 (8), 1021. https://doi.org/10.3390/nu10081021.

Koh, Y.C., Ho, C.T., Pan, M.H., 2020. Recent advances in cancer chemoprevention with phytochemicals. J. Food Drug Anal. 28 (1), 14–37. https://doi.org/10.1016/j.jfda.2019.11.001.

Kubczak, M., Szustka, A., Rogalińska, M., 2021. Molecular targets of natural compounds with anti-cancer properties. Int. J. Mol. Sci. 22, 13659. https://doi.org/10.3390/ijms222413659.

Lu, J.J., Wang, Y.T., 2020. Identification of anti-cancer compounds from natural products. Chin. J. Nat. Med. 18 (7), 481–482.

Luqman, S., Pezzuto, J.M., 2010. NFkappaB: a promising target for natural products in cancer chemoprevention. Phytother. Res. 24 (7), 949–963. https://doi.org/10.1002/ptr.3171.

Maher, T., Ahmad Raus, R., Daddiouaissa, D., Ahmad, F., Adzhar, N.S., Latif, E.S., et al., 2021. Medicinal plants with anti-leukemic effects: a review. Molecules 26, 2741. https://doi.org/10.3390/molecules26092741.

Neergheen, V.S., Bahorun, T., Taylor, E.W., Jen, L.S., Aruoma, O.I., 2010. Targeting specific cell signaling transduction pathways by dietary and medicinal phytochemicals in cancer chemoprevention. Toxicology 278, 229–241.

Newman, D.J., Cragg, G.M., 2009. Microbial antitumor drugs: natural products of microbial origin as anticancer agents. Curr. Opin. Investig. Drugs 10, 1280–1296.

Newman, D.J., Cragg, G.M., 2020. Plant endophytes and epiphytes: burgeoning sources of known and 'unknown' cytotoxic and antibiotic agents. Planta Med. 86, 891–905.

Pan, L., Chai, H., Kinghorn, A.D., 2010. The continuing search for antitumor agents from higher plants. Phytochem. Lett. 3, 1–8.

Ranjan, A., Ramachandran, S., Gupta, N., Kaushik, I., Wright, S., Srivastava, S., et al., 2019. Role of phytochemicals in cancer prevention. Int. J. Mol. Sci. 20 (20), 4981. https://doi.org/10.3390/ijms20204981.

Ren, Y., Kinghorn, A.D., 2019. Natural product triterpenoids and their semisynthetic derivatives with potential anticancer activity. Planta Med. 85 (11–12), 802–814.

Revankar, H.M., Bukhari, N.A., Kumar, G.B., Qin, H.L., 2017. Coumarins scaffolds as COX inhibitors. Bioorg. Chem. 71, 146–159.

Rosen, R.H., Gupta, A.K., Tyring, S.K., 2011. Dual mechanism of action of ingenol mebutate gel for topical treatment of actinic keratoses: rapid lesion necrosis followed by lesion-specific immune response. J. Am. Acad. Dermatol. 66, 486–493.

Safe, S., Kasiappan, R., 2016. Natural products as mechanism-based anticancer agents: Sp transcription factors as targets. Phytother. Res. 30 (11), 1723–1732.

Salehi, B., Zucca, P., Sharifi-Rad, M., Pezzani, R., Rajabi, S., Setzer, W.N., et al., 2018. Phytotherapeutics in cancer invasion and metastasis. Phytother. Res. 32 (8), 1425–1449. https://doi.org/10.1002/ptr.6087.

Sever, R., Brugge, J., 2015. Signal transduction in cancer. Cold Spring Harbor Perspect. Med. 5, a006098.

Soundararajan, P., Kim, J.S., 2018. Anti-carcinogenic glucosinolates in cruciferous vegetables and their antagonistic effects on prevention of cancers. Molecules 23 (11), 2983. https://doi.org/10.3390/molecules23112983.

Stähelin, H.F., von Wartburg, A., 1991. The chemical and biological route from podophyllotoxin glucoside to etoposide: Ninth Cain Memorial Award Lecture. Cancer Res. 51, 5–15.

Tiwari, P., Bae, H., 2022. Endophytic fungi: key insights, emerging prospects, and challenges in natural product drug discovery. Microorganisms 10 (2), 360.

Wall, M.E., Wani, M.C., 1995. Camptothecin and taxol: discovery to clinic—Thirteenth Bruce F. Cain Memorial Award Lecture. Cancer Res. 55, 753–760.

10

Antimicrobial Natural Products

INTRODUCTION

Preparations from traditional medicines form the basis of many anti-infective medicines used to cure topical and systemic infections caused by microbes, and there is an enormous body of primary literature supporting modern and historical uses of plants to treat infections.

Plant compounds have antibacterial, antifungal, antiprotozoal, antiviral and anthelminthic properties—often several of these in a broad spectrum of activity. Each of the following sections is necessarily a brief introduction, with a summary of targets and mechanisms by which antimicrobial agents (of all types) act, and where plant compounds are of historical, current or potential therapeutic importance. The Further Reading list is longer than usual because there are many pathogenic microbes to discuss, and research moves rapidly in this area.

ANTIBACTERIAL ACTIVITY

The current crisis of antibiotic resistance has generated renewed interest in plant products to provide alternatives: to reduce the use of antibiotics; act as antiseptic agents for environmental and personal use; and increasingly, as bacterial resistance-modifying agents taken alongside antibiotics to prevent or delay resistance.

Traditionally, topical infections and wounds were treated with a poultice of fresh or dried herb, or an extract incorporated into an ointment, often with honey and aromatic oils. These preparations were intended to prevent microbial (mainly bacterial) growth and promote wound repair by stimulating cellular growth. Wound healing and repair still respond well to topical phytotherapy, and the antibacterial properties of, for example, essential oils remain crucial to the development of safe personal antiseptic and cosmetic products, including hand gels, mouthwashes and soaps. These are discussed in Chapter 27. A significant advantage of these essential oil compounds is the low potential for microbial resistance and their pleasant odour, but toxicity when taken internally may limit their use.

Antifungal agents are widely produced by plants in response to attack by pathogens, and topical fungal infections may respond to broad-spectrum antimicrobials (see later). However, for systemic infections and in immune-compromised patients, no efficacious plant products are yet available.

Antiprotozoal agents, for treatment of malaria, leishmaniasis, amoebic dysentery and other serious protozoal infections, are almost all derived from natural products and continue to provide new leads for development.

Antiviral plant compounds are under intense scrutiny, and many theoretical herbal treatments have been suggested in the context of severe acute respiratory syndrome (SARS)-COVID (see Chapter 21, The Respiratory System). Herbs used in the treatment of colds and influenza have been subjected to extensive preclinical and clinical investigation: some have direct antiviral effects (elderberry, pelargonium, andrographis), whereas others are taken for their immune-stimulating effects (e.g. echinacea, astragalus).

Intestinal worm infestations have been treated with medicinal plants, such as wormseed and wormwood (*Artemisia* spp.), and tannin-containing herbs, but the most effective and least toxic anthelmintic drugs at present are synthetic and will not be covered here. However, it is worth noting that tannins are of agricultural interest as a means of nematode control, when given in animal feed. Plants rich in tannins, currant leaves (*Ribes* spp.) and legumes, such as sainfoin (*Onobrychis viciifolia),* carob *(Ceratonia siliqua)* and *Acacia* spp., have been shown to decrease the nematode burden in livestock in a more ecologically balanced way and avoiding drug resistance.

PLANT BROAD-SPECTRUM ANTIMICROBIALS

Antimicrobial plant products are produced as a normal part of the plant's chemistry but also when they are under attack from microbes, herbivores and insects. These are called phytoalexins and are very quickly synthesised by the plant, and they display antimicrobial properties against a wide range of bacteria and fungi.

Plant compounds are very different in their chemistry and mechanisms of antimicrobial action, compared with existing antibiotics, which are usually derived from fungi, such as the β-lactams (e.g. penicillins from *Penicillium* species), or from different classes of bacteria, such as the tetracyclines and macrolides (the erythromycins), from Actinobacteria such as *Streptomyces*. Antibiotics are discussed briefly in Chapter 6 (Natural Product Chemistry).

Recent research has highlighted another aspect to plant anticancer (and other therapeutic) compounds: their production from commensal organisms such as bacteria, lichens, fungi and other plants. Just as humans and other mammals host a diverse range of microorganisms in the gut and other organs, plants too host a vast microbiota, both on (epiphytes) and within (endophytes) their structure, which synthesise biologically active molecules. Epiphytic bacteria synthesise the anticancer macrolide maytansine (see Chapter 9).

Bacteria within plants are the source of components producing biological effects. For example, *in vitro* studies using *Echinacea purpurea* showed that bacterial lipoproteins and lipopolysaccharides (LPSs) from endophytes present in the plant material were responsible for most of the macrophage activation detected.

Most herbal drugs are at least dried and stored before they reach the patient, and most are subjected to more elaborate processing before they become (ingredients of) finished herbal medicinal products. The effects of these stages on the quantity, range and viability of plant endophytic bacteria are not known, but some impact is to be expected. In some instances, fresh plant material is used in the preparation of herbal medicinal products, particularly by herbal practitioners, and this material may contain a more intact plant microbiota. Plants typically are harvested at specific times, often during flowering, relating to the profile of active constituents. It is not yet understood how this relates to the microbiome profile and the downstream effects on production of bioactive compounds.

Plant-derived antimicrobials act through a variety of mechanisms, many of which are poorly understood. A summary of examples which

TABLE 10.1 Natural Antimicrobials: Mechanisms and Examples

Mechanism of Action	Examples
Structural disruption of the bacterial cell wall and membrane and increase in cell permeability and leakage of cell constituents	Monoterpenes, thymol, carvacrol, berberine, flavonoids, polyphenolic acids, tannins, curcumin, α-bisabolol, nerolidol, isothiocyanates, allyl sulfides, arbutin
Inhibition of biofilm formation and/or inactivation of mature biofilms, reducing extracellular polysaccharide activity; interference with quorum sensing	Essential oils of lavender, eucalyptus, and citrus, gingerols, allyl sulfides, thymol, polyphenols, anthraquinones, thymoquinone
Inhibition of protein biosynthesis associated with bacterial cell growth and cleavage (e.g. dihydrofolate)	Berberine, sanguinarine, nobiletin, allicin, sophoraflavanone G, baicalein, tannins, liquorice flavones, polyphenols, tannins
Prevention of microbial adhesion to epithelium	Polyphenols, anthocyanins
Inhibition of production of bacterial virulence factors (lipases, proteases, toxins)	Polyphenols, flavonoids
Disruption of the cytoplasmic membrane, binding to deoxyribonucleic acid (DNA), and inhibition of the microbial respiratory chain	Anthraquinones, polyphenols

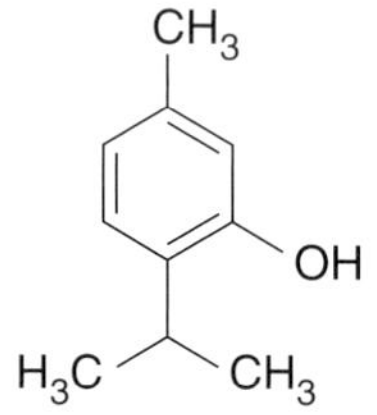

Fig. 10.1 Thymol.

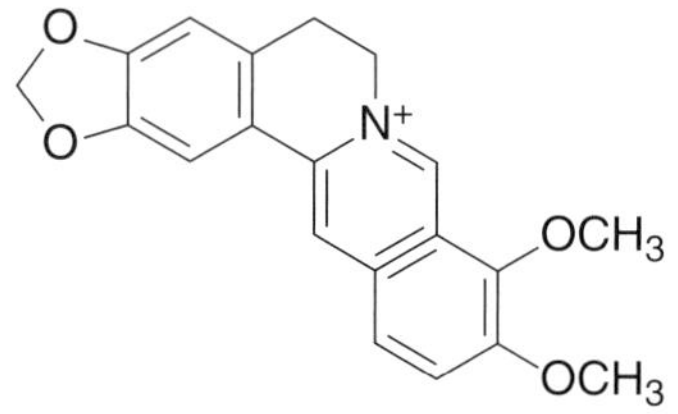

Fig. 10.2 Berberine.

have some evidence of interaction mechanisms is shown in Table 10.1. It is quite usual for one compound to act via more than one mechanism: this is a distinct advantage, making resistance less likely to arise. Antifungal mechanisms are not as well investigated as antibacterial activity, but cell wall and membrane effects are likely to be common. This variety of mechanisms makes plant-derived antimicrobials a valuable resource in reducing the use of conventional antibiotics by providing alternatives for treating mild chronic infections (e.g. urinary, respiratory) and for control of methicillin-resistant *Staphylococcus aureus* (MRSA).

Essential Oils: Monoterpenes and Phenylpropanoids

The most commonly used plant-derived antimicrobials are essential oils and their components, the monoterpenes and phenylpropanoids (phenolic monoterpenes). The activity of an essential oil depends on its chemical constituents and their concentrations: each compound may exhibit a different mechanism of antibacterial action, which may vary because of bacterial architecture; Gram-positive and Gram-negative bacteria differ in their cell membrane compositions. Thymol (Fig. 10.1) has a wide range of antibacterial and antifungal properties and is a popular oral and skin antiseptic (see Chapter 27 (Topical Phytotherapy)). The phenolic hydroxy group, as with thymol and carvacrol, confers increased antimicrobial activity to a monoterpene structure (see Chapter 6, Fig. 6.26), although most essential oil components have intrinsic antimicrobial activity. Their decongestant properties also make them useful in the symptomatic relief of upper respiratory infections (see Chapter 21, The Respiratory System). The long history of the use of aromatic and essential oil-containing plants in the diet, not only for digestive and flavouring purposes, is based on their ability to reduce microbial spoilage and preserve food. This remains a primary focus for these plants as food additives, especially as many culinary herbs contain other antimicrobial agents, such as polyphenolic acids and flavonoids. Systemic toxicity limits the use of some essential oils, such as tea tree, clove and eucalyptus oils, and isolated components such as thymol and carvacrol, except as topical

agents; these are discussed in Chapter 27. Their mechanisms of action include disrupting the cell membrane and inhibiting biofilm formation by quenching quorum sensing (QS; see under Natural Products as Resistance-Modifying Agents). 6-Gingerol (from ginger, *Zingiber officinale;* see Chapter 18, Fig. 18.10) has shown QS-inhibiting effects, as have the garlic allyl sulfides, and these are of particular interest given their wide dietary consumption and safety profile.

Essential oils have a wide spectrum of antifungal and antiyeast activity; this is due mainly to the same mechanisms of action as antibacterial activity (disruption of the fungal cell membrane), and compounds such as thymol and carvacrol have a similarly potent effect. Garlic and clove extracts inhibit the growth of *Candida*; eugenol (present in many essential oils, and the major constituent of clove oil) causes permanent injury to the cells of *Candida albicans*. Essential oils penetrate and disrupt the fungal cell wall and protoplasm membranes and inhibit the synthesis of deoxyribonucleic acid (DNA), ribonucleic acid (RNA), proteins and polysaccharides.

Alkaloids

Isoquinoline, aporphine, quinolone and phenanthrene alkaloids have a wide range of antibacterial properties, in addition to specific effects on protozoa and viruses. Their mechanism of action is thought to be due to inhibition of DNA synthesis and repair mechanisms by intercalating with nucleic acids. Berberine (Fig. 10.2) is a benzylisoquinoline alkaloid found in many medicinal plant species, such as *Coptis chinensis* Franch. (Ranunculaceae), and species of *Berberis, Mahonia, Hydrastis* and *Phellodendron*. It has antidiabetic and many other effects in addition to its antimicrobial properties. Berberine has potent antibacterial effects against, for example, *S. aureus*, but it is readily extruded by multidrug resistance (MDR) pumps, leading to resistance. However, several *Berberis* species also synthesise a separated compound, 5′-methoxyhydnocarpin (5′-MHC), which has no antimicrobial activity alone, but strongly potentiates the action of berberine by its inhibiting MDR-dependent efflux from *S. aureus* cells.

Sulfur-Containing Compounds

Allyl Sulfides

Garlic, *Allium sativum* and other *Allium* spp. (Amaryllidaceae) have a very long history in antiinfective preparations used topically and systemically. The many other acclaimed health benefits of garlic are covered in Chapter 19 (The Cardiovascular System). *Alliums* have a long and rich culinary use, with onions, garlic, shallots and chives all showing antimicrobial activity against various bacteria, fungi and viruses. The antimicrobial constituents include allicin (Fig. 10.3), which degrades naturally to form a range of unstable volatile components, including allyl methyl- and propyl sulfides and diallyl sulfides, ajoene and others. These are strongly antimicrobial against *S. aureus*, *Streptococcus* species and even some Gram-negative bacteria, such as *Helicobacter pylori*, the major bacterial causative agent of stomach ulcers. The chemical mechanisms underlying the antimicrobial activity include membrane disruption and inhibition of biofilm formation.

Isothiocyanates

These are widely present in plants including *Brassica* vegetables and condiments such as wasabi, horseradish and mustards. Isothiocyanates (ITCs) are produced via enzymatic hydrolysis of glucosinolates (GLs) by myrosinase. In the intact plant, myrosinase is stored separately from GLs. When plant tissue damage occurs by chopping or chewing, the myrosinase comes into contact with GLs and effects their hydrolysis to ITCs (see Fig. 6.47).

Allyl isothiocyanate (AITC), benzyl isothiocyanate (BITC), phenyl isothiocyanate (PITC), phenyl ethyl isothiocyanate (PEITC) and sulforaphane (SFN) have been tested against food-borne various pathogenic bacteria including *H. pylori*, *Escherichia coli*, *Pseudomonas aeruginosa*, *Salmonella* and *Clostridium* spp. SFN, AITC and BITC seem to be the most potent, but to date, most studies have been in vitro and effects in vivo have not been assessed. ITCs act by at least two mechanisms depending on bacteria species, acting on cell membranes and leakage of cellular metabolites. SFN, for example, inhibits bacterial QS, affects the pyocyanin production and exerts antibiofilm activity against *P. aeruginosa*; BITC inhibits *E. coli* Shiga toxin production and induces the loss of MRSA membrane integrity.

Coumarins

Coumarins such as osthole and scopoletin (see Fig. 6.16, Chapter 6) exert a wide range of properties, including antibacterial and antiviral activities. They are often produced by a plant in response to infection. Their antibacterial activity is mainly due to inhibiting bacterial DNA gyrase, preventing supercoiling. Aegelinol and agasyllin have shown antibacterial effects against Gram-negative and Gram-positive bacteria.

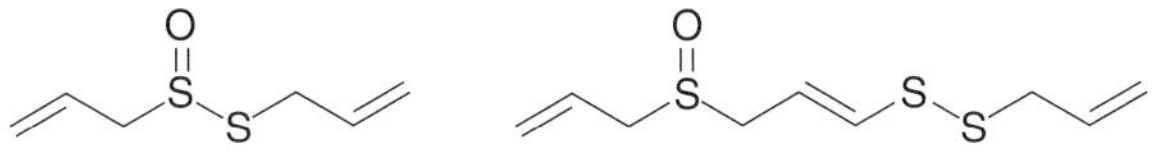

Polyphenols

The term 'polyphenols' as applied here refers to flavonoids, stilbenoids, polyphenolic acids, tannins, anthocyanins and procyanidin oligomers. These have shown many beneficial therapeutic effects, due to their cardiovascular and chemopreventive properties, and many have antibacterial activity, via a range of mechanisms, as shown in Table 10.1. They include **flavonoids** such as chrysin and baicalein (Fig. 10.4); **stilbenes** such as resveratrol; **polyphenolic acids** such as chlorogenic, caffeic and rosmarinic acids; **tannins** including gallic acid and epigallocatechins (Fig. 10.5); **anthocyanins** including delphinidin and cyanidin glucosides; and **proanthocyanin complexes** (PACs) such as those found in cranberry, *Vaccinium macrocarpon*, and blueberry (bilberry), *Vaccinium myrtillus*. These species also contain catechins, flavanols and other phenolics possessing similar antiadhesive activities against uropathogenic bacteria.

Quinones

Arbutin (Fig. 10.6) is the main antimicrobial constituent of Uva-ursi (*Arctostaphylos uva-ursi*) (see Chapter 24). It does not show direct antimicrobial effects but is hydrolysed by bacterial β-glucosidase to hydroquinone. This enzyme exerts strong activity in uropathogens, such as *Enterococcus faecalis*, supporting the specific use of arbutin as a urinary antiseptic. Hydroquinone shows activity against *S. aureus*, MRSA, and extended-spectrum β-lactamase *S. aureus* (ESBL-SA). The action is via disruption of the bacterial cell wall and membrane, increasing permeability and leakage of intracellular contents, and inhibiting protein synthesis.

Thymoquinone (TQ) (Fig. 10.7) is the active ingredient in *Nigella sativa* (black seed; see Chapter 19, The Cardiovascular System) and shows strong antimicrobial effects against *Staphylococcus epidermidis*, *C. albicans* and others, at least partly by inhibiting biofilm activity.

Anthraquinones (AQs) are the active constituents of many medicinal plant genera, including *Frangula*, *Rheum*, *Rumex* and *Senna* species (see Chapter 18, The Gastrointestinal and Biliary System), and they have a wide range of other pharmacological properties, including specific antimicrobial effects.

Research is mainly focused on the properties of emodin, one of the most common aglycones found in all species, but there are many related compounds with similar properties.

The antibacterial activity of emodin (Fig. 10.8) has been shown against various human Gram-positive and Gram-negative pathogens, including *S. aureus*, *S. intermedius*, *E. coli*, *P. aeruginosa*, *Bacillus subtilis*, *Bacillus cereus*, *Vibrio vulnificus*, *Salmonella typhimurium*, *Shigella sonnei* and *Listeria monocytogenes*, most of which are food-borne bacteria. Emodin acts by binding to cell DNA, resulting in cell death, and has antibiofilm properties.

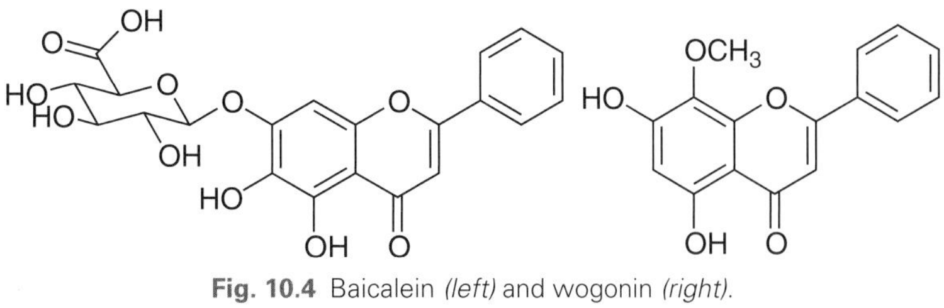

Fig. 10.3 Allicin *(left)* and ajoene *(right)*.

Fig. 10.4 Baicalein *(left)* and wogonin *(right)*.

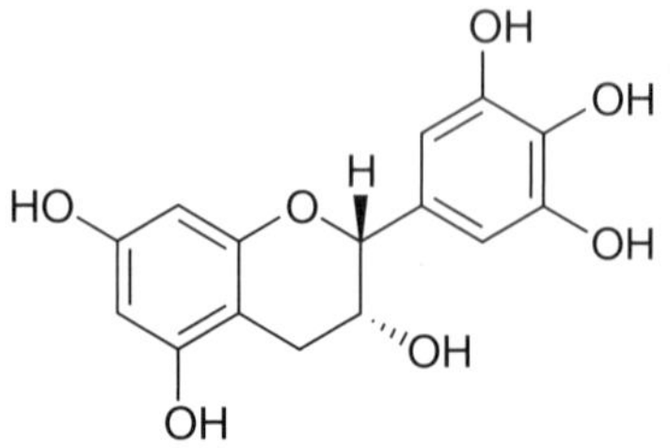

Fig. 10.5 (−)-Epigallocatechin.

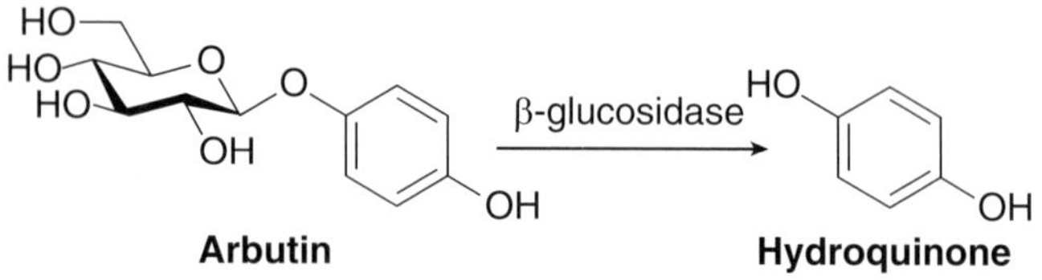

Fig. 10.6 Hydrolysis of arbutin.

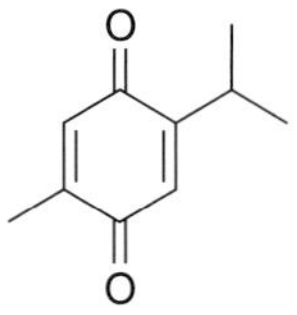

Fig. 10.7 Thymoquinone.

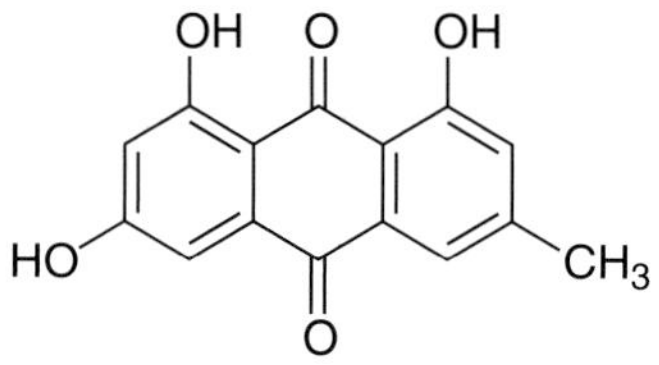

Fig. 10.8 Emodin.

Antifungal activity in vitro has been shown for rhein, physcion, aloe-emodin and chrysophanol, isolated from *Rheum emodi* rhizomes, against *C. albicans*, *Cryptococcus neoformans*, *Trichophyton mentagrophytes* and *Aspergillus fumigatus*. AQs also have antiviral effects, as described later.

Microbial Resistance

Natural resistance may be intrinsic (always expressed in the species) or induced (the genes are naturally present but are only expressed to resistance levels after exposure to an antimicrobial agent). Intrinsic resistance is independent of previous antibiotic exposure, and the most common bacterial mechanisms involved are reduced permeability of the outer membrane and the natural activity of efflux pumps. Multidrug efflux pumps are also a common mechanism of induced resistance. Acquired resistance is achieved through all main routes by which bacteria acquire any genetic material: transformation, transposition and conjugation (horizontal gene transfer (HGT)), and mutations in their own chromosomal DNA; it may be temporary or permanent. Mutations aiding antimicrobial resistance mainly occur in genes encoding drug targets, transporters, and antibiotic-modifying enzymes. The wide use of antibiotics, when used at subinhibitory concentrations, leads to selection of high-level resistance organisms in successive bacterial generations and may increase the ability to acquire resistance to other antimicrobial agents.

Natural Products as Resistance-Modifying Agents

Phytochemicals which exhibit direct antimicrobial effects by disrupting biofilm formation and inhibiting QS (see Table 10.1) also have the potential to act as resistance modifiers.

The most promising strategies for countering antibiotic resistance at present highlight the use of natural efflux pump inhibitors, pyruvate kinase inhibitors and quorum-sensing inhibitors, as shown in Table 10.2, and combinations based on targeting different sites.

Antimicrobial resistance mechanisms are concerned firstly with limiting drug uptake by reducing the cell to exposure of an antimicrobial using physical barriers and by preventing transport into the cell via efflux pumps present in the cell membrane. If absorbed, bacterial

TABLE 10.2 Bacterial Resistance Modifiers From Plants

Mechanism	Structural Class	Examples	Source
Efflux pump inhibition	Alkaloids	Reserpine	*Rauwolfia* spp.
		Harmaline	*Peganum harmala*
		Quinine	*Cinchona* spp.
		Piperine	*Piper* spp.
	Diterpenes (abietane)	Ferruginol	*Chamaecyparis lawsoniana*
		Carnosic acid	*Rosmarinus officinalis*
	Flavolignan	Silyhin	*Silybum marianum*
	Polyphenol	Caffeoylquinic acid	*Artemisia absinthium*
Inhibition of pyruvate kinase	Flavones	Diosmetin	*Citrus* spp.
		Baicalein	*Scutellaria baicalensis*
Inhibition of deoxyribonucleic acid (DNA) gyrase	Coumarins	Aegelinol	*Peudedanum* and other Apiaceae
		Scopoletin	Widespread in plants
	Flavones	Chrysin	*Passiflora*, many other spp.
	Alkaloids	Berberine	*Berberis, Hydrastis, Coptis* spp.
Disruption of biofilm formation; inhibition of quorum sensing	Monoterpenes, phenyl propanoids	Essential oil (e.g. thymol, gingerols)	*Eucalyptus, Lavandula, Thymus. Zingiber* spp., etc.
	Allyl sulfides, isothiocyanates (ITCs)	Allicin, allyl sulfides,	*Allium sativum*
		Allylisothiocyanate, benzylisothiocyanate, sulforaphane, etc. ITC, sulforaphane	*Brassica* spp.
	Quinones, anthraquinones	Arbutin, thymoquinone, emodin	*Arctostaphylos uva-ursi*
			Nigella sativa
			Rheum, Rumex and other spp.

resistance may include inactivation of the drug by inducing metabolic enzymes, such as DNA gyrase and pyruvate kinase, and by modifying the drug target, as with the β-lactamases (see later).

Limiting Drug Uptake

There is a natural difference in the ability of bacteria to limit the uptake of antimicrobial agents. The LPS layer in Gram-negative bacteria provides a barrier to some groups of antimicrobial agents. The mycobacteria have an outer membrane with a high lipid content and are more susceptible to hydrophobic drugs, such as rifampicin and the fluoroquinolones, whereas hydrophilic drugs have limited access to the cell. Bacteria, such as *Mycoplasma*, that do not have a cell wall are therefore intrinsically resistant to all drugs that target the cell wall, including β-lactams and glycopeptides. Polar molecules have difficulty penetrating the cell wall, conferring intrinsic resistance to aminoglycosides.

Bacterial colonisation may involve the formation of a biofilm, a thick, sticky, matrix which contains polysaccharides, proteins, and DNA from the resident bacteria. These biofilms may contain a predominant organism or a wide variety of organisms, as in the biofilm of the normal flora in the gut. A biofilm protects the bacteria from attack by the host immune system, provides physical protection from antimicrobial agents and facilitates horizontal transfer of genes by the proximity of the bacterial cells. To be effective, much higher concentrations of antibiotics are necessary, with the attendant risks of subtherapeutic doses being administered and contributing further to the development of resistance.

Quorum sensing (QS) is a bacterial communication system for coordinating group actions such as forming biofilms and producing virulence factors. Chemical signal molecules called autoinducers (AIs) that regulate gene expression are produced, and these increase in concentration with population density.

Drug Efflux

Efflux pumps function to rid the bacterial cell of toxic substances and transport a large variety of compounds across the cytoplasmic membrane. In this respect they resemble those found in mammalian cells which transport drugs (see Chapter 14, Herbal Medicine Interactions). Bacteria possess encoded genes for efflux pumps, some of which are expressed constitutively, and others which are induced or overexpressed when a suitable substrate is present. Most bacteria possess several types of efflux pumps. Efflux pumps are classified into families, and their structure and function are highly complex (for more detail, see Further Reading).

Efflux Inhibitors From Natural Sources

The first drug shown to reverse an MDR phenotype in *S. aureus* was the alkaloid reserpine, which afforded a fourfold reduction in the minimum inhibitory concentration (MIC) of tetracycline in MRSA. Reserpine has potent pharmacological activities and is too toxic to use internally; since then, other phytochemicals have been identified as MDR inhibitors, as shown in Table 10.2. A significant advantage of several of these—flavonoids, silybin, piperine, polyphenolic acids—is their low toxicity and general health benefits when consumed.

Drug Inactivation and Target Modification

Bacteria inactivate drugs by degradation (e.g. hydrolysis) or by transfer of a chemical group: acetylation occurs with the aminoglycosides, chloramphenicol and the fluoroquinolones, with phosphorylation and adenylation also affecting the aminoglycosides.

Resistance to the β-lactam antibiotics (e.g. penicillins, cefalosporins) by Gram-positive bacteria arises from alterations in the penicillin-binding proteins (transpeptidases involved in the construction of the cell wall), reducing the amount of drug that can bind to that target. β-Lactamases hydrolyse a specific site in the β-lactam ring structure, causing the ring to open and rendering it unable to bind to target proteins. The β-lactamases are drug-hydrolysing enzymes and tetracycline is also inactivated by hydrolysation. An established strategy for counteracting resistance is the pairing of a β-lactamase inhibitor with an antibiotic. These may have weak antimicrobial ability alone but work synergistically in combination with a β-lactam drug. Commonly used combinations include amoxicillin/clavulanic acid and piperacillin/tazobactam. The glycopeptides (e.g. vancomycin) also inhibit cell wall synthesis, and resistance to vancomycin has become a major issue in the enterococci and in MRSA.

For drugs that target DNA synthesis (e.g. fluoroquinolones), resistance may arise from modifications in DNA gyrase in Gram-negative bacteria (or topoisomerase IV in Gram-positive bacteria), resulting in decreased drug binding. Mutations in enzymes such as dihydrofolate reductase (DHFR) cause structural changes which interfere with drug binding. The sulfonamides and trimethoprim are structural analogues of the natural substrates of DHFR (*para*-amino-benzoic acid and dihydrofolate, respectively), and act through competitive binding to mutations in these enzymes but not with that of the natural substrate.

Fig. 10.9 is a simplified schematic diagram of a bacterial cell, showing where phytochemicals have demonstrated the potential for combatting resistance mechanisms. Because this field is still not well understood, it is only a snapshot illustration of current knowledge. Many fields remain unexplored, and mechanisms are still to be elucidated.

ANTIPROTOZOAL AGENTS

Protozoal infections include the most devastating diseases resulting from poverty and deprivation and carry a huge burden of health and especially child mortality. The most important protozoal diseases include malaria (by far the most lethal), trypanosomiasis, Chagas disease, amoebic dysentery, giardiasis and leishmaniasis. Less serious, but also widespread, are toxoplasmosis and trichomoniasis. Many are endemic (but not restricted) to the tropics and involve a nonhuman vector, which may be an insect, larva or snail. Despite being largely preventable by the introduction of clean water, efficient sewerage treatment and reducing mosquito breeding habitats, they remain rife in many parts of the world and especially after environmental and humanitarian disasters, and new antiprotozoal agents are still needed. Chemical methods of controlling these diseases include the use of pesticides (insecticides, molluscicides) to destroy the vector, as well as targeting the parasite.

Pathogenic protozoa are very different in nature and susceptibility to drugs, and their treatment involves different targets according to species. There are effective drugs available for conditions, such as trichomoniasis, amoebic dysentery caused by *Entamoeba histolytica*, and giardiasis (metronidazole is the first line treatment) and for toxoplasmosis (pyrimethamine and sulfadiazine). However, the most serious remain very difficult to treat and resistance to new antiprotozoal agents evolves rapidly and frequently.

Many protozoal infections, apart from malaria, are 'neglected diseases', with little research focused on them. In poor and remote regions, treatment with herbal medicines for protozoal diseases is commonplace, and some cases, such as amoebic dysentery, may be effective. Screening studies for antiprotozoal effects have mainly been carried on plant extracts, with active constituents and mechanisms not investigated. *Leishmania* has been studied more than most, and some active compounds are shown in Table 10.3 with mechanisms if identified.

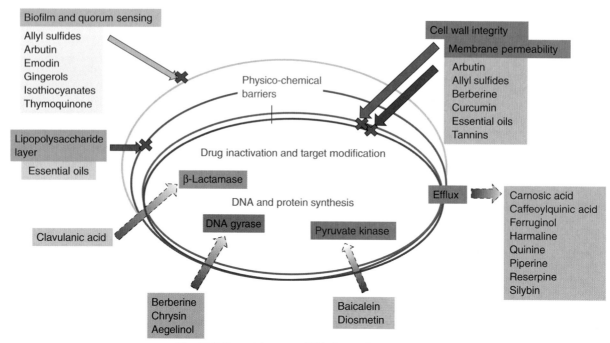

Fig. 10.9 Bacterial targets. *DNA*, Deoxyribonucleic acid.

LEISHMANIASIS

The parasite flagellates *Leishmania donovani*, *L. infantum* and *L. chagasi* are transmitted by the bite of the female sand fly. There are three types of leishmaniasis: the most dangerous is visceral leishmaniasis, also called kala-azar or black fever, characterised by oedema, fatigue, fluid in the peritoneal cavity, enlargement of the spleen, loss of weight, anaemia and greyish skin (hence the name black fever). Cutaneous leishmaniasis, or 'white leprosy' is caused by *L. major*, *L. tropica*, *L. mexicana* and *L. aethiopica* and manifests as lesions on the face, neck and limbs. Mucocutaneous leishmaniasis is caused by *L. braziliensis*, and symptoms include face deformation and damage of soft tissues, cartilage and nasal bones.

Leishmania targets that have been investigated include:
- Inhibition of parasite topoisomerases, enzymes necessary for DNA replication;
- Targeting enzymes involved in parasite metabolism including squalene synthase, cysteine proteases, methionine aminopeptidases and protein kinases;
- Disruption of parasite mitochondrial membrane, leading to cell apoptosis;
- Activation of macrophages.

Known antileishmanial compounds are shown in Table 10.3, with mechanisms identified where possible; however, information in area this sparse.

Trypanosoma cruzi causes Chagas disease and is transmitted by triatomine bugs. African trypanosomiasis (sleeping sickness) is caused by *Trypanosoma brucei gambiense* and *Trypanosoma brucei rhodesiense* and is transmitted by the tsetse fly. Both are susceptible to certain antileishmania compounds and to artemisinins but are outside the scope of this brief introduction.

MALARIA

Medicinal plants, phytochemicals, and their semisynthetic derivatives have provided the source of the most significant antimalarial drugs used today. Malaria is widespread, endemic and lethal, and it is difficult to eradicate because of drug resistance and the susceptibility of the parasite at different stages of its life cycle. Malaria is a mosquito-borne protozoal infection caused by *Plasmodium* species. Currently, five species are known: *Plasmodium falciparum*, *P. ovale*, *P. malariae*, *P. vivax* and *P. knowlesi*. When an infected female *Anopheles* mosquito ingests blood, sporozoites are injected into the host's bloodstream and rapidly reach the liver, where they infect hepatocytes and develop into liver schizonts. These divide to produce infective merozoites, which are released into the bloodstream and invade red blood cells. There they undergo several cycles of replication and develop into ring-stage parasites, which become trophozoites and then multinucleated schizonts. Schizonts produce another wave of merozoites that invade new erythrocytes, and the cycle starts again. The erythrocytic phases of the parasite cause the clinical symptoms of fever, chills and fatigue, that can lead to death.

Some of the merozoite population evolves into sexual gametocytes which are transferred to another mosquito in the blood meal. Here, they develop into gametes that reproduce sexually to form the zygote that evolves to oocyst. The oocyst liberates thousands of sporozoites that migrate to mosquito salivary glands and are injected into the next host, completing the parasite lifecycle.

In some species of *Plasmodium*, sporozoites in the liver persist as dormant forms called hypnozoites, which can reactivate to produce infective merozoites, causing malaria relapse.

Antimalarial drugs target different stages of the parasite lifecycle, with the liver stages of the disease the most difficult to eradicate. Combination therapy, using drugs which target different stages of the lifecycle, is the recommended best strategy for combatting resistance. For the treatment and prophylaxis of malaria, World Health Organization (WHO) guidelines are available which consider emerging resistance in different parts of the world.

Natural products form the basis of modern antimalarial drugs, with quinine being the first effective antiplasmodial drug. It is isolated from *Cinchona* bark and derivatives have been developed which are more potent, less toxic and less likely to lead to resistance; however, resistance is almost inevitable and has already been observed for almost all drugs in use.

TABLE 10.3 Plant Antileishmanial Compounds

Class of Compound and Example	Identified Mechanism(s)
Naphthoquinones	
Diospyrin	Interaction with parasite topoisomerase I, stabilising the enzyme–deoxyribonucleic acid (DNA) complex
Lapachol	
Plumbagin	Induction of topoisomerase II-mediated DNA cleavage
Anthraquinones	
Aloe-emodin, emodin	Activation of host macrophages
Polyphenolics	
Quercetin, luteolin	Inhibition of parasite DNA synthesis and promotion of apoptosis mediated by topoisomerase II
Licochalcone A	Inhibition of parasite mitochondrial dehydrogenases and respiratory chain
Alkaloids	
Quinoline, Isoquinoline	
Berberine, anonaine, liriodenine	Targeting mitochondrial enzymes, triggering caspase-independent cell death
Indole	
Harmaline	Intercalation with DNA, inhibition of aromatic amino acid metabolism
Iridoids	
Amarogentin	Inhibition of topoisomerase I
Sesquiterpene Lactones	
Artemisinin	Increasing messenger ribonucleic acid (mRNA) expression of iNOS, enhancing release of IFN-γ
Triterpenes	
Dihydrobetulinic acid	Targeting both DNA topoisomerases, preventing DNA cleavage and inducing apoptosis
Ursolic acid	Enhancing phagocytic activity of macrophages
18β-Glycyrrhetinic acid	Triggering of Th1 cytokine response and production of iNOS
Saponins	
Hederagenin	Disruption of parasite membrane integrity
Acetogenins	
Annonacin A	Inhibition of parasite respiratory chain

IFN-γ, Interferon gamma; *iNOS*, inducible nitric oxide synthase; *Th1*, type 1 T helper.

An overview of the mosquito lifecycle is shown in Fig. 10.10, with targets for current antimalarial drugs, and Table 10.4 shows the most important currently used antimalarial drugs and their natural product origins.

Traditional medicines for malaria are still widely used and investigated for their additional affects and future molecular leads; for more detail, see Further Reading.

The most significant of these to date are sweet wormwood, cinchona bark and lapacho.

Sweet Wormwood (Qinghaou), *Artemisia annua* L.

Artemisia annua L. (Asteraceae) has been used for thousands of years in China for fevers and disorders of the liver. The discovery of artemisinin as an antimalarial marks a milestone in natural product research, and, in 2015, the achievements of Prof. Youyou Tu (China) were rewarded with the Nobel Prize in Medicine/Physiology. Derivatives of artemisinin are the most recent antimalarials to be introduced to treat multiple drug-resistant strains of *P. falciparum* malaria.

Constituents

The herb contains sesquiterpene lactones, the most important of which is artemisinin (qinghaosu; Fig. 10.11), as well as the arteannuins A–O, artemisitine, artemisinic acid, hydroarteannuin and others. There is also a volatile oil-containing artemisia ketone, cadinene and others, and flavonoids including artemetin.

Therapeutic Uses

Artemisinin is one of the most rapidly acting antiplasmodial compounds known. Several more stable and effective derivatives, such as artemether, arteether and artesunate, have been developed and are being used clinically for both the prophylaxis and treatment of malaria. There is evidence that the whole extract of the aerial parts may be superior to isolated artemisinin because the flavonoids have been linked to inhibition of CYP450 enzymes responsible for the metabolism of artemisinin in the body.

Cinchona, *Cinchona* Spp.

Bark from the trees of the genus *Cinchona* (Rubiaceae) is used as a source of quinine (Fig. 10.12). Red cinchona, *C. pubescens* Vahl (syn.: *C. succirubra* Pav. ex Klotzsch); yellow cinchona, *C. calisaya* Wedd. and other species and hybrids are used. Originally called Peruvian bark, from the country of origin, and Jesuit's bark because it was originally introduced into Europe by Jesuit missionaries, its journey to becoming a widely used global medicine is fascinating (see Chapter 6). Native to mountainous regions of tropical America, it is now cultivated in South-East Asia and parts of Africa. The external surface of the bark is brownish grey, usually fissured, with characteristic greyish-white or greenish patches due to the presence of epiphyte lichens and mosses.

Constituents

The actives are fluorescent quinoline alkaloids, the major being quinine (see Fig. 10.12), with quinidine, cinchonine, cinchonidine, epi- and hydro-derivatives of these, quinamine and others. The total alkaloid content of the bark should be not less than 6.5%, with 30%–60% being of the quinine type.

Therapeutic Uses

The bark was formerly used as a febrifuge, tonic, orexigenic, spasmolytic and astringent, but it is only used now for the extraction of the alkaloids. Both quinine and quinidine have antimalarial activity, and both are cardiac antiarrhythmic agents, which limits their usefulness as antimalarials. Quinine salts were formerly used for the prevention of night cramps and in low doses is an ingredient of some analgesic and cold and flu remedies. Chronic overdosage can result in the condition known as cinchonism, which is characterised by headache, abdominal pain, rashes and visual disturbances.

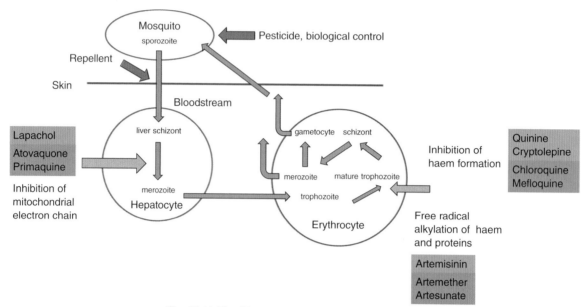

Fig. 10.10 The *Plasmodium* lifecycle and drug targets.

TABLE 10.4	Plant Compounds That Have Provided Leads for Drug Development		
Compound	**Semisynthetic Derivatives**	**Skeleton Type**	**Mechanism**
Artemisinin	Artemether, artesunate, dihydroartemisinin	Sesquiterpene lactone endoperoxide	Free radical alkylation of haem and proteins
Lapachol	Atovaquone	Naphthoquinone	Inhibition of parasite mitochondrial electron transport chain
Quinine	Chloroquine, mefloquine	4-Aminoquinoline	Bind to haem, blocking conversion of haem to haemozoin
	Primaquine, pamaquine	8-Aminoquinoline	Inhibition of mitochondrial electron chain

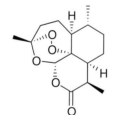

Fig. 10.11 Artemisinin.

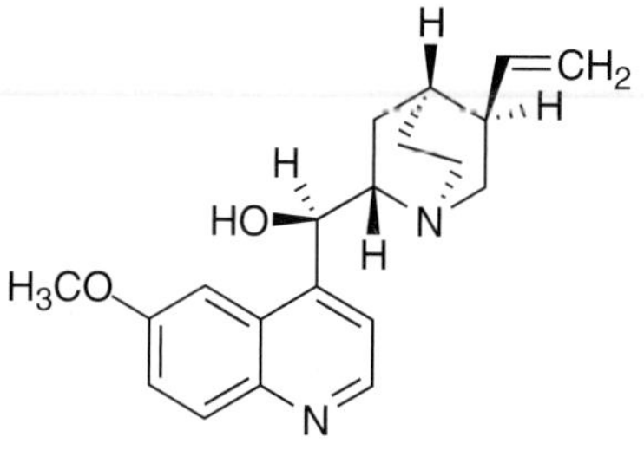

Fig. 10.12 Quinine.

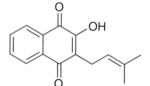

Fig. 10.13 Lapachol.

indigenous to South America. Lapacho is used traditionally for infectious diseases, including protozoal, bacterial, fungal and viral infections, to enhance immune function and for treating various cancers. Lapachol (Fig. 10.13) is antiprotozoal against *Leishmania*, *Trypanosoma* and *Schistosoma* spp., as previously discussed, as well as being antiinflammatory.

Constituents

The active constituents are naphthoquinones, the most important being lapachol (see Fig. 10.13), with deoxylapachol, α- and β-lapachone and others. It also contains AQs, benzoic acid and benzaldehyde derivatives.

Therapeutic Uses

Lapacho has cytotoxic and antitumour activities in vitro and in vivo. Semisynthetic derivatives of lapachol (see Table 10.4) have increased antiparasitic activity with reduced toxicity.

Antiviral Natural Products

A virus consists of nucleic acid (either DNA or RNA, but not both) encased in a protein coat (the capsid); some have a lipid or glycoprotein

Lapacho (Taheebo, Pau D'Arco), *Tabebuia* spp.

Lapacho is obtained from the bark of tropical trees of the genus *Handroanthus* (Bignoniaceae), including *H. impetiginosus* (Mart. ex DC.) Mattos. (syn.: *Tabebuia avellanedae* Lorentz ex Griseb.), *H. serratifolius* (Vahl) S.O. Grose (syn.: *T. serratifolia* (Vahl) G. Nicholson) and others envelope. Therefore, unlike bacteria, fungi and protozoa, there is no cellular structure and metabolic processes which can be targeted and disrupted in the same way. Viruses are not, strictly speaking, living organisms at all because they cannot generate the energy for their own metabolic processes to synthesise proteins and reproduce. Despite this, they are highly adapted parasites of the plant and animal kingdoms and a serious human health threat, and their simplicity and liability to mutation makes them difficult to kill once inside a host cell.

Antiviral effects have been described for many plant extracts; fewer investigations have been carried out for isolated phytochemicals or mechanisms of action. Plant extracts contain ubiquitous compounds which deactivate virus particles; for example, tannins complex with proteins, and therefore screening crude extracts in vitro is likely to produce many positive results but must be treated with caution.

Working with mammalian pathogenic viruses is fraught with dangers and only carried out in specialist institutions at enormous expense. Thus research is restricted to the highest priority and most urgent therapeutic options. Phytochemicals do not currently fit this pattern but may have a potential role as single or adjunctive therapies (see Chapter 21 (The Respiratory System) for a brief account of their proposed use in managing SARS-CoV-2 infection).

Antiviral Mechanisms

Viral infection involves the entry of viral RNA (vRNA) or DNA into a host cell, replication of the viral genome and releasing the new viruses. The six steps of viral replication are attachment, penetration (invasion), uncoating, replication, assembly and release and are outlined as follows and in Fig. 10.14. Antiviral drugs target different stages of infection and replication, by:

1. Inactivating extracellular virus particles
   This is also the mode of action of virucides, which may be toxic to mammalian cells if taken internally
2. Preventing attachment to the host cell membrane and/or entry
   The virus attaches to a host cell, via surface receptors CXCR4 and CCR5
3. Preventing uncoating of the virus after entry
   The virus coating (capsid) is removed, allowing release of vRNA; these processes include deproteinisation
4. Preventing replication of the viral genome
   This is the transcription phase, which converts vRNA into viral DNA (vDNA). Reverse-transcriptase, or RNA-dependent DNA-polymerase, transcribes the vRNA into vDNA, and integrase inserts this vDNA into the cellular DNA.
5. Preventing synthesis of new viral proteins including DNA
   This is the translation phase, involving enzymes including proteases, DNA polymerases, helicases and many others.
6. Inhibiting assembly of new viruses and preventing release
   The host cell releases the newly created viruses, either through the breakage of the cell (cell death) or by budding off through the cell membrane. Neuraminidase enzyme inhibits binding of virion to host cell, allowing release and spread.

Interferons are produced by the host cell in response to infection and their stimulation be part of the mode of action of an antiviral: they upregulate genes involved in the immune response and increase host resistance.

These processes are well beyond the scope of this book but are summarised in Fig. 10.14, which shows a highly simplified scheme of how a virus enters a cell and replicates itself and is released to infect further mammalian cells. Targets for antiviral therapies and the drugs which act at them, and natural products with effects at these targets, are shown. Because this field is relatively new, these are not comprehensive but illustrate enzymes and processes which have been shown to date to interact with these targets.

As is obvious, many targets have not yet been explored for their potential therapeutic applications, and phytochemicals have not been subjected to many studies at all: some are illustrated in Table 10.5.

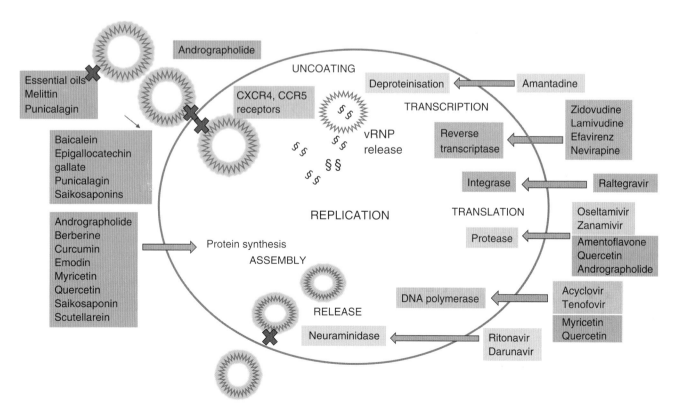

Fig. 10.14 Viral cell entry and drug targets. *DNA*, Deoxyribonucleic acid.

TABLE 10.5 Phytochemicals With Antiviral Effects

Compound	Antiviral Effects Reported	Mechanism of Action
Amentoflavone	SARS-CoV	SARS-CoV 3CL protease inhibitor
Andrographolide	DENV, influenza, HBV, HCV, HSV1, EBV, HIV, SARS-CoV	Inhibits attachment via CXCR4, CCR5
Baicalin	EV 71, DENV, HBV, influenza, RSV	Impedes viral adsorption onto the host cell; inhibits viral replication post entry
Berberine	DENV, EV-71, HBV, HCV, influenza, RSV, ZIKV	Reduces viral RNA and protein synthesis, via numerous signalling pathways (JNK, PI3KIII, AKT signalling)
Chebulagic acid	HSV-1, RSV	Inactivates free virus particles; interferes with binding and post-infection spread
Curcumin	Influenza, HBV, HCV, ZIKV, NOR, HIV, HPV, hCMV, EV71, DENV-2	Inhibits HCV replication via suppressing Akt-SREBP-1 pathway
Emodin	HBV, HSV-1 SARS-CoV	Inhibits DNA replication of HBV inhibits alkaline nuclease activity of HSV-1, blocks interaction of SARS-CoV spike protein with angiotensin-converting enzyme-2
Epigallocatechin gallate	EV 71, HCV	Interferes with viral replication. inhibits viral entry
Meliacine	HSV-2	Induces TNF-α and IFN-γ production
Melittin	HIV-1	Inactivates virus through disruption of the lipid envelope
Myricetin	HIV, influenza, SARS-CoV	DNA helicase inhibitor
Punicalagin	HSV-1, RSV	Inactivates free virus particles; interferes with binding and post-infection spread
Quercetin	JEV, influenza A, EBV, RV, HCV	Inhibits viral replication but not viral attachment and entry
Saikosaponins A, B2, C, D	HBV, HCoV-229E	Inhibits attachment and penetration Saikosaponin C inhibits HBV DNA replication
Scutellarein	SARS-CoV	DNA helicase inhibitor
Silymarin	HCV	Enhancement of the IFN-associated JAK-STAT pathway
Tellimagrandin I	HCV	Penetration inhibitor

AKT, Protein kinase B; *DENV*, dengue virus; *EBV*, Epstein–Barr; *EV 71*, enterovirus 71; *FMDV*, foot and mouth disease; *HBV*, hepatitis B; *hCMV*, human cytomegalovirus; *HCoV-229E*, human coronavirus 229E; *HCV*, hepatitis C; *HIV*, human immunodeficiency virus; *HPV*, human papilloma virus; *HSV*, herpes simplex; *IFN-γ*, interferon gamma; *JAK-STAT*, Janus kinase-signal transducer and activator of transcription; *JEV*, Japanese encephalitis virus; *JNK*, c-Jun N-terminal kinase; *MV*, measles; *NOR,* Norovirus; *RSV*, respiratory syncytial virus; *RV,* Rhinovirus; *SARS-CoV*, coronavirus; *SREBP*, sterol regulatory element binding protein; *TNF-α*, tumour necrosis factor α; *VZV*, varicella zoster; *ZIKV*, Zika virus.

Antiviral Herbal Medicines

Traditional herbal medicines with some clinical evidence to support their use are summarised as follows: the best known include *Andrographis paniculata, Sambucus nigra* and *Pelargonium* spp. These are widely used in upper respiratory viral infections, such as colds and influenza, and are discussed in Chapter 21. The active constituents of *Andrographis*, andrographolide and its derivatives, have been extensively studied for their antiviral mechanisms and several identified (see Table 10.5). The active compounds in *Sambucus* and *Pelargonium* are polyphenolics such as flavonoids and anthocyanins.

The isoquinoline alkaloids such as berberine (Fig. 10.2) are present in medicinal plants traditionally used to treat viral infections (particularly hepatitis); these include *Berberis* spp., *C. chinensis, Hydrastis canadensis, Phellodendron* spp. and *Chelidonium majus.* Berberine has many antimicrobial effects (see earlier), making it a potentially useful but complicated therapy option due to its other pharmacological properties.

AQs, including the hypericins, found in St John's wort, *Hypericum perforatum* (used as an antidepressant, see Chapter 22) and emodin (see Fig. 10.8), which has already been described for its other antimicrobial effects, have well-documented antiviral properties and are being further explored for their potential.

FURTHER READING

NB: This section is extended to provide an entry into this vast and complex field.

Ayaz, M., Ullah, F., Sadiq, A., Ullah, F., Ovais, M., Ahmed, J., et al., 2019. Synergistic interactions of phytochemicals with antimicrobial agents: potential strategy to counteract drug resistance. Chem. Biol. Interact. 308, 294–303.

Ben-Shabat, S., Yarmolinsk, L., Porat, D., Dahan, A., 2020. Antiviral effect of phytochemicals from medicinal plants: applications and drug delivery strategies. Drug Deliv. Transl. Res. 10, 354–367.

Berillo, D., Kozhahmetova, M., Lebedeva, L., 2022. Overview of the biological activity of anthraquinones and flavanoids of the plant *Rumex* species. Molecules 27 (4), 1204. https://doi.org/10.3390/molecules27041204.

Cui, X., Lü, Y., Yue, C., 2021. Development and research progress of anti-drug resistant bacteria drugs. Infect. Drug Resist. 14, 5575–5593. https://doi.org/10.2147/IDR.S338987.

Dong, X., Zeng, Y., Liu, Y., You, L., Yin, X., Fu, J., et al., 2020. Aloe-emodin: a review of its pharmacology, toxicity, and pharmacokinetics. Phytother Res. 34 (2), 270–281. https://doi.org/10.1002/ptr.6532.

Fernandez-Alvaro, E., Hong, W.D., Nixon, G., O'Neill, P.M., Calderón, F., 2016. Antimalarial chemotherapy: natural product inspired development of preclinical and clinical candidates with diverse mechanisms of action. J. Med. Chem. 59, 5587–5603.

Ferreira, J.F., Luthria, D.L., Sasaki, T., Heyerick, A., 2010. Flavonoids from *Artemisia annua* L. as antioxidants and their potential synergism with artemisinin against malaria and cancer. Molecules 15 (5), 3135–3170.

Ghodsian, S., Taghipour, N., Deravi, N., Behniafar, H., Lasjerdi, Z., 2020. Recent researches in effective antileishmanial herbal compounds: narrative. Parasitol. Res. 19, 3929–3946.

Gibbons, S., 2008. Phytochemicals for bacterial resistance – strengths, weaknesses and opportunities. Planta Med. 74, 594–602.

Gómez Castellanos, J.R., Prieto, J.M., Heinrich, M., 2009. Red Lapacho (*Tabebuia impetiginosa*) – a global ethnopharmacological commodity? J. Ethnopharmacol. 121 (1), 1–13.

Hoste, H., Torres-Acosta, J.F.J., Sandoval-Castro, C.A., Mueller-Harvey, I., Sotiraki, S., Louvandini, H., et al., 2015. Tannin-containing legumes as a model for nutraceuticals against digestive parasites in livestock. Vet. Parasitol. 212 (1–2), 5–17.

Jiang, M., Sheng, F., Zhang, Z., Ma, X., Gao, T., Fu, C., et al., 2021. *Andrographis paniculata* (Burm.f.) Nees and its major constituent andrographolide as potential antiviral agents. J. Ethnopharmacol. 272, 113954. https://doi.org/10.1016/j.jep.2021.113954.

Jothi, R., Hari, P.N., Gowrishankar, S., Pandian, S.K., 2021. Bacterial quorum-sensing molecules as promising natural inhibitors of *Candida albicans* virulence dimorphism: an in silico and in vitro study. Front. Cell. Infect. Microbiol. 11, 781790.

Khameneh, B., Eskin, N.A.M., Iranshahy, M., Fazly Bazzaz, B.S., 2021. Phytochemicals: a promising weapon in the arsenal against antibiotic-resistant bacteria. Antibiotics (Basel) 10 (9), 1044. https://doi.org/10.3390/antibiotics10091044.

Klongsiriwet, C., Quijarda, J., Williams, A.R., Mueller-Harvey, I., Williamson, E.M., Hoste, H., 2015. Synergistic inhibition of *Haemonchus contortus* exsheathment by flavonoid monomers and condensed tannins. Int. J. Parasitol Drugs. Drug Resist. 5 (3), 127–134.

Kumar, A., Ekavali., Chopra, K., Mukherjee, M., Pottabathini, R., Dhull, D.K., 2015. Current knowledge and pharmacological profile of berberine: an update. Eur. J. Pharmacol. 761, 288–297.

Li, J., Liu, D., Tian, X., Koseki, S., Chen, S., Ye, X., et al., 2019. Novel antibacterial modalities against methicillin resistant *Staphylococcus aureus* derived from plants. Crit. Rev. Food Sci. Nutr. 59 (Suppl. 1), S153–S161.

Lin, L.T., Hsu, W.C., Lin, C.C., 2014. Antiviral natural products and herbal medicines. J. Trad. Complement. Med. 4, 24–35.

Ma, C., He, N., Zhao, Y., Xia, D., Wei, J., Kang, W., 2019. Antimicrobial mechanism of hydroquinone. Appl. Biochem. Biotechnol. 189 (4), 1291–1303.

Marchese, A., Barbieri, R., Sanchez-Silva, A., Daglia, M., Nabavi, S.F., Jafari, N.J., et al., 2016. Antifungal and antibacterial activities of allicin: a review. Trends Food Sci. Technol. 52, 49–56.

Morais, M.C., Souza, J.V., da Silva Maia Bezerra Filho, C., Dolabella, S.S., Sousa, D.P., 2020. Trypanocidal essential oils: a review. Molecules 25, 4568. https://doi.org/10.3390/molecules25194568.

Munita, J.N., Arias, C.A., 2016. Mechanisms of antibiotic resistance. Microbiol. Spectr. 4 (2). https://doi.org/10.1128/microbiolspec.

Nass, J., Efferth, T., 2018. The activity of Artemisia spp. and their constituents against trypanosomiasis. Phytomedicine 47, 184–191.

Newman, D.J., Cragg, G.M., 2020. Plant endophytes and epiphytes: burgeoning sources of known and 'unknown' cytotoxic and antibiotic agents. Planta Med. 86, 891–905.

Pugh, N.D., Jackson, C.R., Pasco, D.S., 2013. Total bacterial load within *Echinacea purpurea*, determined using a new PCR-based quantification method, is correlated with LPS levels and in vitro macrophage activity. Planta Med. 79 (01), 9–14.

Pugh, N.D., Tamta, H., Balachandran, P., Wu, X., Howell, J., Dayan, F.E., et al., 2008. The majority of in vitro macrophage activation exhibited by extracts of some immune enhancing botanicals is due to bacterial lipoproteins and lipopolysaccharides. Int. Immunopharmacol. 8, 1023–1032.

Reygaert, W.C., 2018. An overview of the antimicrobial resistance mechanisms of bacteria. Microbiology 4 (3), 482–501.

Romeo, L., Iori, R., Rollin, P., Bramanti, P., Mazzon, E., 2018. Isothiocyanates: an overview of their antimicrobial activity against human infections. Molecules 23 (3), 624. https://doi.org/10.3390/molecules23030624.

Semwal, R.B., Semwal, D.K., Combrinck, S., Viljoen, A., 2021. Emodin – a natural anthraquinone derivative with diverse pharmacological activities. Phytochemistry 1 (190), 112854. https://doi.org/10.1016/j.phytochem.2021.112854.

Stermitz, F.R., Lorenz, P., Tawara, J.N., Zenewicz, L.A., Lewis, K., 2000. Synergy in a medicinal plant: antimicrobial action of berberine potentiated by 5′-methoxyhydnocarpin, a multidrug pump inhibitor. Proc. Natl. Acad. Sci. (U. S. A) 97 (4), 1433–1437.

Tajuddeen, N., Van Heerden, F.R., 2019. Antiplasmodial natural products: an update. Malar. J. 18 (1), 404.

Tariq, S., Wani, S., Rasool, W., Shafi, K., Bhat, M.A., Prabhakar, A., et al., 2019. A comprehensive review of the antibacterial, antifungal and antiviral potential of essential oils and their chemical constituents against drug-resistant microbial pathogens. Microb. Pathog. 134, 103580. https://doi.org/10.1016/j.micpath.2019.103580.

Tu, Y., 2016. Artemisinin – a gift from traditional Chinese medicine to the world (Nobel Lecture). Angew. Chem. 55 (35), 10210–10226.

Ungogo, M.A., Ebiloma, G.U., Ichoron, N., Igoli, J.O., de Koning, H.P., Balogun, E.O., 2020. A review of the antimalarial, antitrypanosomal, and antileishmanial activities of natural compounds isolated from Nigerian flora. Front. Chem. 8, 617448.

Waditzer, M., Bucar, F., 2021. Flavonoids as inhibitors of bacterial efflux pumps. Molecules 26 (22), 6904. https://doi.org/10.3390/molecules26226904.

Warowicka, A., Nawrot, R., Goździcka-Józefiak, A., 2020. Antiviral activity of berberine. Arch. Virol. 165, 1935–1945.

Wright, C., 2007. Recent developments in naturally derived antimalarials: cryptolepine analogues. J. Pharm. Pharmacol. 59, 899–904.

Zeng, B., Wei, A., Zhou, Q., Yuan, M., Lei, K., Liu, Y., et al., 2022. Andrographolide: a review of its pharmacology, pharmacokinetics, toxicity and clinical trials and pharmaceutical researches. Phytother Res. 36 (1), 336–364.

SECTION 4

Herbal Medicinal Products

11

The Complex Pharmacology of Herbal Medicines

Herbal medicines are complex mixtures of phytochemicals, even if composed of only one plant species, and the preparation, whether as the dried or processed herb, an extract or finished herbal product (defined in Chapter 12, Table 12.1), influences the composition of the herbal medicine and thus its therapeutic properties.

The spectrum of botanical products ranges from 'health' foods, nutraceuticals and herbal supplements composed of benign and innocuous compounds, to more potent herbal medicines; some contain toxic compounds and should not be used (see Chapter 13). Highly potent drugs (e.g. anticancer natural products, see Chapter 9) are used as single chemical entities since the dose needs to be very precise. These isolated compounds from plant species are not usually considered to be herbal drugs.

Interactions between constituents of herbal mixtures, especially in traditional formulae, are expected and considered positive, enhancing efficacy, and reducing the incidence and severity of side effects. Conversely, 'incompatible' herbal combinations are documented in many traditions, based on disease theory and empirical experience. The same principles and mechanisms apply to all interactions, whether relating to herbal or synthetic drugs, as discussed in Chapter 14.

If the active principles (constituents) of herbal medicines are generally considered safe, the natural mixture found in a plant extract may have benefits conferred by the presence of a range of components. Although many extracts are characterised phytochemically, their mechanisms of action are complex and some still unknown. Increasingly, extracts of known composition (standardised to a range, or more than one class of compounds) are designated the 'active pharmaceutical ingredient (API)' and used in clinical and preclinical research, in the same way as is a single-entity drug.

MEASURING SYNERGISTIC, ADDITIVE AND ANTAGONISTIC EFFECTS

Constituents in a herbal medicine may interact with several different pharmacologic targets, as well as each other, in a complex network. Herbal medicine has been described as the 'herbal shotgun' approach, as opposed to the 'silver bullet' of conventional medicine.

The general understanding of synergy is that it is an effect seen by a combination of substances which is greater than would have been expected from a consideration of individual contributions. The combination index (CI) and isobole methods are commonly used for identifying synergy, and systems biology for investigating multitarget synergy (Williamson, 2001; Wagner & Ulrich-Merzenich, 2009; Zhou et al., 2016).

The Combination Index (CI)

This is a quantitative determination of synergistic effects: a CI less than 1 indicates synergy, a CI equal to 1 indicates an additive effect and a CI

greater than 1 indicates antagonism. It is the most conclusive and practical method for demonstrating synergy and has no limitations regarding the number of ingredients in the tested combination. However, it requires determination of the dose responses of each individual constituent and the combination.

The Isobole Method

An old and established method, this is independent of the mechanism of action of the agents. An isobole is an 'iso-effect' curve, in which a combination of ingredients (d_a, d_b) is represented by a point on a graph, the axes of which are the dose axes of the individual agents (D_a and D_b). If there is no interaction, the isobole (the line joining the points representing the combination to those on the dose axes representing the individual doses with the same effect as the combination) will be a straight line. If synergy is present, the dose of the combination needed to produce the same effect will be less than that for the individual components and the curve will be 'concave up'. The opposite applies for antagonism, which produces a 'concave down' isobole, as shown in Fig. 11.1. It is most suited to two-component mixtures, especially compounds in the same plant.

SINGLE-HERB PREPARATIONS

Individual herbs with multiple pharmacological effects are often used alone, especially in modern phytotherapy and for self-medication. Interaction between constituents is still expected and has been documented in many herbs. Determination of synergy between components of a mixture is time-consuming and not carried out routinely to prove efficacy. For regulation and patent protection, it is more important to justify the safety and efficacy of the API, but there are published reports of synergy being shown for specific multiherb preparations.

Ginkgo, *Ginkgo biloba* L.

The constituents of ginkgo have complementary as well as synergistic effects. For example, the terpene lactones (ginkgolides) are platelet-activating factor (PAF) antagonists, a mechanism of antiinflammatory activity, with a synergistic interaction between them. The ginkgoflavones have an effect on the overall activity: they are also antiinflammatory; the combination being considered additive and possibly synergistic in increasing blood circulation to the brain. Ginkgo extracts are usually standardised to both terpene lactone and ginkgoflavone content (see Chapter 12, Fig. 12.6.1). Clinical studies have shown ginkgo to be effective in improving cognitive function and, when taken in combination with other herbal preparations such as ginseng (*Panax ginseng* C.A. Mey.), ginkgo also shows synergistic-like interactions (Scholey & Kennedy, 2002).

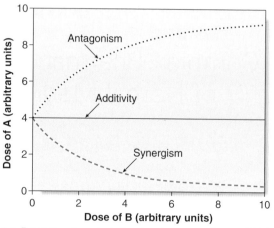

Fig. 11.1 Example of an isobole showing synergism, additivity and antagonism.

Cannabis, *Cannabis* sativa L.

Cannabis extracts and isolated constituents, notably cannabidiol (CBD) and tetrahydrocannabinol (THC), have potential as therapeutic agents in chronic conditions, such as rheumatoid arthritis, infection, multiple sclerosis and others. Extensive pharmacological research has been carried out on isolated cannabinoids and characterised herbal extracts (reviewed by Bonini et al., 2018; Pisanti & Bifulco, 2019), with extracts showing qualitative and quantitative differences in effect to that of isolated cannabinoids (e.g. Wilkinson et al., 2003). The presence of CBD in an extract can modify the effects of THC, for example, by attenuating the anxiogenic effects produced by THC alone; the ratio of THC to CBD is carefully controlled in licensed cannabis products, according to therapeutic indication, and forms the basis of the API of each product.

CBD has become an option for treating a range of conditions, the most important being intractable epilepsy in children, and as an adjunctive therapy with other antiepileptics. It is a subject of intense interest for other applications, including topical use for inflammatory skin conditions, such as psoriasis and eczema.

The constituents of cannabis interact with multiple targets: THC binds to cannabinoid receptors (CBRs) 1 and 2: modulation of CBR 1 confers psychoactive effects, and with CBR 2 mediates inflammatory and immune responses, although both are involved in many other pathways. However, CBD has very low affinity for both CBR 1 and 2, exerting its multiple effects (e.g. analgesic, antiinflammatory and behavioural) via other mechanisms. These include modulation of transient receptor potential (TRP) channels, activation of peroxisome proliferator activated receptor γ (PPARγ) and 5-hydroxytryptamine 1A (5HT1A) receptors, G protein–coupled receptor 55 (GPR55), and antagonism and inhibition of adenosine reuptake (reviewed by Williamson et al., 2020). The minor cannabinoids are being investigated for their pharmacologic properties, and cannabis holds promise for many more therapeutic developments.

Willow Bark, *Salix alba* L.

Standardised extracts of willow bark are used for the treatment of inflammatory diseases, such as osteoarthritis, and it is usually assumed that the effect is due to the salicin (and therefore salicylic acid) content. However, the gastrointestinal side effects commonly encountered with nonsteroidal antiinflammatory drugs, including aspirin, have not been seen with willow extracts and the concentration of salicin appears insufficient to explain efficacy. No effect on cyclooxygenase-1 (COX-1) has been found, but COX-2 and lipoxygenase, involved in pain and inflammation, are inhibited (reviewed by Williamson, 2001). This shows that herbal medicines do not necessarily work in the same way as isolated constituents and suggests that other constituents modify their effects.

Ispaghula, *Plantago ovata* Forssk.

Ispaghula, or psyllium husk, is effective in treating both constipation and diarrhoea. The fibre acts as a bulk laxative when taken with plenty of water and absorbs water from the intestinal lumen to reduce diarrhoea if taken with minimal liquid. However, ispaghula may be more effective in chronic constipation than are other types of fibre due to the presence of gut-stimulating constituents, mediated partly through cholinergic activation. Ispaghula also contains antiamoebic constituents, supporting its traditional use in dysentery (Gilani & Rahman, 2005).

Ispaghula has also been shown to improve glycaemic control in patients with type 2 diabetes (Gibb et al., 2015), again attributed to the fibre content, which delays the absorption of dietary carbohydrates from the gut.

Liquorice, *Glycyrrhiza* Species

Liquorice root is used in many systems of medicine and has a wide range of therapeutic indications, particularly inflammatory conditions, mediated via multiple pathways and constituents. Whole extracts of liquorice inhibit angiogenesis, granuloma formation and fluid exudation in inflammation, as does isoliquiritin, whereas glycyrrhizin and glycyrrhetinic acid tend to promote angiogenesis. The isolated flavonoids inhibit COX and lipoxygenase, and glycyrrhizin attenuates Lipopolysaccharide (LPS)-induced acute lung injury by inhibiting COX-2 and inducible nitric oxide synthase expression (reviewed by Hosseinzadeh & Nassiri-Asl, 2015; Williamson, 2001). The chemical standards for liquorice, the processed root and extracts intended for different purposes, including flavouring, are slightly different and are reflected in pharmacopoeial monographs for quality control (see Fig. 12.9).

MULTIHERB PREPARATIONS

In traditional medicine systems, medicinal plants are often combined according to empirical observation as well as ancient principles, with some combinations supported by more recent evidence. In Ayurveda, long pepper (*Piper longum* L.) and black pepper (*Piper nigrum* L.) are added to many formulae, and the constituent alkaloid piperine has many useful pharmacological activities (antiinflammatory, antiallergic, digestive) that can add to the effects of the other ingredients in the formula. Piperine also increases the bioavailability of other drugs by enhancing absorption via modulation of the drug transporter P-glycoprotein and inhibition of cytochrome P450 (CYP-450) drug-metabolising enzymes (Najar et al., 2010). It is often formulated with turmeric, to enhance the bioavailability of curcumin in antiinflammatory products.

Assessing multifactorial effects in mixed formulae is being addressed in the studying of interactions in traditional Chinese medicine multiingredient herbal formulations. A pragmatic approach is to link published preclinical and clinical evidence showing a rationale for the inclusion of each medicinal plant in the formula, with new targeted pharmacologic tests relevant to the therapeutic indication. In the case of the Chinese herbal medicine PHY 906, an adjunctive agent used in cancer chemotherapy, each plant ingredient was shown to contribute to the overall effect, which was to enhance efficacy and reduce side effects of conventional treatment (Liu & Cheng, 2012). A study on the fixed herbal combination STW5 (Iberogast), used to treat irritable

---

BOX 11.1   A strategy for examining synergistic and other interactions: the example of Iberogast, a 9-herb formula for irritable bowel syndrome and functional dyspepsia

A. Summary of the Contribution of Individual Herbs in the Formula STW5 (Iberogast)

Herb	EFFECTS IN PRECLINICAL GASTROINTESTINAL STUDIES				
	Acid regulation	Mucosal protection	Inflammation	Spasmolytic effects	Gastric emptying
Iberis amara	▓				▓
Melissa officinalis			▓	▓	
Matricaria recutita	▓	▓	▓		
Carum carvi		▓	▓	▓	▓
Mentha piperita	▓			▓	
Angelica archangelica		▓			▓
Chelidonium majus	▓			▓	▓
Silybum marianum			▓		
Glycyrrhiza glabra	▓	▓			

B. Synergy Between Specific Extracts

Synergistic, antagonistic and additive interactions in two *in vitro* models: inhibition of release of interleukin-8 (IL-8) in human oesophageal epithelial cells, an indicator of antiinflammatory effects, and release of Ca^{2+} in intestinal smooth muscle cells, a marker for gastric motility. Inflammation was induced with capsaicin.

Herbal ingredient	Inhibition of IL-8 release	Stimulation of Ca^{2+} release
Whole extract	▓	▓
Carum carvi + Angelica archangelica	▓	
Silybum marianum + other partners	▓	
Melissa officinalis		▓

Note:

Shaded areas denote activity

- Inhibition of Il-8 release shown by the whole mixture STW5, with *Silybum marianum* the most important partner for IL-8 reduction. *Angelica archangelica* with *Carum carvi* showed synergism.
- Stimulation of Ca^{2+}-release shown by mixture STW5, whereas only *Melissa officinalis* showed activity alone
- The original investigation was more complicated than implied here, with other interesting interactions and apparent contradictions (see Ulrich-Merzenich et al, 2019)

Modified from Ulrich-Merzenich, G., Welslau, L., Aziz-Kalbhenn, H. et al. Synergy quantifications to identify individual contributions of combination partners to the overall activity - the example of STW 5. *Phytomedicine* 60 (July):153013.

---

bowel syndrome and functional dyspepsia, identified synergistic interactions between medicinal plant ingredients and pharmacological effects which complement each other, and is shown as an example in Box 11.1 (adapted from Ulrich-Merzenich et al., 2019).

IMPLICATIONS OF MULTIFACTORIAL EFFECTS

- **Identification of actives**

Extraction of medicinal plants with a view to finding the chemical compound(s) responsible for the effects may lead to inconclusive results for several reasons. If a combination of substances is needed for the effect, then bioassay-led investigation, which narrows activity down to a fraction and, eventually, a single compound, is unlikely to yield useful results. A clinically successful Chinese formula, used to treat eczema in children, was investigated phytochemically and

pharmacologically; however, activity was lost during the fractionation procedure and was only present with the mixture (reviewed by Williamson, 2001).

- **Unstable constituents**

Other components present, which may include antioxidants, may 'protect' the actives from decomposition. This is thought to occur with valerian (*Valeriana* spp.), garlic (*Allium sativum* L.), ginger (*Zingiber officinale* Roscoe) and hops (*Humulus lupulus* L.).

- **Unknown active constituents**

For some herbs, even those that are widely used, the actives may not have been completely identified. This is in fact very common and, as can be seen from the example of liquorice discussed earlier, even for medicinal plants with a very long history of use. Examples include chasteberry (*Vitex agnus-castus* L.), passionflower (*Passiflora incarnata* L.) and hawthorn (*Crataegus* spp.).

- **A range of actives identified**

It is unusual for a plant to contain only one active constituent. Even in cannabis, where there is only one significant psychoactive ingredient, its effects are modified by the presence of other constituents. This is reflected in the analytical methods used in pharmacopoeial monographs to ensure quality, as discussed in Chapter 12.

Systems Biology

Computational and mathematical modelling, based on experimental data, is used for predicting and understanding networks of components and protein/gene targets. It requires large data sets of chemical, genetic and pharmacological data and generates information on potential targets and metabolites of the herbal ingredients. It is a powerful research tool for investigating mechanisms of action of combinations and identifying key active components, prodrugs and novel targets and is being particularly applied to Chinese herbal medicine (e.g. Cai et al., 2018).

REFERENCES

Bonini, S.A., Premoli, M., Tambaro, S., Kumar, A., Maccarinelli, G., Memo, M., et al., 2018. *Cannabis sativa*: a comprehensive ethnopharmacological review of a medicinal plant with a long history. J. Ethnopharmacol. 227, 300–315.

Cai, F.F., Zhou, W.J., Wu, R., Su, S.B., 2018. Systems biology approaches in the study of Chinese herbal formulae. Chin. Med. 13, 65. https://doi.org/10.1186/s13020-018-0221-x. PMID: 30619503.

Gibb, R.D., McRorie Jr., J.W., Russell, D.A., Hasselblad, V., D'Alessio, D.A., 2015. Psyllium fiber improves glycemic control proportional to loss of glycemic control: a meta-analysis of data in euglycemic subjects, patients at risk of type 2 diabetes mellitus, and patients being treated for type 2 diabetes mellitus. Am. J. Clin. Nutr. 102 (6), 1604–1614.

Gilani, A.H., Rahman, A.U., 2005. Trends in ethnopharmacology. J. Ethnopharmacol. 100 (1–2), 43–49.

Hosseinzadeh, H., Nassiri-Asl, M., 2015. Pharmacological effects of *Glycyrrhiza* spp. and its bioactive constituents: update and review. Phytother. Res. 29 (12), 1868–1886.

Liu, S.H., Cheng, Y.C., 2012. Old formula, new Rx: the journey of PHY906 as cancer adjuvant therapy. J. Ethnopharmacol. 140 (3), 614–623.

Najar, I.A., Sachin, B.S., Sharma, S.C., Satti, N.K., Suri, K.A., Johri, R.K., 2010. Modulation of P-glycoprotein ATPase activity by some phytoconstituents. Phytother. Res. 24 (3), 454–458.

Pisanti, S., Bifulco, M., 2019. Medical cannabis: a plurimillennial history of an evergreen. J. Cell. Physiol. 239, 8342–8351.

Scholey, A.B., Kennedy, D.O., 2002. Acute, dose-dependent cognitive effects of *Ginkgo biloba, Panax ginseng* and their combination in healthy young volunteers: differential interactions with cognitive demand. Hum. Psychopharmacol. 17 (1), 35–44.

Ulrich-Merzenich, G., Welslau, L., Aziz-Kalbhenn, H., Kelber, O., Shcherbakova, A., 2019. Synergy quantifications to identify individual contributions of combination partners to the overall activity – the example of STW 5. Phytomedicine 60, 153013.

Wagner, H., Ulrich-Merzenich, G., 2009. Synergy research: approaching a new generation of phytopharmaceuticals. Phytomedicine 16 (2–3), 97–110.

Wilkinson, J.D., Whalley, B.J., Baker, D., Pryce, G., Constanti, A., Gibbons, S., et al., 2003. Medicinal cannabis: is Δ-9 THC responsible for all its effects? J. Pharm. Pharmacol. 55 (2), 1687–1694.

Williamson, E.M., 2001. Synergy and other interactions in phytomedicines. Phytomedicine 8 (5), 401–409.

Williamson, E.M., Liu, X., Izzo, A.A., 2020. Trends in use, pharmacology, and clinical applications of emerging herbal nutraceuticals. Br. J. Pharmacol. 177 (6), 1227–1240. https://doi.org/10.1111/bph.14943.

Zhou, X., Seto, S.W., Chang, D., Kiat, H., Razmovski-Naumovski, V., Chan, K., et al., 2016. Synergistic effects of Chinese herbal medicine: a comprehensive review of methodology and current research. Front. Pharmacol. 7, 201.

12

Production, Quality Control and Standardisation of Herbal Medicines

PRODUCTION

Herbal drugs, extracts and preparations, as defined in Box 12.1, are sold directly to consumers or used as starting materials for the manufacture of herbal medicines. Varying degrees of extraction, refinement and standardisation are involved and need to be monitored throughout the process. Suitable standards and methods are provided by pharmacopoeial monographs.

High-quality herbal products can only be made with good-quality plant starting material. The discovery of toxic pyrrolizidine alkaloids in St John's wort (*Hypericum perforatum* L.) products in 2015, due to contamination with weeds such as *Senecio* species, illustrates this very well. Traceability is becoming increasingly important in assuring quality and starts with cultivation under Good Agricultural and Collection Practices (GACP) (see World Health Organization (WHO), 2003). Wild-collected plants are still widely used but present extra challenges of authentication and/or possible contamination with other species, in addition to concerns about sustainability and conservation. Endangered species and expensive herbs, such as wild ginseng and saffron, are even more liable to adulteration or falsification. Quality assurance monitoring continues during processing and manufacture of the herbal product according to 'Good Manufacturing Practice' (GMP) and 'Guidelines on Good Herbal Processing Practices' (GHPP) for herbal medicines (see WHO, 2007a, 2018), 'Quality Control Methods for Herbal Materials' (WHO, 2011), 'Guidelines for Assessing Quality of Herbal Medicines with Reference to Contaminants and Residues' (WHO, 2007b) and 'Guideline for Selecting Marker Substances of Herbal Origin for Quality Control of Herbal Medicines' (WHO, 2017). Each stage of the process is directed by following pharmacopoeial methods and meeting standards specified in either general or individual herbal monographs. Quality assurance extends through packaging and sale, ending with postmarketing surveillance and pharmacovigilance, as shown in Fig. 12.1. Pharmacovigilance for herbal medicinal products is discussed further in Chapter 15.

Herbal drugs may be sold loose, or in teabags, and are sometimes referred to as *crude drugs*. They are usually dried and cut, but otherwise untreated, although in traditional medicine further processing may be applied. They are used to make extracts for manufacturing other dosage forms, such as liquids, capsules, tablets and granules. These extracts are of varying degrees of chemical characterisation, as shown in Box 12.1. The extraction process and influences on composition of extracts are shown in Fig. 12.2. Pure compounds isolated from plant drugs are not considered to be herbal medicines.

Ensuring and Measuring Quality During Production: The Role of World Health Organization Guidelines and Pharmacopoeial Monographs

Contamination can be introduced to herbal medicines at any stage, from growing the crop, harvesting, and during storage, extraction, and the manufacturing process. There are many forms of adulteration, both deliberate and accidental, and these are summarised in Box 12.2.

Quality standards, usually from an official source, such as a pharmacopoeia, are applied at different stages of manufacture and are legally enforceable. They provide the means for an independent judgement as to the overall quality and apply throughout the shelf life of a product. Inclusion in a pharmacopoeia does not indicate that a substance is either safe or effective for the treatment of any disease; it gives guidance only on quality.

If the plant has been grown according to GACP, checking its botanical identity should be straightforward, and if a crop has been grown organically, and is certified as such, it is not necessary to carry out pesticide residue testing, unless contamination is suspected. This illustrates an important point: herbal material sold as being of pharmacopoeial quality does not have to be subjected to every test routinely; however, it must conform to those standards and is expected to pass the tests if carried out. Pharmacopoeial methods are accepted by regulatory authorities and, if different procedures are used to assure quality, these must be validated.

Many countries publish an official National Pharmacopoeia. The European Pharmacopoeia (Ph. Eur.) is the result of a collaboration between countries in Europe, including the United Kingdom, and all its monographs are incorporated into National Pharmacopoeias. This has the advantage of making quality control (QC) a more harmonious process throughout Europe with validated methods available to all. National Pharmacopoeias include additional herbal drugs and extracts that are only used in a particular country or region. These may be derived from Ph. Eur. herbal drugs, but occasionally the starting material is not the subject of a monograph, but as the extracts are controlled this is not deemed necessary.

Other reputable sources, such as the American Herbal Pharmacopoeial (AHP) monographs, are not official but recognised as comprehensive and well referenced.

The WHO has published monographs on medicinal plants and good practice guidelines, and pharmacopoeial tests appropriate to each stage of production are shown in Fig. 12.1. The following summary discusses these tests in the order in which they are covered in a typical herbal monograph.

Herbal Drug Names

A medicinal plant, herbal medicine or botanical product may be referred to in different terms at different stages during the long supply chain that eventually leads to the patient or consumer. This is complicated by language issues, geographical sources, local common names, medical perspectives and the reassigning of species by plant taxonomists. To harmonise definitions of herbal drugs, pharmaceutical names may be applied; these are Latin translations derived from the plant organ Table 12.1 and part or all of a species name. When used

BOX 12.1   Definitions of Herbal Drugs and Preparations

Herbal Drugs

Herbal drugs are mainly whole, fragmented or broken plants or parts of plants in an unprocessed state, usually in dried form but sometimes fresh. In this general monograph, the word 'plant' is used in the broader sense to also include algae, fungi and lichens. Certain exudates that have not been subjected to a specific treatment are also considered to be herbal drugs. Herbal drugs are precisely defined by the botanical scientific name according to the binomial system (genus, species, variety and author).

The term *herbal drug* is synonymous with the term *herbal substance* used in European Community legislation on herbal medicinal products.

Dried Herbal Drugs

Dried herbal drugs are obtained from cultivated or wild plants. Suitable collection, cultivation, harvesting, drying, fragmentation and storage conditions are essential to guarantee their quality.

Dried herbal drugs are, as far as possible, free from impurities such as soil, dust, dirt and other contaminants such as fungal, insect and other animal contaminations. They are not rotten.

Fresh Herbal Drugs

A fresh herbal drug is one that is intended to be processed into a herbal drug preparation (e.g. essential oil, juice, tincture) within a relatively short period of time after harvesting. Under these circumstances, the extensive analysis prescribed for dried herbal drugs is not appropriate, provided that processing takes place within a validated time period after harvesting.

Processed Herbal Drugs

Traditional processing methods have the potential to alter the physical characteristics and/or chemical constituents of a herbal drug. Traditional processing methods may require the addition of processing aids to the herbal drug, for example, honey, vinegar, wine, milk and salt.

Herbal Drug Preparations

Homogeneous products are obtained by subjecting herbal drugs to treatments such as extraction, distillation, expression, fractionation, purification, concentration or fermentation. Herbal drug preparations include, for example, extracts, essential oils, expressed juices, processed exudates, and herbal drugs that have been subjected to size reduction for specific applications, for example, herbal drugs cut for herbal teas or powdered for encapsulation.

Extracts

Herbal drug extracts are liquid (liquid extraction preparations), semisolid (soft extracts and oleoresins) or solid (dry extracts) preparations using suitable solvents.

Standardised extracts are adjusted to a defined content of one or more constituents with known therapeutic activity. This is achieved either by adjusting the extract with inert excipients or by blending batches of the extract.

Quantified extracts are adjusted to one or more active markers, the content of which is controlled within a limited, specified range. Adjustments are made by blending batches of the extract.

Other extracts are not adjusted to a particular content of constituents. For control purposes, one or more constituents are used as analytical markers. The minimum content for these analytical markers is given in an individual monograph.

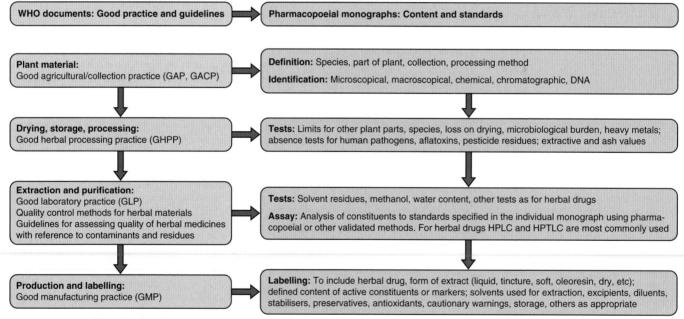

Fig. 12.1 Regulatory processes for the quality assurance of herbal drugs, extracts and preparations. *HPLC,* High-performance liquid chromatography; *HPTLC,* high-performance thin-layer chromatography.

in the context of a monograph, these titles define very precisely the species and part of plant to which the monograph refers but may not reflect the current botanical name. Although Latinised, these titles are not italicised by convention, as is the binomial scientific name, and the two should not be confused.

A comprehensive table of herbal drugs that are included in the European Pharmacopoeia is provided in the Annex, together with an explanation of terms.

Identification

Botanical identification. A pharmacopoeial monograph provides standards for botanical identification of herbal material, for the macroscopic appearance (i.e. that visible to the unaided eye or with a hand lens) and also its microscopic characteristics. Most herbal drugs are supplied in cut form, and may be difficult to identify, and in such cases, microscopy can help to confirm identity. It is also useful for powdered samples, although most powders are much more easily

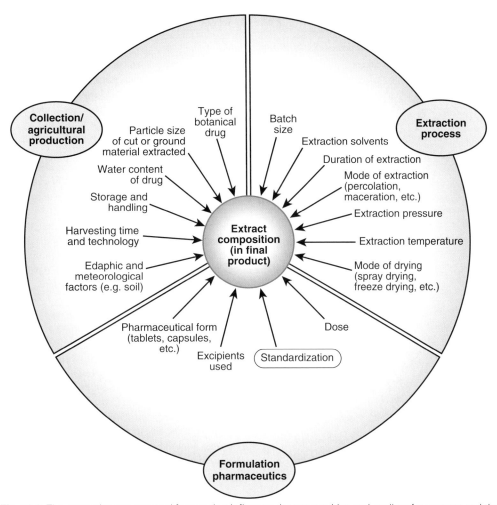

Fig. 12.2 The extraction process and factors that influence the composition and quality of an extract and the final product.

degraded and commercial trade tends to be in cut and dried samples or extracts. Microscopy is often overlooked as an analytic tool; however, with some very basic equipment and a small amount of training it is possible to gain a great deal of information quickly and easily. It is useful for picking out microcontamination, such as the presence of sand, fungal hyphae, insect parts and animal hairs, as these may be too small to see with the unaided eye but are very obvious when viewed under a microscope.

Microscopy is also useful for distinguishing from which part of a plant a powdered substance originates. It may be difficult to distinguish a leaf from a whole herb powder by just looking at it, but the botanical material can be identified because of the presence of large amounts of stem (which are limited in leaf drugs) as well as elements of the flower and seed. Pollen grains are useful for identifying medicinal plants and may also be present in good leaf samples because pollen is ubiquitous.

Plant cell structures as diagnostic features. Certain plant cell types are found in all plant tissues, for example, parenchyma, the 'basic' cell type and also xylem (water-conducting tissue), but their abundance is important. For example, bark is composed of mainly cork and phloem, with its associated parenchyma and fibres, but little xylem tissue because it has been removed from the outer surface. Heartwood contains almost only xylem elements, together with its associated parenchyma and fibres. Other cell types occur only in particular organs, for example, epidermis, trichomes (hairs, both covering and glandular) and stomata in plant parts, such as the leaf

and flower, which are in contact with the atmosphere. Cell inclusions, such as starch, are highly diagnostic of storage organs such as roots and rhizomes, as well as seeds and fruits, which often have a high content of oils and proteins. A summary of the types of cells that may be seen—or not seen—under the microscope for different plant parts is shown in Table 12.1

Examples of characteristics in powdered herbal drugs are illustrated in Figs 12.3–12.5, but this is not a comprehensive list, and there is insufficient space here to cover microscopic techniques and the diagnostic characteristics of individual herbal drugs. Further detailed information can be obtained from most pharmacopoeias, the AHP 'Microscopic Characterisation of Botanical Medicines' (Upton et al., 2011), and the classic 'Atlas of Microscopy of Medicinal Plants, Culinary Herbs and Spices', republished in 2005 and available online (Jackson & Snowden, 2005). These publications include guidelines for slide preparation and clearing and staining techniques as well as contain illustrations of powdered herbal drugs. Photographs can also be viewed in the AHP and on the websites of many pharmacopoeias.

The following overview of leaf characteristics (which are crucial for identifying herbaceous plant material), lignified tissues (which are important diagnostic features in most herbal drugs and especially barks, roots, seeds and other woody materials), and some cell inclusions illustrates the application of microscopy to identification.

Epidermis characteristics. Fragments of the epidermis indicate the presence of leaf, stem, fruit or flower parts. The epidermis is a waterproof layer of cells and contains pores (known as stomata)

BOX 12.2   How Contamination Arises and Carries Through the Production Process

Environmental growing conditions
Soil, light, rain, temperature, infection, infestation
Contamination with human pathogens (e.g. from sewage)

Harvesting
Wrong time of growing cycle, part of plant, late harvest
Excess soil or gravel in underground plant parts

Drying and storage
Fungal and microbial spoilage due to incomplete drying, including aflatoxin content
Animal and insect infestation (e.g. rodents, beetles)

Production
Use of inferior plant material (e.g. Chamomile, deteriorated flower-heads; Ginkgo, high ginkgolic acid varieties)
'Exhausted' (extracted and re-dried) (Gentian, water-soluble extractive)
Falsification, substitution with cheaper product (e.g. liquorice for ginseng, safflower for saffron)
Introduction of other components ('spiking') in natural extract (e.g. terpenes in essential oils)
Photodecomposition (e.g. essential oils, anthraquinone and cardiac glycosides)
Atmospheric oxidation (resinification of essential oils, rancidification of fatty oils)

that open and close to allow passage of air and water, which are usually more abundant on the lower surface of the leaf. The shape of the cell walls and arrangement of the cells and also the stomata are characteristics of plant families and sometimes individual species. Some epidermises have a striated waxy cuticle that can be seen as faint lines on the cell surface, and some have thickened cell walls, giving a beaded appearance. Trichomes (hairs) may be present and are useful characteristics for identifying a plant family, genus and even species. There are two types, covering and glandular trichomes, but within these types there is a wide variety of shapes and sizes, from unicellular to highly organised multicellular structures, and they may have thin or thick walls and a warty appearance. The epidermis of the flower petals (corolla) has similar structures but does not contain chlorophyll.

Some examples of microscopic leaf features that can be seen in powdered herbal leaf drugs are shown in Fig. 12.3. The trichomes and arrangement of stomata are particularly diagnostic; some are unique to one species (e.g. cannabis glandular trichomes).

Herbal drugs consisting of the whole plant or aerial parts contain more fragments of stem, flower and fruit, and more lignified tissue than leaves.

Lignified tissue. Lignified (woody) cells are present in older plants and organs that need strength to support the plant, as with stems and tree trunks, and to confer protection, as in seeds and fruits. Lignified cells include fibres that are long, narrow, tapered, thick-walled cells found in groups and adjacent to specialised cells, such as phloem and xylem, to provide strength with flexibility. In a few cases (notably ginger rhizome), the fibres are not lignified, but this is unusual. Xylem (water-conducting) elements are also usually lignified, especially in older tissues, and parenchyma cells may also become lignified through age and where extra supporting strength is required. Sclereids are thick-walled cells, and if the walls are very thick indeed, these are called stone cells. They are mainly isodiametric, but

TABLE 12.1   Plant Tissues, Organs, Exudates and Characteristic Cell Types Seen Under the Microscope

Organ	Predominant Cell Types and Contents	Absent or Sparse Tissues	Useful Diagnostic Features: Abundance and Morphology
Leaf	Epidermis, stomata, parenchyma, xylem, collenchyma, calcium oxalate	Lignified tissue, starch, protein, fat	Epidermal cell walls, arrangement of stomata, covering and glandular trichomes, cuticular striations, calcium oxalate crystals
Stem	As leaf, but with more abundant xylem, collenchyma, parenchyma, fibres and lignified tissue	Starch, protein, fat	Xylem tissue thickening and lignification, epidermis and stomata or bark, fibres, calcium oxalate crystals
Flower	Calyx and bracts: as leaf Corolla: epidermis, papillae, trichomes, secretory cells, anther, pistil, pollen grains	Starch, protein, fat	Glandular and covering trichomes, stomata, pollen. Others dependent on stage of flower and part used, for example, bud (Sophora, cloves), flowerhead (chamomile), petal (calendula), stigma (saffron)
Aerial parts 'herb'	Leaf, flower, stem, occasionally fruits or seeds	Starch, protein, fat	Epidermis and glandular trichomes of leaf and corolla, pollen, calcium oxalate crystals, fibres
Fruit and seed	Fruit pericarp, seed testa and endosperm, secretory tissue	Depending upon type, maturity, whether peeled or divided, presence of seed	Abundant starch, protein, inulin, oil, fat, trichomes of epicarp, stone cells and lignified fibres, calcium oxalate, secretory tissue, residual pollen
Bark	Cork, phloem sieve tubes, parenchyma, fibres, secretory tissue	Xylem. Peeled bark (e.g. cinnamon) has no cork layer	Starch, lignified parenchyma, fibres and stone cells, calcium oxalate crystals, secretory tissue
Root and rhizome	Cork, parenchyma, xylem, phloem, secretory tissue	Peeled root has no cork layer	Abundant starch, protein, lignified parenchyma, fibres and stone cells, calcium oxalate crystals, secretory tissue
Woods	Xylem, parenchyma, secretory tissue, calcium oxalate	Phloem, cork, starch	Exclusively xylem vessels and tracheids, and parenchyma, highly lignified
Exudates	Oleoresin, balsams, gum-resins, latex, wax	Cellular structures	Amorphous masses, may contain characteristic epidermal fragments from scraping

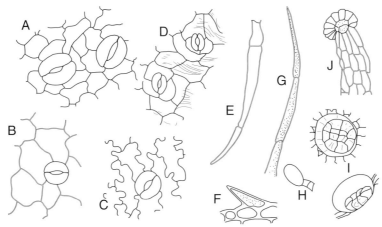

Fig. 12.3 Leaf epidermal tissues in powdered botanical drugs (varying magnifications). (A) Leaf epidermis with anomocytic stomata (i.e. no particular arrangement); (B) epidermis with thickened ('beaded') walls; (C) wavy-walled epidermis; (D) straight-walled epidermis with anisocytic stomata (i.e. one much smaller adjacent cell) and cuticular; (E) multicellular covering trichome with smooth walls; (F) unicellular conical trichome; (G) multicellular covering trichome with thick, warty walls; (H) small glandular trichome with unicellular head; (I) glandular trichome characteristic of the mint family, surface and side view; (J) unusual glandular trichome, unique to cannabis.

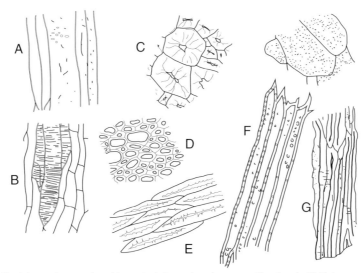

Fig. 12.4 Lignified tissue in powdered botanical drugs (varying magnifications). (A) Xylem vessels, bordered pitted; (B) xylem vessels, reticulately thickened; (C) thick-walled stone cells; (D) isodiametric stone cells from seed testa; (E) thick-walled sclereids; (F) thin-walled fibres; (G) thick-walled fibres.

sometimes with projections; for example, giving a stellate appearance. They usually occur in groups and confer hardness in a tissue without the long fracture associated with fibres (in other words, they snap rather than bend) and are very common in bark and seeds, as well as the 'stones' of soft fruit. As lignin is waterproof, they have pores or gaps in the thickening to allow passage of water and air to other parts of the organ, and these patterns of thickening may also help in identification of plant material. Lignin can be identified by staining, as explained by Upton et al. (2011) and Jackson and Snowden (2005). Some of the most common types of lignified tissue, from different medicinal plants showing their different types of thickening, are illustrated in Fig. 12.4.

Cell inclusions. Substances such as starch, calcium oxalate, protein, inulin, silica, calcium carbonate and oils and fats are stored in cells and can be used as diagnostic tools. Calcium oxalate crystals occur in various shapes and sizes: tiny particles known as microsphenoids or crystal sand; cluster or rosette crystals; needle crystals or raphides;

and prism crystals, which are often found alongside fibres as a crystal sheath (see Fig. 12.5). They can be viewed under polarised light to confirm their identity.

Starch is extremely common in plant storage organs and occurs as simple and compound grains. It can be stained with iodine solution (it goes dark blue) or viewed under polarised light, where it shows a light on dark cross pattern. Starch must be viewed before the slide is cleared to look for other cell features.

Chemical identification. The main analytical technique used is chromatographic fingerprinting using high-performance thin-layer chromatography (HPTLC) (Reich, 2007; Wagner et al., 2011). Monographs give details as to how to conduct the analysis, with descriptions and illustrations of the acceptable results. Chemical methods for identifying herbal drugs are discussed in Chapter 7.

Tests. General tests in pharmacopoeia apply to all herbal drugs, although exceptions and additional tests are introduced depending on liability to specific contamination (Box 12.3).

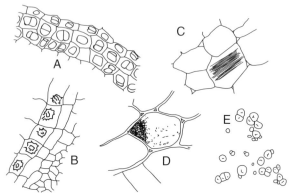

Fig. 12.5 Cell inclusions in powdered herbs (varying magnifications). (A) Calcium oxalate prisms arranged in a crystal sheath; (B) calcium oxalate cluster crystals; (C) calcium oxalate needle crystals; (D) calcium oxalate microsphenoids or crystal sand; (E) starch grains, simple and compound.

Related species may be subject to an absence test; for example, adulteration of star anise, *Illicium verum* Hook. f., with Japanese star anise, *Illicium anisatum* L., has caused deaths in infants given anise tea to soothe colic. Microscopical differentiation of species is unreliable, so a chemical test is added to show the absence of the neurotoxin anisatin.

Foreign matter (see Box 12.3) is specified in the British Pharmacopoeia (BP) and Ph. Eur. as not more than 2%, unless otherwise specified. It is measured simply by weighing 100 g to 500 g of the herbal material, spreading it out in a thin layer, examining it with the unaided eye or a lens (6× magnification), separating out foreign matter, weighing it and calculating its percentage.

Foreign inorganic matter measures the amount of dust, sand or soil present in the herbal material and is mainly applied to underground organs such as roots, rhizomes and tubers. It is measured as an *Ash value*, calculated by incinerating a sample of the herbal drug. However, plants naturally contain inorganic substances (especially calcium salts), so to differentiate these, the *Total ash* can be dissolved in weak acid, leaving the *Acid insoluble ash* as a measure of the soil and sand content.

Water content, if too high, may result in spoilage by bacteria and moulds and enzymatic degradation. It is usually measured as '*loss on drying*' or (less often) by chemical methods. For high volatile oil-containing plants (>1% oil), distillation methods are used instead.

Other tests: in some cases, usually when newer methods are unavailable, older tests are performed on specific herbal drugs. For example, the *Extractable matter* shows if herbal material has been 'exhausted' (i.e. previously extracted) and is a simple test to perform. The *Swelling index* is used for mucilage-containing herbal drugs and bulk laxatives (such as ispaghula husk), as the swelling properties are the reason for its effect. The *Bitterness value* is used for gentian and is related to its traditional use as a bitter tonic, for stimulating the appetite during debility.

BOX 12.3 Pharmacopoeial Tests Applied to Herbal Drugs, Dried and Fresh

Herbal Drugs: Tests (Abridged) (Ph. Eur. 1433; Ph. Eur. Test Methods)

Foreign matter (*2.8.2*) Carry out a test for foreign matter, unless otherwise prescribed or justified and authorised. The content of foreign matter is not more than 2% *m/m*, unless otherwise prescribed or justified and authorised. An appropriate specific test may apply to dried herbal drugs liable to be adulterated.

Loss on drying (*2.2.32*) Carry out a test for loss on drying, unless otherwise justified.

Water (*2.2.13*) A determination of water content may be carried out instead of a test for loss on drying for dried herbal drugs with a high essential-oil content.

Pesticides (*2.8.13*) Dried herbal drugs comply with the requirements for pesticide residues. The requirements take into account the nature of the plant, where necessary the preparation in which the plant might be used, and where available the knowledge of the complete treatment record of the batch of the plant.

Heavy metals (*2.4.27*) Unless otherwise stated in an individual monograph or otherwise justified:
  —*cadmium*: maximum 1.0 ppm
  —*lead*: maximum 5.0 ppm
  —*mercury*: maximum 0.1 ppm.
  Where necessary, limits for other heavy metals may be required.
  Where necessary, dried herbal drugs comply with other tests, such as the following, for example.
Total ash (*2.4.16*)
Ash insoluble in hydrochloric acid (*2.8.1*)
Extractable matter
Swelling index (*2.8.4*)
Bitterness value (*2.8.15*)
Aflatoxin B$_1$ (*2.8.18*). Where necessary, limits for aflatoxins may be required.
Ochratoxin A (*2.8.22*). Where necessary, a limit for ochratoxin A may be required.
Radioactive contamination

In some specific circumstances, the risk of radioactive contamination is to be considered.
Microbial contamination
Where a dried herbal drug is used whole, cut or powdered as an ingredient in a medicinal product, the microbial contamination is controlled (*5.1.8, 5.1.4*).

Assay
Unless otherwise justified, dried herbal drugs are assayed by an appropriate method.

Storage
Protected from light.

Fresh Herbal Drugs
A fresh herbal drug is intended to be processed (e.g. into essential oil, juice, tincture) within a short period of time after harvesting. The following analytical requirements are considered suitable, provided that processing takes place within a validated time period.
(1) For a fresh herbal drug that has been cultivated from seeds, cuttings, etc., whose origin and traceability can be demonstrated, and where the complete history from planting to harvesting is documented:
   — macroscopic identification of the plant and plant parts to be processed.
   — compliance with a suitable limit test for foreign matter.
(2) Where the information on life cycle from seed to harvesting is incomplete, the same analytical requirements apply, as well as any additional tests that may be necessary depending on potential or known quality issues.
(3) For wild-crafted herbal drugs, the analytical requirements should be assessed depending on the ease of identification and potential adulterants, as well as the method of processing.

When handling and processing fresh herbal drugs, it is necessary to ensure, by visual inspection or other suitable means, the absence of unwanted fermentation, the presence of which may alter the quality of the preparation, including possible mycotoxin production.

Microbial Contamination of Herbal Drugs

Some level of microbial burden is unavoidable, and limits are set for total aerobic microbial count (TAMC) and the total combined yeasts/moulds count (TYMC). The limits vary slightly according to the purpose of the herbal drug or extract. Contamination with human pathogens (mainly from sewage), such as *Escherichia coli* and *Salmonella* spp., is tested for specifically: *E. coli* levels have limits, and *Salmonella* must be absent.

Microbial Toxins and Mycotoxins

Fungal infection (usually from incomplete drying) can produce carcinogenic, mutagenic, teratogenic and hepatotoxic compounds, such as the aflatoxins and ochratoxin A, produced by *Aspergillus* species. Limit tests are included in some herbal drug monographs, such as ochratoxin A in liquorice. Aflatoxin levels above 2 µg/kg (measured as aflatoxin B$_1$) should not be present in any herbal drug.

Specific Plant Toxins

Certain well-known compounds, such as aristolochic acids and pyrrolizidine alkaloids, are tested to see if there is any likelihood of their being present due to contamination with weeds, confusion of nomenclature, or as part of a traditional formula.

Heavy Metals

Contamination (with lead, arsenic, mercury, cadmium, etc.) may arise from environmental pollution. Metals accumulate in some plants and are further concentrated during processing. Lead and arsenic have also been found in imported herbal products, where they have been included as part of a traditional formula.

Unless otherwise stated, the limits are cadmium, 1.0 ppm; lead, 5.0 ppm; mercury, 0.1 ppm.

Pesticide Residues

The most important are the persistent chlorinated and organophosphate insecticides. Many of these are banned globally, but poor agricultural practices and lack of traceability may lead to occurrences.

Assay

An assay is included except in unusual circumstances (such as where the chemical composition of the plant is incompletely known, or a validated method is proving difficult to develop). Work usually continues on incomplete monographs and an assay is added as soon as possible. The assay is usually High-performance liquid chromatography (HPLC)-based. In some older monographs it may be colorimetric. It is intended to measure at least one of the active substances, if known! The techniques involved are discussed in Chapter 7.

Monographs for Traditional Herbal Medicines

The increase in global use of traditional herbal medicinal products (THMPs), now classified as medicines under EU Directive 2004/24/EC, has led to a surge in efforts to define their quality. The same standards are required for THMPs as for any other herbal drug, but monographs may also cover aspects such as traditional processing methods, which may require the addition of processing aids, for example, honey, vinegar, wine, milk and salt, and may also involve heat treatment by stir-baking or roasting. See Zhao et al. (2010) for more information.

EXTRACTS

Herbal products often use extracts rather than raw material to provide a more concentrated form of the active constituent(s). Extracts are prepared from starting material that complies with the monograph for that herbal substance and are subjected to similar quality-control

analysis, although their identification does not involve botanical characters, of course. In addition, tests for residues are included for extracts that have been produced using organic solvents.

The method of extraction, for example, infusion in hot water (herbal tea or tisane), decoction (boiling in water), percolation (repeated extraction with hot solvent), maceration (soaking), and pressing of fresh plant material (for expressed juice, oils or fats) depends on the type of raw material and the finished herbal product required. Leaf drugs are more suitable for infusion, whilst hard and woody drugs such as barks and roots may require decoction or percolation.

The Drug–Extract Ratio

The *drug–extract ratio (DER)* gives information on *the amount of extract obtained from the herbal drug*. A DER of 4:1 (maceration, 70% ethanol) means that 4 units of the herbal drug have yielded 1 unit of dried extract. The DER varies considerably depending on the herbal drug and the solvents used. Chamomile flowers (*Matricaria chamomilla* L.), extracted in water produce a DER in the range of 6–8:1 (meaning that 6–8 kg of herbal drug produces 1 kg extract), whereas for turmeric (*Curcuma longa* L.), extracted with 96% ethanol, the DER typically is in the range of 20–50:1. In other words, for chamomile, a large amount of extract can be obtained (12%–18%), but for turmeric, only a very small amount (2%–5%) is produced.

Types of Extract

As shown in Box 12.1, extracts are prepared that exert varying degrees of control over the concentration of the active ingredients.

Standardised Herbal Extracts

Standardisation is an attempt to produce consistent quality in an extract by defining concentrations of compounds or groups of compounds. It is important for the safe use of potent medicinal plants and for conducting clinical studies. It also enables a dose regimen to be defined so patients can purchase herbal products and self-medicate. There are monographs for standardised extracts for *Senna, Digitalis, Belladonna, Ipecacuanha* and others in the BP and Ph. Eur., reflecting their well-known chemical composition and potent effects.

Standardisation may be related to one compound or a range:

Defined single content: for example, for *Ipecacuanha liquid extract, standardised*, the content of total alkaloids is stated as [1.80%–2.20%], calculated as emetine. The acceptable tolerance is usually within the range ±5% to ±10%.

Defined range of content: for *Frangula bark dry extract, standardised*, the content of assayed constituents is stated as [15.0%–30.0%]—much broader than for *Ipecacuanha*.

Special extracts. Production of a standardised extract can include combining batches to give a consistent product and/or removing unwanted constituents to give a more concentrated product. It does not include the addition of isolated substances, of herbal or other origin, or anything not normally found in the plant, unless as part of a finished herbal product and stated on the label.

Quantified extracts. Some extracts are assayed, but the contents are not adjusted, and their content must be within the values given in the definition section of an individual monograph. If a plant is grown and processed under controlled conditions, then the resulting extracts will have a certain amount of batch-to-batch uniformity.

Refined extracts. Extracts may be processed to remove unwanted constituents. One example is *Ginkgo*, which is sometimes refined to limit the concentrations of ginkgolic acids (considered to be allergenic) to less than 5 ppm (see Fig. 12.6). A refined extract is usually further characterised as a *Refined and standardised extract*, as for Bilberry, or a *Refined and quantified extract*, as for *Ginkgo*.

GINKGO LEAF (*Ph. Eur. 1828*)
DEFINITION
Whole or fragmented, dried leaf of *Ginkgo biloba* L.
Content
Not less than 0.5% of flavonoids, expressed as flavone glycosides (dried drug).

REFINED AND QUANTIFIED GINKGO DRY EXTRACT (*Ph. Eur. 1827*)
DEFINITION
Refined and quantified dry extract produced from Ginkgo leaf.
Content
— *flavonoids, expressed as flavone glycosides*: 22.0–27.0% (dried extract);
— *bilobalide*: 2.6–3.2% (dried extract);
— *ginkgolides A, B and C*: 2.8–3.4% (dried extract);
— *ginkgolic acids*: maximum 5 ppm (dried extract);
PRODUCTION
The extract is produced from the herbal drug by an appropriate procedure using organic solvents and their mixtures with water, physical separation steps as well as other suitable processes.

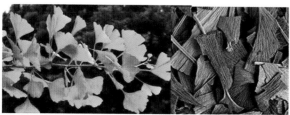

Starting material: Ginkgo leaf

Fig. 12.6 Ginkgo monographs.: Ginkgo, monographs. Ph. Eur. Suppl. Strasbourg, France: Council of Europe; 2021. Available online at https://pheur.edqm.eu/

SENNA PODS (*Ph. Eur. 0207*)
Alexandrian Senna Fruit
DEFINITION
Dried fruit of *Senna alexandrina* Mill.
(syn. *Cassia acutifolia* Delile and *Cassia angustifolia* Vahl).
Content: Minimum 2.0% of total hydroxyanthracene glycosides, expressed as sennoside B ($C_{42}H_{38}O_{20}$) (dried drug).

SENNA TABLETS BP
DEFINITION
Senna Tablets contain the powdered pericarp of Senna Fruit, Alexandrian or Tinnevelly.
Content of total sennosides, calculated as sennoside B, 85.0–115.0% of the stated amount

STANDARDISED SENNA GRANULES BP
DEFINITION
Standardised Senna Granules contain Alexandrian Senna Fruit in powder form with suitable excipients. The granules contain 0.55% w/w of sennosides, calculated as sennoside B.

SENNA LIQUID EXTRACT BP
DEFINITION
Senna Fruit Alexandrian or Tinnevelly, crushed 100 g; Coriander Oil, 6 mL; Ethanol (90%), 250 mL; Purified water: a sufficient quantity
TESTS*
Ethanol content: 21–24% v/v; Dry residue:17–25% w/v., Relative density: 1.02 to 1.09

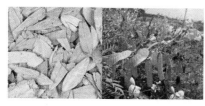

Starting material: Senna fruit and leaf

SENNA LEAFLET (*Ph. Eur. 0206*)
Senna Leaf
DEFINITION
Dried leaflets of *Senna alexandrina* Mill.
(syn. *Cassia acutifolia* Delile and *Cassia angustifolia* Vahl).
Content
Minimum 2.0% of total hydroxyanthracene glycosides, expressed as sennoside B ($C_{42}H_{38}O_{20}$) (dried drug).

STANDARDISED SENNA LEAF DRY EXTRACT (*Ph. Eur. 1261*)
DEFINITION
Standardised dry extract produced from Senna Leaf (*0206*)
Content
5.5–8.0% hydroxyanthracene glycosides, expressed as sennoside B ($C_{42}H_{38}O_{20}$) (dried extract). The measured content does not deviate from the value stated on the label by more than ± 10%.
PRODUCTION
The extract is produced from the herbal drug by a suitable procedure using ethanol (50–80% *V/V*).

Fig. 12.7 Senna monographs: Ph. Eur. and BP

Figs 12.6–12.11 show examples of where specific tests are applied in the BP and Ph. Eur. The 'parent' monograph of the starting material is linked to preparations derived from it (overlapping boxes), which include standardised extracts (Senna, Peppermint, Liquorice, see Figs 12.7–12.9) and refined and quantified extracts (Ginkgo, Fig. 12.6). Some preparations, although derived from Ph. Eur. materials, are only found in national pharmacopoeias (see Senna, Cinnamon (Fig. 12.10), Peppermint, Star Anise and Aniseed (Fig. 12.11), Liquorice) and some must be extemporaneously prepared (see Anise, Cinnamon). Occasionally, the raw material is not the subject

PEPPERMINT LEAF *(Ph. Eur. 0406)*
DEFINITION
Whole or cut, dried leaf of *Mentha × piperita* L.
Content:
Essential oil content: for the whole drug, 12 mL/kg
(anhydrous drug); for the cut drug, 9 mL/kg

PEPPERMINT LEAF DRY EXTRACT *(Ph. Eur. 2108)*
DEFINITION
Dry extract produced from *Peppermint* leaf (0406).
Content:
Minimum 0.5% of rosmarinic acid ($C_{18}H_{16}O_8$;) (dried extract).
PRODUCTION
The extract is produced from the herbal drug by a suitable procedure using
ethanol (30–50% *V/V*) or water at minimum 60°C.

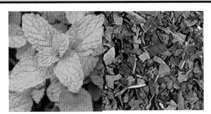

Starting material: Peppermint leaf

FRESH PEPPERMINT LEAF
No official monograph is available for fresh leaf

PEPPERMINT OIL *(Ph. Eur. 0405)*
DEFINITION
Essential oil obtained by steam distillation from the fresh aerial parts
of *Mentha × piperita* L.

PEPPERMINT GASTRO-RESISTANT CAPSULES BP
DEFINITION
Peppermint Oil Gastro-resistant Capsules contain Peppermint
Oil. They are covered with a gastro-resistant coating.

Fig. 12.8 Peppermint monographs. Peppermint, monographs. Ph. Eur. Suppl. Strasbourg, France: Council of
Europe; 2021. Available online at https://pheur.edqm.eu/

LIQUORICE DRY EXTRACT FOR FLAVOURING PURPOSES *(Ph. Eur. 2378)*
DEFINITION
Dry extract produced from *Liquorice* root (0277)
Content
5.0–7.0% 18β-glycyrrhizic acid ($C_{42}H_{62}O_{16}$; M_r 823) (dried extract).
PRODUCTION
The extract is produced from the cut herbal drug by a suitable procedure
using water.
TESTS*
Loss on drying,
Ochratoxin A: Maximum 80 µg per kilogram of extract.

LIQUORICE *(Ph. Eur. 0277)*
Liquorice root
DEFINITION
Dried, unpeeled or peeled, whole or cut, root and stolons of
Glycyrrhiza glabra L. and /or *G. inflata* Bat. and/or. *G. uralensis*
Fisch.
TESTS*
Loss on drying, Total ash (unpeeled and peeled drug)
Acid insoluble ash (unpeeled peeled drug).
Ochratoxin A: Maximum 20 µg per kilogram of herbal drug

LIQUORICE LIQUID EXTRACT BP
DEFINITION
Liquorice Liquid Extract is produced from Liquorice. It contains not less than 1.4% w/v of 18β-
glycyrrhizic acid, $C_{42}H_{62}O_{16}$.
PRODUCTION
The liquid extract is produced by extraction with water, precipitation of unwanted constituents,
concentration of the extraction liquors and the addition of sufficient ethanol (96%) and water to
produce the required volume. The liquid extract must stand for a minimum of 4–8 weeks prior
to decantation of the clear supernatant liquid.
TESTS*
Loss on drying, Total ash, Acid insoluble ash.
Ochratoxin A: Maximum 20 µg per kilogram of herbal drug

Liquorice: starting material

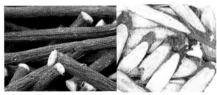

LIQUORICE ROOT FOR USE IN TCM BP
DEFINITION
Dried, unpeeled root and rhizome of *Glycyrrhiza uralensis*
Fisch. and/or of *Glycyrrhiza inflata* Bat. and/
or *Glycyrrhiza glabra* L. collected in spring and autumn,
separated from the rootlets and dried in the sun.
It contains not less than 2.0% of glycyrrhizic acid.
TESTS*
Loss on drying: Total ash: Acid insoluble ash,
Ochratoxin A: Not more than 2 ppb

PROCESSED LIQUORICE ROOT FOR USE IN TCM BP
Content
Not less than 2.0% of glycyrrhizic acid ($C_{42}H_{62}O_{16}$) calculated with reference to the
dried material.
PRODUCTION
Liquorice Root for use in TCM is cleaned, softened thoroughly, sliced transversely or
longitudinally to form uniform pieces and dried.
TESTS*
Loss on drying, Total ash, Acid insoluble ash.
Ochratoxin A: Maximum 20 µg per kilogram of herbal drug

Fig. 12.9 Liquorice monographs: Ph. Eur. and BP

CINNAMON BARK *(Ph. Eur. 0387)*
Ceylon Cinnamon
DEFINITION
Dried bark, freed from the outer cork and the underlying parenchyma, of the shoots grown on cut stock of *Cinnamomum verum* J.Presl.
Content:
Minimum 12 mL/kg of essential oil.

CEYLON CINNAMON BARK OIL *(Ph. Eur. 1501)*
Cinnamon Oil
DEFINITION
Essential oil obtained by steam distillation of the bark of the shoots of *Cinnamomum verum* J.Presl.

CONCENTRATED CINNAMON WATER BP
DEFINITION
Cinnamon Oil 20 mL;
Ethanol (90%), 600 mL;
Purified water: a sufficient quantity to produce 1000 mL
Extemporaneous preparation.
TESTS
Ethanol content: 52–56% v/v,
Weight per mL 0.914–0.922 g

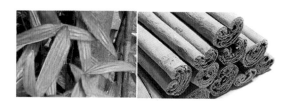

Starting material: Cinnamon Bark and Leaf

CINNAMON LEAF
No official monograph for leaf as starting material. It is a by-product used only to produce essential oil, which is not the same as cinnamon bark oil, and is less expensive.

CEYLON CINNAMON LEAF OIL *(Ph. Eur. 1608)*
Cinnamon Oil
DEFINITION
Oil obtained by steam distillation of the leaves of *Cinnamomum verum* J.Presl.

Fig. 12.10 Cinnamon monographs: Ph. Eur. and BP

STAR ANISE *(Ph. Eur. 1153)*
DEFINITION
Dried composite fruit of *Illicium verum* Hook.f.
Content:
Minimum 70 mL/kg essential oil (anhydrous drug)
Minimum 86.0% of *trans*-anethole in the essential oil.
TESTS*
Illicium anisatum (= *I. religiosum*) and other *Illicium* spp.

STAR ANISE OIL *(Ph. Eur. 2108)*
DEFINITION
Essential oil obtained by steam distillation of the dry ripe fruits of *Illicium verum* Hook.f.

CONCENTRATED ANISE WATER BP
DEFINITION
Anise or Star Anise Oil 20 mL;
Ethanol (90%), 700 mL;
Purified water, freshly boiled and cooled:
a sufficient quantity to produce 1000 mL
Extemporaneous preparation.
TESTS
Ethanol content: 60–64% v/v,

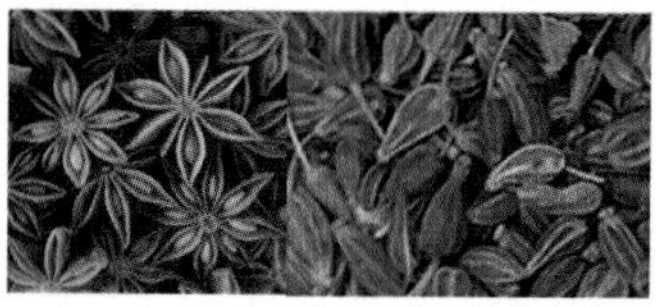

Starting material: Star Anise and Aniseed

ANISEED *(Ph. Eur. 0262)*
Anise
DEFINITION
Whole, dry cremocarp of *Pimpinella anisum* L.
Content:
Minimum 20 mL/kg essential oil (anhydrous drug)

ANISE OIL *(Ph. Eur. 0804)*
Aniseed Oil
DEFINITION
Oil obtained by steam distillation of dry ripe fruits of *Pimpinella anisum* L.

Fig. 12.11 Star Anise and Aniseed monographs: Ph. Eur. and BP

of a monograph, but its preparations are (Cinnamon leaf, and fresh Peppermint leaf, used to distil the essential oil). As an underground organ, *Acid insoluble ash* is specified for Liquorice, which is subject to different monographs with varying limits, depending on its purpose and processing method. All its preparations include a limit test for the mycotoxin ochratoxin A.

Specific absence tests for toxic-related species are exemplified by Star Anise and illustrate the need to have botanical and chemical identification tests in some cases. The monograph excerpts show the variety of tests needed to assure the quality of herbal drugs, generally and specifically.

NEW METHODS FOR QUALITY ASSURING HERBAL PRODUCTS

Herbal medicines are so complex that no current methods are ideal for assuring their quality. However, given the importance of correct identification of the plant species, which cannot be done in the same way as for single-entity drugs, improving authentication is a good place to start. Botanical identification is unique to herbal medicines and can now be determined genetically in addition to morphologically.

DNA Barcoding Methods for Identification

Reliable methods of identifying plant species are now available using their DNA profiles, although the appropriate use of these methods is not always understood. In 2015, the US Attorney General published a report on herbal products suggesting that 'in a large number of the tested products, there was no detectable plant DNA whatsoever', which was widely criticised on scientific grounds, not least because extracts do not contain DNA (see Tyler, 2015).

Advantages of DNA-Based Methods

- DNA profiles are highly accurate and diagnostic, if used in context.
- DNA-based methods are ideal for routine screening once the method is set up.
- They are highly sensitive when discriminating between closely related species.

Limitations of DNA-Based Methods

- DNA profiles provide only information about the botanical identity of the plant, not the quality of the herbal material, which is affected by environmental factors (see Fig. 12.2).
- DNA analysis does not give information on the part of plant included.
- DNA-based methods cannot be used in extracts from which the plant material has been removed.
- Processing methods may destroy the DNA.
- DNA will not pick up contamination with any plant that is not actively being looked for.
- It is complicated to use these techniques on multiherbal formulae.
- There is a high risk of contamination of with environmental or other samples of DNA.

The first DNA-based method in the BP was introduced to distinguish *Ocimum tenuiflorum* L. (tulsi) from related species of *Ocimum* (basil). The BP method uses short regions of DNA with species-specific sequences as barcodes for recognition, and these are published as part of the monograph. DNA barcoding is of great potential use in identifying toxic species, for example, pyrrolizidine alkaloid-containing plants (Kalantar & Williamson, 2022). General guidance on how to conduct DNA-based identification methods for herbal drugs is also included in the BP 2020.

CONCLUSIONS

Quality assurance of herbal products can only be guaranteed by taking care throughout the entire process, from growing the medicinal plant to its eventual administration to a patient. Pharmacopoeial standards and guidelines for good practice are there to assist at all stages, for the benefit of the manufacturer, who has a responsibility to ensure that the product is safe and of good quality, and for the benefits of the consumer, who also needs that assurance. Monographs are drafted by the secretariat of the Pharmacopoeial Commission, supported by analytical laboratories and in collaboration with independent experts.

Many herbal producers, especially those making Traditional Herbal Registration products, carry out additional tests that are not mandatory according to the pharmacopoeial monograph and assist in the work of the pharmacopoeia by seconding staff as members of expert groups, sharing analytical methods, taking part in collaborative trials,

and testing new methods, usually at no charge. This may benefit the company in that its own methods are included, but it does not confer a monopoly since other methods can be used if validated.

It should be noted that if an official monograph is available for any herbal drug or preparation, compliance with such a monograph is usually essential for inclusion of that herbal substance in a registered product. Even so, meeting existing standards may not accurately reflect the therapeutic activity, and monographs are continually revised and updated to reflect new information and new techniques. Biological assays have long been used in drug analysis and, more recently, strategies using quality markers based on biological activity have been applied to Chinese medicine, as reviewed by Wu et al. (2018).

FURTHER READING

Council of Europe, 2021. European Pharmacopoeia. Council of Europe, Strasbourg. Available at: http://www.edqm.eu.

Jackson, B.P., Snowden, D., 2005. Atlas of Microscopy of Medicinal Plants Culinary Herbs and Spices. CBS Publishers & Distributors, New Delhi.

Kalantar Zadeh, M., Williamson, E.M., 2022. Pyrrolizidine Alkaloids in Herbal Medicines and Food: A Public Health Issue. Ch 3 in Advances and Challenges in Pharmacovigilance for Herbal Medicines. Ed Barnes J. Springer pp 27-40.

Medicines and Healthcare Products Regulatory Agency (MHRA), 2021. British Pharmacopoeia. MHRA, London. Available online: https://www.pharmacopoeia.com.

Reich, E., 2007. High-performance Thin-Layer Chromatography for the Analysis of Medicinal Plants. Springer-Verlag, Berlin.

Tyler, S., 2015. The supplement saga: a review of the New York Attorney General's herbal supplement investigation. HerbalGram 106, 44–55. Available at: www.herbalgram.org.

Upton, R., Graff, R., Jolliffe, G., Länger, R., Williamson, E.M. (Eds.), 2011. American Herbal Pharmacopoeia: Microscopic Characterization of Botanical Medicines. CRC Press, Boca Raton.

Wagner, H., Bauer, R., Melchart, D., Xiao, P.-G., Staudinger, A., 2011. Chromatographic Fingerprint Analysis of Herbal Medicines. Thin-Layer and High Performance Liquid Chromatography of Chinese Drugs, second ed. Springer Verlag, Berlin.

World Health Organization (WHO), 2003. Guidelines on Good Agricultural and Collection Practices (GACP) for Medicinal Plants. WHO, Geneva. Available at: http://apps.who.int/medicinedocs/en/d/Js4928e/#Js4928e.

World Health Organization (WHO), 2007a. Guidelines on Good Manufacturing Practices (GMP) for Herbal Medicines. WHO, Geneva. Available at: http://apps.who.int/medicinedocs/en/m/abstract/Js14215e/.

World Health Organization (WHO), 2007b. Guidelines for Assessing Quality of Herbal Medicines With Reference to Contaminants and Residues. WHO, Geneva. Available at: http://apps.who.int/medicinedocs/en/m/abstract/Js14878e/.

World Health Organization (WHO), 2011. Quality Control Methods for Herbal Materials. WHO, Geneva. Available at: http://apps.who.int/medicinedocs/en/m/abstract/Jh1791e/.

World Health Organization (WHO), 2017. Guideline for Selecting Marker Substances of Herbal Origin for Quality Control of Herbal Medicines. WHO Technical Report Series, No. 1003, 2017. Annex 1. http://apps.who.int/medicinedocs/documents/s23240en/s23240en.pdf.

World Health Organization (WHO), 2018. Guidelines on Good Herbal Processing Practices (GHPP) for Herbal Medicines. WHO Technical Report Series, No. 1010, 2018. https://www.who.int/traditional-complementary-integrative-medicine/publications/trs1010_annex1.pdf.

Wu, X., Zhang, H., Fan, S., et al., 2018. Quality markers based on biological activity: a new strategy for the quality control of traditional Chinese medicine. Phytomedicine 44, 103–108.

Zhao, Z., Liang, Z., Chan, K., et al., 2010. A unique issue in the standardization of Chinese materia medica: processing. Planta Med. 76 (17), 1975–1986.

13

Toxicity of Herbal Constituents

OCCURRENCE IN HERBAL MEDICINES

Toxic plant species provide some of our most important drugs but are not normally used as herbal medicines (HMs). Some other plants, which are used as HMs, have shown toxicity which outweighs any therapeutic benefit, but their use persists in some traditional medicine systems. More commonly, these herbal substances occur as contaminants or adulterants of other medicinal plant species and are avoidable with good agricultural and collection practices (GACPs), as discussed in Chapter 12. Traditional use is not a reliable indication of safety: toxicity resulting from chronic use or manifesting long after use may make connections difficult.

Some toxic compounds, including pyrrolizidine alkaloids (PAs) and aristolochic acids (AAs), are present as both contaminants and as ingredients of traditional formulas and still pose potential serious risks. Allergic reactions can be elicited by any drug, and idiosyncratic responses are not restricted to plant medicines. However, some plant families, especially the daisy family (Asteraceae), are notorious for causing allergic reactions. New integrated approaches are being advocated to examine more subtle forms of herbal toxicity (e.g. Williamson et al., 2014).

Pyrrolizidine Alkaloids

PAs that are unsaturated at the 1,2-position (e.g. senecionine; Fig. 13.1) cause venoocclusive disease as well as being hepatocarcinogenic, and their effects are cumulative (Xu et al., 2019). The European Medicines Agency (EMA) has concluded that there is no level of PA ingestion that is without risk, and environmental exposure should be reduced to as low as reasonably practicable (EMA, 2016).

PAs occur mainly in the plant families Boraginaceae, Asteraceae and Fabaceae and pose a public health problem because they can contaminate foods, including flours, honey and even eggs, as well as being found in some traditional medicines (see Kalantar-Zadeh & Williamson 2022 for review). HMs containing PAs include butterbur (*Petasites hybridus* (L.) G. Gaertn., B. Mey. & Scherb.), coltsfoot (*Tussilago farfara* L.) and comfrey (*Symphytum* spp.), although the more commonly used medicinal variety, *Symphytum × uplandicum*, contains very low concentrations of PAs, and external use of comfrey is considered safe (Kuchta & Schmidt, 2020). In China, hepatic sinusoidal obstruction syndrome associated with oral intake of PAs causes abdominal distension, pain, ascites, jaundice and hepatomegaly (Zhuge et al., 2019). Worryingly, PAs have been found in a variety of unrelated HMs in Europe (Letsyo et al., 2017), and even in products with a Traditional Herbal Registration (THR) in European countries, such as some St John's wort (*Hypericum perforatum* L.) products, due to contamination with weeds. This happens during the collecting process, but interspecific transfer of PAs has been shown to occur when ragwort (*Jacobaea vulgaris* Gaertn., syn. *Senecio jacobaea* L.) is used as a mulch for growing chamomile or parsley (Nowak et al., 2016), emphasising the importance of GACPs and traceability of plant material.

Aristolochic Acids

Most species of birthwort (*Aristolochia*, known as snakeroot) and related genera, including *Asarum* (Aristolochiaceae), contain AAs (Fig. 13.2) and aristolactams. These cause kidney failure and urothelial malignancies, known as aristolochic acid nephropathy (AAN). Although banned in many parts of the world, species from the genus are used as traditional medicines, especially in the treatment of gastrointestinal complaints, snake bites, poisoning and gynaecologic conditions, including the treatment of sexually transmitted diseases (STDs) (Heinrich et al., 2009). A much wider spectrum of toxicity in related compounds is found in other genera of the Aristolochiaceae, including *Asarum*, and their safety may need to be revisited (Michl et al., 2016; Liu & Wang, 2021).

Contamination of HMs with *Aristolochia* species has caused illness and death. More than 100 patients from a Belgian clinic suffered kidney failure after the intake of weight-loss pills containing *Aristolochia fangchi* Y.C. Wu ex L.D. Chow & S.M. Hwang. In the first report (1993), the plant was stated to be *Stephania tetrandra* S. Moore, or 'hang fang ji', but *A. fangchi*—'guang fang ji'—had been used instead. Whether this was accidental or deliberate is not clear, but pharmacopoeial tests for *S. tetrandra* now include a specific test for the absence of *Aristolochia* species. Contamination of foods with *Aristolochia* is also major concern in some parts of the world: AAN has been reported in China, Bangladesh and in central Europe, where it is known as Balkan endemic nephropathy (Heinrich et al., 2009).

Essential Oil Constituents

Most monoterpenes and sesquiterpenes found in essential oils (see Chapter 6 for structures) are considered safe in normal culinary, flavouring and medicinal use, although undiluted distilled oils may be toxic even at low doses and cause irritation and allergic reactions when applied externally. They are easily absorbed through the skin, and some terpenes, such as limonene, are used as penetration enhancers to aid the transdermal delivery of drugs in adhesive patches. Individual compounds have shown carcinogenic, genotoxic and neurotoxic effects, but in medicinal plants that are formulated as decoctions, boiling may reduce the concentration of these constituents.

β-Asarone

β-Asarone and its oxidation products and metabolites are known to be genotoxic (Hermes et al., 2021). It is present in the essential oil of *Acorus calamus* L., but low β-asarone-containing varieties can be used. *Acorus* species are widely used in traditional medicine and, in China, *Acorus tatarinowii* Schott is used to treat dementia and amnesia.

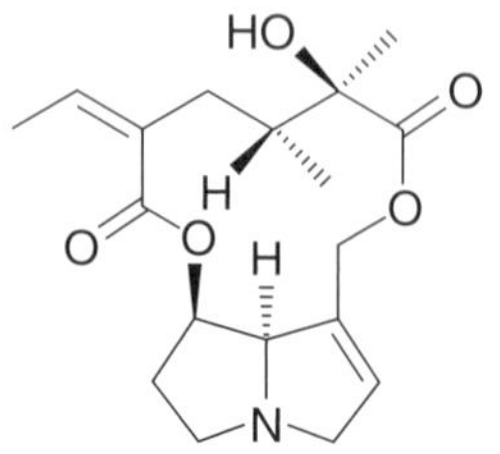

Fig. 13.1 Senecionine.

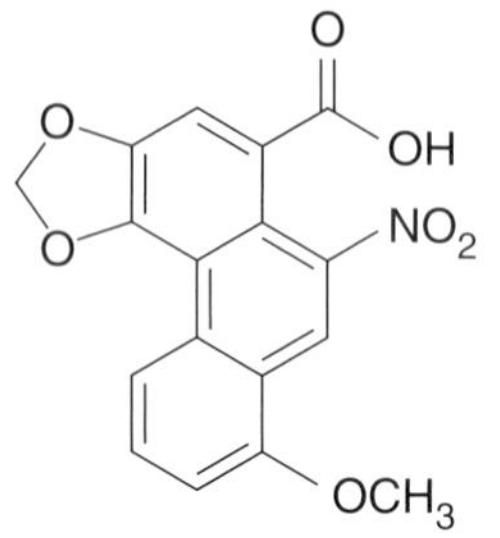

Fig. 13.3 Anisatin.

Fig. 13.2 Aristolochic acid.

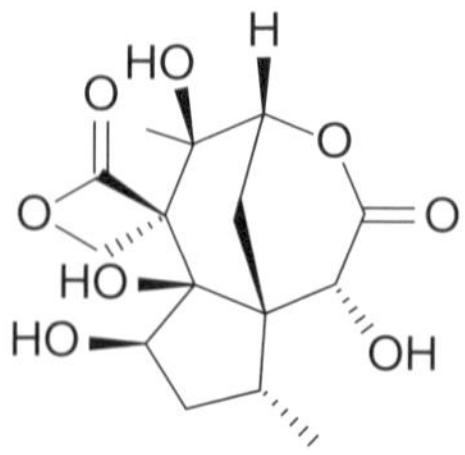

Recent studies suggest a potential use of β-asarone in degenerative cognitive disorders (Li et al., 2021) via modulation of autophagic activity. Many species of *Asarum* contain asarones and the phenylpropanoids discussed later, in addition to AAs (Liu & Wang, 2021), raising further concerns for their safety.

Safrole, Methysticin and Methyleugenol

Safrole is the main constituent of *Sassafras* oil, which is no longer used medicinally due to concerns about its potential carcinogenicity, and is found in smaller quantities in nutmeg, *Myristica fragrans, Houtt.* which also contains methysticin. Both phenylpropanoids are potential metabolic precursors of the psychoactive drug methylene dioxymethamphetamine (MDMA) and have been used as starting materials for illicit chemical synthesis. Methyl eugenol is found in many essential oils, although it has limits imposed on acceptable safe concentrations when used as a flavouring agent. Many *Asarum* species contain safrole, myristicin and methyleugenol as major components of their volatile oils (Liu & Wang, 2021).

Thujone

Thujone, present in wormwood (*Artemisia absinthium L.*), is toxic in large doses and may cause convulsions and hallucinations. The liqueur absinthe, distilled from wormwood and other herbs, was popular in Paris in the late 1800s and early 1900s and its use was associated with writers and artists, including Ernest Hemingway, Oscar Wilde, Marcel Proust, Picasso and Van Gogh. It was eventually banned in many countries. However, the amounts of thujone found in the drink are now considered to be too low to cause 'absinthism', and the symptoms thought more likely to be due to the high alcohol content and common adulterants. Absinthe is now legally produced, especially with low-thujone content, and is increasing in popularity. Thujone is a component of sage (*Salvia officinalis L.*) essential oil and many other commonly used herbs.

Camphor

Camphor is a cyclic monoketone present in many essential oils, including rosemary (*Rosmarinus officinalis Spenn.*) herb and originally obtained from *Cinnamomum camphora* wood. In large doses it causes nausea, vomiting, headache, dizziness, convulsions, delirium, and even death. Camphor inhibits nicotinic receptors and is an agonist at several transient receptor vanilloid potential (TRVP, or capsaicin receptor) channels. Formerly used as an expectorant, camphor is still found in topical applications for muscle sprain and to relieve skin irritation and itching, for example from insect bites, and as an inhaled decongestant in coughs and colds, as part of multiingredient preparations. It can be effective in these indications but should be used with caution because it is absorbed very easily through the skin.

Sesquiterpene Lactones

These are commonly present in plants in the Asteraceae family and are often responsible for the biologic activity of the herb. Some sesquiterpene lactones, such as anthecotulide, are highly allergenic, and misidentification of mayweed (*Anthemis cotula L.*) instead of chamomile (*A. nobilis L.* or *Matricaria chamomilla L.*) is addressed in the quality assurance of these floral herbs.

Anisatin (Fig. 13.3) is a neurotoxin occurring in the fruits of shikimi fruit, *Illicium anisatum L.*, which may occur as adulterants of star anise, *I. verum* Hook.f. (see Wang et al., 2011 for review). Symptoms of anisatin poisoning include diarrhoea, vomiting, stomach pain, seizures, loss of consciousness and respiratory paralysis. This is particularly dangerous in infants who are given a star anise infusion for colic, consisting of a single fruit in water. If this fruit is toxic, the result can be fatal. An absence test for *I. anisatum* is included in the monograph for star anise (Chapter 12).

Diterpene Esters

The phorbol, daphnane and ingenol esters found in the Euphorbiaceae and Thymelaeaceae are highly proinflammatory and are known to activate protein kinase C, as well as having tumour-promoting (cocarcinogenic) activity. The most important is tetradecanoyl phorbol acetate (phorbol myristate acetate; Fig. 13.4), which is a tumour promoter and an important biochemical research tool. Some of these plants were formerly used as drastic purgatives (e.g. croton oil, from *Croton tiglium L.*, Euphorbiaceae) but should now be avoided in herbal products.

Plant Lectins and Agglutinins

Castor beans, which are used to produce castor oil for use in medicines and cosmetics, contain a highly toxic lectin, ricin, which is denatured during manufacture of the oil, but the oil, and the seed cake remaining (which is used as animal feed), should not be used without heat processing. Pokeweed (*Phytolacca americana L.*), which is sometimes used as an antiinflammatory herb, contains phytoagglutinins called pokeweed mitogens. These have been known to cause gastrointestinal upset when taken in the fresh herb, but because they are heat labile they may denature on processing. They are also used as biochemical tools in immunology research.

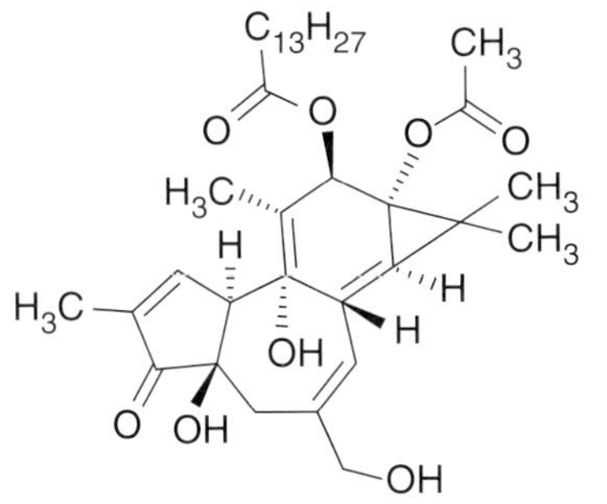

Fig. 13.4 Tetradecanoyl phorbol acetate.

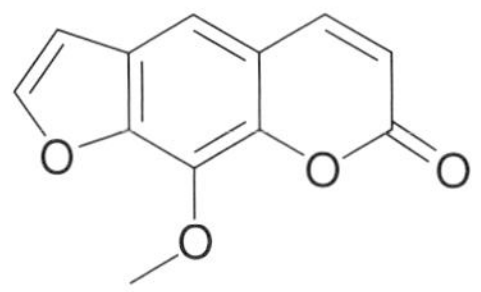

Fig. 13.5 Xanthotoxin.

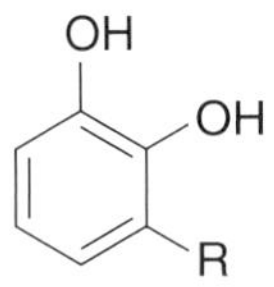

Fig. 13.6 Urushiols.

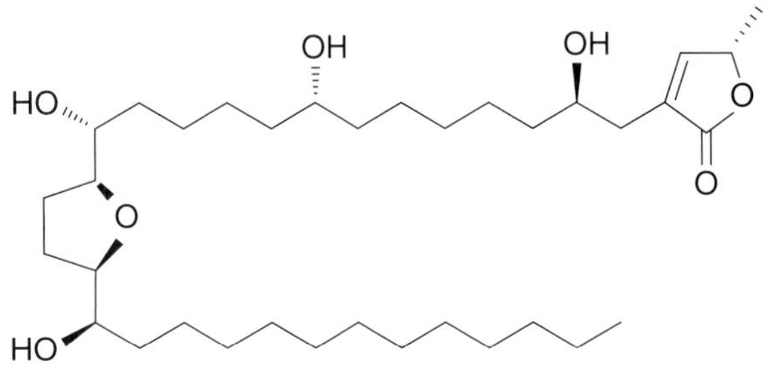

Fig. 13.7 Annonacin 1.

Fig. 13.8 Amygdalin.

Furanocoumarins

Some furanocoumarins (e.g. imperatorin, psoralen and xanthotoxin (Fig. 13.5)), found in giant hogweed (*Heracleum mantegazzianum Sommier & Levier*) and other umbelliferous plants and citrus peels, are phototoxic and produce photodermatitis on contact. Psoralen plus UV-A radiation (PUVA therapy) is occasionally used in the treatment of psoriasis, in specialist hospital clinics.

Urushiol Derivatives

The urushiols (Fig. 13.6), anacardic acids and ginkgolic acids are phenolic compounds with a long side chain. The uroshiols are found in poison ivy (*Toxicodendron radicans (L.) Kuntze*) and poison oak (*Toxicodendron quercifolium (Michx.) Greene*) and cause severe contact dermatitis. The anacardic acids, which are found in the liquor surrounding the cashew nut (*Anacardium occidentale L.*), are less toxic. The ginkgolic acids are reputed to cause allergic reactions; however, they are present in *Ginkgo biloba L.* fruit rather than the leaf, which is the medicinal part.

Annonacins

Soursop (also known as graviola) is used as an unproven cancer treatment, and, although consumption of the fruit and juice is widespread and considered safe, there are neurotoxic acetogenins, the annonacins (Fig. 13.7), which are also the anticancer compounds, in the leaf and bark. In countries such as Guadeloupe, where the leaf and bark are consumed as HMs (and not only for cancer), there is a significantly higher incidence of atypical Parkinson disease (PD) than elsewhere. The annonacins cause atypical PD in animal models by destroying dopaminergic neurons and so this treatment cannot be recommended (Champy et al., 2009).

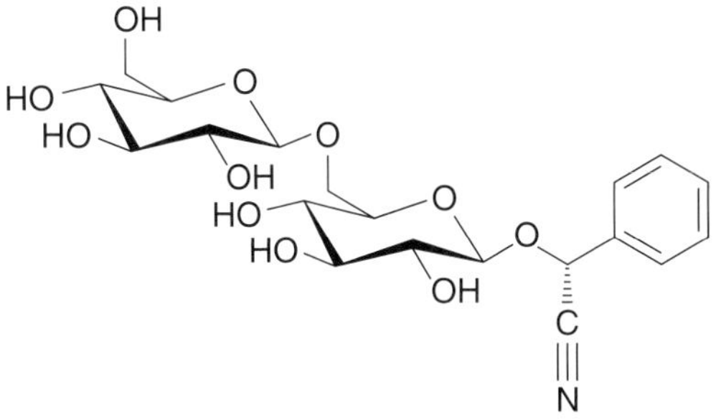

Cyanogenetic Glycosides

Cyanogenetic glycosides, such as amygdalin (Fig. 13.8), are present in many foods and herbs, including nuts, such as almonds. They are so-called because they release hydrogen cyanide when crushed, via the action of various enzymes, and also generate flavour compounds, such as benzaldehyde. Their presence in small amounts in fruits and nuts is not a concern. However, herbal remedies containing high concentrations of cyanogenetic glycosides or laetrile (synthesised from amygdalin by hydrolysis) are promoted as alternative cancer treatments. In some cases, simply ingesting crushed apricot kernels (*Prunus armeniaca L.*) is recommended, and this practice has resulted in documented hospital admissions.

PROCESSING AS A MEANS OF DETOXIFICATION

Chemical and physical methods are used in traditional medicine systems to detoxify herbal materials, but they are not infallible, and reports of intoxication still occur. These have been more fully discussed in the context of traditional Chinese medicine (TCM) by Liu et al. (2014), but the species most often involved in reports of toxicity is aconite (*Aconitum* spp.), reviewed briefly next.

Aconitine

The tubers and roots of *Aconitum* spp. (Ranunculaceae) have been used medicinally for centuries in TCM for the treatment of syncope, rheumatic fever, painful joints, gastroenteritis, diarrhoea, oedema, bronchial asthma, tumours and other medical conditions. The material contains aconitine (Fig. 13.9) and related diterpene alkaloids, which can be denatured by special processing. The improper use of *Aconitum* in India, Japan and especially China has caused numerous deaths (Chan, 2015). In China, only the processed (i.e. detoxified) tubers and roots of *Aconitum* are allowed to be administered orally or adopted as raw materials for pharmaceutical manufacturing. More than 70 techniques are applied for processing *Aconitum* roots to lower toxic alkaloid concentrations to below a certain threshold, a principle that is not accepted in Europe.

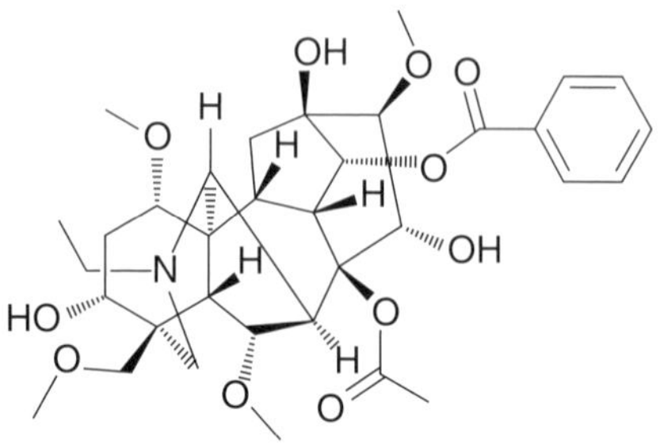

Fig. 13.9 Aconitine.

REFERENCES

Champy, P., Guérineau, V., Laprévote, O., 2009. MALDI-TOF MS profiling of annonaceous acetogenins in *Annona muricata* products for human consumption. Molecules 14, 5235–5246.

Chan, T.Y.K., 2015. Incidence and causes of aconitum alkaloid poisoning in Hong Kong from 1989 to 2010. Phytother. Res. 29 (8), 1107–1111.

EMA, 2016. Public statement on contamination of herbal medicinal products/traditional herbal medicinal products with pyrrolizidine alkaloids. Available at: http://www.ema.europa.eu/docs/en_GB/document_library/Public_statement/2016/06/WC500208195.pdf.

Heinrich, M., Chan, J., Wanke, S., Neinhuis, C., Simmonds, M.S., 2009. Local uses of Aristolochia species and content of nephrotoxic aristolochic acid 1 and 2 – a global assessment based on bibliographic sources. J. Ethnopharmacol. 125 (1), 108–144.

Hermes, L., Römermann, J., Cramer, B., Esselen, M., 2021. Quantitative analysis of β-Asarone derivatives in *Acorus calamus* and herbal food products by HPLC-MS/MS. J. Agric. Food Chem. 69 (2), 776–782.

Kalantar-Zadeh, M., Williamson, E.M., 2022. Pyrrolizidine alkaloids in herbal medicines and food: a public health issue. In: Barnes, J. (Ed.), Herbal Pharmacovigilance. Springer-Verlag.

Kuchta, K., Schmidt, M., 2020. Safety of medicinal comfrey cream preparations (*Symphytum officinale* s.l.): the pyrrolizidine alkaloid lycopsamine is poorly absorbed through human skin. Regul. Toxicol. Pharmacol. 118, 104784. https://doi.org/10.1016/j.yrtph.2020.104784.

Letsyo, E., Jerz, G., Winterhalter, P., Lindigkeit, R., Beuerle, T., 2017. Incidence of pyrrolizidine alkaloids in herbal medicines from German retail markets: risk assessments and implications to consumers. Phytother. Res. 31 (12), 1906–1909. https://doi.org/10.1002/ptr.5935.

Li, Z., Ma, J., Kuang, Z., Jiang, Y., 2021. β-Asarone attenuates Aβ-induced neuronal damage in PC12 cells overexpressing APPswe by restoring autophagic flux. Front. Pharmacol. 12, 701635. https://doi.org/10.3389/fphar.2021.701635.

Liu, H., Wang, C., 2021. The genus Asarum: a review on phytochemistry, ethnopharmacology, toxicology and pharmacokinetics. J. Ethnopharmacol. 282, 114642. https://doi.org/10.1016/j.jep.2021.114642.

Liu, X., Wang, Q., Song, G., Zhang, G., Ye, Z., Williamson, E.M., 2014. The classification and application of toxic Chinese Materia Medica. Phytother. Res. 28 (3), 334–347.

Michl, J., Kite, G.C., Wanke, S., Zierau, O., Vollmer, G., Neinhuis, C., et al., 2016. LC-MS- and (1)H NMR-based metabolomic analysis and in vitro toxicological assessment of 43 aristolochia species. J. Nat. Prod. 79 (1), 30–37.

Nowak, M., Wittke, C., Lederer, I., Klier, B., Kleinwächter, M., Selmar, D., 2016. Interspecific transfer of pyrrolizidine alkaloids: an unconsidered source of contaminations of phytopharmaceuticals and plant derived commodities. Food Chem. 213, 163–168.

Wang, G.W., Hu, W.T., Huang, B.K., Qin, L.P., 2011. *Illicium verum*: a review on its botany, traditional use, chemistry and pharmacology. J. Ethnopharmacol. 136 (1), 10–20.

Williamson, E.M., Chan, K., Xu, Q., Nachtergael, A., Bunel, V., Zhang, L., et al., 2014. Evaluating the safety of herbal medicines: integrated toxicological approaches. Science 347 (6219 Suppl. l), S47–S49.

Xu, J., Wang, W., Yang, X., Xiong, A., Yang, L., Wang, Z., 2019. Pyrrolizidine alkaloids: an update on their metabolism and hepatotoxicity mechanism. Liver Res. 3 (3–4), 176–184. https://doi.org/10.1016/j.livres.2019.11.004.

Zhuge, Y., Liu, Y., Xie, W., Zou, X., Xu, J., Wang, J., et al., 2019. Expert consensus on the clinical management of pyrrolizidine alkaloid-induced hepatic sinusoidal obstruction syndrome. J. Gastroenterol. Hepatol. 34 (4), 634–642. https://doi.org/10.1111/jgh.14612.

14

Herbal Medicine Interactions

INTRODUCTION

Herbal medicines (HMs), including those sold as nutritional/dietary/food supplements, are widely used to maintain health, prevent disease and treat chronic and refractory diseases, and are often taken alongside conventional medicines (referred to as 'drugs' in this context) by self-medication. This has the potential to cause drug interactions that could, in the most serious cases, lead to toxicity (with increased drug plasma concentrations) or treatment failure (with a decrease to subtherapeutic concentrations).

Herb–drug interactions (HDIs) may have a beneficial outcome by improving absorption of poorly orally bioavailable drugs, but harmful HDIs are understandably a higher priority in terms of public health. The herbal medicine most frequently cited in HDI reports is St John's wort (*Hypericum perforatum*), and its concomitant use with immunosuppressive, antiretroviral, cardiac or antineoplastic agents and hormonal oral contraceptives may result in reduced plasma concentrations of these drugs and, therefore, reduced efficacy (Russo et al., 2014; Nicolussi et al., 2020).

Herbal drugs may also interact with each other, and, in traditional formulae, components are selected to increase efficacy and attenuate toxicity according to traditional principles governing combinations. HMs are taken to enhance the effects of conventional drugs and to reduce side effects. For example, *Schisandra sphenanthera* is used in liver transplant patients taking the immune suppressant tacrolimus: the herbal–drug combination increases the oral bioavailability of tacrolimus, reduces some of its side effects and improves liver function (Wei et al., 2013). The herbal medicine PHY 906, based on an ancient Chinese formula, is used in cancer chemotherapy to improve outcomes and reduce side effects (Liu & Cheng, 2012). There are many other examples of the adjunctive use of traditional Chinese medicine throughout cancer treatment (e.g. Qi et al., 2015).

Under-reporting of cases of suspected adverse effects associated with HMs is a known problem (see Chapter 15), and physicians often also fail to ask their patients about their use of HMs and other 'supplements'. Therefore, no overall reliable information on the frequency of clinically relevant HDIs is available, and many individual reports are poorly detailed (Izzo et al., 2016). However, even well-documented case reports may not be able to establish a cause-and-effect relationship, especially with a multidrug regimen.

MECHANISMS OF HERBAL MEDICINE INTERACTIONS

Pharmaceutical Incompatibility

HMs are often formulated from liquid extracts, and some components, if mixed with other drugs or extracts prior to administration, may be chemically or pharmaceutically incompatible. This can take the form of complexation, such as between polyphenols or metals with proteins, causing precipitation and leading to reduced solubility and absorption, or as chemical degradation to inactive or toxic metabolites.

This incompatibility can be resolved by changing the dosage regimen, but true drug interactions involve physiological processes and cause changes in therapeutic outcomes. These interactions may be synergistic or additive, where the effect is increased, or antagonistic, where it is decreased. They occur via *pharmacodynamic* and *pharmacokinetic* mechanisms. An overview of these processes is shown in Fig. 14.1.

Pharmacodynamic Interactions

Pharmacodynamic (PD) mechanisms are involved when two agents interact due to their intrinsic pharmacological effects and include receptor-binding effects, when two drugs may have agonist, antagonist, partial and/or inverse agonist activity. At a systemic level, biochemical changes induced by drug treatment, such as hypokalaemia due to diuretics and laxatives, may increase toxicity of another drug. The disease state of the patient may affect drug clearance, for example, in kidney failure and liver disease.

Pharmacokinetic Interactions

Pharmacokinetic (PK) interactions occur when drug Absorption, Distribution, Metabolism or Excretion (ADME) are altered by another drug.

Absorption is influenced by transit time through the gut (e.g. excessive laxative use may reduce transit time sufficiently to reduce absorption). The pH of the gut determines whether a drug is present in an ionised or nonionised form, with nonionised drugs being more lipophilic and more easily absorbed. Chemical complexation may also take place, reducing solubility.

Distribution, after absorption by the gut, and thus bioavailability, is mediated via drug transporters such as P-glycoprotein (P-gp) or multidrug resistance protein 1 (MDR1), organic anion transporters (OATs), tissue depot and serum binding. P-gp transports many important drugs, and in the intestinal epithelium it pumps these back into the gut lumen. In the liver, P-gp excretes drugs into the bile duct; in the kidney, it excretes them into the urine; and in the blood–brain barrier and blood–testis barrier, it pumps them back into the capillaries. *Increased* intestinal expression of P-gp reduces absorption of drugs, so plasma concentrations may be too low, whereas *decreased* P-gp elevates blood concentrations, which in some circumstances can lead to toxic concentrations of the drug. Some cancer cells express large amounts of P-gp, making them multidrug resistant. P-gp is inhibited by some natural compounds (e.g. quercetin and curcumin), which may provide a means of delaying resistance or improving drug bioavailability.

Metabolism of drugs in phase 1 takes place mainly via cytochrome P450 (CYP) enzymes, which are found in hepatocytes and other cells. Of currently prescribed drugs 70%–80% are metabolised by CYP enzymes. Over 50 are known, but only 6 are responsible for metabolising most drugs, the 2 most significant being CYP3A4 and CYP2D6 (Cho & Yoon, 2015).

CYP enzyme induction: if enzyme activity is increased, the metabolism of another substrate drug will also be increased, leading to reduced

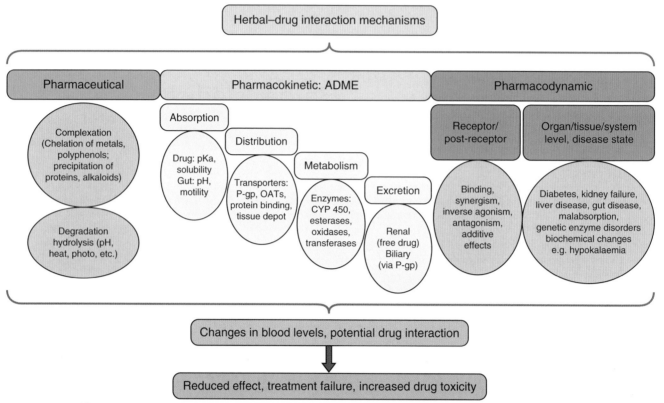

Fig. 14.1 Herbal–drug interactions: chemical and physiological mechanisms involved. *ADME,* Absorption, distribution, metabolism or excretion; *OATs,* organic anion transporters; *P-gp,* P-glycoprotein.

plasma drug concentrations and even treatment failure (unless the substrate drug is a prodrug, in which case, the increased metabolism will lead to increased concentrations of the active metabolite). *CYP enzyme inhibition:* if enzyme activity is inhibited, the metabolism of another substrate drug will be decreased, leading to increased plasma levels and possible toxicity.

Other enzymes that may be involved in drug interactions include esterases and oxidases, and in phase 2 metabolism, transferases, which conjugate nonpolar drugs into more water-soluble forms for excretion by the kidney.

Excretion takes place via the kidney and biliary systems. In the kidney, glomerular filtration and tubular secretion and reabsorption occur before excretion in the urine, but this applies only to the free drug and not protein-bound forms. In biliary excretion, drugs and metabolites are excreted by the liver into the gall bladder, and via bile duct into the intestine, to be excreted in the stool. The gut flora may metabolise drugs and hydrolyse conjugates, which may be reabsorbed in the enterohepatic cycle. P-gp is involved in the process of biliary excretion, and inhibition reduces the amount of drug or metabolite eliminated via this route.

The expression of CYP enzymes (including 3A4), transferases and drug transporters (Pg-p, OATs) is regulated via the pregnane X receptor (PXR) and the constitutive androstane receptor (CAR). These nuclear receptors play a crucial role in all drug metabolism, and inhibitors and activators have been identified in HMs (Yu et al., 2011).

PHARMACOGENOMICS AND PHARMACOGENETICS

Pharmacogenomics (genetic variations in individuals and populations) and *pharmacogenetics* (single drug–gene interactions) influence drug response. Taking genetic factors into account when prescribing treatment is now termed 'personalised medicine'. In traditional

and complementary medicine, individualised medicine is not a new approach at all, with both physical and psychological aspects (rather than a genetic profile) considered in addition to disease symptoms.

The phenomenon of pharmacogenetics was first described by Pythagoras (ca 510 BCE), when he linked fava bean consumption with haemolytic anaemia ('favism') in some individuals, which was later found to be due to a deficiency of the enzyme glucose-6-phosphate dehydrogenase. Individuals can also be broadly categorised according to their speed of metabolism, ranging from 'ultra-rapid' to 'poor' metabolisers. The major genetic polymorphisms involve CYP2D6, 2C19 and 2C9. In ultrarapid metabolisers they may result in treatment failure, and in poor metabolisers, toxicity (Samer et al., 2013).

EVALUATING HERBAL MEDICINE INTERACTIONS

Protocols and standards used for the evaluation of interactions of HMs are similar to those used for other drug interactions and for reporting adverse events (see Chapter 15). The pharmaceutical quality of HMs is rarely as high as that of licensed medicines, and they are subject to wide variations in composition, which may be important with respect to their potential for drug interactions, for example, through variable effects on CYP enzymes. HMs also have the potential for long and unsupervised consumption, which may be important with respect to the potential for drug interactions to occur.

Individual herbal ingredients may interact through more than one mechanism. For example, in conjunction with other antidepressants, St John's wort may lead to a serotonergic syndrome by PD mechanisms, whereas taken with ciclosporin it reduces blood concentrations via PK processes. It induces several CYP enzymes, as well as P-gp, via induction of the PXR, making it susceptible to several different mechanisms of interaction. Most other HMs do not pose the same danger, but St John's wort provides an example of how experimental results

TABLE 14.1 Common Herbal Drugs and Their Interaction Studies in Humans

Herbal Drug	Prescribed Drug	Effects Found in Human Studies and Case Reports
Astragalus, Milkvetch or Huangqi. Root *Astragalus membranaceus* (Fisch.) Bunge	Docetaxel	No interaction
Dan shen, Red sage. Root. *Salvia miltiorrhiza* Bunge	Theophylline Clopidogrel, fexofenadine, warfarin	No interaction Reduced plasma concentrations of drug
Echinacea. Root, herb, juice Purple/narrow-leaved/pale coneflower. *E. purpurea* (L.) Moench./*E. angustifolia* DC./*E. pallida* (Nutt.) Nutt.	Caffeine, digoxin, docetaxel, etravirine, lopinavir/ ritonavir, midazolam, warfarin Darunavir Etoposide	No interaction Reduced blood concentrations of darunavir in some individuals Increased toxicity of etoposide (1 case)
Ginger. Rhizome *Zingiber officinale* Roscoe	Warfarin Nifedipine	No interaction Enhanced antiplatelet effect
Ginkgo. Leaf. Maidenhair tree. *Ginkgo biloba* L.	Anastrozole, aspirin, atorvastatin, cilostazol, donepezil, letrozole, simvastatin, tamoxifen, warfarin Phenytoin, valproate	No interaction Single case reports suggest decreased blood concentrations
Ginseng. Root Asian/Korean ginseng *Panax ginseng* C.A. Mey.	Fexofenadine, lopinavir/ritonavir, warfarin Imatinib, lamotrigine, midazolam	No interaction Single case reports suggest increased toxicity of imatinib and lamotrigine; possible reduced effect of midazolam
Milk thistle. Fruits. *Silybum marianum* (L.) Gaertn.	Indinavir, nifedipine, midazolam, dextromethorphan, caffeine drug probe cocktail	No interaction
St John's wort. Herb. *Hypericum perforatum* L.	Carbamazepine, ibuprofen, prednisone, repaglinide, mycophenolate Alprazolam, amitriptyline, ciclosporin, digoxin, gliclazide, imatinib, indinavir, irinotecan, midazolam, nevirapine, nifedipine, omeprazole, oral contraceptives, tacrolimus, verapamil, warfarin, zolpidem Paroxetine, venlafaxine	No interaction Decreased blood concentrations, leading to treatment failure, for example, rejection episodes in transplant patients on ciclosporin, and breakthrough bleeding with hormonal contraception. Serotonin syndrome, due to additive effects with selective serotonin reuptake inhibitors.
St John's wort low-hyperforin extract	Caffeine, dextromethorphan, digoxin, tolbutamide drug probe cocktail	No interaction
Schisandra, Magnolia vine. Wu Wei Zi. Fruit *Schisandra chinensis* (Turcz.) Baill., *S. sphenanthera* Rehder & E.H. Wilson	Midazolam, paclitaxel, tacrolimus, talinolol	Blood concentrations increased and bioavailability improved. May be beneficial but monitoring required

can reflect patient risk. The most important mechanisms have been well-reviewed by Butterweck and Nahrstedt (2012), Cho and Yoon (2015) and Gurley et al. (2012). In most traditional and complementary medicine systems, preparations containing multiple medicinal plants are used more commonly than single herbal substances, which introduces further complexity, and the combination must be treated as the active ingredient.

Table 14.1 illustrates the interaction profiles of popular medicinal plants, taken from human studies. Mechanistic studies carried out to elucidate their mechanisms of action are shown in Table 14.2. 'Negative' findings, i.e. those demonstrating a lack of activity, are highlighted in bold. These are equally useful in evaluating the safety of herbal drugs, if less exciting for researchers.

RISK FACTORS ASSOCIATED WITH HERBAL MEDICINE INTERACTIONS

As shown in Box 14.1, risk factors for HDIs arise from the nature of the herbal substance and the drug, and the susceptibility of the patient, and both are usually involved. HMs are widely used by older adults (Agbabiaka et al., 2017) and are administered to children. Older patients have a generally slower metabolism and are more likely to be

taking multiple medications, whereas infants and children do not have the same range of enzymes, and these processes develop at different rates.

Patients with serious and chronic diseases, such as cancer and HIV, are more likely to use complementary therapies of all types, including HMs and nutritional supplements. These patients are becoming increasingly aware of HDIs, and studies show a general trend towards caution with their supplement use (e.g. Alsanad et al., 2016).

Pregnant and lactating women are usually prescribed only essential drugs (e.g. for epilepsy) but their use of HMs is rarely monitored, and some herbal products are used specifically at these times. The most widely used include raspberry leaf tea (*Rubus idaeus* L.) and ginger (*Zingiber officinale* Roscoe) during pregnancy and fenugreek (*Trigonella foenum-graecum* L.), fennel (*Foeniculum vulgare* Mill.) and ginger during breast-feeding. These have not been associated with increased risk of HDIs, but complete safety has not been established.

CONCLUSIONS

The use of herbal and nutritional supplements is increasing, and the practice of integrated medicine is becoming more widely accepted. Western-trained health professionals may have received little or no training in

TABLE 14.2 Constituents and Effects of Herbal Drugs on Metabolic Enzymes and Drug Transporters

Medicinal Plant	Major Constituents	EFFECTS ON ENZYMES		EFFECTS ON TRANSPORTERS		Clinical Interactions Overview (Details as Reported in Table 14.1)
		Inhibition	Induction	Inhibition	Induction	
Astragalus *Astragalus membranaceus*	Triterpene saponins, (astragalosides), isoflavones	CYPs 1A2, 3A4	—	—	—	Potentially reduced clearance of some drugs but no clinical reports.
Dan Shen *Salvia miltiorrhiza*	Diterpenoids (tanshinones), phenolics (salvianolic acids)	CYPs 2C9, 2C19, 3A4, UGT, carboxylesterases	—	OAT1, OAT3	P-gp	Reduced plasma concentrations of drugs transported via P-gp. Potential for interaction with ester prodrugs.
Echinacea *Echinacea* spp.	Alkylamides (root), caffeic acid derivatives, polysaccharides	No effect on CYPs 2D6, 1A2	CYP3 AA4 (weak)	—	P-gp	Clinical studies and case reports show weak interaction potential. Isolated case reports are unconfirmed.
Ginger *Zingiber officinale*	Phenolic gingerols/shogaols, mono- and sesquiterpenes	—	—	Pg-p (weak)	—	Clinical and *in vivo* studies suggest low interaction profile.
Ginkgo leaf *Ginkgo biloba*	Diterpene lactones (ginkgolides, bilobalide), flavone glycosides	CYPs 1A2, 2C8, 2C9, 2E1	CYPs 3A4, 2C19	Pg-p	—	Generally low potential for interaction but additive effects (e.g. antiplatelet) may be involved.
Ginseng root *Panax ginseng*	Triterpene saponins, (ginsenosides, GS), polyacetylenes, etc.	CYPs 2C9, 2C19, 2D6 UGT	CYP 3A4	Pg-p (high-dose GS)	—	Clinical tests show overall low potential for interaction but isolated cases suggest caution.
Milk thistle *Silybum marianum*	Flavonolignans, mixture known as silymarin	No effect on CYP1A2, CYP2B6, CYP2C9, CYP2C19, CYP3A4	—	OATP1B1, OATP1B3, OATP2B1	—	No significant effects, including on indinavir pharmacokinetics.
St John's wort *Hypericum perforatum*	Naphthodianthrones (hypericins); phloroglucinols (hyperforins) flavonols	CYP1A2	CYPs 3A4, 2C9, 2C19, 2E1	—	P-gp, strong	Mechanistic studies show that strong inhibition, especially via two mechanisms, increases likelihood of clinical interaction.
St John's wort low-hyperforin extract	Naphthodianthrones (hypericins); flavonols	No effect on CYP1A2, CYP2B6, CYP2C9, CYP2C19, CYP3A4	—	No effect on P-gp	—	Drug cocktail probes in human studies show no interaction for low-hyperforin SJW extract.
Schisandra *Schisandra* spp.	Lignans, the schisandrins and schisandrols (gomisins, wuweizus)	CYP3A4	—	P-gp	—	Inhibition of P-gp improves oral bioavailability of some drugs and may be of therapeutic benefit.

CYP, Cytochrome; *OATs*, organic anion transporters; *P-gp*, P-glycoprotein.

BOX 14.1 Risk Factors Associated With Herbal Medicine Interactions

Properties of Drug/Herb	Patient Susceptibility
• Strong enzyme inducers or inhibitors	• Genetic polymorphism
• Strong inducers of P-glycoprotein	• Multiple medication regime
• Narrow therapeutic index of drug	• Impaired absorption from gut
• Steep dose–response curve of drug	• Reduced metabolism in liver disease
• Oral administration route	• Reduced excretion in kidney failure
• Long-term treatment	• Inappropriate self-medication

the appropriate use of HMs, which predisposes them to advise patients against them. However, if an individual has been taking a combination without perceiving any harm, they may decide that the prescriber has a lack of expertise in this area and not inform them of their HM use. Pharmacists are ideally placed to advise patients on HDIs if they have information available and are easily approached by patients, especially if they are also dispensing their prescribed medicines. It is not possible to list all potential HDIs here, so an up-to-date reference should always be consulted. When possible, registered herbal products should be recommended as these are certified as good quality. They also include patient information leaflets that give more details about combinations to avoid.

REFERENCES

Agbabiaka, T.B., Wider, B., Watson, L.K., Goodman, C., 2017. Concurrent use of prescription drugs and herbal medicinal products in older adults: a systematic review. Drugs Aging 34, 891–905.

Alsanad, S.M., Howard, R.L., Williamson, E.M., 2016. An assessment of the impact of herb-drug combinations used by cancer patients. BMC Complementary Alternat. Med. 16, 393.

Butterweck, V., Nahrstedt, A., 2012. What is the best strategy for preclinical testing of botanicals? A critical perspective. Planta Med. 78 (8), 747–754.

Cho, H.J., Yoon, I.S., 2015. Pharmacokinetic interactions of herbs with cytochrome p450 and p-glycoprotein. Evid. Based Complement. Alternat. Med. 2015, 736431.

Gurley, B.J., Fifer, E.K., Gardner, Z., 2012. Pharmacokinetic herb–drug interactions (part 2): drug interactions involving popular botanical dietary supplements and their clinical relevance. Planta Med. 78 (13), 1490–1514.

Izzo, A.A., Hoon-Kim, S., Radhakrishnan, R., Williamson, E.M., 2016. A critical approach to evaluating clinical efficacy, adverse events and drug interactions of herbal remedies. Phytother. Res. 30 (5), 691–700.

Liu, S.-H., Cheng, Y.-C., 2012. Old formula, new Rx: the journey of PHY906 as cancer adjuvant therapy. J. Ethnopharmacol. 140 (3), 614–623.

Nicolussi, S., Drewe, J., Butterweck, V., Meyer Zu Schwabedissen, H.E., 2020. Clinical relevance of St. John's wort drug interactions revisited. Br. J. Pharmacol. 177 (6), 1212–1226.

Qi, F., Zhao, L., Zhou, A., Zhang, B., Li, A., Wang, Z., et al., 2015. The advantages of using traditional Chinese medicine as an adjunctive therapy in the whole course of cancer treatment instead of only terminal stage of cancer. Biosci. Trends 9 (1), 16–34.

Russo, E., Scicchitano, F., Whalley, B.J., Mazzitello, C., Ciriaco, M., Esposito, S., et al., 2014. *Hypericum perforatum*: pharmacokinetic, mechanism of action, tolerability, and clinical drug–drug interactions. Phytother. Res. 28, 643–655.

Samer, C.F., Lorenzini, K.I., Rollason, V., Daali, Y., Desmeules, J.A., 2013. Applications of CYP450 testing in the clinical setting. Mol. Diagn. Ther. 17 (3), 165–184.

Wei, H., Tao, X., Di, P., Yang, Y., Li, J., Qian, X., et al., 2013. Effects of traditional Chinese medicine Wuzhi capsule on pharmacokinetics of tacrolimus in rats. Drug Metab. Dispos. 41, 1398–1403.

Yu, C., Chai, X., Chen, S., Zeng, S., 2011. Identification of novel pregnane X receptor activators from traditional Chinese medicine. J. Ethnopharmacol. 136 (1), 137–143.

15

Regulation and Pharmacovigilance for Herbal Medicines

As discussed in Chapter 1, herbal medicines (HMs) are available in several forms, including as dried plant material (herbal drugs), extracts of herbal drugs formulated as finished products (dosage forms such as tablets and capsules) and marketed as herbal medicinal products (HMPs), dietary supplements and/or fortified health foods. Isolated chemical entities are also extracted from plant material but are not considered to be HMs. These products are used for health benefits, yet herbal starting materials and finished products can be of variable quality, and some products can cause adverse drug reactions (ADRs). Thus, it is important that HMs are regulated (i.e. comply with accepted standards) so that there are assurances on their quality, safety and effectiveness. Equally, it is essential that there is ongoing surveillance (pharmacovigilance) of HMPs.

CHARACTERISTICS OF REGULATION FOR HERBAL MEDICINES

In many countries, legislation is provided only for products to be regulated as medicines (with 'licensed' indications for use) or as foods (without health claims). In most countries, conventional medicines are required to hold a marketing authorisation (MA) or product licence (PL), which may be granted by a competent authority for regulating medicines following an application by the manufacturer/sponsor. MAs/PLs are granted where products meet stringent requirements for quality, safety and efficacy in relation to *specific indications for use*. Once authorised, manufacturers have ongoing obligations with respect to their products, including safety monitoring, and MAs/PLs can be suspended or withdrawn. In principle, there is no reason why manufacturers could not apply for an MA for a specific indication for an HMP; however, in practice, due to the chemical complexity of HMs (and other reasons), it is extremely difficult for manufacturers to meet the exacting requirements set out for conventional medicines.

At the same time, HMs are used to treat and prevent medical conditions and symptoms and for health maintenance, which (mostly) distinguishes their use from that of foods. The barriers inherent for HMPs in attempting to meet medicines legislation requirements, and the unsuitability of 'food legislation' as a regulatory framework for HMs, meant that, in many countries, herbal products were—and, in some cases, remain—essentially unregulated. However, even in countries where there are no specific regulations for HMs, a herbal product could breach legislation if, for example, therapeutic claims are made for a product that is not authorised as a medicine.

Simplified Regulatory Frameworks

Over the last two decades, many countries have introduced new regulatory frameworks for HMPs and for other types of 'natural health' products. Typically, these are simplified regulatory systems for 'low-risk' products used for minor, self-limiting conditions suitable for self-treatment; they usually apply to HMPs sold in retail outlets and are not intended to control HMs administered or supplied by traditional medicine (TM) practitioners. These frameworks usually require

manufacturers to meet pharmaceutical quality standards for their products, as discussed in Chapter 12.

Evidence of traditional use, i.e. *documented* use, of that product or one that is materially similar, for a minimum specified period, usually 2–3 generations or 30–50 years, depending on the regulatory framework, is accepted in lieu of evidence from new clinical trials, which are not required. Assessment of safety is often limited to a bibliographic review and/or inclusion of permitted ingredients from an approved list. The inclusion (or not) of ingredients on these lists is usually determined using a risk-based approach. Permissible ingredients may be subject to use for specific purposes (e.g. as an excipient only or as an active ingredient) and restrictions relating to maximum concentration or quantity, method of preparation, route of administration, addition of label warnings and so forth. There are usually some mandatory pharmacovigilance requirements for manufacturers of products marketed under these regulatory schemes (see later).

The regulation of HMs is complex and, not surprisingly, varies from country to country even where a similar 'risk-based' approach is taken. Initiatives aimed at harmonising regulation have been successful in some regions, notably the European Union (EU), with the implementation of the Traditional Herbal Medicinal Products Directive (THMPD) 2004/24/EC in 2004. The THMPD provides a mechanism whereby manufacturers/sponsors can apply for a Traditional Herbal Registration (THR) for HMs that meet requirements for quality (as discussed in Chapter 12), safety (bibliographic review) and traditional use. Traditional use requires evidence that the HMP is derived from the same plant and prepared in a similar way, and has been used for at least 30 years, of which at least 15 years are in the EU. This allows for restricted medicinal claims.

In the UK and EU, HMPs are regulated separately to homoeopathic products and 'food supplements', whereas other Western countries regulate HMs together with these other types of products. For example, in Australia, Canada and the United States, these products are regulated collectively as 'complementary medicines', 'natural health products' and 'dietary supplements', respectively. The scope and types of products covered in these regulatory frameworks are summarised in Table 15.1.

Terminology used in relation to the different regulatory frameworks varies and terms are not synonymous across countries. For example, in the UK, HMs that meet the requirements of the THR scheme are granted a Traditional Herbal *Registration*. In Australia, most complementary medicines are available as '*listed*' medicines, with a small number of other products having met the stringent criteria to be a '*registered*' medicine. Thus, 'registration' (UK) and 'registered' (Australia) have entirely different meanings and requirements. In Canada, natural health products that meet the relevant regulatory requirements are granted a 'product licence', whereas in the UK, 'product licences' are granted only to medicinal products (typically, conventional medicines) that have met the requirements for an MA based on the full dossier of chemical, pharmaceutical, pharmacological, toxicological and clinical data. That said, some 'licensed' HMPs do exist in the UK: these

TABLE 15.1   Scope of Selected Regulatory Frameworks for Complementary Medicines, Natural Health Products and Dietary Supplements

Country	Regulatory Framework	Scope
Australia	Therapeutic Goods Act 1989	'Complementary medicines' include vitamin, mineral, herbal, aromatherapy and homoeopathic products.
Canada	Natural Health Product Regulations 2003	'Natural health products' include vitamins, minerals, herbal remedies, homoeopathic medicines, traditional medicines (e.g. traditional Chinese and Ayurvedic (East Indian) medicines), probiotics, amino acids, essential fatty acids and others.
United States	Dietary Supplements Health and Education Act 1994	'Dietary supplements' are vitamins, minerals, herbs/other botanicals, amino acids, or ... a concentrate, metabolite, constituent, extract or combination of any of these ingredients.

products were initially granted a 'product licence of right' because they were already on the market when the licensing system was introduced in the 1970s. They have not necessarily undergone stringent testing, but their popularity and long history of use have not raised significant safety concerns.

Regulations in some countries allow more than one pathway for HMPs to achieve a registration/licence/listing/authorisation. In Canada, manufacturers may apply through a pathway for licensing *traditional medicines*, or for natural health products making 'modern health claims'. The evidence criteria are different: for the 'modern health claims' pathway, these are more substantive for products considered to pose a medium or high risk of harm. In Australia, in 2018, a new route to achieve 'listed' status—known as the 'assessed-listed' pathway—was introduced, whereby herbal/complementary medicines are included in the Australian Register of Therapeutic Goods (ARTG) following self-certification of the safety and quality of the product, and *premarket assessment* by the Therapeutic Goods Administration (TGA) *of efficacy evidence (based on finished product) supporting the proposed indications*. This new category was introduced to allow manufacturers to make higher level claims where they are adequately supported by evidence and to motivate manufacturers to invest in clinical research to support their products; it is intended to bridge the (substantial) gap between 'listed' and 'registered' categories in terms of the evidence-base required. In the EU, the 'well-established use' directive (99/83/EC) was introduced to allow greater flexibility on the use of bibliographic data to demonstrate safety and efficacy, but interpretations vary between EU member states and this directive is not a widely accepted route to marketing.

In Brazil, HMPs may be authorised as HMs, based on clinical evidence and consistent quality, or as traditional herbal products, based on traditional use and formulations including only low-risk ingredients. Both categories are subject to regulation relating to both simplified and regular MA processes.

Plants Used in Traditional Medicine Systems

Regulations for natural health products/complementary medicines may, as in Australia and Canada, specifically include many plants and other substances used in TM systems, including Traditional Chinese Medicine (TCM), Ayurvedic Medicine and Ethnomedicine of the First Nations (Canada), on their 'permitted ingredients/substances' lists. In contrast, the implementation of the THMPD (see earlier) effectively meant that non-EU TM products (with few exceptions) could not meet the traditional use requirements as many had been introduced for sale only in the 1990s.

Outside Europe, countries with a very long heritage of TM use and intrinsic acceptance and integration of these ancient TM systems as part of contemporary healthcare have comprehensive approaches to governance of these systems. For example, in India, where Ayurvedic medicine has been used for thousands of years (see Chapter 16.3),

the Department of Ayurveda, Yoga & Naturopathy, Unani, Siddha and Homoeopathy (AYUSH) within the Ministry of Health & Family Welfare regulation and improvement of quality standards for herbal drugs used in Ayurvedic medicine, among other functions related to these traditional medical systems. Similarly, in China, TCM 'drugs' are regulated by the National Medical Products Administration (NMPA, formerly the China Food and Drug Administration), which also regulates Western medicines and medical devices. TCM drugs include Chinese materia medica, raw herbal and nonherbal drugs, processed and sliced herbal drugs (also known as TCM decoction pieces), which are prepared according to TCM principles, and Chinese 'patent' medicines (CPMs), which are manufactured products often containing multiple ingredients based on a traditional formula. All these types of products are included in the Chinese Pharmacopoeia. CPMs in particular are subject to specific regulations regarding their manufacture and evaluation; TCM decoction pieces are used as ingredients for CPMs and should also be prepared according to GMP guidance and to meet Chinese pharmacopoeial standards.

Despite an increased awareness globally of quality and safety issues that can arise with HMPs, some countries are still without specific regulations for them. For example, in New Zealand (NZ), HMs (and homoeopathic remedies) are defined in the NZ Medicines Act 1981, but are exempt from requirements to obtain premarket approval with respect to quality, safety and efficacy provided they meet certain criteria (e.g. materials are subject to simple processing only and are marketed without health claims). As there are no specific regulations for HMs and other natural health products, these products are captured as 'dietary supplements' under the Dietary Supplement Regulations 1985 and the Food Act 1981. These regulations do not require adherence to GMP standards nor any premarket assessment or approval, but they do provide some restrictions on ingredients permitted in dietary supplements, such as substances classified as prescription only, and therapeutic claims are not permitted.

Isolated Chemical Entities from Medicinal Plants

Isolated compounds from plants are not considered to be HMs for regulatory purposes. In many countries, such compounds are treated as new chemical entities and need to be authorised in the same way as synthetic drugs. However, some of the simplified regulatory frameworks mentioned earlier allow for isolated chemical compounds from plants—and even their metabolites—to be included as the sole ingredient, or as an additional ingredient, in 'natural health products or dietary supplements (see Table 15.1). For example, in Canada, the alkaloid cytisine, a nicotinic acetylcholine receptor agonist that occurs in parts of the common laburnum (*Laburnum anagyroides* Medik., Fabaceae) and some other species and is used in smoking cessation, is permitted as an ingredient in natural health products. Synthetic derivatives of naturally occurring chemicals are also (currently) permitted in some countries. For example, in the United States, there are 'dietary supplements' containing the vinca alkaloid derivative vinpocetine, a synthetic derivative of apovincamine, from the leaves of the lesser periwinkle *Vinca minor* L. (Apocynaceae).

Classification of Ingredients

The regulatory frameworks described earlier are largely intended for 'low-risk' products used for minor, self-limiting conditions suitable for use in self-treatment. Independent of whether a country has a specific regulatory framework for HMs, usually there is a separate system for classification of medicinal product ingredients, sometimes referred to as 'scheduling'. High-risk substances are classified as 'prescription-only' medicines (POM) and may only be supplied on the prescription of an authorised prescriber. Many conventional medicines, particularly those new to the market, and isolated chemical entities that originated from plant material (e.g. digoxin) are classified as prescription-only medicines. Likewise, potentially hazardous plants can also be classed as POM, although in many countries it is extremely unlikely that prescribers would use these plants. Some plants are classed as 'pharmacy-only' medicines (P), and certain others may be subject to dose (but not duration of treatment) and route of administration restrictions.

Introducing, or changing, the classification status of a substance or product is a way of implementing additional controls, particularly where a safety concern has arisen. This is illustrated by an incident in New Zealand involving a herbal product containing an extract of *Artemisia annua* L. (Asteraceae) marketed as an unauthorised (unregulated) dietary supplement for joint health and mobility. A series of ADR reports of hepatotoxicity was received by the NZ Pharmacovigilance Centre and, ultimately, Medsafe (the competent authority) sought classification of *A. annua* as a prescription medicine so that it could not be included as an ingredient in HMPs for self-treatment. Similar actions were taken in the UK and other countries following reports of ADRs associated with *Aristolochia* species (Aristolochiaceae) and kava (*Piper methysticum* G. Forst., Piperaceae): in these cases, *Aristolochia* species as well as some other plants that can be confused with *Aristolochia* species, and *P. methysticum*, were prohibited in unlicensed medicines, effectively removing them from the market.

Herbal Medicines Supplied by Herbal and Other Traditional Medicine Practitioners

The regulatory frameworks discussed earlier do not usually include products compounded and supplied by herbalists and other TM practitioners. Again, the approach to this differs across countries and is complex, since it concerns the regulation of both the practitioners themselves and the products they prepare and supply.

In some countries, herbal and TM practitioners are educated through university programmes, have a high level of professional organisation and are subject to statutory professional regulation. For example, in Australia, there is statutory regulation of Chinese medicine practitioners, where the Chinese Medicine Board of Australia works with the Australian Health Practitioner Regulation Agency to implement the regulatory framework. In other instances, the extent and quality of education and training can be highly variable, there may be little or no professional organisation, neither self- nor statutory regulation, nor any requirements to practice in accordance with a code of ethics or standards.

In Australia, Canada, New Zealand, the UK and some other countries, herbal and TMs that are extemporaneously prepared, for a specific patient following consultation, are exempt from regulations; this allows herbalists and other TM and natural-health practitioners to prepare individualised treatments. The prescribing and supply of certain herbal preparations may also be restricted to specific categories of registered TM practitioners. And others can only be prescribed by a medically qualified practitioner (i.e. doctor) and sold or supplied by a pharmacist (see Classification of Ingredients).

PHARMACOVIGILANCE FOR HERBAL MEDICINES

Pharmacovigilance is the science and practices concerning with identifying, evaluating and interpreting information on adverse reactions associated with the use of medicines and other healthcare products and is an essential public health function.

The safety profile of most HMs has not been subject to the comprehensive scientific scrutiny that is applied to assessing the safety of conventional drugs, so pharmacovigilance is very important in the context of HMs. A history of safe use in traditional HM can provide limited assurance about (lack of) acute toxicity, but cannot provide reliable information on many other aspects of safety, such as the effects of long-term use, latent adverse reactions, use in contemporary medical conditions (e.g. HIV infection) and concurrent use with conventional medicines. Preparing certain traditional HMs in particular ways (e.g. 'cooking' or boiling certain herbs used in TCM) is used to reduce toxicity, as with *Aconitum* spp., but these practices need to be underpinned by scientific evidence, and universally adopted if effective. Incomplete processing of Aconite still leads to numerous fatalities annually.

While the public health risk of HMs needs to be kept in perspective, serious adverse reactions, include hepatic and renal toxicity, associated with the use of certain herbal preparations have been reported. In some cases, these are due to the toxicity of constituents of the plant material used, as discussed in Chapter 13 (Toxicity of Herbal Constituents); in other instances, the adverse reaction may have occurred due to failures in quality, such as contamination of the plant material with toxic weeds or other plant species, microorganisms or pesticides (see Chapter 12). The potential for drug interactions to occur between plant medicines and conventional medicines taken concurrently is of increasing concern, and is discussed in Chapter 14 (Herbal Medicine Interactions).

Regulatory Pharmacovigilance for Herbal Medicines

The regulatory frameworks described earlier place obligations on manufacturers to undertake pharmacovigilance activities for products marketed under these regulations. In the UK, manufacturers of (the small number of) licensed HMs and those of herbal products with a THR have the same obligations regarding pharmacovigilance as do MA holders for conventional medicines, including mandatory requirements for handling ADR reports received from patients and health practitioners, and the timely submission of these to the Medicines and Healthcare Products Regulatory Agency. The only exception is that THR holders are not usually required to submit periodic safety update reports (PSURs) for their THR products.

Elsewhere, there are similar (but not identical) requirements. In Australia, manufacturers/sponsors of medicines registered or listed on the ARTG are required to comply with the Australian Therapeutic Goods Administration's guidance on pharmacovigilance responsibilities. For 'listed' medicines (most herbal and other complementary medicines in Australia are 'listed' medicines), the mandatory requirements include submission of all serious ADR reports for their products to the TGA within 15 calendar days and informing the TGA of any significant safety issues within 72 hours of identification. Similar requirements were enacted in the Natural Health Product Regulations (2003) in Canada, whereas in the United States, since 2007, manufacturers have been mandated to report serious suspected 'adverse events' associated with 'dietary supplements' (which, in the United States, includes herbal medicines; see Table 15.1) to the Food and Drug Administration (FDA) Center for Food Safety and Applied Nutrition (CFSAN) Adverse Event Reporting System (CAERS) within 15 business days of first receiving notification.

There are many countries that do not yet have specific regulations for HMs, meaning that there are no obligations on manufacturers to submit any information on reports they receive about ADRs associated with their products, including serious reactions, to a national competent authority. Pharmacovigilance for these unregulated products relies on the submission of spontaneous reports of suspected ADRs associated with HMs being submitted to the national pharmacovigilance centre by product users, or health professionals informed about such reactions by their patients. Since there is generally a lack of awareness among the public and health professionals of the need for pharmacovigilance for HMs, as well as substantial under-reporting of ADRs associated with these products, only low numbers of reports are received and it is possible that safety concerns may go undetected.

Spontaneous Reporting Schemes for Herbal Medicines

Formalised pharmacovigilance systems for health practitioners to report suspected ADRs were first introduced in a few countries in the 1960s. Initially, these spontaneous ADR reporting schemes involved reporting for authorised medicinal products only, which essentially excluded HMs as many were, or remain, unauthorised/unregulated products. Today, more than 170 member and associate member countries contribute their national ADR report data to the WHO Programme for International Drug Monitoring, maintained by the Uppsala Monitoring Centre in Sweden. Many countries do undertake pharmacovigilance for at least some types of herbal and TMs, but several have not so far integrated these HMs into their pharmacovigilance systems, or do not yet have such a system.

An important development in pharmacovigilance with relevance to HMs has been the introduction of direct patient reporting of suspected ADRs to national reporting schemes. Since HMs are used mostly in self-treatment, the introduction of direct patient reporting could be particularly important as a method of stimulating ADR reporting for these products. ADR reporting forms are being revised to include the collection of data relating to HMs. There are also examples of dedicated spontaneous reporting schemes for HMs: in Italy, an online 'phytovigilance' scheme was introduced in 2002 to stimulate and collect spontaneous reports of suspected ADRs associated with food supplements, herbal products and compounded preparations containing herbal ingredients. This is separate to the medicines pharmacovigilance system that collects reports of ADRs associated with conventional drugs and authorised/registered HMPs.

Despite these initiatives, reports of suspected ADRs associated with HMs submitted to national pharmacovigilance centres represent a very small proportion of the total number of reports received. One exception to this is China, where around 10%–15% of reports of suspected ADRs are for TCM drugs, often with allergic reactions associated with injectable CPMs.

Safety Signal Detection for Herbal Medicines

Due to the low numbers of reports received, apart from at the international level, statistical methods for signal detection are rarely used for HMs. Rather, signals are usually identified manually through an increase in the number of reports for a specific herbal substance, or some other change in the reporting pattern. Reports then undergo clinical review and causality assessment to aid identification of 'signals'. This approach has identified several safety issues, including hepatotoxicity associated with black cohosh (*Actaea racemosa* L.; syn.: *Cimicifuga racemosa* L.) root/rhizome extracts, green tea (*Camellia sinensis* (L.) Kuntze) and supercritical carbon dioxide extracts of *A. annua* L. herb, and drug interactions associated with St John's wort (*Hypericum perforatum* L.).

Beyond spontaneous reporting of ADRs, many other methods, such as intensive monitoring and other observational study designs, including those using 'real-world' data, are used for conventional medicines to investigate their harms profile. However, these methods have hardly been applied to examining HMs beyond a research context, if at all. Many important challenges in pharmacovigilance for HMs remain and greater engagement with users of HMs, as well as with herbal and TM practitioners, is likely to be pivotal to improving pharmacovigilance for these products.

FURTHER READING

Barnes, J. (Ed.), 2022. Pharmacovigilance for Herbal and Traditional Medicines. Advances, Challenges, and International Perspectives. Springer (in press).

Barnes, J., 2012. Adverse drug reactions and pharmacovigilance of herbal medicines. In: Talbot, J., Aronson, J. (Eds.), Stephens' Detection and Evaluation of Adverse Drug Reactions, sixth ed. Wiley, Chichester, pp. 645–683.

de Smet, P.A.G.M., 1997. An introduction to herbal pharmacovigilance. In: De Smet, P.A.G.M., Keller, K., Hansel, R., Chandler, R. (Eds.), Adverse Effects of Herbal Drugs, vol. 3. Springer-Verlag, Berlin, pp. 1–13.

Ernst, E., De Smet, P.A., Shaw, D., Murray, V., 1998. Traditional remedies and the 'test of time'. Eur. J. Clin. Pharmacol. 54 (2), 99–100.

Reddy, K.J., Alex, M.J., Thomas, A. (Eds.), 2017. Regulations for Herbal Medicine – Worldwide: A Focus on Current Regulations and Their Requirements. Lambert Academic Publishing.

Uppsala Monitoring Centre. The WHO Programme for International Drug Monitoring. Available at: https://who-umc.org/about-the-who-programme-for-international-drug-monitoring/.

WHO, 2004. WHO Guidelines on Safety Monitoring of Herbal Medicines in Pharmacovigilance Systems. WHO, Geneva.

WHO, 2013. WHO Traditional Medicine Strategy: 2014–2023. WHO, Geneva.

World Health Organization, 2019. WHO Global Report on Traditional and Complementary Medicine 2019. World Health Organization, Geneva.

World Health Organization, 2019. Pharmacovigilance and Traditional and Complementary Medicine in South-East Asia. A Situation Review.

Zhang, L., 2018. Pharmacovigilance of herbal and traditional medicines. In: Bate, A. (Ed.), Evidence-Based Pharmacovigilance. Clinical and Quantitative Aspects. Humana Press, New York, pp. 37–65.

16

Plants in Traditional Medicine Systems

INTRODUCTION

Most countries have their own systems of traditional medicine (TM) which remain an important part of healthcare. TM modalities are no longer limited to the country, culture or region in which they originated: many are now practised globally.

The World Health Organization defines TM as 'the sum total of the knowledge, skill, and practices based on the theories, beliefs, and experiences indigenous to different cultures, whether explicable or not, used in the maintenance of health as well as in the prevention, diagnosis, improvement or treatment of physical and mental illness'. An important feature is that the traditional knowledge and practices are handed down from generation to generation, orally or in writing.

TM includes an array of practices and approaches, incorporating traditional herbal preparations and formulae, spiritual therapies, manual techniques and exercises, applied alone or in combination. The WHO also sees TM to be an important element of primary healthcare, as highlighted in the Astana Declaration: 'We support broadening and extending access to a range of health care services through the use of high-quality, safe, effective and affordable medicines, including, as appropriate, traditional medicines, vaccines, diagnostics and other technologies' (WHO, 2018).

Most TMs are based on plant material, but in some systems, especially traditional Chinese medicine (TCM), natural ingredients not of plant origin (e.g. insects, animal parts and minerals) are included. These are outside the scope of this book.

The WHO TM strategy 2014–2023 recognises the continued and global use and practice of TM; its economic, social and cultural importance; and advances in regulation and standards. Their remit is 'to support WHO member states in:

- harnessing the potential contribution of TM to health, wellness and people-centred healthcare;
- promoting the safe and effective use of TM by regulating, researching and integrating TM products, practitioners and practice into health systems, where appropriate'.

The WHO has published numerous monographs and guidelines relating to TM, including good agricultural and collection practices for medicinal plants, safety monitoring in pharmacovigilance systems, development of consumer information and, most recently, herb–drug interactions. All are available at the WHO website (www.who.org).

GLOBAL EXTENT OF MEDICINAL PLANT USE

Almost 18,000 plant species are recorded as used in medicines, and a substantial proportion of these relate to use in TM. The materia medica of TCM, for example, uses over 3000 plant species. Not surprisingly, trade in raw materials used in TM is vast. Unreliable supply chains and unsustainable and/or illegal trade in endangered plant (and animal) species for medicinal purposes have contributed to their extinction risk.

The extent of use of herbal medicines is difficult to estimate since it involves several points of access (e.g. self-treatment, consultations with TM practitioners) and because studies often conflate TM with other herbal medicines and natural health products. In developing countries in particular, a substantial proportion of the population (up to 80% in parts of Africa) relies on the use of TM and traditional healers as their only, or main, source of healthcare. The extent to which individuals consult different types of traditional or complementary medicine practitioners varies across different countries, ethnic populations and patient groups. However, market research data indicate that sales of herbal and other complementary medicines are substantial and increasing; for example, sales in the United States in 2017 were over US$ 8.8 billion, and in China in 2016, the market was worth US$ 100–120 billion (reviewed in WHO, 2021).

THE EVIDENCE BASE FOR TRADITIONAL MEDICINE

In the region from which a TM originates, there is usually a firm confidence and cultural acceptance as a healthcare option, whereas outside the area, general uncertainty about the practice and effectiveness is common. Scientific evidence to support or refute the philosophical concepts of a TM system is virtually impossible but evidence relating to the safety and efficacy of a TM product or treatment can be obtained through good clinical trials. Many studies with traditional Chinese, Ayurvedic and other TMs have been carried out, but have not always met high standards of methodological quality. The Cochrane Library contains over 100 systematic reviews of clinical trials of Chinese herbal medicines, which provide limited evidence of efficacy, but typically conclude that 'further, more rigorous, studies' are required.

The safety of TM has not been subject to the comprehensive scrutiny applied to conventional medicines. A history of safe use in TM can provide a limited degree of assurance about the (usually, lack of) acute toxicity, but not on many other aspects of safety, such as the effects of long-term use, latent adverse reactions, use in contemporary medical conditions (e.g. HIV and coronavirus infection), and concurrent use with conventional medicines.

While the public health risk of using TMs needs to be kept in perspective, serious adverse reactions associated with certain preparations have been reported. Many countries in which TM use is most prevalent do not have established or well-resourced drug safety monitoring systems, and these are not easily applied to collecting data on TMs, some of which contain up to 15 or more ingredients of plant or other origin. The preparation and its components may be named ambiguously, or even unidentified. Even in countries with well-established pharmacovigilance systems, reports from traditional practitioners of suspected adverse reactions are scarce, as discussed in Chapter 15.

HERBAL MEDICINE USE IN MINOR DISORDERS AND SERIOUS DISEASE

The treatment of minor or self-limiting disorders, and chronic or serious disorders, is approached differently in TM. Minor disorders include aches and pains, diarrhoea, wounds or injuries, and facilitation of childbirth, for which a common remedy will be taken, usually an indigenous plant or one easily obtainable from a local market, and well known within the community. Serious disorders may be life-threatening, debilitating, or conditions that cannot be diagnosed by indigenous healers, such as metabolic diseases, epilepsy and psychiatric conditions: in some TM systems they are considered to have a supernatural component. Plant remedies will be used, but may have a more ritualistic purpose. Practices such as divination, incantation and even sacrifice may be included, to appease the supernatural entity.

CORRELATION OF TRADITIONAL USE WITH SCIENTIFIC EVIDENCE

The purpose of a medicinal plant, as viewed within a TM system, influences the way it is investigated scientifically. Dose is difficult to assess with natural materials due to their variability, so highly potent plants were rarely used as traditional herbal medicines and some plants that we now find useful were considered dangerous. For example, the foxglove, a source of the cardiac glycoside digoxin, has no historical documentation as a herbal medicine, due to the narrow therapeutic index of the drug. It was necessary to develop a standardised preparation, assayed biologically, and compressed into a tablet, before *Digitalis* gained widespread acceptance.

Medicines for common ailments usually contain specific classes of compounds. Antipyretic or analgesic compounds, such as salicylates and sesquiterpene lactones, may be found in a medicinal plant known as a cure for fever, and haemostatic and astringent substances, such as tannins in a plant used to staunch bleeding and for diarrhoea. However, if ritual is more often involved in the use of a particular plant, it is almost impossible to surmise what compounds may be present; this approach is therefore much less useful. The plant may be a treasure trove of useful compounds, but the traditional use will not provide any information about it.

Thus, there may be a correlation between traditional usage and pharmacological action, such as the isolation of antipyretic principles from a 'fever' remedy, but, even so, the results may turn out to be different to our expectations, as with *Cinchona*. The bark was traditionally used in South America for 'fever', but in many tropical countries 'fever' really means 'malaria'. Quinine is antipyretic to some extent, but it has a much more relevant property, which is to kill the malaria parasite *Plasmodium*. Therefore, plants based on traditional usage are usually subject to a battery of tests, since some important modern drugs have been developed from plants used for a different purpose entirely. For example, in the Caribbean the periwinkle *Catharanthus* (*Vinca*) *rosea* (L.) G. Don (originally from Madagascar) was used traditionally for treating diabetes, but on further investigation it yielded the powerful anticancer alkaloids vincristine and vinblastine.

TMs have yielded many useful modern drugs, although not as many as those yielded by poisonous species. Toxic plants are well known to the healers and may also be used for nefarious purposes, in witchcraft or as 'ordeal' poisons, as with the Calabar bean (*Physostigma venenosum* Balf.), which is the source of the anticholinesterase physostigmine (eserine).

COMMONALITY OF SPECIES USED GLOBALLY

The following sections discuss TM in the West, Asia, China, Japan, Indonesia, Australasia and Oceania. In this revised edition, details of some TM concepts have been condensed to make room for more detail on the medicinal plants most prominent in those systems, in the form of tables. When collating these for each traditional system, certain species or genera appear in almost every list, and it is striking that, even with the disparity in philosophies and principles behind their inclusion, these plants are used for very similar therapeutic indications (Table 16.0.1). The reasons for this commonality are varied. Medicinal plants and spices are used as food and medicine, and global trade has contributed to their incorporation into regional TM systems, which may be far from where the plant originates. Tropical species such as ginger, turmeric, pepper, aloe, cinnamon and many others are widely used in temperate countries. Related species and genera, containing similar phytochemical constituents, tend to be used for similar medicinal purposes in all TM systems, presumably based on observational evidence obtained independently. Berberine and related alkaloid-containing plants (from the genera *Berberis, Coptis, Hydrastis,*

TABLE 16.0.1 Species and Genera Used in Many Systems of TM for Similar Purposes[a]

Botanical Name	Common English Names
Acacia spp.	Acacia
Allium sativum	Garlic
Aloe spp.	Aloe
Artemisia spp.	Wormwood
Atropa, Datura, Scopolia, Solanum etc.	Nightshade
Azadirachta indica	Neem
Berberis, Coptis, Hydrastis, Mahonia	Barberry, mahonia, etc.
Capsicum spp.	Chilli, cayenne pepper
Carica papaya L.	Pumpkin
Centella asiatica	Gotu kola, Indian pennywort
Cinnamomum spp.	Cinnamon, cassia bark
Curcuma longa	Turmeric
Dioscorea spp.	Yam
Ficus spp.	Fig
Glycyrrhiza spp.	Liquorice
Lawsonia inermis	Henna
Lobelia spp.	Lobelia
Mentha spp.	Mint
Momordica charantia	Karela, bitter melon
Ocimum spp.	Basil
Piper spp.	Pepper
Punica granatum	Pomegranate
Rheum spp.	Rhubarb
Syzygium aromaticum	Clove
Trigonella foenum-graecum	Fenugreek
Vitex spp.	Chaste tree
Zingiber officinale	Ginger

[a]These purposes, and more information about the medicinal plant, can be seen in the individual entries for each type of TM.

Mahonia, Sanguinaria, etc.), are used globally, and whereas species in the 'New World' (the Americas, Oceania) may be different, they are all used for diabetes, diarrhoea and dysentery, infections, inflammation and liver disorders, similarly with the tropane alkaloid-containing medicinal plants (like from the genera *Atropa, Datura, Scopolia, Solanum* and others). See also Chapter 4 (Plant Families Yielding Important Medicines).

Other individual species have become widely used based on research evidence, reputation, availability and population migration. Table 16.0.1 is a selected 'shortlist' of species and genera used in different systems of medicine for similar purposes. These have generally been well investigated, and pharmacological activity has been found that supports their traditional use. They are discussed in more detail in Part B.

FURTHER READING

Barnes, J., 2012. Adverse drug reactions and pharmacovigilance of herbal medicines. In: Talbot, J., Aronson, J. (Eds.), Stephens' Detection and Evaluation of Adverse Drug Reactions, sixth ed. Wiley, Chichester, pp. 645–683.

Booker, A., Johnston, D., Heinrich, M., 2012. Value chains of herbal medicines – research needs and key challenges in the context of ethnopharmacology. J. Ethnopharmacol. 140 (3), 624–633.

Kew, R.B.G., 2016. The State of the World's Plants Report, 2016. Royal Botanic Gardens, Kew, London.

WHO, 2013. WHO Traditional Medicine Strategy: 2014–2023. WHO, Geneva. Available at: http://apps.who.int/iris/bitstream/10665/92455/1/9789241506090_.

WHO, 2016. WHO Uppsala Monitoring Centre. Monitoring of Herbal Medicines. WHO, Geneva. Available at: http://www.who-umc.org/DynPage.aspx?id=105337&mn1=7347&mn2=7252&mn3=7322&mn4=7492.

WHO, 2018. Declaration of Astana (Global Conference on Primary Health Care. WHO, Geneva, Switzerland. Astana, Kazakhstan, 25 and 26 October 2018).

WHO, 2021. Key Technical Issues of Herbal Medicines with Reference to Interaction with Other Medicines. World Health Organization, Geneva. Licence: CC BY-NC-SA 3.0 IGO.

16.1 Western Herbal Medicine and Phytotherapy

Western herbal medicine, or medical herbalism, traces its historical traditions back to Galen (a Greek physician of the 2nd century AD) whose model comprised 'bodily humours' (blood, black bile, yellow bile, phlegm), their 'temperaments' (e.g. hot, cold, damp), and the belief that illness resulted from an imbalance in these humours. Medicinal plants were used to correct these imbalances and were often described as, for example, 'heating' or 'cooling'; a 'cooling' herb, such as peppermint (*Mentha* × *piperita* L.), would be used to treat a 'hot' condition, such as fever. A significant evolution in the development of medical herbalism occurred with the publication of 'Culpeper's Herbal' in 1652, one of the first comprehensive compilations of medical and pharmaceutical knowledge on plant medicines. Western herbalism has also drawn on other traditions, such as the use of medicinal plants in North America after Samuel Thomson, although Thomson was himself influenced by herbalism in Europe. This is discussed in Chapter 2.

MODERN HERBALISM

Today, medical herbalism continues to draw on traditional knowledge, but increasingly this is interpreted and applied in a modern context. Herbalists are trained in basic health sciences in addition to phytochemistry and pharmacology, as well as the therapeutic use of medicinal plants, and frequently work with patients already under conventional medical treatment and with a diagnosed condition. There is an increasing emphasis, particularly among professionally organised medical herbalists, on using evidence from modern clinical trials to support the use of traditional herbal medicines. 'Western' herbal medicine is also highly developed in countries such as Australia, New Zealand, United States and Canada, which also have their own TM systems, used by indigenous peoples. Herbal practice covers a wide spectrum: from traditionalists, who refer mainly to the older philosophies and herbal formulae, to those who prefer a 'modern' rational or scientific approach, often referred to as phytotherapy. Most herbalists use elements of both and adapt their practice to include new medicines highlighted by modern research.

The following are important aspects of modern herbalism:

- It is holistic: psychological and emotional well-being, as well as physical symptoms, are considered when treatment is prescribed.
- Medicinal plants are selected on an individual basis for each patient; thus it is likely that even patients with the same physical symptoms will receive a different combination of medicinal plants.
- Herbalists aim to identify the underlying cause (e.g. stress) of a patient's illness and to address this in the treatment plan.
- Medicinal plants may be used to stimulate the body's healing capacity, to 'strengthen' bodily systems and to 'balance' disturbed body functions rather than to treat symptoms directly.
- Medicinal plants are used frequently with the general aim of 'eliminating toxins' or 'stimulating' the circulation; these are contentious claims not accepted by many scientists.
- The intention is to provide long-term relief from the health/medical condition.

In phytotherapy, the chemical constituents of a medicinal plant are seen as acting together to produce the therapeutic effect, as discussed in Chapter 11, or the effects of one constituent may reduce the likelihood of adverse effects due to another. Thus, herbalists believe it is important to use plant material as a whole (or refined) extract, as opposed to isolating a specific chemical constituent. Similarly, combinations of different medicinal plants are expected to interact in beneficial ways to produce the overall effect.

CONDITIONS TREATED BY HERBALISTS

Medical herbalists treat a wide range of diseases, and all patient groups, including pregnant women, breast-feeding mothers, children and older patients. Conditions treated are often long-term or debilitating, or where conventional treatment is unsuccessful or not acceptable to the patient. These include: autoimmune conditions, such as Crohn's disease, lupus and rheumatoid arthritis; infections of the upper respiratory and urinary tracts; exhaustion, fatigue and fatigue syndromes; conditions relating to fertility, pregnancy, childbirth and breast-feeding; digestion and nutrition; skin disorders, including acne, eczema and dermatitis; heart and circulatory issues; musculoskeletal problems; emotional and mental health conditions, including anxiety and depression; other issues such as menstrual problems, migraine and sleep disorders.

The herbalists' approach to treatment is multifaceted and may involve the use of medicinal plants to relieve symptoms, and to reduce inflammation generally, 'strengthen' the immune system, aid 'detoxification' or hormonal balance, and to support the body and specific organs in a manner not expected of conventional medicines.

HERBALISTS' CONSULTATIONS AND PRESCRIPTIONS

A first consultation may last for an hour or more, during which the herbalist will take a full case history, including perhaps a family medical history, with detailed symptoms of the illness, diet and lifestyle; the herbalist may also employ or arrange for diagnostic tests and examinations (e.g. blood pressure, blood and urine glucose, urine protein analysis for infection) depending on the nature of the presenting illness and whether the patient already has a conventional clinical diagnosis. The practitioner can then develop a treatment plan, typically comprising herbal medicines as well as dietary advice and recommendations for nutritional supplements where appropriate. Generally, a combination of several different medicinal plants (usually four to six) is prescribed for the treatment of a particular patient. Treatment is reviewed regularly and is typically changed according to the response.

Herbalists usually prescribe tinctures and/or fluid extracts, and where a prescription requires several medicinal plants, tinctures and fluid extracts may be blended. Some herbalists prepare their own stock material and others purchase from specialist suppliers. Many dispense their own prescriptions and commercial products, such as herbal teas, tablets, capsules and topical preparations including creams, lotions and ointments, may also be prescribed.

MODERN 'PHYTOTHERAPY'

In contrast to traditional medical herbalism, modern or 'rational' phytotherapy is the practice of evidence-based herbal medicine. Herbal medicines are selected on the basis of their known phytochemistry and clinical pharmacology in the same way as conventional medicines and single-herbal preparations are commonly prescribed. Originating in Germany, it is generally more acceptable to medical practitioners everywhere and is the main basis of marketing 'over-the-counter' (nonprescription) herbal medicines for self-treatment.

The same medicinal plants are used in both approaches (see Table 16.1.1, and Part B for further information on each), but the formulations used may be very different. For example, St John's wort (*Hypericum perforatum* L.) is used in both traditional medical herbalism and rational phytotherapy; however, whereas traditional medical herbalists may use tinctures, fluid extracts and extemporaneously prepared mixtures that are not necessarily standardised to any particular

TABLE 16.1.1   Important Medicinal Plants in Western Herbal Medicine

Indication	Common Name[a]	Botanical Name[b] and Plant Part(s)
Digestive and liver disorders	Artichoke	*Cynara cardunculus* L., leaf
	Gentian	*Gentiana lutea* L., root
	Ginger	*Zingiber officinale* Roscoe, rhizome
	Liquorice	*Glycyrrhiza glabra* L., root and rhizome
	Milk thistle	*Silybum marianum* (L.) Gaertn., fruit
	Peppermint	*Mentha* × *piperita* L., leaf and oil
Constipation	Frangula	*Frangula* spp., bark
	Ispaghula	*Plantago ovata* Forssk., seed and seed husk
	Senna	*Senna alexandrina* Mill. (syn.: *Cassia senna* L.), fruit and leaf
Anxiety, depression, insomnia, stress	Chamomile (German)	*Matricaria chamomilla* L., flowers
	Hops	*Humulus lupulus* L., strobiles
	Passiflora	*Passiflora incarnata* L., herb
	St John's wort	*Hypericum perforatum* L., herb
	Valerian	*Valeriana officinalis* L., root
Pain, fever, inflammation	Devil's claw	*Harpagophytum procumbens* (Burch.) DC. ex Meisn., root
	Feverfew	*Tanacetum parthenium* (L.) Sch. Bip., herb
	Rosehip	*Salix* spp., bark
	Turmeric	*Rosa canina* L., fruit
	Willow bark	*Curcuma longa* L., rhizome
Skin irritation, inflammation and wound healing	Arnica	*Arnica montana* L., flower
	Calendula	*Calendula officinalis* L., flower
	Centella	*Centella asiatica* (L.) Urb., herb
	Witch hazel	*Hamamelis virginiana* L., bark and leaf
Upper respiratory infections	Echinacea	*Echinacea* spp., juice, herb, root
	Elder flower and berry	*Sambucus nigra* L., flower and fruit
	Ivy	*Hedera helix* L., leaf
	Pelargonium	*Pelargonium sidoides* DC., *P. reniforme* (Andrews) Curtis, root
	Sage	*Salvia officinalis* L., herb
Urinary infections	Bearberry	*Arctostaphylos uva-ursi* (L.) Spreng., leaf
	Cranberry	*Vaccinium macrocarpon* Aiton, juice
Cardiovascular disorders	Butcher's broom	*Ruscus aculeatus* L., rhizome
	Garlic	*Allium sativum* L., bulb
	Hawthorn	*Crataegus* spp., leaf and fruit
	Horse chestnut	*Aesculus hippocastanum* L., seed
	Red vine leaf	*Vitis vinifera* L., leaf

TABLE 16.1.1 Important Medicinal Plants in Western Herbal Medicine—cont'd

Indication	Common Name[a]	Botanical Name[b] and Plant Part(s)
Cognitive enhancement	Ginkgo	*Ginkgo biloba* L., leaf
	Ginseng	*Panax* spp., root
	Rosenroot	*Rhodiola rosea* L., rhizome
Female hormonal disorders and pregnancy	Agnus castus	*Vitex agnus-castus* L., fruit
	Black cohosh	*Actaea racemosa* L., rhizome
	Raspberry leaf	*Rubus idaeus* L., leaf
	Red clover	*Trifolium pratense* L., herb
	Soya	*Glycine max* (L.) Merr., seed
Male hormonal disorders	Nettle	*Urtica dioica* L., root and leaf
	Pumpkin seed	*Cucurbita pepo* L., seed
	Pygeum bark	*Prunus africana* (Hook.f.) Kalkman, bark
	Saw palmetto	*Serenoa repens* (W. Bartram) Small, fruit

[a]Common names given are English versions; there are simply too many regional and colloquial names to list.
[b]Latin names have been checked using the Medicinal Plant Names Service, Royal Botanic Gardens, Kew (https://mpns.science.kew.org/) and are as current as possible. Synonyms may also need to be checked when reviewing the literature.

conventional dosage forms, such as tablets or capsules. A comparison of the main features of both approaches is provided in Table 16.1.2.

EVIDENCE OF SAFETY AND EFFICACY

There is a substantial body of clinical evidence on the potential benefits and harms associated with the use of specific herbal medicines (see Part B). Much of this information relates to the use of specific phytomedicines and there has been very little investigation of the efficacy and safety of phytotherapy as used by traditional medical herbalists. Although illustrated in case studies, robust scientific evaluation of the efficacy and safety of herbalism as a treatment approach requires evaluation.

In most countries, medical herbalists are not recognised as state-registered health professionals, and there is no legal requirement for

TABLE 16.1.2 Comparison of Herbalism and Rational Phytotherapy

Herbalism	Rational Phytotherapy
Assumes synergistic or additive effects occur between chemical constituents of plants	Seeks evidence of synergy or additive effects to support use
Holistic, individualistic prescribing	Symptom- or condition-based prescribing
Preparations mainly formulated as tinctures or fluid extracts	Preparations formulated as tinctures and as solid dosage forms (tablets or capsules)
Mainly uses combinations of medicinal plants	Single-plant products often used
Standardisation of preparations optional	Uses standardised extracts of plants or plant parts
Not always scientifically evaluated	Science-based approach

medical herbalists to have completed specific education and training programmes. To become a member of most professional organizations, it is necessary to have successfully completed a recognised training programme, although these are becoming increasingly unavailable in Western countries.

FURTHER READING

Barnes, J., Ernst, E., 1998. Traditional herbalists' prescriptions for common clinical conditions: a survey of members of the National Institute of Medical Herbalists. Phytother. Res. 12, 369–371.
Denham, A., Green, J., Hawkey, S., 2011. What's in the bottle? Prescriptions formulated by medical herbalists in a clinical trial of treatment during the menopause. J. Herb. Med. 1, 95–101.
Mills, S.Y., Bone, K., 2000. Principles and Practice of Phytotherapy. Churchill Livingstone, Edinburgh.
Nissen, N., Evans, S., 2012. Exploring the practice and use of Western herbal medicine: perspectives from the social science literature. J. Herb. Med. 2 (1), 6–15.
Owen, N., 2011. An herbal therapeutic approach to food intolerance and immune dysfunction: an illustrative case history. J. Herb. Med. 1 (2), 53–63.
Tobyn, G., Denham, A., Whitelegg, M., 2010. Illustrated by Marije Rowling. The Western Herbal Tradition: 2000 Years of Medicinal Plant Knowledge. Churchill Livingstone/Elsevier, Edinburgh.

16.2 Traditional Chinese Medicine and Kampo

TCM originated in China, with Kampo originally derived from ancient TCM, merged with indigenous Japanese practices and culture. TCM is now used globally, and increasingly in the West. There are many good, standard references (e.g. see WHO website resources) available for the study of TCM and these are not listed here. Kampo, however, is less widely known, despite its popularity and integration into the health system, and its similarities to TCM, so selected references are provided for Further Reading.

TRADITIONAL CHINESE MEDICINE

Our understanding of TCM is based on a complex set of documents and records, as well as their historical, medical, philosophical and anthropological interpretations, stretching back well over 5000 years. At that time, none of the knowledge was written down, apart from primitive inscriptions of prayers for the sick on pieces of tortoise carapace and animal bones, so a mixture of superstition, symbolism and fact was passed down by word of mouth for centuries. TCM still contains very many remedies selected for their symbolic significance rather than proven effects, and the use of animal products from endangered species or from cruel practices has overshadowed the perception of TCM outside China. TCM herbal products are much more widely used and are relatively well researched and accepted globally. As a holistic therapy which considers all aspects of an illness, including physical, emotional and spiritual, the concept of balance and harmony is supremely important in TCM. Early records were discussed in Chapter 2, but additional historical milestones show the evolution of TCM into what it is today.

Shen Nong, the legendary Chinese emperor, is credited with the discovery of herbal medicine in around 2800 BCE, and he is also reputed to have defined the opposing, yet complementary, principles eventually known as **yin** and **yang**. **Confucius** (551–479 BCE) is celebrated as China's greatest sage. He established a code of rules and ethics based on the premise that there is an order and harmony to the universe resulting from a delicate balance of yin and yang forces. Humans should cultivate the five virtues of benevolence, justice, propriety, wisdom and sincerity, in order to exert their own life force in this cycle.

Food and medicine became interrelated and in TCM, still are. Herbal medicine was initially the domain of shamans and mountain recluses, who believed that the mountain mists contained high concentrations of **qi**, the vital essence of life. They practised the 'way of long life', which involved a herbal diet and medicine combined with martial arts—a link that continues today. The principles of TCM became consolidated and a search for the 'elixir of life' began to obsess the Chinese aristocracy. In TCM, drugs to rejuvenate and increase longevity are still prized.

The Han dynasty (206 BCE–CE 220) saw remedies (including veterinary) recorded in handy booklets or Gansu, which were strips of bamboo or wood bound together. Herbal medicines were collected in the *Shen Nong Ben Cao Jing* (The Pharmacopoeia of Shen Nong) and classified into three categories:
- **Upper**: drugs that nurture life.
- **Middle**: drugs that provide vitality.
- **Lower**: 'poisons' used for serious disease.

The most noted physician of these times was **Zhang Zhogjing**, who divided diseases into 'yin' or 'yang'. His prescriptions aimed to correct any imbalances of these forces. He also contributed to acupuncture by drawing a map of meridians along which the body's vital energy (qi) is said to flow. During this period, the theory of the circulation of the blood was described, and anaesthetics were used, based mainly on *Datura*. By the end of the Han dynasty all the elements we regard as vital to TCM were in place, and refinement went on throughout the Tang, Song and Ming dynasties. During the **Ming dynasty**, **Li Shizhen** (CE 1518–1593) produced the classic herbal encyclopaedia *Ben Cao Gang Mu*. It took 27 years to compile and consists of 52 volumes containing 1892 medicines. It was translated into Japanese, Korean, English, French, German and other languages, and marked the beginning of a cultural exchange between Chinese and Western medicine.

In the **20th century**, TCM had a turbulent period; missionary doctors translated Western medical journals into Chinese, and many Chinese doctors who had studied abroad turned against TM. However, after the 1949 revolution, the new People's Republic of China reinstated TCM and set up new medical colleges. The Third (or Cultural) Revolution of 1966–1976 brought science and medicine to a standstill, and 'barefoot doctors' with little training were sent to rural areas to replace the denounced 'intellectual' Westerners. Today, both systems coexist and even Western-style medical schools teach students the basics of TCM and acupuncture. Research into TCM has evolved using new methods and concepts (e.g. metabolomics) which are appropriate for evaluating complex effects (see Chapter 11) and is now highly sophisticated.

Concepts in Traditional Chinese Medicine
Qi, the Essential Life Force

Qi permeates everything. It is transferable. For example, digestion extracts qi from food and drink and transfers it to the body; and breathing extracts qi from the air and transfers it to the lungs. These two forms of qi 'meet' in the blood and form 'human qi', which circulates through the body. It is the quality, quantity and balance of qi that determines your state of health and lifespan. Therefore, diet and breathing exercises are very important. It is thought that the original vital energy, **yuan qi**, is gradually dissipated throughout life, and should be conserved using diet, exercise (e.g. Tai chi, kung fu) and herbal medicine.

Yin and Yang

The theory of yin and yang still permeates all aspects of Chinese thought. Their attributes are:
- **Yin**: negative/passive/dark/female/water.
- **Yang**: positive/active/bright/male/fire.

Yin is considered to be the stronger: fire is extinguished by water, and water is 'indestructible'. So yin is always mentioned before yang; however, they are always in balance. Consider the well-known symbol (Fig. 16.2.1): where yin becomes weak, yang is strong and vice versa. Both contain the seed of each other: their opposites within themselves.

The Five Elements

The elements are wood, fire, earth, metal and water. They dominate everything on earth, and each is associated with a vital organ of the body:
- Heart: fire.
- Liver: wood.
- Spleen: earth.
- Lungs: metal.
- Kidneys: water.

The Vital Organs

Until the 20th century, cutting up a human body was considered a grave insult to the individual and the ancestors, rarely carried out, and applied in most cultures. The vital organs in most TM systems, and of TCM, do not correspond to our organs exactly. Precise anatomy was not considered particularly important since it was the relationship between the organs, the five elements, qi, and yin and yang that mattered.

The organs are also considered to be yin or yang and are paired. Coupled organs are connected by meridians, or energy channels, through which qi flows. Meridians are not associated with the nervous system and cannot be seen physically. They are stimulated with

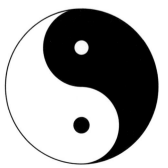

Fig. 16.2.1 The yin–yang symbol.

medicinal plants and by acupuncture and will have a direct effect on a particular organ as well as a toning effect on the system.

Causes of Disease

Bacteria, viruses and chemicals are not considered to be causes. If an organ is weak, it may be attacked, and, therefore, the weakness is the cause and must be rectified. It may be the result of external forces and internal emotional factors. The external 'cosmological' forces are called the **six excesses:**

- Wind.
- Cold.
- Summer heat.
- Dampness.
- Dryness.
- Fire.

Most people, if healthy, are not affected by the six excesses but, if the body is deficient in qi or weather conditions are abnormal, then this may cause imbalance and ill health.

The Seven Emotions

These are considered the major internal causes of disease. Excessive emotional activity causes a severe yin/yang imbalance, blockage of qi in the meridians and impairment of vital organ function. This leads to damage of the organs and allows disease to enter from outside, or a minor weakness from inside to develop. The seven emotions are:

- Joy.
- Anger.
- Anxiety.
- Concentration.
- Grief.
- Fear.
- Fright.

Once physical damage has occurred, by whatever cause, it will need more than emotional factors to cure it and medicines will be used. There are a few other causes, and include epidemics, insect and animal bites, worm infestation and hereditary diseases.

Diagnosis

Various methods are used:
- **Examination of the tongue:** shape, colour, coating, markings
- **Pulse diagnosis**: more than one pulse will be taken, depending on the pressure exerted
- **Palpation of internal organs**: to determine consistency and tone
- **Massage**: to detect temperature and knotted muscles or nerves
- **Interviewing**: sleep patterns, tastes in food and drink, stool and urine quality, perspiration and sexual activity.

Treatment

The purpose is to rectify harmony, restore qi and the yin/yang balance. For example, 'cold' diseases, such as cold in the lungs, coughs, vomiting and nausea are considered to be a deficiency of yang and treatment would be with a warming medicinal plant such as ginger (see examples in Table 16.2.1). A list of common medicinal plants and their indications is given in Table 16.2.2. Once the prescription has been formulated, the patient may be given a crude medicinal plant mixture with written instructions on how to prepare it at home, usually as an infusion (tea) or decoction. Pastes and pills are prepared by the herbalist and may take several days to complete. Slow-release preparations are made using beeswax pills; tonic wines, fermented dough (with medicinal plants in) and external poultices are also common.

KAMPO

Kampo (also known as 'kanpo') is Japanese herbal medicine. It is part of Japanese TM, along with acupuncture and acupressure (shiatsu), and has been practised for around 1500 years. Kampo has retained similarities with TCM, such as holistic diagnostic patterns of disease and individualised prescriptions, but it has also continued to evolve through practice in Japan (Kurihara et al., 2018).

As with other forms of TM, Kampo recognises the relationship between the human body and its environment and views disease as resulting from imbalance in the patient's normal state or equilibrium. The aim of treatment is to restore this balance, based on a patient's 'Sho', the symptom pattern or Kampo diagnosis. The Sho is often named in terms of a specific treatment formula; thus, the pathological condition is directly associated with the prescription. The same formula may be used to treat several different conditions, and many different formulae may be indicated for a particular condition (Kuchta & Cameron, 2021). Many ingredients are included for their immunomodulatory properties.

A Kampo formula typically comprises five to nine medicinal plants; most are included in the older *Shang Han Za Bing Lun* and described in modern books. A well-known Kampo medicine, 'Sho-saiko-to', is used for the treatment of acute fever, pneumonia, bronchitis, influenza, gastrointestinal disorders, chronic hepatitis and other liver diseases, and comprises seven herbal drugs: *Bupleurum falcatum* root; *Pinellia ternata* tuber; *Scutellaria baicalensis* root; *Ziziphus jujuba* fruit; *Panax ginseng* root; *Glycyrrhiza uralensis* root; and *Zingiber officinale* rhizome. These are all included in Table 16.2.2.

Today, Kampo is widely practised in Japan and is fully integrated into the healthcare system. It is formally recognised by the Japanese government, and this has also influenced practice. Kampo medicine can only be practised by conventional doctors in Japan, without

TABLE 16.2.1 Treatment of Disease in Traditional Chinese Medicine According to the Nature of Disease and the Remedy					
Type of Disease	**Example of Disease**	**Nature of Disease**	**Nature of Remedy**	**Example of Remedy**	**Desired Effect**
Cold	Nausea, vomiting	Yin	Yang	*Zingiber officinale* Roscoe	Warming
Hot	Malaria, fever	Yang	Yin	*Artemisia annua* L.	Cooling
Empty	Fatigue, diabetes	Yin, yang, qi deficiency	Tonic	*Panax ginseng* C. A. Mey.	Nourishing
Full	Congestion in chest	Yang	Yin	*Scutellaria baicalensis* Georgi	Cooling
Internal	Weak pulse	Yin	Yang	*Aconitum carmichaelii* Debeaux	Warming
External	Psoriasis	Yang	Yin	*Arctium lappa* L.	Cooling

TABLE 16.2.2   Some Important Herbs in Traditional Chinese and Japanese Medicine and Their Uses

Botanical Name	English Name	Chinese Name	Nature	Medical Use
Aconitum carmichaelii Debeaux	Aconite root	Chuan wu tou	Very pungent and hot	Heart tonic, diarrhoea, analgesic. Highly toxic; use contentious
Angelica sinensis (Oliv.) Diels	Chinese angelica root	Dang gui	Sweet, pungent, warm	Menstrual disorders, analgesic
Arctium lappa L.	Great burdock fruit, gobo	Niu bang zi	Pungent, bitter, cold	Sore throat, pneumonia, psoriasis
Artemisia annua L.	Sweet wormwood, sweet sagewort	Qing hao	Bitter, cold, yin	Malaria, fever
Asparagus cochinchinensis (Lour.) Merr.	Chinese asparagus root	Tian men dong	Sweet, bitter, cold	Chronic cough with phlegm, constipation
Astragalus propinquus Schischkin, A. mongholicus Bunge	Milkvetch root	Huang qi	Sweet, slightly warm	Strengthen the immune system in infections
Atractylodes lancea (Thunb.) DC.	Atractylodes root	Bai zhu	Pungent, acrid, bitter, warm	Gastrointestinal bloating, indigestion, diarrhoea
Bupleurum falcatum L., *B. chinense* DC.	Chinese thorowax herb	Chai hu	Pungent, bitter, cooling	Liver tonic
Cinnamomum cassia (L.) J. Presl	Chinese cinnamon. Cassia bark	Rou gui	Pungent, sweet, very hot	Diarrhoea, tonic, dysmenorrhoea
Coix lacryma-jobi L., *C. lacryma-jobi* var. *ma-yuen* (Rom.Caill.) Stapf	Job's tears, seeds	Yi yi ren	Sweet, plain, slightly cold	Dysentery, painful joints, diuretic
Coptis chinensis Franch. and related spp.	Golden thread root	Huang lian	Bitter, cold	Diabetes, dysentery, eczema, infections
Cyperus rotundus L.	Nut grass root	Xiang fu	Pungent, sweet, neutral	Liver disorders, amenorrhoea, sedative
Ephedra sinica Stapf	Ephedra herb	Ma huang	Pungent, slightly bitter, warm	Bronchial asthma, hay fever
Gastrodia elata Blume	Gastrodia root	Tian ma	Sweet, neutral	Hypertension, cognitive impairment, CNS disorders
Glycyrrhiza uralensis Fisch. ex DC.	Chinese liquorice root and rhizome	Gan cao	Sweet, neutral	Asthma, bronchitis, ulcers, steroid activity
Lonicera japonica Thunb.	Japanese honeysuckle flower	Jin yin hua	Sweet, cold	Fever, throat infections, ulcers
Lycium barbarum L.	Goji, wolfberry	Gou qi zi	Sweet, neutral	Abdominal pain, dry cough, fatigue, dizziness, headache
Paeonia lactiflora Pall.	Chinese white peony root	Bai shao yao	Bitter, slightly cold, yin	Fever, haemostatic antiinflammatory
Panax ginseng C.A. Mey.	Ginseng root	Ren shen	Sweet, neutral	Tonic, aphrodisiac, appetite stimulant
Perilla frutescens (L.) Britton	Beefsteak plant, leaf, seed	Zi su	Pungent, warm, yang	Allergic reactions, fever
Pinellia ternata (Thunb.) Makino	Green dragon, Pinellia tuber	Ban xia	Warm, acrid	Nausea, morning sickness, pain, swelling, anxiety, depression. Only used processed
Rehmannia glutinosa (Gaertn.) DC.	Chinese foxglove root	Di huang	Sweet, bitter, cold	Rheumatoid arthritis, asthma, urticaria, chronic nephritis
Rheum palmatum L.	Rhubarb root	Da huang	Bitter, cold	Constipation, burns, diarrhoea, jaundice
Salvia miltiorrhiza Bunge	Red sage root	Dan shen	Bitter, cold	Menstrual disorders, chest pain, blood clots
Schisandra chinensis (Turcz.) Baill., *S. sphenanthera* Rehder & E.H. Wilson	Schisandra, magnolia vine fruit	Wu wei zi	Sour, warm	Diarrhoea, thirst, asthma, cough
Scutellaria baicalensis Georgi	Baical skullcap herb	Huang qin	Bitter, cold	Dysentery, jaundice
Sophora flavescens Aiton	Sophora root	Ku shen	Bitter, cold	Dysentery, jaundice, asthma, parasites, skin disease
Styphnolobium japonicum (L.) Schott (syn.: *Sophora japonica* L.)	Pagoda tree flower bud	Huai hua	Bitter, slightly cold	Blood disorders, clots, reduces cholesterol
Tribulus terrestris L.	Caltrops, puncture vine fruit	Ci ji li	Sweet, warm	Liver and kidney tonic, lumbago, tinnitus
Wolfiporia cocos (F.A. Wolf) Ryvarden & Gilb. (syn.: *Poria cocos* (Schw.) Wolf	Poria mushroom, hoelen	Fu ling	Sweet, neutral	Fatigue, anxiety, CNS disorders, inflammation
Zingiber officinale Roscoe	Ginger	Gan jiang	Pungent, sweet, very hot	Nausea, vomiting, colds, diarrhoea.
Ziziphus jujuba Mill.	Chinese jujube	Suan zao ren	Sweet, sour, neutral	Liver and heart tonic

specific training or a licence to do so, although many medical universities now include Kampo in their curriculum. Some Kampo medicines are included in Japanese clinical practice guidelines, and approved formulae are covered by national health insurance.

Modern Kampo uses around 200 recognised formulae, and most access to Kampo is through use of manufactured products. Some Kampo prescriptions may have the same name as TCM formulae, but the ingredients could be different. The Japanese Pharmacopoeia XIV included over 100 crude herbal medicines, animal and mineral products used in Kampo medicine, which is relatively limited compared to TCM.

There are over 350 randomised controlled trials of Kampo medicines in Japan, although these studies have not always used a Kampo diagnosis. Adverse drug reactions, including allergic reactions, gastrointestinal effects, fever, headache and haematuria, have been reported following the use of Kampo medicines and there is also the potential for drug interactions to occur.

FURTHER READING

Borchers, A.T., Sakai, S., Henderson, G.L., 2000. Shosaiko-to and other Kampo (Japanese herbal) medicines: a review of their immunomodulatory activities. J. Ethnopharmacol. 73 (1–2), 1–13.

Kurihara, Y., Han, C., Harada, Y., Kobayashi, H., 2018. General introduction to kampo medicine – the nuts and bolts of kampo. Junt. Med. J. 64 (4), 258–263. https://doi.org/10.14789/jmj.2018.64.JMJ18-R09.

Kuchta, K., Cameron, S.B., 2021. Tradition to pathogenesis: a novel hypothesis for elucidating the pathogenesis of diseases based on the traditional use of medicinal plants. Front. Pharmacol. 12, 2788. https://doi.org/10.3389/fphar.2021.705077.

Motoo, Y., Arai, I., Tsutani, K., 2014. Use of Kampo diagnosis in randomized controlled trials of Kampo products in Japan: a systematic review. PLoS One 9 (8), e104422 e104422.

Yu, F., Takahashi, T., Moriya, J., Kawaura, K., Yamakawa, J., Kusaka, K., et al., 2006. Traditional Chinese Medicine and Kampo: a review from the distant past for the future. J. Int. Med. Res. 34, 231–239.

16.3 Asian Traditional Medicine: Ayurveda, Siddha, Jamu and Unani

Ayurveda is the most ancient system of medicine still in use today, and it has influenced many other types of TM, such as Siddha, Jamu and Unani medicine. Many remedies are common to all systems, and also to TCM (see Table 16.2.2), although the philosophical rationale for their application may be a little different.

AYURVEDA

Ayurveda, an ancient system of sacred Hindu medicine, originating in India, as well as being an oral tradition, is also well documented. Over 5000 years ago, the great seers (or 'rishis') organised the 'fundamentals of life' into what became known as Ayurveda, and this has evolved and adapted over the years whilst still retaining the philosophical basis on which it was founded. It now accommodates modern science, especially in relation to the testing of medicines, and research and adaptation are actively encouraged. Like other forms of holistic medicine, Ayurveda considers the patient as an individual and 'normality' as what is appropriate for that person. The patient is therefore subject to unique imbalances, unlike Western medicine, where populations are generalised and 'normal' means what is applicable to the majority. Eastern thought values subjectivity, and considers it a vital addition to objectivity, the goal in Western medicine.

Prana, the Life Energy

Prana is the life energy which activates both body and mind. Nutrient prana from the air gives energy to the vital prana in the brain, via respiration, and is thus the equivalent of qi in Chinese medicine. In the body, prana is centred in the head, and governs emotions, memory, thought and other functions of the mind. Prana kindles the bodily fire, or **agni**, and governs the functioning of the heart, entering the bloodstream from where it controls the vital organs or **dhatus**.

Bhutas, the Five Elements

The ether (space), air, fire, water and earth are considered to be the basic elements, or manifestations of cosmic energy. They are related to the five senses (hearing, touch, vision, taste and smell) and their resultant actions. As an example, ether is related to hearing, since sound is transmitted through it to the ear, the associated sense organ, leading to speech, from the organs of action, the tongue and vocal cords. Likewise, fire is associated with the eyes as sense organs, leading to an action such as walking, by an organ of action, such as the feet.

Tridosha: Vata, Pitta and Kapha—the Three Humours

Ether, air, fire, water and earth (the five basic elements) are manifest in the human body as three basic principles or humours known as the '**tridosha**', which is unique to Ayurveda. The three humours, known as **vata, pitta** and **kapha** (individually called **doshas**), govern all biological, psychological and physiopathological functions of the body and mind. The primary requirement for the diagnosis and treatment of disease is to understand the relationship between these. If the tridosha works in harmony, the result is health and a feeling of well-being in the individual. However, in cases of imbalance and disharmony, the result is illness. The tridosha affects the creation, maintenance and destruction of bodily tissues and the elimination of toxins (**ama**) from the body. It is also responsible for basic human emotions such as fear, anger and greed, and more complicated sentiments such as understanding, compassion and love, and as such is the foundation of the psychosomatic nature of man.

The tridosha (vata, pitta and kapha) has recently been defined as an equilibrium, balance and coordination between the three vital body systems: the central nervous system (CNS) corresponding to vata, the endocrine system to pitta and the immune axis to kapha, operating

TABLE 16.3.1   Determining the Human Constitution According to the Tridosha

Aspect of Constitution	Vata Character	Pitta Character	Kapha Character
Bodyweight	Low	Moderate	Overweight
Skin	Dry Rough Cool	Soft Oily Warm	Thick Oily Cool
Eyes	Small Dark Dull	Sharp Green Grey	Large Blue
Hair	Dry Dark Curly	Oily Fair	Oily Thick Dark or fair
Appetite	Poor Variable	Good Excessive	Steady
Thirst	Variable	Excessive	Scanty
Mind	Restless Active	Aggressive Intelligent	Calm Slow
Emotional temperament	Insecure Unpredictable	Irritable Aggressive	Calm Greedy
Speech	Fast	Penetrating	Slow
Physical activity	Very active	Moderate	Lethargic
Sleep	Interrupted	Little sound	Heavy Long

To find the Ayurvedic constitution, just tick the most relevant description, and count up the ticks in each column to determine the dominant type. It may not just show one pure type, but, for example, vata-pitta or pitta-kapha. Then the best diet for a particular constitution can be found. Foods that aggravate a particular dosha should not be taken in excess by a person of that type; for example, a vata person should not take excessive amounts of lamb, cabbage, potatoes or dried fruits. However, eggs, rice, cooked vegetables and sweet fruits would be beneficial to someone of vata constitution. It can also be used to decide which type of food to eat in different seasons. For example, in summer, pitta predominates, and those foods that aggravate pitta should be avoided; but winter is the season of kapha, so seafood, melon and cows' milk products are not recommended then. Autumn is the season of vata, and spring is kapha-pitta.

with both positive and negative feedback. To try to correlate this ancient philosophy with modern science is difficult, but some analogies can be drawn. The tridosha can be considered to govern all metabolic activities: catabolism (vata), metabolism (pitta) and anabolism (kapha). When vata is out of balance, the metabolism will be disturbed, resulting in excess catabolism, which is the breakdown or deterioration process in the body; excess would, therefore, induce emaciation. When anabolism is greater than catabolism (excess kapha), there is an increased rate of growth and repair of organs and tissues. Excess pitta disturbs metabolism generally. The tridosha can be described further:

- **Vata**, affiliated to air or ether (space), is a principle of movement. It can be characterised as the energy controlling biological movement and is thus associated with the CNS, and governs functions such as breathing, blinking, all forms of movement, the heartbeat and nervous impulses.
- **Pitta** is affiliated to fire and water and governs bodily heat and energy. It, therefore, controls body temperature; is involved in metabolism, digestion, excretion and the manufacture of blood and endocrine secretions; and is also involved with intelligence and understanding.
- **Kapha** is associated with water and earth. It is responsible for physical structure, biological strength, regulatory functions, including that of immunity, the production of mucus, synovial fluid and joint lubrication and assists with wound healing, vigour and memory retention.

Prakruti, the Human Constitution

Humans can also be divided into personality types, and the constitution of an individual (prakruti) is determined by the state of the parental tridosha at conception (unlike astrology, which depends on time of birth). Most people are not completely one type or another, but can be described as vatapitta or pittakapha, for example. Table 16.3.1 shows some of the characteristics of each dosha, and how constitution is determined and used to suggest a suitable diet. This is purely for illustration and not a tool for self-diagnosis!

In addition to the vata, pitta and kapha type of personalities, three attributes provide the basis for distinctions in human temperament, individual differences, and psychological and moral dispositions. In Ayurveda, a state of health exists when the digestive fire (**agni**) is in a balanced condition and the bodily humours (vata-pitta-kapha) are in equilibrium. The three waste products (**mala**), which are urine, faeces and sweat, should be produced at usual levels, the senses functioning normally, and the body, mind and consciousness working in harmony. When the balance of any of these systems is disturbed, the disease process begins.

Agni, the Digestive Fire

Agni governs metabolism and is essentially pitta in nature. An imbalance in the tridosha will impair agni and, therefore, affect metabolism. Food will not be digested or absorbed properly, and toxins will be produced in the intestines, and may find their way into the circulation. These toxins are known as ama and are the root cause of disease.

TABLE 16.3.2 Effect of Different Foods on the Tridosha

DOSHA	VATA		PITTA		KAPHA	
Food Type	Aggravates	Balances	Aggravates	Balances	Aggravates	Balances
Meat	Lamb, pork, venison	Beef, eggs, turkey white meat, chicken	Beef, lamb, pork, egg yolk	Chicken, turkey, egg white	Beef, lamb, pork, seafood	Chicken, turkey dark meat, rabbit, eggs
Cereals	Rye, barley	Oats, rice, wheat	Barley, oats, brown rice	White rice, wheat, barley, oats	Oats, rice, wheat	Barley, rye, corn
Vegetables	Raw vegetables, cauliflower, sprouts, cabbage, aubergine, mushrooms, onion, peas, potatoes	Cooked vegetables, carrots, garlic, green beans, cucumber, avocado, courgettes	Carrots, aubergine, garlic, onion, spinach, tomatoes, hot peppers	Broccoli, sprouts, lettuce, peas, cauliflower, mushrooms, courgettes	Cucumber, tomatoes, courgettes	Cauliflower, sprouts, cabbage, carrots, aubergine, lettuce, mushrooms, onions, peas, potatoes
Fruit	Dried fruit, apples, pears, watermelon	Sweet fruits, apricots, peaches, bananas, cherries, grapes, citrus	Sour fruits, peaches, bananas, grapes, lemons, oranges, pineapple	Sweet fruits, apples, melon, coconut, raisins, prunes	Bananas, coconut, grapefruit, grapes, lemon, orange, melon, pineapple	Apples, apricots, peaches, pears, cherries, raisins, prunes
Dairy	All OK	All OK	Buttermilk, cheese, yogurt,	Butter, milk	None	Goats milk
Oils	All OK	All OK	Corn, sesame, almond	Sunflower, soya, olive	None	None
Condiments	All OK	All OK	Most	Coriander, fennel, turmeric	All	Salt

Overactive ama is also detrimental in that over combustion of nutrients may occur, leading to vata disorders and emaciation.

Malas, the Three Waste Products

These are the faeces, urine and sweat, and production and elimination of these are vital to health. Their appearance and properties can give many indications of the state of the tridosha and, therefore, health. As an example, the colour of urine depends on the diet, and, if the patient has a fever or jaundice (pitta disorders), it may be darker. Substances such as coffee and tea, which stimulate urination, also aggravate pitta and render the urine dark yellow.

Dhatus, the Seven Tissues

The human body consists of seven basic tissues or organs (constructing elements) or dhatus. When there is a disorder in the balance of the tridosha, the dhatus are directly affected. The dhatus do not correspond to our definition of anatomy but are more a tissue type than an individual organ.

Gunas, the Attributes

Ayurveda encompasses a subtle concept of attributes or qualities called gunas. These attributes contain potential energy while their associated actions express kinetic energy. Vata, pitta and kapha each have their own attributes, and substances having similar attributes will tend to aggravate the related bodily humour. Through the understanding of these attributes, the balance of the tridosha may be maintained. The diseases and disorders ascribed to vata, pitta and kapha are treated with the aid of medicines of the opposite attribute, to try to correct the deficiency or excess. Vata disorders are corrected with the aid of sweet (**madhur**), sour (**amla**) or saline

and warm (**lavana**) medicines. 'Aggravation' of pitta is controlled by sweet (madhur), bitter (**katu**) or astringent and cooling (**kashaya**) herbs. Kapha disorders are corrected with pungent (**tikta**), bitter (katu) or astringent and dry (kashaya) herbs. There is often little distinction between foods and medicines, and controlling the diet is an integral part of Ayurvedic treatment. Foods are also described according to their properties, such as their taste (**rasa**) and physical and chemical properties (**guna**); these affect the tridosha (Table 16.3.2).

APPLICATION OF AYURVEDA

Diagnosis

Taking a case history involves astrological considerations, and a thorough medical examination where the appearance of the tongue, properties of the urine, sweat and sputum will also be examined. **Karma**, the good and bad effects across incarnations, is also considered.

Treatment

This may involve diets, bloodletting, fasting, skin applications and enemas, which are used to cleanse the system. Medicines may then be given to bring the dhatus into balance again. These include herbal treatments as well as minerals, and there are thousands in use. In addition, yogic breathing and other techniques are used. Some of the most popular medicinal plants used in Ayurveda, together with their properties, are shown in Table 16.3.3. Further important medicinal plants used in Ayurveda, and also Siddha medicine, are shown in Table 16.3.4.

In modern Indian herbal medicine, the Ayurvedic properties are described together with the conventional pharmacological and phytochemical data. Drugs are prepared as tinctures, pills, powders and

TABLE 16.3.3   Examples of Ayurvedic Medicinal Plants and Their Effects on the Tridosha

English Name	Ayurvedic Name	Effect on Dosha	Medical Use
***Acorus calamus* L.** Sweet flag	Vacha	Pacifies vata and kapha	Nerve stimulant, digestive
***Adhatoda vasica* Nees (now classed as *Justicia adhatoda* L.)** Malabar nut	Vasaka	Pacifies pitta and kapha	Respiratory disorders, fevers
***Aegle marmelos* (L.) Corrêa** Bengal quince	Bael, bel	Promotes pitta	Antidysenteric, digestive, tonic
***Andrographis paniculata* (Burm.f.) Nees** Green chiretta, chirata	Kalmegh	Pacifies kapha and pitta	Liver protectant, jaundice
***Eclipta prostrata* (L.) L. (syn.: *Eclipta alba* (L.) Hassk.)** Trailing eclipta	Bhringaraja	Pacifies kapha and pitta	Skin and hair disorders
***Embelia ribes* Burm.f.** Embelia	Viranga	Pacifies kapha and vata	Vermifuge, contraceptive
***Ocimum tenuiflorum* L. (syn: *O. sanctum* L.)** Holy basil	Tulsi	Pacifies kapha and vata	Expectorant, febrifuge, immunomodulatory
***Phyllanthus emblica* L. (syn.: *Emblica officinalis* Gaertn.)** Indian gooseberry	Amla	Balances tridosha	Improves memory and intelligence, tonic
***Phyllanthus niruri* L.** Stone breaker	Bhumyamalaki	Pacifies kapha and pitta	Diabetes, jaundice, liver protectant
***Picrorrhiza kurroa* Royle ex Benth.** Kutki, yellow gentian	Katurohini	Pacifies kapha and pitta	Hepatoprotective, immunomodulator
***Piper nigrum* L.** Black pepper	Kali mirch	Pacifies vata and pitta	Digestive, respiratory disorders
***Swertia chirayita* (Roxb.) H. Karst.** Chiretta	Chirayita	Balances tridosha	Appetite stimulant, liver disorders
***Terminalia arjuna* (Roxb. ex DC.) Wight & Arn.** Arjun myrobalan	Arjuna	Pacifies pitta and kapha	Heart tonic, angina, hypertension
***Terminalia chebula* Retz.** Black myrobalan	Haritaki	Balances tridosha	Digestive, blood tonic, antiasthmatic
***Tribulus terrestris* L.** Caltrops	Gokhru	Pacifies vata and pitta	Digestive, diuretic, aphrodisiac
***Withania somnifera* (L.) Dunal** Winter cherry	Ashwagandha	Pacifies kapha and vata	Analgesic, sedative, rejuvenator

some formulae unique to Ayurveda (Table 16.3.5). Ayurveda is very metaphysical and practitioners view it as a way of life as opposed to a career.

Rasayana

Rasayana are remedies considered to have diverse action and, therefore, affect many systems of the body, leading to a positive effect on health—panaceas in other words. The most important are *Asparagus racemosus* (**shatavari**), *Phyllanthus emblica* (**amla**), *Piper longum* (**pimpli**), *Terminalia chebula* (**haritaki**), *Tinospora cordifolia* (**guduchi**) and *Withania somnifera* (**ashwagandha**). They are included in many recipes and are used to strengthen the tissues of the body. In general, modern research has found them to have antioxidant, immunomodulating and various other attributes.

SIDDHA

Siddha (Tamil) medicine is based on a combination of ancient medicinal practices, alchemy and spiritual disciplines. It is thought to have developed during the Indus civilisation, 2500–1700 BCE and is part of Tamil culture, and widely practised in South India and Sri Lanka.

TABLE 16.3.4 Important Medicinal Plants Used in Ayurveda, Siddha and Unani Medicine

Herb[a] and Part(s) Used	Common English Names[b]	Traditional Indications[c]
Abrus precatorius L. Leaf, seed	Jequirity bean, rosary pea	Convulsions, vomiting, contraception. Seeds highly toxic
Acacia nilotica (L.) Willd. ex Delile Leaf, bark, seed, root, gum, young pods	Babul, Egyptian acacia, thorny acacia, gum Arabic tree (https://en.wikipedia.org/wiki/Vachellia_nilotica - cite_note-5)	Diabetes, dysentery, diarrhoea, infections, pain, inflammation
Asparagus racemosus Willd. Root	Sparrow grass, wild asparagus, shatavari	Reproductive and postpartum conditions in women, gastrointestinal disorders
Azadirachta indica A. Juss. Leaf, bark, seed, oil	Neem, Indian lilac, margosa	Head lice, fleas, as insecticide and repellent, inflammation, infections
Bacopa monnieri (L.) Wettst. Herb.	Water hyssop, thyme-leaved gratiola	Memory enhancement, inflammation, anxiety, stress
Berberis aristata DC. Root, root bark, stem	Indian barberry	Dysentery, bitter tonic, jaundice, fever
Boerhaavia diffusa L. Leaf, fresh leaf juice, stem, root	Spreading hogweed, pigweed	Pain, gastrointestinal, respiratory, urinary, cardiovascular and liver disorders
Boswellia serrata Roxb. ex Colebr., *B. sacra* Flueck. Gum-resin	Indian frankincense, olibanum, guggul	Arthritis, inflammation, inflammatory bowel disease, asthma
Caesalpinia bonduc (L.) Roxb. Seed, bark.	Bonduc nut, nicker nut, fever nut	Fever, worms, skin disorders, diarrhoea, inflammation
Cedrus deodara L (Roxb. ex D. Don.) G. Don Heartwood, bark, leaf, oil	Himalayan cedar, deodar	Fever, headache, skin disease, insecticide
Centella asiatica (L.) Urb. (syn.: *Hydrocotyle asiatica* L.) Herb	Gotu kola, hydrocotyle, Indian pennywort	Skin conditions, wound healing, memory enhancement
Cissus quadrangularis L. Stem, leaf, root	Bone setter	Bone healing, dyspepsia, colic
Commiphora wightii (Arn.) Bhandari, *C. mukul* (Hook. ex Stocks) Engl. Resin	Guggul	High cholesterol, arteriosclerosis, skin disorders, weight loss, diabetes
Crataeva nurvala Buch.-Ham. Stem bark, root, leaf	Three-leaved caper	Kidney stone, urinary infection
Cuminum cyminum L. Fruit (seed)	Cumin	Gastrointestinal disorders, diabetes
Cyperus rotundus L. Rhizome	Nut grass, nut sedge, coco-grass, Java grass	Gastrointestinal disorders, diarrhoea, diabetes, fever, inflammation
Elettaria cardamomum (L.) Maton Fruits (pods), seeds	Cardamom	Gastrointestinal, cardiovascular disorders
Euphorbia hirta L. Herb	Pill-bearing spurge, asthma plant, snakeweed	Asthma, respiratory disorders, dysentery, infections
Ficus religiosa L. Leaf, stem bark	Sacred fig, bodhi, peepul, pipal tree	Gastric ulcer, diabetes, skin disease, infections
Fumaria indica (Hausskn.) Pugsley Herb	Fumitory	Inflammation, infections, liver disorders, diarrhoea
Gossypium herbaceum L. Bark, root bark, seed	Cotton	Contraception, dysmenorrhoea, dysentery, skin disease
Gymnema sylvestre (Retz.) R. Br. ex Sm. Leaf, root	Periploca of the wood	Diabetes
Hemidesmus indicus (L.) R. Br. ex Schult Root	Indian sarsaparilla	Diabetes, pain, inflammation, diarrhoea, debility, skin disorders, infections
Holarrhena pubescens Wall. ex G. Don (syn.: *H. antidysenterica* Wall.) Seed, bark	Tellicherry, kurchi	Diabetes, dysentery, fever, skin disorders, jaundice
Lawsonia inermis L. Bark, leaf	Henna	Jaundice, skin disease, wound healing, bleeding disorders

Continued

TABLE 16.3.4   Important Medicinal Plants Used in Ayurveda, Siddha and Unani Medicine— cont'd

Herb[a] and Part(s) Used	Common English Names[b]	Traditional Indications[c]
Leptadenia reticulata (Retz.) Wight & Arn. Leaf root	Leptadenia	Stimulant, tonic, skin conditions, infections
Mangifera indica L. Fruit, seed, stem bark, root, leaf	Mango	Diarrhoea, asthma, cough, inflammation
Momordica charantia L. Fruit, leaf	Bitter melon, bitter gourd, karela	Diabetes, hypercholesterolaemia
Moringa oleifera Lam. Leaf, stem	Drumstick tree, horseradish tree	Diabetes, inflammation, nutrient source
Murraya koenigii (L.) Spreng. Leaf	Curry leaf tree	Diabetes, diarrhoea, dysentery, skin conditions
Nelumbo nucifera Gaertn. Leaf, flower, fruit, seed, root	Sacred lotus, Indian lotus	Gastric and cardiovascular and gastric disorders, bleeding, bruising, cancer
Nigella sativa L. Seed, oil	Black seed, black cumin, black caraway	Diabetes, hypertension, skin conditions, allergies
Picrorriza kurroa Royle ex Benth. Root, rhizome	Kutki, yellow gentian	Liver disorders fever, inflammation
Plumbago zeylanica L. Root, leaf	White leadwort, chitra	Inflammation, dysentery, diarrhoea
Punica granatum L. Fruit, rind, leaf, root	Pomegranate	Worms, diarrhoea, bleeding disorders, dysmenorrhoea
Rubia cordifolia L. Roots and stems	Common or Indian madder	Dysentery, inflammation, skin disorders, infections
Semecarpus anacardium L. f. Fruit, gum, oil	Marking nut tree	Inflammation, skin disorders, anorexia
Senna alata (L.) Roxb. (syn.: *Cassia alata* L.) Leaf	Ringworm bush, candle bush	Skin fungal infections, laxative
Sesamum indicum L. Leaf, seed, oil	Sesame	Diarrhoea, catarrh, female conditions for phytoestrogenic activity
Sida cordifolia L. Seed, leaf, root	Country mallow, Indian common mallow	Weight loss, asthma, nasal congestion, cough, fluid retention, inflammation
Solanum nigrum L. Herb, fruit	Black nightshade	Liver disorders, jaundice, inflammation
Syzygium aromaticum (L.) Merr. & L.M. Perry (syn.: *Eugenia caryophyllata* Thunb.) Unopened flower bud, oil	Clove	Coughs, colds, infections, toothache, fatigue, digestive disorders
Syzygium cumini (L.) Skeels Leaf, seed, fruit, bark	Malabar plum, Java plum, jamun, jambolan	Diabetes, skin conditions, gastrointestinal disorders, diarrhoea, worms
Tinospora sinensis (Lour.) Merr. (syn.: *T. cordifolia* (Willd.) Miers. Root, stem, leaf	Heart-leaved moonseed	Diabetes, arthritis, infections, allergies, gastrointestinal disorders
Trachyspermum ammi (L.) Sprague ex Turrill (syn.: *Ammi copticum* L.). Fruit (seeds)	Ajowan, ajwain, carom	Infections, cardiovascular conditions, digestive disorders
Trigonella foenum-graecum L. Seed	Fenugreek	Diabetes, hypercholesterolaemia, inflammation, eczema, ease childbirth, enhance lactation, menstrual pain
Vitex negundo L. Leaf, seed, root	Horseshoe/five-leaved/Chinese/chaste tree, nisinda	Inflammation, oedema, skin disease

[a]Latin names have been checked using World Flora Online (www.worldfloraonline.org) and are as current as possible, Some synonyms, widely used for the commercial product, are given, but there are many more which need to be checked when reviewing the literature.
[b]Common names given are English versions; there are simply too many regional and colloquial names to list.
[c]These are selective and may vary in different regions.

TABLE 16.3.5 Methods of Preparing Ayurvedic Medicines

Formulation	Method of Production
Juice (swaras)	Cold-pressed plant juice
Powder (churna)	Shade-dried, powdered plant material
Cold infusion (sita kasaya)	Herb/water 1:6, macerated overnight and filtered
Hot infusion (phanta)	Herb/water 1:4, steeped for a few minutes and filtered
Decoction (kathva)	Herb/water 1:4 (or 1:8, 1:16 then reduced to 1:4), boiled
Poultice (kalka)	Plant material pulped
Milk extract (ksira paka)	Plant boiled in milk and filtered
Tinctures (arava, arista)	Plant fermented, macerated or boiled in alcohol
Pills or tablets (vati, gutika)	Soft or dry extracts made into pills or tablets
Sublimates (kupipakva rasayana)	Medicine prepared by sublimation
Calcined preparations (bhasma)	Plant or metal is converted into ash
Powdered gem (pisti)	Gemstone triturated with plant juice
Scale preparations (parpati)	Molten metal poured on leaf to form a scale
Medicated oils or ghee (sneha)	Plant heated in oil or ghee
Medicated linctus/jam (avaleha)	Plant extract in syrup

According to the Siddha system, there are five elements: earth, water, fire, air and ether. Three of these—air, fire and water—form the fundamental components or humours—*vata, pitta,* and *kapha,* as with Ayurveda. Their proportions govern an individual's physical and mental disposition and form the connecting link between the microcosm (the human) and the macrocosm (the earth).

*Siddhar*s believe *vata* to be identical to divine energy, therefore imbalance can be the root cause of any disease. Siddha medicine uses conjunctive treatment with plants and minerals to a greater extent than Ayurveda. For simple ailments, the Siddha practitioner initially uses medicinal plants, and if not effective, mineral and animal products are added.

UNANI

Unani medicine is the TM system of the Middle East and Arabia. It is also referred to as Unani Tibb, Greco-Arab and Islamic medicine. Its origin is in the teachings of the Greek physicians Hippocrates and Galen and, later, by the great Persian philosopher, scientist and writer Ibn Sina (Avicenna), and other Islamic scholars and physicians (see Chapter 2). Unani has been influenced by other traditions from China, India, Egypt and the Middle East, and by Islamic teachings and writings, and evolved over time. Today, Unani medicine is practised widely in India, Pakistan and Middle Eastern countries, and with many regional variations throughout Central Asia (e.g. traditional Uighur medicine). In India, Unani medicine is recognised by the government, and taught in medical colleges.

Unani takes a holistic view of health, and an individualistic approach to treatment, focussing on the underlying cause of illness rather than just symptoms, and part of the approach is to effect lifestyle changes to improve health and quality of life. Unani refers to the galenical model of four bodily 'humours' ('akhlat'), as with early Western herbalism:

phlegm ('balgham')

blood ('dam')

yellow bile ('safra')

black bile ('sauda')

Each person is believed to have a unique humoral constitution, the composition of which determines the person's temperament ('mizaj'), depending on the dominant humour: 'balghami' (phlegmatic), 'damvi' (sanguine), 'safravi' (choleric) or 'saudavi' (melancholic); individuals can also be assigned a combination of temperaments. The humours are linked to the four elements, similar to the concept of the bhutas or elements in Ayurveda. Unani medicine links phlegm with water, blood with air, yellow bile with fire, and black bile with earth; the elements are believed to be present in these body fluids and if their equilibrium is disturbed, this leads to pathological changes and the manifestation of clinical symptoms. Management of the condition requires diagnosing the disease, eliminating the cause, and normalising the humours, tissues and organs. The approach may comprise pharmacotherapy with Unani medicines, dietary modification and use of concurrent non-drug therapies.

The Unani pharmacopoeia is vast and comprises over 2000 substances from herbal, mineral and animal sources, many of which are also used in Ayurveda, Western herbal medicine and TCM. Unani medicines can be single-ingredient preparations, or, more usually, multi-ingredient preparations comprising several ingredients. Powdered toxic metals including mercury and arsenic were included, but these are now largely prohibited. Access to treatment can be through a Unani practitioner or 'hakim', and manufactured Unani medicinal products available online.

Prophetic medicine, al-Tibb al-nabawi, is advice given by the prophet Muhammad in the *hadith* and is distinct from Unani. Certain medicines are highly prized due to their place in the hadith and the Quran; they include black seed (*Nigella sativa*), fenugreek seed and leaf (*Trigonella foenum-graecum*), henna leaf (*Lawsonia inermis*), senna leaf and fruit (*Senna* spp.), honey, olives and olive oil, and dates.

JAMU

Jamu (or Jammu) is the TM practised in Indonesia and other parts of South-East Asia, including Malaysia and Singapore. It originated in central Java and has influences from Ayurveda and TCM, and from Arab countries and Chinese regions, because of the importance of Java as a centre of trade in spices. Jamu has a less structured approach to healing, and the remedies (also known as jamu) are passed down through generations, with local Indonesian plants as the main ingredients. Jamu preparations used to maintain health, and as preventive and curative medicines, they are taken frequently, and long term.

Traditionally, herbal medicines are taken as an infusion, usually prepared in the home, from a mixture of fresh or dried medicinal plants. Preparation of these home remedies has evolved into 'jamu gendong', whereby 'jamu women' sell home-made jamu on the streets. These are usually freshly prepared liquid formulations and are taken daily as a health tonic, and for the treatment of minor ailments. In jamu, as with other TM, there is an emphasis on maintaining vitality, increasing virility and aiding recovery after childbirth. Today, the production of jamu is a major industry, particularly in Indonesia, and preparations are available in numerous

TABLE 16.3.6 Popular South-East Asian Traditional Medicinal Plants Used in Jamu

Botanical Species and Part(s) Used	Common Name	Traditional Use
Abelmoschus moschiatus Medik. Herb, seed, oil	Ambrette, musk mallow	Antispasmodic, aphrodisiac
Alpinia galanga (L.) Willd., and related spp. Rhizome	Greater galangal	Antiinflammatory, antitumour, antimicrobial, gastroprotective
Alstonia scholaris (L.) R. Br. Stem bark	Devil's tree	Dysentery, malaria, antiparasitic
Anacardium occidentale L. Stem bark	Cashew tree	Antiinfective, antihypertensive. stomachic
Cinnamomum burmannii (Nees & T.Nees) Blume Bark, oil	Indonesian cassia	Antimicrobial, antidiabetic, antiinflammatory
Curcuma xanthorrhiza Roxb. Rhizome (fresh and dried)	Javanese ginger/turmeric	Gastrointestinal disorders, antiinflammatory, tonic
Cymbopogon citratus (DC.) Stapf Leaf, oil	Lemon grass	Antispasmodic, antiinflammatory, skin disorders. Insecticide (oil, topical use).
Eurycoma longifolia Jack Leaf, bark, root	Tongkat Ali	Sexual dysfunction, anxiety, appetite stimulant, general tonic
Garcinia mangostana L. Fruit (rind)	Mangosteen	Antibacterial, anticancer, memory enhancement.
Kaempferia galanga L. Rhizome	Resurrection lily, sand ginger	Antiinflammatory, antihypertensive, cough
Morinda citrifolia L. Fruit, juice	Noni, Indian mulberry	Antiinflammatory, immune support, cardiovascular health, general tonic
Orthosiphon aristatus (Blume) Miq. Leaf	Java tea, cat's whiskers	Antiinflammatory, antimicrobial, antihypertensive, diuretic
Psidium guajava L. Leaf	Guava	Antiinflammatory, antiinfective, antidiabetic, cardiovascular health

pharmaceutical forms, including solid dose forms such as tablets and pills, powders and tonics for internal use, and creams, ointments and so forth for external use.

'Jamu-jamu majun' are medicines formulated as pills for enhancing male vitality. Traditional 'majun' are large soft pills prepared from powdered ingredients kneaded with honey and fat and shaped into the soft pills; these are increasingly available formulated as capsules.

Safety problems resulting from poor-quality jamu products have been reported, especially with the use of jamu medicines adulterated with synthetic drugs. Aflatoxins have been detected in commercial jamu products, and substantial microbial contamination of jamu gendong raw materials and finished products has been reported.

Table 16.3.6 shows some important South-East Asian traditional medicinal plants used in jamu. These are in addition to many pantropical species already discussed in other TM systems.

FURTHER READING

Elfahmi, H.J., Woerdenbag, O.K., 2014. Jamu: Indonesian traditional herbal medicine towards rational phytopharmacological use. J. Herbal Med. 4 (2), 51–73.

Govindarajan, R., Vijayakumar, M., Pushpangadan, P., 2005. Antioxidant approach to disease management and the role of rasayana herbs of ayurveda. J. Ethnopharmacol. 99, 165–178.

Lad, V., 1990. Ayurveda the Science of Self-Healing. Lotus Press, Wisconsin.

Limyati, D.A., Juniar, B.L., 1998. Jamu Gendong, a kind of traditional medicine in Indonesia: the microbial contamination of its raw materials and endproduct. J. Ethnopharmacol. 63 (3), 201–208.

Pole, S., 2012. Ayurvedic Medicine: The Principles of Traditional Practice. Pub' Singing Dragon. ISBN-13 978-184819113.

Sairam, T.V., 2000. Home Remedies, vols. I–III. Penguin, India.

Sathasivampillai, S.V., Rajamanoharan, P.R.S., Munday, M., Heinrich, M., 2017. Plants used to treat diabetes in Sri Lankan siddha medicine–an ethnopharmacological review of historical and modern sources. J. Ethnopharmacol. 198, 531–599.

Tuschinsky, C., 1995. Balancing hot and cold – balancing power and weakness: social and cultural aspects of Malay jamu in Singapore. Soc. Sci. Med. 41 (11), 1587–1595.

Williamson, E.M. (Ed.), 2002. Major Herbs of Ayurveda. Churchill Livingstone, Edinburgh.

16.4 Traditional African Medicine

The cultural and climatic diversity of Africa has resulted in a variety of different TM systems. In North Africa (Egypt, Morocco, Tunisia), TM is linked to that of southern Europe and Unani medicine and is well documented. **Traditional African medicine (TAM)** however, refers to sub-Saharan Africa and is a mainly oral tradition with few written records. TAM assumes the existence of supernatural forces in the cause of disease, to a greater extent than most other systems, and employs magic and divination. These and some of the more exotic practices, which include the use of animal parts, especially in the religion vodun (voodoo) in West Africa, have undermined its credibility. However, these aspects are an important part of TAM and it is necessary to understand the context in which a herbal medicine is used, which may not necessarily reflect its pharmacological activity, to evaluate any contribution to medicine. The African flora remains a huge resource for the discovery of new bioactive compounds: from an estimated biodiversity of ~45,000 plant species, only 5000 have documented medicinal use.

CONCEPTS IN TRADITIONAL AFRICAN MEDICINE

The causes of disease, defined culturally, are essential for an understanding of TAM. In African thought, all living things are connected to each other and to the gods and ancestral spirits. If harmony exists between all of these, then good health is enjoyed, but, if not, misfortune or ill-health will result. Forces can be directed at humanity by displeased gods, ancestors and also by witches, resulting in disharmony, which must be resolved before good health can be restored. Treatment may also involve much more than medicine; practices such as divination and incantation may be carried out to help with diagnosis, and sacrifices may be needed to placate the supernatural entity. The traditional healer is likely also to be a religious leader, since health and spirituality are closely intertwined in TAM. Apart from physical examination, the diagnosis may also involve several other forms of diagnosis and treatment:

- **Confessions** may be extracted. These are thought to be both healing and prophylactic. In the case of a child, the mother may need to examine her previous behaviour, since the sins of the mother can be visited on the child. (This compares with ideas in Christianity and other religions.)
- **Divination** may be required and may involve throwing objects and interpreting the pattern in which they fall. This is a consistent feature of many cultures and still persists in Europe in such forms as the 'reading of tea leaves'.

In TAM, serious illness is considered due to supernatural influences to a greater extent than are everyday aches and pains and digestive disorders, and treatment is consequently more concerned with ritual, including incantation and sacrifice, than with minor disorders. Herbal medicines may form part of the ritual rather than contributing any pharmacological activity. The treatment of disease is based on mind–body dualism and examines the whole lifestyle of the patient. The spiritual emphasis of TAM is important and can be rationalised with respect to modern life to some extent. If stress is caused by, for example, breakdown in relationships, loss of status and financial stability, disobedience of religious laws or behaviour causing guilt and shame, lowered immune resistance and ill-health may ensue. We now recognise the importance of psychosomatic factors: the placebo effect demonstrates this very well.

In TAM, medicinal plants are used in two ways, only one of which corresponds to the Western perception of drug therapy. The traditional healer will, however, use medicinal plants not only for their pharmacological properties, but also for their power to restore health as supernatural agents, based on two further assumptions:

- Plants are living and it is thought that all living things generate a vital force, which can be harnessed. This belief is rather similar to that held by some people that uncooked vegetables, particularly items such as sprouting beans, also contain a life-force.
- The release of the force may need special rituals and preparations such as incantations to be effective. This scenario is reflected in the cultivation of the 'bedside manner' and other reassuring measures used to instil confidence in health professionals.

The method of administration of a medicinal plant preparation is essential for understanding TAM. In conventional medicine, some form of absorption of the drug must take place. It can be orally, rectally, parenterally, topically or by inhalation. In TAM, this is not necessarily important (although it will happen in many instances) as ingredients can be encapsulated and worn as an amulet, necklace or around the wrist or ankle. They may not even come into contact with the patient at all; perhaps being placed above the door, or under a mat or pillow, to ward off evil spirits which may be causing disease.

The choice of plant may have been made on a basis that has no scientific rationale; for example, a plant that bears many fruits may be used to treat infertility, as with the ancient 'Doctrine of Signatures', where a plant was thought to display features indicating its use. This is a recurrent theme in the history of medicine throughout the world.

Nevertheless, effective strategies for using TAM herbal knowledge are available, for example, from studies of antimalarial plants used by Nigerian healers. An important consideration is the division between those plant species used as medicines and those employed for more nefarious purposes. Highly poisonous species are rarely used for healing because it is not possible to accurately control the dose. Paradoxically, these have more often led to the development of modern drugs than relatively innocuous species. For example, *Physostigma venenosum* Balf., the Calabar bean, which yields the alkaloid physostigmine (eserine) and its derivatives neostigmine (used for myasthenia gravis) and rivastigmine (used for Alzheimer disease), has no traditional medical use. It was an ordeal poison in Nigeria, administered to those accused of witchcraft, where death indicated guilt. Other African species yielding important drugs include the Madagascar periwinkle, *Catharanthus roseus* (L.) G. Don, which contains vincristine and vinblastine (used for leukaemias and Hodgkin lymphoma) and the Cape bushwillow, *Combretum caffrum* (Eckl. & Zeyh.) Kuntze, which yields the combretastatins, currently under investigation as antiangiogenic agents.

Some of the most widely used African medicinal plants are listed in Table 16.4.1. They do not include toxic species used as sources of potent drugs. Their indications (dysentery, fever, inflammation) reflect the everyday health problems which are treated with TM in Africa. Popular herbal medicines from African species which are now used globally include Devil's claw, from the root of *Harpagophytum* species, Umckaloabo, from the root of *Pelargonium* species, yohimbe, from the bark of *Pausinystalia johimbe* and the *Hoodia* 'cactus', *Hoodia gordonii*. Other pantropical and temperate species, such as ginger

TABLE 16.4.1   Examples of Widely Used African Medicinal Plants

Species	Common Names	Traditional Uses
Aframomum alboviolaceum (Ridl.) K. Schum. (syn.: *A. latifolium* (Afzel.) K. Schtum) (Zingiberaceae) Fruit, seed, rhizome	Ginguenga, Heaven fruit	Pain, fever, inflammation, infections, worms
Aframomum melegueta K. Schum. (Zingiberaceae) Leaf, fruit, seed	Grains of heaven, Melegueta pepper	Pain, inflammation, infections, diarrhoea
Agathosma betulina Berg. Pillans and other spp. (Rutaceae) Leaf	Buchu	Urinary infections, prostatitis, respiratory and gastric disorders
Aloe ferox Mill. [Xanthorrhoeaceae] Leaf exudate, leaf mucilage/gel	Cape aloe, aloes, aloe vera gel	Gastrointestinal disorders, inflammation, skin disease, infections
Aspalathus linearis (Burm.f.) R. Dahlgren (Fabaceae) Leaf, fermented	Rooibos, red bush, bush tea	General health support, diabetes, alternative to caffeine-containing teas
Boophone disticha (L.f.) Herb. (Amaryllidaceae) Bulb	Century plant	Pain, wound healing; hallucinogen
Brucea antidysenterica J. F. Mill. (Simaroubaceae) Leaves, roots, seeds	Waginos	Diarrhoea, dysentery, indigestion, skin problems, leprosy
Cajanus cajan (L.) Millsp. (Fabaceae) Leaves, seeds, roots	Pigeon pea	Sickle-cell anaemia, hypertension
Carica papaya L. (Caricaceae) Seed	Pumpkin	Contraception, male urinary disorders
Catha edulis (Vahl.) Endl. (Celastraceae) Leaf, root, bark	Khat, bushman's tea	Respiratory disease, stimulant
Catharanthus roseus (L,) G. Don (syn.: *Vinca rosea* L.) (Apocynaceae) Herb	Madagascar periwinkle	High blood pressure, cancer
Cola nitida (Vent.) Schott. & Endl., *C. acuminata* (P. Beauv.) Schott. & Endl. (Malvaceae) Seed	Cola nut	Fatigue, dysentery, diarrhoea, migraine
Combretum micranthum G. Don (Combretaceae) Leaf	Kinkeliba	Hypertension, weight loss, pain
Cryptolepis sanguinolenta (Lindl.) Schltr. (Apocynaceae) Root	Ghana quinine, nibima	Malaria
Cyclopia intermedia E. Mey. (Fabaceae) Leaf, stem, fermented	Honeybush tea	General health, cardiovascular disease, diabetes
Diospyros mespiliformis Hochst. ex A.DC. (Ebenaceae) Leaf, bark, root.	Jackalberry	Dysentery, diarrhoea, parasitic infections
Euphorbia drupifera Thonn. (syn.: *Elaeophorbia drupifera* (Thonn.) Stapf (Euphorbiaceae) Leaf, bark, latex	Kankan, toro	Worms, purgative, respiratory disorders, skin conditions
Ficus obliqua G. Forst. (Moraceae) Root bark, sap, leaves, fruit	Small-leaved fig	Dysentery, diarrhoea, pain and inflammation
Garcinia kola Heckel (Clusiaceae) Seed	Bitter kola, koluviron	Pain, inflammation, arthritis, infections
Harpagophytum procumbens (Burch.) DC. ex Meisn. (Pedaliaceae) Root	Devil's claw, grapple plant	Pain, inflammation, arthritis
Hibiscus sabdariffa L. (Malvaceae) Flower	Roselle	Weight loss, hypertension, high cholesterol
Holarrhena floribunda (G. Don) T. Durand & Schinz (Apocynaceae) Bark	Kurchi	Dysentery, fever, colitis
Hoodia gordonii (Masson) Sweet ex Decne. (Apocynaceae) Stem	Hoodia cactus	Weight loss, appetite suppressant
Hunteria umbellata (K. Schum.) Hallier f. (Apocynaceae) Bark, root, seed	Abeere	Diabetes, bleeding disorders, fever, inflammation, worm infestation

TABLE 16.4.1 Examples of Widely Used African Medicinal Plants—cont'd

Species	Common Names	Traditional Uses
Hypoxis hemerocallidea Fisch, C.A. Mey. & Avé-Lall. (syn.: *H. rooperi* T. Moore (Hypoxidaceae) Tuber (corm)	African potato, African star grass	Male urinary problems, lung disease. arthritis
Kigelia africana (Lam.) Benth. (Bignoniaceae) Fruit, bark, root	Sausage tree	Infectious diseases, skin disorders, inflammation
Pausinystalia johimbe (K. Schum.) Pierre ex Beille (Rubiaceae) Bark	Yohimbe	Sexual dysfunction, weight loss
Pelargonium sidoides DC., *P. reniforme* (Andrews) Curtis Root	Pelargonium, Umckaloabo	Respiratory infections
Piper guineense Schumach. & Thonn. (Piperaceae) Fruit, roots, leaves	West African pepper	Oedema, cough, inflammation, digestive disorders
Prunus africana (Hook.f.) Kalkman (Rosaceae) Bark	Pygeum bark	Male urinary problems, pain, fever, inflammation
Rauvolfia vomitoria Afzel. (Apocynaceae) Root, stem bark	Poison devil's pepper	Sedative, psychosis, diarrhoea, jaundice, fever, high blood pressure, inflammation
Ricinus communis L. (Euphorbiaceae) Seed oil	Castor bean	Infections, diarrhoea, contraception, laxative, skin conditions
Sutherlandia frutescens (L.) R. Br (Fabaceae) Leaf, young stem	Cancer bush	Viral infections, cancer, gastrointestinal disorders, pain and inflammation
Vernonia amygdalina Delile (Asteraceae)[a] Leaf, root	Bitter leaf	Fever, diarrhoea, dysentery, hepatitis
Voacanga africana Stapf Bark	Small-fruit wild frangipani	Worm infestations, sexual enhancement
Xylopia aethiopica (Dunal) A. Rich. (Annonaceae) Fruit	Ethiopian pepper	Respiratory disease, pain, inflammation, digestive disorders oedema

[a]*Vernonia amygdalina* is one of very few documented chimpanzee medicinal plants, in addition to *Lippia plicata* (Verbenaceae). These species are self-selected and eaten for treating intestinal nematode (worm) infections.

(*Zingiber* species), turmeric (*Curcuma* species), basil (*Ocimum* species) and wormwoods (*Artemisia* species), are also widely used throughout Africa.

FURTHER READING

Kahumba, J., Rasamiravaka, T., Okusa, P.N., Bakari, S.A., Bizumukama, L., Kiendrebeogo, M., et al., 2015. Traditional African medicine: from ancestral knowledge to a modern integrated future? Science 350 (6262), S61–S63.

Neuwinger, H.D., 2000. African Traditional Medicine. Medpharm, Stuttgart.

Okpako, D.T., 1999. Traditional African medicine: theory and pharmacology explored. Trends. Pharm. Sci. 20, 482–484.

Sofowara, A. (Ed.), 1979. African Medicinal Plants: Proceedings of a Conference. University of Life Press, Nigeria.

Thomas, O.O., 1989. Perspectives on ethno-phytotherapy of Yoruba medicinal herbs and preparations. Fitoterapia 60, 49–60.

Van Wyk, B.E., 2015. A review of commercially important African medicinal plants. J. Ethnopharmacol. 176, 118–134.

16.5 Indigenous Medicine of the Americas

In the American nations, there is a wide range of TM practices, including those maintaining a strong indigenous element. In many Central American and some Caribbean and South American countries, healthcare at all levels remains limited and poorly supported, making it accessible only for wealthy individuals; herbal medicines are, therefore, still widely used by many people. The North and South American continents are huge, and diverse in so many ways—geographically, botanically, ethnically—and culturally the

societies have been shaped by a long series of dramatic external interventions. Consequently, it is impossible to summarise all TM practices here, and this chapter provides references to direct further investigation.

Until the European invasion of the 'New World' in 1492, American medicine was developed through small local networks, relying on local resources in diverse ecozones. After the Spanish and Portuguese conquests, indigenous medicinal and toxic plants produced important contributions to world medicine and science. In 1552, Martín de la Cruz wrote the 'Little Book of the Medicinal Herbs of the Indians' (*Libellus de Medicinalibus Indorum Herbis*), which increased interest in the use of American medicinal plants. Numerous other books followed promoting the discoveries from the 'New World', including the *Florentine Codex*, compiled by Fray Bernardino de Sahagún (ca. 1545–1590)—the first ethnographic study in México systematically inquiring about traditional practices, including the medicines used. There is a long tradition of exchange between the Americas and other continents and the long colonial rule resulted in the development of medicines from these becoming widely available globally (Table 16.5.1). At the same time, many European, African and other herbal medicines have become important elements of American 'traditional' medicine.

Today, in Canada and the United States, TM is less often practised by indigenous groups, in contrast to most regions of South/Central America, México and the Caribbean, for example. In many regions

TABLE 16.5.1   American Medicinal Plants Yielding Important Herbal Drugs and Natural Products

Common Name	Species	Plant Part	Geographical Origin	Constituents Where Known	Medicinal Use
Black/wild Cherry	*Prunus serotina* Ehrh.	Bark	North America	Cyanogenetic glycosides (amygdalin, prunasin)	Bronchitis, colds, coughs, fevers
Beth root	*Trillium erectum* L.	Root	Mid and Western USA	Steroidal saponins (bethogenins)	Astringent, to stem bleeding in haemorrhage and after childbirth
Boldo	*Peumus boldus* Molina	Leaf	Chile	Alkaloids (boldine); tannins (catechin)	Digestive, liver disease, diuretic
Cascara	*Frangula purshiana* (DC.) A.Gray ex J.G. Cooper	Bark	USA	Anthraquinone glycosides (cascarosides)	Laxative, purgative (Chapter 18)
Cinchona	*Cinchona pubescens* Vahl, *C. calisaya* Wedd.	Bark	South America	Quinoline alkaloids (quinine)	Fever, malaria (Chapter 10)
Coca	*Erythroxylum coca* Lam.	Leaf	Bolivia, Peru, Colombia	Tropane alkaloids (cocaine)	CNS stimulant (Chapter 22)
Cohosh, black	*Actaea racemosa* L.	Root	North America	Triterpene glycosides (actein)	Female disorders (Chapter 24)
Condurango	*Marsdenia cundurango* Rchb.f.	Bark	Peru, Ecuador	Pregnane glycosides (condurangin)	Indigestion, cancer
Cranberry	*Vaccinium macrocarpon* Aiton	Berry	North America	Polyphenolics (proanthocyanidins)	General health, urinary disorders (Chapter 24)
Damiana	*Turnera diffusa* Willd. ex Schult.	Leaf	Southern USA, Mexico	Cyanogenetic glycosides, hydroquinones (arbutin)	Aphrodisiac, tonic (Chapter 25)
Echinacea	*Echinacea* spp.	Herb, root, juice	USA, Canada	Alkylamides, caffeic acid derivatives	Immune stimulant, colds, flu (Chapter 21)
Evening primrose	*Oenothera biennis* L.	Leaf, seed oil	USA	Polyunsaturated fatty acids (*cis*-linoleic, *cis*-γ-linolenic)	Inflammatory skin conditions (Chapter 27)
Grape, Oregon	*Berberis aquifolium* Pursh	Root, berries	Western USA	Benzylisoquinoline alkaloids (berberine)	Inflammatory skin conditions (psoriasis), jaundice, dysentery, infections (Chapter 10)
Goldenseal	*Hydrastis canadensis* L.	Root	Canada, Eastern USA	Benzylisoquinoline alkaloids (hydrastine, berberine)	Jaundice, dysentery, infections (Chapter 10)
Guarana	*Paullinia cupana* Kunth	Berry	Brazil	Xanthines (e.g. caffeine)	Stimulant, tonic (Chapter 22)
Ipecacuanha	*Carapichea ipecacuanha* (Brot.) L. Andersson	Root	Brazil	Isoquinoline alkaloids (emetine)	Antiamoebic, dysentery, emetic (Chapter 21)
Lapacho	*Handroanthus* (*Tabebuia* spp.)	Bark	South America	Naphthoquinones (lapachol)	Antiinfective, anticancer (Chapter 10)
Lemon verbena	*Aloysia citriodora* Palau	Herb	Chile, Peru	Essential oil (neral, geranial,	Digestive disorders, sedative, antimicrobial, insect repellent
Lobelia	*Lobelia inflata* L.	Herb	Northern USA, Canada	Pyridine alkaloids (lobeline)	Stimulant
Mate	*Ilex paraguayensis* A. St.-Hil.	Leaf	Paraguay	Xanthines (e.g. caffeine)	Stimulant, tonic (Chapter 22)
May apple	*Podophyllum peltatum* L.	Root	Eastern USA, Canada	Lignans (podophyllotoxin)	Emetic, vermifuge, cancer (Chapter 9)

TABLE 16.5.1   American Medicinal Plants Yielding Important Herbal Drugs and Natural Products—cont'd

Common Name	Species	Plant Part	Geographical Origin	Constituents Where Known	Medicinal Use
Quassia	*Picrasma excelsa* (Sw.) Planch., *Quassia amara* L.	Wood	Central and tropical South America	Quassinoids (quassin)	Insecticide, vermifuge, amoebicide (Chapter 27)
Sarsaparilla	*Smilax ornata* Lem., *S. aristolochiifolia* Mill.	Root	Central America, Mexico, Jamaica	Steroidal saponins based diosgenin, smilagenins	Rheumatism, skin disorders, steroidal precursor (Chapter 6)
Saw palmetto	*Serenoa repens* (W. Bartram) Small	Berry	Southern USA	Phytosterols (β-sitosterol), fatty acids	Male urinary disorders (Chapter 25)
Witch hazel	*Hamamelis virginiana* L.	Bark, leaf	Eastern USA, Canada	Gallotannins (hamamelitannins)	Astringent, topical skin and ocular inflammation (Chapter 27)
Yam, wild	*Dioscorea villosa* L.	Root	Southern USA	Steroidal saponins based on diosgenin, diarylheptanoids	Rheumatism, colic, menopausal symptoms. Steroid precursor (Chapter 6)
Yew, pacific	*Taxus baccata* L.	Bark	Western USA	Diterpenes (taxol)	Cancer (Chapter 9)

people both in rural and urban regions heavily rely on herbal medicines, and state governments actively promote the development and use of these products.

Many American psychoactive plants have become globally famous. Starting in the mid-20th century, neuropharmacology has benefited from the study of hallucinogenic plants and mushrooms. In some regions of rural México, important species, such as Mexican morning glory (*Turbina corymbosa* (L.) Raf.), and mushrooms, such as *Psilocybe* spp. (Agaricales), and peyote, *Lophophora williamsii* (Lem) J.M. Coult. have been used for centuries. Phytochemical investigations of the Amazonian Ayahuasca brews have contributed to a better understanding of the effects of tryptamine hallucinogens. Dimethyltryptamine (DMT), found in *Psychotria viridis* Ruiz & Pav. and other species, is rapidly metabolised by monoamine oxidase (MAO) in the body; however, traditionally, it is taken together in admixtures with *Banisteriopsis caapi* (Spruce ex Griseb.) C.V. Morton which contains MAO inhibitors, and this prevents the breakdown of active constituents. The study of these psychoactive mixtures has been described in detail and demonstrates the comprehensive medical understanding of Amazonian practitioners of TMs.

Such traditional knowledge is now being identified and investigated for its potential to treat mental health conditions: psilocybin, for example, may have a place in treating depression. Similarly, ayahuasca is being actively explored for the treatment of various forms of addiction.

The Americas cover all geographical zones, and plants used, and people using them, are thus extraordinarily varied. It is not possible to summarise the principles of such diverse cultural beliefs, but the role of medicines and natural products derived from American plants in modern use is testament to both the history and diversity of these continents, and of the continued need for plant-based healthcare in many countries and regions of the Americas.

FURTHER READING

Arnason, J.T., Harris, C.S., Guerrero-Analco, J.A., 2022. Phytochemistry in the ethnopharmacology of North and Central America. Front. Pharmacol. 13, 815742. https://doi.org/10.3389/fphar.2022.815742.

Daws, R.E., Timmermann, C., Giribaldi, B., Sexton, J.D., Wall, M.B., Erritzoe, D., et al., 2022. Increased global integration in the brain after psilocybin therapy for depression. Nat. Med. 28 (4), 844–851. https://doi.org/10.1038/s41591-022-01744-z.

Geck, M.S., Cristians, S., Berger-González, M., Casu, L., Heinrich, M., Leonti, M., 2020. Traditional herbal medicine in Mesoamerica: toward its evidence base for improving universal health coverage. Front. Pharmacol. 11, 1160. https://doi.org/10.3389/fphar.2020.01160.

Heinrich, M., Frei Haller, B., Leonti, M., 2014. A perspective on natural products research and ethnopharmacology in Mexico: the eagle and the serpent on the prickly pear cactus. J. Nat. Prod. 201477 (3), 678–689. https://doi.org/10.1021/np4009927.

16.6 Traditional Medicine in Australasia

AUSTRALIAN ABORIGINAL TRADITIONAL MEDICINE

Traditional Aboriginal medicine is the TM system of Australian Aborigines, the indigenous people of Australia. Like many other indigenous systems of medicine, it is an oral tradition (i.e. the traditional knowledge is handed down by word of mouth and, for example, through song and dance). An Aboriginal pharmacopoeia has been published, which brings together traditional knowledge from the Northern Territory (Barr 1988), but, unfortunately, much of the Aboriginal traditional medical use knowledge has been lost (Stack, 1989).

As with some other indigenous systems of medicine, Aborigines attributed serious illness and death to malevolent spirits or sorcery.

Spiritual 'doctors' of great wisdom, power and standing would be summoned to determine the cause of death or illness and, through performing sacred rites, to cure the illness; these esteemed healers were also believed to hold the power to inflict illness, or a 'death curse', as punishment (Byard, 1988).

The Aboriginal concept of the 'Dreaming' is fundamentally linked to Aborigines' beliefs about causes of illness and the healing power of plants. The concept describes Aboriginal beliefs about the formation of the universe and encompasses the belief that some of the spiritual Ancestors were transformed into plants (and others into humans, animals and so forth). Some Ancestor spirits transformed into rocks, or watering holes, and these 'Dreaming' locations are also considered sacred (Clarke, 2011). There are strong beliefs among Aborigines that disturbances of the power of 'Dreaming' locations can also cause serious illness. Aborigines see strong connections between people and plants (since both originate from spiritual Ancestors) and so they have substantial cultural significance. Some plants, or sites in the physical landscape where certain plants grow, are considered sacred. From an Aboriginal perspective, plants have great powers, and are used in rituals, as medicines, intoxicants and stimulants, and there is not necessarily clear, or even any, distinction between these uses.

With respect to minor ailments, due to the nomadic nature of their existence, initially all Aborigines used plants and other substances (such as animal fats and oils, earth, mud, clay and sand) as treatments essential for their survival. The Australian flora is unique, and many of the medicinal plant species used by Aborigines are different to those used by indigenous people elsewhere. In addition to using plants and other natural substances, blood-letting or cutting (to allow pain to 'escape'), massage, wearing of amulets, chants and ceremonies also played a role in treating injury and disease. Most medicinal plants were prepared as ointments or pastes composed of crushed plant parts mixed with animal fats or oils, and applied externally; infusions of leaves or bark were also applied to the body, or sometimes taken internally. Some plants were burnt over a fire and the vapour inhaled.

Aboriginal medicine is still practised today by Aboriginal tribes in central and northern Australia; its practice varies widely in other regions (Oliver, 2013). The practice has evolved, and modalities such as blood-letting are unlikely to be used; however, the belief that serious illness results from bad spirits and sorcery remains.

Medicinal plants ('bush medicines') remain an important component for treating minor ailments, such as coughs and colds, boils and other skin disorders, bites and stings, burns and other wounds. The plants most commonly used are those that are easily accessible and require minimal preparation. The traditional remedies selected, indications for use and methods of preparation differ across different Aboriginal tribes and areas. In some tribes, only certain individuals are permitted to reveal the location of the native plants and describe their uses, although all members of the tribe would have the knowledge (Stack, 1989). In some instances, special rituals, including singing of special songs, are performed during collection of plants, and this is believed to be important for the medicinal value of the remedies. Some important traditional medicines are listed in Table 16.6.1. Some native plants used by indigenous Australians, such as the volatile oils (tea tree oil) from the Australian tea tree *Melaleuca alternifolia* (Maiden & Betche) Cheel and eucalyptus oil from the eucalyptus tree (*Eucalyptus* spp.), have an important place in the Australian community, being used for antimicrobial activity and respiratory conditions, respectively (Barnes et al., 2016).

Improving Aboriginal health in Australia is among government priorities for future policy development and investment, including in medical and health research relating to indigenous medicine. The National Aboriginal and Torres Strait Islander Health Plan 2013–2023 of the Australian Government (Commonwealth of Australia, 2013) notes 'the significance of culture to well-being, and therefore good health, is also demonstrated by using traditional knowledge and the practices of traditional healers, which are adapted by many people for complementary use with western science in an integrated health care system'. At present, there are some examples of state-funded access to *ngangkari* (one of the Aboriginal names for traditional indigenous healers), and of use of traditional healers and traditional medicine both alone and in combination with Western healthcare (Oliver, 2013).

In Australia there is substantial interest in exploring the potential medicinal value of traditional Aboriginal plant medicines through a combined approach comprising understanding the traditional knowledge relating to use of plants by Aborigines with rigorous scientific investigation, with the ultimate aim of identifying potential new therapeutic compounds (Locher et al., 2013; Simpson et al., 2013). Such activities need to be approached with the necessary engagement with local indigenous communities (and, optimally, driven by them), benefit-sharing arrangements, and protection of traditional knowledge in place.

RONGOĀ MĀORI

The traditional medical system of the indigenous people (known as Māori) of Aotearoa New Zealand is Rongoā Māori. Like many other indigenous systems of medicine, it is an oral tradition (i.e. the traditional knowledge is handed down by word of mouth), and pays particular attention to spiritual aspects of a person's health. To Māori, Rongoā Māori is a cultural treasure (*taonga*) and is an essential component of a culturally appropriate way of life that acknowledges the connections of all things and involves the health and well-being of the people as well as that of their environment. *Te Tiriti o Waitangi* (the Treaty of Waitangi), the founding document of New Zealand, sets out protections for Rongoā Māori practices.

Historically, Māori believed that some illnesses were caused by supernatural forces, and the tohunga (Māori traditional healers) were believed to be the earthly conduit of the spirits that controlled all aspects of life. As with other traditional systems, illness was believed to result from some sort of disharmony or imbalance with nature: the role of tohunga was to determine the nature of this discord, and to use plant, physical (e.g. massage) and spiritual treatments to correct it (Anon, 2008; Jones, n.d.).

The arrival of European settlers to New Zealand in the 1800s brought new diseases and other challenges for Māori that had a devastating effect on the health of Māori. Also, due to the emergence of 'quack' practitioners, the Tohunga Suppression Act 1907 was passed (along with a Quackery Prevention Act in 1908 in response to 'quack' European doctors). The Tohunga Suppression Act was rarely enforced. However, it caused the practice of Rongoā Māori to become secretive and discussed only among Māori communities; despite this, the traditional knowledge relating to Rongoā thrived and developed during this time (Anon, 2008). The Act was repealed in 1962.

Today, Rongoā Māori involves the use of traditional herbal medicines (*rongoā rākau*) and some other substances of natural origin, massage (*mirimiri*) and prayer (*karakia*) and is a holistic system of healthcare incorporating physical, social, cultural, emotional, family (*whānau*) and spiritual aspects of health; each aspect is important to ensure full recovery of the patient.

The use of native plant medicines is a key component of Rongoā Māori; these plants are typically collected from the wild by Māori

TABLE 16.6.1   Some Important Medicinal Plants of Australian Aboriginal Medicine and Selected Uses

Scientific Name; Family[a]	Common Names[b]	Preparation and Administration	Traditional Medical Uses
Acacia melanoxylon R. Br.; Fabaceae, s.l.	Blackwood	Bark, infusion used externally	Painful joints
Carpobrotus glaucescens (Haw.) Schwantes; Aizoaceae	Pigface	Leaf juice	Ant bites
Dodonaea polyandra Merr. & L. M. Perry; Sapindaceae	Uncha	Leaves, applied to tooth or cavity	Toothache
Duboisia hopwoodii (F. Muell.) F. Muell.; Solanaceae		Leaves, prepared as pituri;[c] chewed	Intoxicant, euphoric, narcotic
Eremophila alternifolia R. Br.; Scrophulariaceae	Narrow leaf fuchsia bush, native honeysuckle	Leaves, infusion used internally and externally	As decongestant, expectorant, analgesic, colds, influenza, fever, headache, septic wounds
Eremophila longifolia (R. Br.) F. Muell.; Scrophulariaceae	Fuchsia bush, weeping emu bush		Coughs, colds
Eremophila freelingii F. Muell.; Scrophulariaceae	Rock fuchsia bush	Leaves, decoction applied as wash	Aches, pains, including headache
Eucalyptus spp.; Myrtaceae	Gum tree	Leaves, infusion Bark, poultice applied externally	Pain relief
Ficus opposita Miq.; Moraceae		Leaves, infusion applied to skin	Scabies
Ipomoea pes-caprae (L.) R. Br.; Convolvulaceae	Beach convolvulus	Leaves, heated and applied to wound Juice	Analgesia, skin infections, green ant bites, insect stings, scabies Diuretic, laxative
Planchonia careya (F. Muell.) R. Knuth; Lecythidaceae	Cocky apple tree	Inner bark, liquid applied externally	Sores, boils, burns
Solanum laciniatum Aiton, *Solanum aviculare* G. Forst.; Solanaceae	Kangaroo apple	Fruit; poultice	Joint swellings

[a]Latin names have been checked using the Medicinal Plant Names Service, Royal Botanic Gardens, Kew (https://mpns.science.kew.org/) and/or the Australian Plant Name Index/Australian Plant Census (https://biodiversity.org.au/nsl/services/search/name-check), and are as current as possible. Synonyms may also need to be checked when reviewing the literature.
[b]Common names given are mostly English versions; there are simply too many regional and colloquial names to list.
[c]Small dried fragments of plant material mixed with alkaline wood ash.
Compiled from Barr (1988), Byard (1988), Clarke (2011), Stack (1989).

traditional healers, often from specific locations only, and have specific methods of collection and preparation in accordance with customs (*tikanga*), and to reduce potential toxicity. The remedies are usually crude water or ethanol extracts of crushed, fresh or dried plant material, sometimes boiled, and taken orally as an infusion. With some plants, the leaves or shoots are chewed, or these and other plant parts are made into poultices or compresses for topical use. Māori traditional medicines are used to treat a range of conditions, often minor ailments, including wounds and other skin conditions, gastrointestinal disorders, aches and pains, and upper respiratory tract infections. Māori may also access rongoā to help with chronic medical conditions, such as diabetes and mental health issues, in part because of a lack of response to conventional medicine, or because they feel that rongoā better addresses all their needs as a patient. Some important medicinal plants of Rongoā Māori and selected uses are listed in Table 16.6.2.

Māori traditional healers have an essential role in the practice of Rongoā Māori. The practice of Rongoā Māori and use of medicinal plants vary between rongoā practitioners and in different regions, and treatment of patients and conditions is also individualised (Anon, 2008). Practitioners learn through the oral transmission of knowledge by respected tribal elders (*kaumātua*) and/or through an 'apprenticeship' with a practising tohunga; more formalised training programmes and qualifications are becoming available.

In line with the WHO's strategic goals with respect to traditional medicine, the New Zealand Ministry of Health introduced several initiatives, including the publication of standards for traditional Māori healing (Ministry of Health, 1999) and a Rongoā development plan for how Rongoā Māori (Ministry of Health, 2006) will be made available and supported within the health and disability sector in New Zealand. The Ministry of Health in New Zealand now funds a number of Rongoā Māori providers to provide some Rongoā services.

Information on the traditional uses, chemical constituents and other scientific information on New Zealand's medicinal plants has been collated, though, in general, there has been limited scientific study of the *clinical* pharmacology of Māori plant medicines.

TABLE 16.6.2   Some Important Medicinal Plants of Rongoā Māori and Selected Uses

Botanical Name; Family	Māori Name(s); Other Common Names	Preparation and Administration	Traditional Medical Uses
Kunzea spp.; Myrtaceae	Kānuka;[a] white tea tree, white mānuka	Bark; decoction	Diarrhoea, dysentery
Kunzea ericoides (A. Rich.) Joy Thomps. (syn.: *Leptospermum ericoides* A. Rich.) and *L. scoparium* J. R. Forst. & G. Forst.; Myrtaceae	Mānuka, kahikatoa; red tea tree	Bark; decoction Gum; topical Seedpods; decoction Seedpods; chewed	Mouthwash, diarrhoea, dysentery, back pain Burns Dysentery Diarrhoea
Macropiper excelsum (G. Forst.) Miq.; Piperaceae	Kawakawa, kawa; Māori pepper tree	Leaves, pulped, applied as poultice Leaves; decoction Leaves, root; chewed	Toothache, boils Boils, other skin disorders, bruises, wounds, stomach pains, gonorrhoea Toothache, dysentery
Phormium tenax J. R. Forst. & G. Forst.; Asphodelaceae	Harakeke, korari; flax	Gum; topical	Burns, scalds, wounds
Pomaderris kumeraho A. Cunn. ex Fenzl; Rhamnaceae	Kūmarahou, pāpapa; gumdigger's soap, poverty weed, golden tainui	Leaves; boiled Rhizome; poultice Root; decoction Root juice; lotion	Asthma, bronchitis, coughs, colds, mild laxative, tuberculosis Boils Constipation, wounds Ringworm

[a]The name kānuka is in common use today, but in early records, the name mānuka was used, thus records for mānuka are also relevant here. Manaaki Whenua—Landcare Research (2022) Ngā Rauropi Whakaoranga. https://RauropiWhakaoranga.landcareresearch.co.nz. Accessed 2021–12-03

REFERENCES

Barnes, J., McLachlan, A., Sherwin, C., Enioutina, E.Y., 2016. Herbal medicines: challenges in the modern world. Part 1. Australia and New Zealand. Expert. Rev. Clin. Pharmacol. 9 (7), 905–915.

Barr, A., 1988. Traditional Bush Medicines: an Aboriginal Pharmacopoeia. Greenhouse Publications, Richmond, Vic.

Byard, R., 1988. Traditional medicine of aAboriginal Australia. CMAJ (Can. Med. Assoc. J.) 139 (8), 792–794.

Clarke, P.A., 2011. Aboriginal People and Their Plants. Rosenberg, Dural, NSW.

Commonwealth of Australia, 2013. National aboriginal and Torres Strait Islander health plan, 2013–2023. http://www.health.gov.au/NATSIHP. (Accessed 3 December 2021) last accessed 03.12.21.

Locher, C., Semple, S.J., Simpson, B.S., 2013. Traditional Australian aboriginal medicinal plants: an untapped resource for novel therapeutic compounds? Future Med. Chem. 5 (7), 733–736.

Oliver, S.J., 2013. The role of traditional medicine practice in primary health care within aboriginal Australia: a review of the literature. J. Ethnobiol. Ethnomed. 9, 46

Simpson, B.S., Claudie, D.J., Smith, N.M., McKinnon, R.A., Semple, S.J., 2013. Learning from both sides: experiences and opportunities in the investigation of Australian aboriginal medicinal plants. J. Pharm. Pharm. Sci. 16 (2), 259–271.

Stack, E.M., 1989. Aboriginal Pharmacopoeia. The Third Eric Johnston Lecture. Northern Territory Library Service, Darwin.

Rongoā Māori

Anon, 2008. Demystifying Rongoā Māori: traditional Nāori healing. Best Pract. J. 32 (13), 32–36. Available at: http://www.bpac.org.nz/magazine/2008/may/docs/bpj13_rongoa_pages_32-36_pf.pdf.

Jones, R., Rongoā – medicinal use of plants – understanding rongoā. Te Ara – the Encyclopedia of New Zealand. http://www.TeAra.govt.nz/en/rongoa-medicinal-use-of-plants/pages1-7. (Accessed 6 December 2021) accessed 06.12.21.

Ministry of Health Manatu Hauora, 1999. Standards for Traditional Māori Healing. Ministry of Health, Wellington, New Zealand.

Ministry of Health, 2006. Taonga Tuku Iho – Treasures of Our Heritage: Rongoā Development Plan. Ministry of Health, Wellington, New Zealand.

FURTHER READING

Australian Aboriginal Traditional Medicine Clarke, P.A., 2011. Aboriginal People and Their Plants. Rosenberg, Dural, NSW.

Brooker, S.G., Cambie, R.C., Cooper, R.C., 1987. New Zealand Medicinal Plants. Heinemann, Auckland.

Mark, G., Boulton, A., Kerridge, D., 2019. Rongoā māori is not a complementary and alternative medicine: rongoā māori is a way of life. Int. J. Hum. Rights Educ. 3 (1) Article 12.

Ministry of Health. Rongoā Māori: traditional Māori healing. Ministry of Health, Wellington, New Zealand. https://www.health.govt.nz/our-work/populations/maori-health/rongoa-maori-traditional-maori-healing [accessed December 6, 2021].

Ngā Ngā Tipu Whakaoranga – Māori Plant Use Database. Available at: http://maoriplantuse.landcareresearch.co.nz.

Robin, A., Rongoā Māori. Health Navigator New Zealand. https://www.healthnavigator.org.nz/health-a-z/r/rongo%C4%81-m%C4%81ori/#Overview. (Accessed 6 December 2021) (accessed 6 December 2021).

17

Complementary, Alternative and Integrative Plant Therapies

Medicinal plants are widely used in conventional medicine, and even more in traditional medicine (TM), complementary therapies and as alternatives to conventional treatment. These diverse approaches, collectively known as complementary and alternative medicine (CAM), are based on philosophies fundamentally different to scientific thought (Box 17.1). CAM includes many nondrug therapies, such as acupuncture, chiropractic, osteopathy, hypnotherapy, massage, reflexology, meditation and yoga, which are outside the scope of this book. Others, such as homoeopathy, aromatherapy and anthroposophical medicine, involve the use of plant-derived substances (Box 17.2) and will be briefly discussed. Traditional medical systems are also sometimes considered as CAM, especially outside their geographical or cultural origin; these are discussed in Chapter 16.

HOMOEOPATHY

History

Homoeopathy was developed around 200 years ago by Samuel Hahnemann, a German physician and apothecary. His development of the principles of this controversial approach to treatment needs to be considered against the background of medical practice at the time, when the use of leeches, bloodletting, strong purgatives and emetics, and preparations containing toxic heavy metals, such as arsenic and mercury, was widespread. Hahnemann was dissatisfied with these harsh therapeutic strategies, and this led him to give up the practice of medicine. During this period, he experimented with cinchona bark (which was used to treat malaria) and found that, with high doses of the substance, he experienced similar symptoms to those of malaria. Hahnemann used this approach (which he called a 'proving') with healthy volunteers who were given substances to build up a 'symptom picture' for each, and based on his findings, outlined three basic principles of (classical) homoeopathy:

1. A substance which, in large doses, causes symptoms in a healthy person can be used to treat the same symptom(s) in a person who is ill. Thus Coffea, a remedy prepared from the coffee bean (main constituent, caffeine, a central nervous system stimulant), is used to treat insomnia. This is the 'like cures like' concept, or 'Similia similibus curentur'.
2. The minimum dose should be used to prevent side effects. Initially, Hahnemann used high doses of substances, which often led to toxic effects, so these were diluted in a stepwise manner and subjected to vigorous shaking at each step. This process is called potentisation, and it is claimed that the more dilute the remedy, the stronger it is.
3. Only a single remedy or substance should be used in a patient at any one time.

Modern Homoeopathy

Despite the controversies, homoeopathy has spread widely and is a very popular form of healthcare in many Asian and Western countries. Hahnemann's principles of homoeopathy still form the basis of modern practice, apart from the single remedy rule which is ignored by many in favour of multiple prescribing. Today, around 1200 homoeopathic remedies are commonly used. Homoeopaths still rely on Hahnemann for guidance, although modern-day provings involving healthy volunteers are sometimes undertaken. Homoeopaths also claim that:

- The signs and symptoms of disease represent the body's attempt to restore order.
- Homoeopathic remedies work by stimulating the body's own healing activity (the 'vital force') rather than by acting directly on the disease process.
- The 'vital force' is expressed differently in each individual, so treatment must be chosen on an individual basis and thus needs to be holistic.

In choosing a remedy for a particular patient, a homoeopath will consider the patient's physical, mental and emotional symptoms, as well as personal characteristics, likes and dislikes, in order to select the homoeopathic remedy with a 'symptom picture' most closely matching that of the patient. Computerised repertories (databases of homoeopathic remedy symptom pictures) are now available that facilitate this process.

Homoeopathic and Herbal Medicines

Homoeopathic and herbal medicines are often confused and/or deemed to be similar, but there are fundamental differences between the two types of preparation:

- Homoeopathic remedies are (mostly) highly dilute, whereas herbal medicines are used at material strengths. However, since homoeopathic preparations are extracted from raw material and then diluted, there is a borderline group including 'mother tinctures' and lower potencies (less diluted), that may contain clinically relevant concentrations of active ingredients.

> **BOX 17.1 Complementary and Alternative Medicines**
>
> Several of these therapies involve the administration (internally or externally) of plant-derived preparations, such as essential oils. In homoeopathy, other substances are also used (e.g. minerals), and they are administered in a highly diluted form ('potentiation'), an approach that as such differentiates homoeopathy from biomedicine. Several of these approaches, such as **homoeopathy**, are described as 'a holistic' or complete systems of healing in that they proffer a philosophy for health and illness, together with a distinct approach to the diagnosis and treatment of a wide range of complaints and disorders. In addition to the therapies listed above, CAM includes acupuncture, chiropractic, massage, osteopathy, reflexology and other therapies.
>
> It should be noted that individuals with a scientific interest in herbal medicines do not consider the rational use of herbal preparations (i.e. science-based phytotherapy) to be part of CAM (see Chapter 16, Regulation and Pharmacovigilance for Herbal Medicines).

- Many homoeopathic remedies (around 65%) originate from plants, whereas by definition all herbal medicines originate from plants (for examples of plant-based homoeopathic preparations, see Table 17.1).

Many plant species used in homoeopathy are also used as herbal medicines; others are poisons unless highly diluted. Other natural materials used in the preparation of homoeopathic remedies include animal and insect parts, venoms and secretions, chemicals and minerals.

The starting point for the production of most homoeopathic remedies is the 'mother tincture', usually an alcohol/water extract of crude plant material. The mother tincture is then diluted according to either the decimal (dilution steps of 1 in 10; D or X) or centesimal (dilution steps of 1 in 100; C) scale to produce the required potency as shown in Table 17.2. The centesimal scale goes as far as M (1 in 10^{2000} dilution, i.e. 2000 centesimal dilution steps) and 10 M (1 in $10^{20,000}$) dilutions. There are also LM potencies, which involve serial dilutions of 1 in 50,000. Higher potencies are prepared robotically and used by specialists rather than for self-medication.

Some plant species are classified as prescription-only medicines at lower potencies, although higher dilutions are considered suitable for self-medication and are very popular. Examples include most of the herbs in Table 17.1, and also Croton (*Croton tiglium* L.), Hyoscyamus (*Hyoscyamus niger* L., henbane) and Nux vomica (*Strychnos nux-vomica* L.)

Potentisation

According to Hahnemann's second principle, the more dilute the preparation, the stronger the medicine. The potency is enhanced with each succussion step, so although 2X and 1C preparations are the same concentration, 2X is considered to be more potent because it has undergone two steps of succussion, whereas a 1C has undergone only one. Homoeopaths have put forward several arguments to explain how highly dilute homoeopathic remedies could work, the most well-known of which is the 'memory of water' theory. Proponents claim that the process of succussion somehow alters the solvent molecules such that they become rearranged to form 'imprints' of molecules of the original starting material.

Evidence of Efficacy

Many controlled clinical trials have investigated the efficacy of homoeopathic interventions, including, increasingly, studies assessing individualised homoeopathy, and in specific health conditions. Despite this, their efficacy remains disputed and controversial. For historical and other details, see Further Reading.

BOX 17.2 Characteristics of Complementary and Alternative Medicines Using Medicinal Plants

Homoeopathy also focuses on understanding a patient's psychological, emotional and physical health, but treatment with specially prepared highly diluted ('potentiated') material is used. Thus its philosophical basis and therapeutic approaches are completely different from approaches where biologically active preparations are used.

Anthroposophical medicine also focuses on a holistic understanding of illness in terms of how the four 'bodies' and the functional systems interact with each other. Diagnosis involves conventional tools, the patient's life story and social context and even bodily expressions. It uses an integrated therapeutic programme that includes diet, therapeutic movement (eurythmy), artistic therapies, massage and anthroposophic medicines.

Aromatherapy is the therapeutic use of essential oils, generally distilled from plants and used for therapeutic purposes generally or in order to increase a person's well-being.

Flower remedies of various types are obtained using a very simple extraction procedure used on the flowers of a range of common plant species, and they are widely available for self-treatment.

TABLE 17.1 Examples of Homoeopathic Remedies Originating From Plant Material

Common Name of Remedy	Plant Source	Common Plant Name(s)	Plant Part
Aconite	*Aconitum napellus* L.	Monkshood	Whole plant
Arnica	*Arnica montana* L.	Arnica	Dried flowers
Allium cepa	*Allium cepa* L.	Red onion	Whole fresh plant
Belladonna	*Atropa belladonna* L.	Deadly nightshade	Whole fresh plant
Bryonia	*Bryonia alba* L.	White bryony	Root
Euphrasia	*Euphrasia officinalis* L.	Eyebright	Whole plant
Hydrastis	*Hydrastis canadensis* L.	Goldenseal	Fresh root
Rhus tox	*Toxicodendron pubescens* Mill. (syn.: *Rhus toxicodendron* L.)	Poison ivy	Fresh leaves
Staphisagria	*Delphinium staphisagria* L.	Stavesacre	Seeds
Stramonium	*Datura stramonium* L.	Thorn apple, Jimson weed	Fresh plant

TABLE 17.2 Commonly Used Homoeopathic Potencies and Dilutions

| No of Succussions | DECIMAL (X OR D) | | CENTESIMAL (C) | |
	Potency	Dilution	Potency	Dilution
10	1X	10^{-1}	1C	10^{-2}
30	3X	10^{-3}	3C	10^{-6}
60	6X	10^{-6}	6C	10^{-12}
300	30X	10^{-30}	30C	10^{-40}
2000	200X	10^{-200}	200C	10^{-400}

Safety

It seems unlikely that highly dilute homoeopathic remedies can cause adverse drug reactions, but isolated cases associated with their use have been reported. Pooled data from clinical trials indicate that adverse effects may occur more frequently with homoeopathy than with placebo, but that these are mild and transient (e.g. headaches, tiredness, skin reactions and diarrhoea), and similar for both homoeopathy and placebo.

ANTHROPOSOPHICAL MEDICINE

History

Anthroposophical medicine is a vision of health and disease based on the work of Austrian philosopher Rudolf Steiner (1861–1925), who explored how human beings and the natural world could be described, not only in physical terms, but also in terms of soul and spirit. He called this philosophy 'anthroposophy', and its development resulted in what is now known as anthroposophic medicine. Steiner believed that consciousness could not be defined in physical terms, but nevertheless aimed anthroposophic medicine to be an extension, not an alternative, to conventional medicine. Steiner viewed each person as having four 'bodies' or 'forces':
- A physical body
- An etheric body, or life force
- An astral body, or conscious awareness
- A spiritual body, or self-awareness or ego.
  Individuals have three functional systems:
- The 'sense-nervous' system (the head and spinal column), focusing on 'cooling' and 'hardening' processes (e.g. the development of arthritis).
- The 'reproductive-metabolic' system, which includes parts of the body that are in constant motion (e.g. the limbs and digestive system) and which focuses on warming and softening processes (e.g. fevers).
- The 'rhythmic' system (the heart, lungs and circulation), which balances the other two systems.
  Steiner believed that health is maintained by the harmonious interaction of the three systems, and that cacophonous (inharmonious) interactions between the systems result in illness.

Modern Anthroposophic Medicine

Anthroposophic medicine today is still based on Steiner's philosophy. Diagnosis involves not only conventional history-taking, physical examination and laboratory investigations, but also the patient's life story, body shape, social behaviour and context as well as movement and modes of artistic expression. Practitioners use a range of therapies, including diet, therapeutic movement (eurythmy), artistic therapies and massage, as well as anthroposophic medicines, in a holistic regime. Anthroposophic medicine is particularly well developed in Austria, Germany, Switzerland and the Netherlands, where specialist hospitals as well as general practitioners practise this approach. Anthroposophic medicine is used, under medical supervision, for serious conditions including supportive and adjunctive treatment in cancer. Remedies for the symptomatic relief of minor conditions are available for self-medication.

Anthroposophic Herbal Medicines

Anthroposophic medicines are derived mainly from plants and minerals. Steiner believed that the sizes of different plant organs, such as flowers, leaves and roots, are disproportionate in plants with medicinal properties. Usually, the disproportionately sized part would be used therapeutically: for example, nettle (*Urtica dioica*) produces an abundance of green leaves, whereas the flowers and fruit are insignificant in terms of size, so from an anthroposophic perspective, nettle leaves are deemed to have medicinal properties. They are used to stimulate the assimilation of iron (e.g. in anaemia) and improve blood circulation. However, the whole plant, or a different organ, may be used therapeutically as specific parts are related to each of the systems: roots relate to the 'sense-nervous system', flowers and fruit to the 'reproductive-metabolic system' and leaves to the 'rhythmic system'.

Ingredients are sometimes 'potentised' using the X (D) rather than the C potency series (as discussed earlier in the previous section, Homoeopathy). These are low dilutions, so measurable quantities of plant constituents are present, and they can be considered to be herbal medicines.

A popular therapy derived from an anthroposophical approach is mistletoe (*Viscum album* L.). Based on Steiner's observations of the shape and habit of the plant, it has been developed as a cancer treatment. Mistletoe is a semiparasite, growing on a range of host trees such as apple (*Malus* spp.), pine (*Pinus* spp.) or oak (*Quercus* spp.), and extracts from each type of host are prescribed for patients with different types of cancer. Lectin-standardised mistletoe extracts for injection are widely available, particularly in Germany, and mistletoe therapy is used in complementary medicine outside the anthroposophic system. Mistletoe extracts are used in some TM systems, including Western herbal medicine, mainly for hypertension.

AROMATHERAPY

History

Aromatic plants, their exudates, extracts and distillates, have been used in medicines, cosmetics, insecticides, preservatives, perfumes and for religious purposes, for thousands of years. The foundation of aromatherapy is attributed to Rene-Maurice Gattefosse, a French perfumer chemist, who first used the term aromatherapy in 1928. Gattefosse burnt his hand while working in a laboratory and found that lavender oil helped the burn to heal quickly with little scarring. Jean Valnet developed Gattefosse's ideas of the benefits of essential oils in wound healing and used essential oils more widely in specific medical disorders.

Modern Aromatherapy

Aromatherapy is the therapeutic use of essential oils. These are obtained from plant material (e.g. roots, leaves, flowers and seeds) usually by distillation, although physical expression (using compression and pressure) is used to obtain some, especially those from the rind of citrus fruits. Key aspects of aromatherapy are described below:
- Essential oils can be used not only for the treatment and prevention of disease, but also for positive effect on mood, emotion and well-being.
- As a holistic therapy: an essential oil, or a combination of essential oils, can be selected to suit each client's symptoms, personality and emotional state.
- Essential oils are not only prescribed with reference to reputed pharmacological properties (e.g. antibacterial and antiinflammatory) but also to concepts not recognised in conventional medicine (e.g. 'balancing' and 'energising').
- The constituents of each oil and combinations work synergistically to improve efficacy or reduce adverse effects (described as 'quenching') associated with particular constituents.

Conditions Treated

Aromatherapy is widely used as an approach to relieving stress, promoting relaxation and improving well-being in a wide range of conditions from the relatively minor to adjunctive therapy in serious disease. Aromatherapy is very popular as a complementary therapy in conventional healthcare settings, such as in mental health, palliative and respite care, and in specialised units caring for patients with severe learning and physical disabilities.

An aromatherapist will take a case history, including details of medical history, lifestyle, diet and emotional state, to select essential oils appropriate for the individual. The most common method of application is by massage, where (usually) two to three essential oils are diluted in a vegetable carrier (or base) oil, such as grapeseed, jojoba, wheatgerm or sweet almond oil.

In addition to their aromatherapy properties (calming, stimulating, uplifting, etc.), essential oils are used in mainstream medicine and TM: they are administered topically for dermatological inflammation and infections and musculoskeletal pain; inhaled via steam baths, vapourisers and skin rubs for respiratory congestion and headache; taken internally as spasmolytics and carminatives and as part of indigestion remedies; and to render many pharmaceutical formulations palatable, especially paediatric medicines.

Aromatic plants are used to make teas, but essential oils should never be taken internally if undiluted, and without medical supervision. Some aromatherapists also suggest that essential oils can be administered vaginally or rectally (tampons, suppositories), but this may cause mucosal membrane irritation if not appropriately formulated.

Essential Oils

Typically, an essential oil contains around 100 or more chemical constituents. Some contain one or two major constituents, and the therapeutic and toxicological properties of the oil can largely be attributed to those, but other constituents present at lower concentrations can be significant. The composition of an essential oil varies according to chemotype, environmental and growing conditions, plant part used and the methods of harvesting, extraction and storage. The constituents are volatile, sensitive to light, heat, air and moisture, and are easily oxidised and degraded. The source of essential oils should be referred to by the Latin binomial name of the plant species. The plant part used may need to be specified and, sometimes, the chemotype.

Efficacy and Safety

Essential oils are believed to act by exerting pharmacological effects following their absorption into the circulation, and via the effects of their odour on the olfactory system. There is evidence that they are absorbed into the circulation after topical application (i.e. massage) and after inhalation, although amounts are likely to be very small.

Individual essential oils have been shown to have pharmacological effects in preclinical studies, but there is little good-quality clinical research investigating their efficacy when used as practised by aromatherapists. Clinical trials assessing the effects of inhaled lavender oil on sleep, and peppermint oil or ginger oil for nausea and vomiting, report cautiously positive findings. Tea tree oil applied topically is effective in the treatment of skin infections and inflammation, and is widely used in antibacterial formulations, including cosmetics.

Data regarding the safety of essential oils as used in aromatherapy are limited. Few adverse effects associated with aromatherapy treatment have been reported; most reports relate to cases of contact dermatitis in patients or aromatherapists. Minor transient adverse effects, such as drowsiness, headache and nausea, can occur after aromatherapy treatment. The increasing use of essential oils during pregnancy and childbirth is concerning, and because of uncertainties about their safety, general advice is that the use of essential oils should be avoided during pregnancy, particularly the first trimester. Certain oils should also be avoided by patients with epilepsy (Table 17.3).

TABLE 17.3 Popular Essential Oils Used in Aromatherapy

Essential Oil Common Name	Species Name Used in Commerce (With Accepted Scientific Binomial,[a] If Different)	Aromatherapy Application, With Some Pharmacological Properties
Bergamot	Citrus bergamia	Calming, uplifting
Black pepper	Piper nigrum	Stimulant, warming, antiinflammatory
Chamomile (Roman)	Anthemis nobilis (Chamaemelum nobile (L.) All.)	Soothing, relaxing, antiinflammatory
Clary sage	Salvia sclarea	Uplifting, calming sedative
Cypress	Cupressus sempervirens	Calming, restoring
Eucalyptus	Eucalyptus globulus	Decongestant, antiinflammatory, antiseptic
Fennel	Foeniculum vulgare	Stimulating, restorative, digestive
Frankincense	Boswellia carteri (Boswellia sacra Flück.)	Rejuvenating, calming, antiinflammatory
Geranium	Pelargonium graveolens	Stimulating, uplifting
Ginger	Zingiber officinale	Warming, stimulating, antiinflammatory
Grapefruit	Citrus paradisi	Stimulating, refreshing, uplifting
Juniper	Juniperus communis	Astringent, stimulating, antiinflammatory
Lavender	Lavandula officinalis (Lavandula angustifolia Mill.)	Relaxing, calming, sedative
Mandarin	Citrus reticulata	Calming, restorative, uplifting
Patchouli	Pogostemon patchouli (Pogostemon cablin (Blanco) Benth.)	Calming, uplifting, antiinflammatory
Peppermint	Mentha piperita	Cooling, stimulating, antiinflammatory
Rosemary	Rosmarinus officinalis	Stimulant for circulation, memory, respiration
Tea tree	Melaleuca alternifolia	Decongestant, antiinflammatory, antiseptic
Thyme	Thymus vulgaris	Stimulant, antiinflammatory, antiseptic
Ylang ylang	Cananga odorata	Calming, soothing, relaxing

[a]These names have been checked using World Flora online. However, in commerce, the market for essential oils is dominated by the perfume, cosmetic, food, flavouring and pharmaceutical industries, where traditional names remain in common use.

FLOWER REMEDIES

Bach flower remedies are probably the most well known, although there are many other flower remedies or essences. They are usually derived from native plants of a particular region or country, such as Australian bush flower, rain forest (Brazil) and Alaskan flower essences.

History

Dr Edward Bach (1886–1936) was a physician and homoeopath, who believed that negative states of mind caused physical illness. His approach to maintaining health was focused on the patient's psychological state, and by treating patients' emotional and mental responses to their illness, physical symptoms would be relieved. He identified 38 negative psychological states (including jealousy, hopelessness, guilt and indecision) and sought natural remedies that could be used to 'correct' these negative states of mind. To do this Bach visited the countryside, concentrated on these specific emotional states and was intuitively drawn towards particular wildflowers that he believed could relieve them.

Flower Remedies

Bach developed 37 remedies based on single wildflowers and tree blossoms. He intended each remedy to be used for a specific emotional or mental state, such as:

- Gentian (*Gentianella amarella* (L.) Börner) for despondency
- Holly (*Ilex aquifolium* L.) for jealousy
- Impatiens (*Impatiens glandulifera* Royle) for impatience
- Pine (*Pinus sylvestris* L.) for guilt
- Rock rose (*Helianthemum nummularium* (L.) Mill.) for terror.

He also developed a preparation termed 'Rescue Remedy', which is a combination of five remedies: impatiens, rock rose, star of Bethlehem (*Ornithogalum umbellatum* L.), cherry plum (*Prunus cerasifera* Ehrh.) and clematis (*Clematis vitalba* L.). Bach recommended it for difficult and demanding situations, such as shock, terror and bereavement. It is now popular for exam nerves, performance anxiety, stage fright and many other modern-day dilemmas.

Flower remedies are made from mother tinctures, which are produced by infusing flowers in spring water and either allowing them to stand in direct sunlight for several hours or boiling them for 30 minutes and straining. The filtrate is diluted with an equivalent volume of alcohol (brandy) to make the mother tincture, and the remedies are prepared by adding two drops of mother tincture to 30 mL of grape alcohol, equivalent to a 1 in 100,000 dilution. Flower remedies are usually taken orally (2–4 drops added to a cold drink and sipped), or drops are placed directly under the tongue, and even on the wrist or temples. Rescue Remedy is also available as a cream for external use.

Efficacy and Safety

There is limited research into the effects of flower remedies, and randomised clinical trials have not found evidence of efficacy. Flower remedies are claimed to be completely free from adverse effects, and this is likely, given that they contain only highly dilute material. However, as flower remedies contain alcohol, they may be unsuitable for some individuals.

GENERAL CONCLUSIONS

While evidence for the clinical usefulness of many CAM herbal products is very limited, they remain very popular world-wide, widely discussed in the press, on the Internet and in self-help books. Some CAM therapies, especially aromatherapy, are generally regarded as more beneficial than harmful in improving quality of life and are widely accepted by the medical establishment, patients, scientists and consumers. Essential oils with pleasing aromas tend to be used (more geranium and less garlic), so treatment is generally enjoyable and relaxing, and massage brings its own benefits. Massage, especially with aromatic oils, is a common feature of many TM systems, not to mention modern sports medicine and 'wellness' centres and spas. Other CAMs, such as homoeopathy, anthroposophical medicine and flower remedies, are accepted as being innocuous, if not effective. Our intention is to explain how plants are viewed and applied in CAM systems, and highlight the most important, rather than enter the debate about efficacy.

Health professionals need to know if a patient is using CAM, and if so, whether it is safe with their therapy regime (luckily, most are!). They may be asked for 'approval' or further details about a particular remedy. Pharmacies often market CAM preparations alongside conventional medicines and, if so, should be able to provide impartial advice about *all* the medicines they sell. 'Health food' shop staff are now expected, and trained, to give safe and accurate information.

Many types of CAM use plant species which are toxic or regulated as medicines, and especially in homoeopathy. Depending on the concentration of active constituents, these may be subject to restricted prescribing or sale. Many pharmacopoeias now include specifications for homoeopathic mother tinctures and plant raw materials, as with herbal medicines, but not for potentised remedies. General requirements for quality, safety and health claims apply, as with all manufactured medicinal products, and regardless of philosophy, all plant medicines need to be subject to the same quality assurance and principles of good practice as any other medicine.

FURTHER READING

Buchholzer, M.-L., Werner, C., Knoess, W., 2014. Current concepts on integrative safety assessment of active substances of botanical, mineral or chemical origin in homeopathic medicinal products within the European regulatory framework. Regul. Toxicol. Pharmacol. 68 (2), 193–200.

Buckle, J., 2015. Clinical Aromatherapy, third ed. Churchill Livingstone, London, Elsevier.

Dantas, F., Rampes, H., 2000. Do homeopathic medicines provoke adverse effects? A systematic review. Br. Homeopathy J. 89 (Suppl. 1), S35–S38.

Ernst, E., 2010. Bach flower remedies: a systematic review of randomised clinical trials. Swiss Med. Wkly. 140, w13079.

Lillehei, A.S., Halcon, L.L., 2014. A systematic review of the effect of inhaled essential oils on sleep. J. Altern. Complement. Med. 20 (6), 441–451.

Mathie, R.T., 2015. Controlled clinical studies of homeopathy. Homeopathy 104 (4), 328–332.

Tisserand, R., Young, R., 2013. Essential Oil Safety. A Guide for Health Professionals, second ed. Churchill Livingstone, Edinburgh.

World Health Organization, 2009. Key Technical Issues of Quality Impacting on the Safety of Homeopathic Medicines. WHO, Geneva.

Important Plant Medicines

- Introduction
- Plant derived medicines and their indications
- Annex: naming herbal drugs

Introduction

This part is devoted to plant-derived medicines, arranged into therapeutic categories. Natural anticancer drugs are covered in Chapter 9, and antimicrobials in Chapter 10. Miscellaneous supportive therapies for stress, ageing, cancer and debility are becoming increasingly important globally, and are often of Asian origin; examples include ginseng, ashwagandha, reishi, schisandra and green tea, as discussed in Chapter 26.

Our aim is not to provide a guide to prescribing, a herbal compendium or a pharmacopoeia, but to highlight the most important drugs obtained from plant sources, both historically and in a modern setting, and to aid more detailed literature searching by providing easily available reviews. Entries are not necessarily consistent in length or detail: more emphasis is given to the most important herbal drugs, or those not covered extensively elsewhere. Inclusion in Part B is not an endorsement, but an acknowledgement that these herbal drugs are in use. Instead, we have highlighted the main therapeutic indications, supported by references and further reading, and reviews where available. Both pure compounds and herbal medicines are included; isolated natural products are used mainly in conventional medicine and are treated in the same way as any other drug; examples given include morphine, codeine, digoxin, pilocarpine, atropine and colchicine. Herbal drugs may also be used as extracts, often refined to contain fractions standardised to a desired class of compounds. Many are incorporated into the European/ British Pharmacopoeia (Eur. Ph./BP) and if so, they are marked with the symbol (†).

The Annex 'Naming Herbal Drugs' contains a list of Eur. Ph. monographs, including all of those cited in the text where available, and others which are important, but that we do not have space to cover in detail. Some pharmacopoeias use an official Latin drug name for a herbal preparation, and this is given together with the species to which the monograph applies. Plant material may be referred to in different terms, which may change during the long and complex supply chain leading from the agricultural environment to the product taken by the patient or consumer. It may vary with terms used in trading, local and colloquial names, official national nomenclature, and the reassigning of species by taxonomists.

Plant derived medicines and their indications

Chapter 18: The gastrointestinal and biliary system
Chapter 19: The cardiovascular system
Chapter 20: Weight-loss supplements
Chapter 21: The respiratory system
Chapter 22: The central nervous system
Chapter 23: The musculo-skeletal system
Chapter 24: Female hormonal and reproductive conditions
Chapter 25: The male reproductive system
Chapter 26: Supportive therapies for stress, ageing, cancer and debility
Chapter 27: Topical phytotherapy: skin, hair, eye, ear, nose and throat

Annex Naming herbal drugs: pharmaceutical, common English, and accepted botanical names (binomials), and synonyms.

The Gastrointestinal and Biliary System

INTRODUCTION

Disorders of the gastro-intestinal system (GI), as the point of ingestion and site of first response to xenobiotics, toxins and micro-organisms, are extremely common, and changes in the diet may also cause disruption to normal digestive processes. The acidity of the stomach and digestive enzymes form a natural barrier and destroy some micro-organisms. Transit through the GI may be enhanced to speed up excretion of toxins, manifested as diarrhoea, and emesis (vomiting) may be an immediate response to remove harmful agents from the stomach before they reach the intestines. However, these defences are not always sufficient to prevent further progress through the digestive system, which remains vulnerable to many conditions. Although sickness and diarrhoea serve a vital function, these symptoms may be triggered long after the threat has been dealt with, or they may be inappropriate responses to some forms of treatment such as cancer chemotherapy. Herbal and plant-derived medicines have always been popular remedies for GI disorders, and they still represent some of the most effective therapies for such conditions and side effects of conventional drug treatment.

DIARRHOEA

Diarrhoea of sudden onset and short duration is very common, especially in children. It normally requires no detailed investigation or treatment, as long as the loss of electrolytes is kept under control. However, chronic, serious cases of diarrhoea caused by more virulent pathogens are still a major health threat to the population of poor tropical and subtropical areas. The World Health Organization (WHO) has estimated that approximately 5 million deaths are due to diarrhoea annually (2.5 million in children under 5 years).

The first-line treatment is oral rehydration therapy using sugar–salt solutions, often with added starch, and the use of gruel rich in polysaccharides (e.g. rice or barley 'water') is an effective measure. The polysaccharides of rice (*Oryza sativa*) grains are hydrolysed in the GI tract; the resulting sugars are absorbed because the co-transport of sugar and Na^+ from the GI lumen into the cells and mucosa is unaffected. Rice suspensions thus actively shift the balance of Na^+ towards the mucosal side, enhance the absorption of water and provide the body with energy, and the efficacy of rice starch has been demonstrated in several clinical studies. The treatment of diarrhoea in adults, particularly for travellers, may also include opiates or their derivatives, to reduce GI motility. Many classical antidiarrhoeal preparations contain opium extracts, or the isolated alkaloids morphine and codeine (e.g. kaolin and morphine mixture and codeine phosphate tablets), although these are controlled by law in some countries. Opioid derivatives such as loperamide, which have limited systemic absorption and therefore fewer central nervous system side

effects, have superseded these agents to some extent but the natural substances are still used and are highly effective. Dietary fibre, including that found in bulk-forming laxatives (quantum vis (q.v.)), can also be used to treat diarrhoea; in this case, the fibre is taken with only a small amount of water.

Starch†

Starch is used for rehydration purposes and may be derived from rice (*Oryza sativa* L.), maize (*Zea mays* L.) or potato (*Solanum tuberosum* L.). Giving starch-based foods (like gruels) has been shown to be therapeutically beneficial and is a first-line treatment in minor self-limiting cases. These are also used as excipients for tablet production. Starch particles give a very characteristic microscopic picture, which can be used to differentiate the various types, but chemical analysis is rarely carried out.

Tannin-Containing Drugs

Tannins are astringent, polymeric polyphenols, and are found widely in plant drugs. The most important medicinal plants used in the treatment of diarrhoea include greater burnet (*Sanguisorba officinalis* L.†), black catechu (*Senegalia catechu* (L.f.) P.J.H. Hurter & Mabb.; syn.: *Acacia catechu* (L.f.) Willd.), oak bark (*Quercus robur* L.†), tormentil (*Potentilla erecta* (L.) Raeusch.†), tea and coffee. Tannin-containing drugs are generally safe, but care should be taken with concurrent administration of other drugs since tannins are not compatible with alkalis or alkaloids, and form complexes with proteins and amino acids.

Constipation is often due to an inappropriate diet and lack of physical activity, for example, while being confined to bed during illness, or the result of taking other medication (especially opioids). It is characterised by reduced and difficult bowel movements and is diagnosed when the frequency of bowel movements is less than once in 2 or 3 days. Although the causes are not usually serious in nature, continuous irregularity in bowel movements should be investigated in case there is a risk of malignant disease. The subjective symptoms (straining heavily, hard stools, painful defecation and a feeling of insufficient evacuation) make it one of the most commonly reported health problems. Constipation is often associated with other forms of discomfort such as abdominal cramps, dyspepsia, bloating and flatulence. Alternating diarrhoea and constipation is a symptom of IBS.

CONSTIPATION

Various types of plant-derived laxatives are used: stimulant laxatives (purgatives), which act directly on the mucosa of the GI tract; bulk-forming laxatives, which act mainly via physicochemical effects within the bowel lumen; and osmotic laxatives, which act by drawing water

TABLE 18.1   Swelling Factors of Various Bulk-Forming Laxatives

Common Name	Botanical Source	Swelling Factor (Eur. Ph.)	Notes
Ispaghula seed	*Plantago ovata*	≥9 (seed) ≥40 (testa of the seed)	
Psyllium seed	*Plantago indica* and *P. afra*	≥10	
Linseed	*Linum usitatissimum*	≥4 (entire seed) ≥4.5 (ground seed)	Also rich in fatty acids (in endosperm of seed)
Wheat bran	*Triticum aestivum*	—	Rich in fibre

into the gut and thus softening the stool. Osmotic laxatives may be mineral in origin, for example, magnesium salts, or derived from natural products such as milk sugars.

Patients generally require rapid relief from constipation, and the immediate effect of stimulant and saline purgatives is very well known. Although there is no problem using them occasionally, or on a short-term basis (<2 weeks), or prior to medical intervention such as x-ray (Roentgen) diagnostics, long-term use should be discouraged. The exception is for patients taking opioids for pain management, who may need to use stimulant laxatives routinely. The most important adverse effect of the long-term use of the stimulant laxatives and saline purgatives is electrolyte loss. Hypokalaemia, pathologically reduced levels of potassium (K^+), may even worsen constipation and cause damage to the renal tubules. The risk of hypokalaemia is increased with the administration of some diuretics and hypokalaemia exacerbates the toxicity of the cardiac glycosides (e.g. digoxin), which are often prescribed for elderly patients. Hyperaldosteronism, an excess of aldosterone production, which leads to sodium (Na^+) retention, and again to potassium loss and hypertension, is also a risk. In general, the use of bulk-forming or osmotic laxatives is preferred, unless there are pressing reasons for using a stimulant laxative.

Bulk-Forming Laxatives

These are bulking agents with a high percentage of fibre and are often rich in polysaccharides, which swell in the GI tract. They influence the composition of food material in the GI tract, especially via the colonic bacteria, which are thus provided with nutrients for proliferation. This in turn influences the composition of the GI flora and the metabolism of the food in the tract (including an increase in gas, or flatus). Fibre-rich food is part of a healthy diet, but processed food and modern lifestyles have generally reduced fibre intake. Bulk-forming laxatives are generally not digested or absorbed in the GI tract, but pass through it largely unchanged.

Bulking agents can be distinguished from swelling agents in that bulking material contains large amounts of fibre, whereas swelling material is generally composed of plant material (seeds) with a dense cover of polysaccharides on the outside. Both types of medicinal drugs may swell to a certain degree by the uptake of water, but swelling agents in the strict sense include only medicinal plants that form mucilage or gel. The **swelling factor** (which compares the volume of drug prior to and after soaking it in water) is an indicator of the amount of polysaccharides present in the drug and is generally used as a marker for the quality of bulk-forming laxatives. The European Pharmacopoeia requires a minimal value of the swelling factor for each agent, and the swelling factors of the phytomedicines detailed later are shown in Table 18.1. Preparations of bulk-forming laxatives are always taken with plenty of water. They can, paradoxically, be used to treat diarrhoea if given with very little fluid; they then absorb the fluid from the lumen and increase the consistency of the stool.

Linseed (Flax), *Linum usitatissimum* L.†

Linseeds are the ripe, dried seeds of flax (*L. usitatissimum*, Linaceae), a plant grown for its fibre (used in the clothing industry) and for the seed oil, which is used in paints and varnishes, and to make oilcloth ('linoleum'). Flax, with its characteristic blue flowers, is an annual and has long been under human cultivation. The dark brown (less often yellowish-white) seeds are oblong or ovate with a characteristic pointed end. They are tasteless but slowly produce a mucilaginous feel when placed in the mouth. The outer layer of the seed (testa) is rich in polysaccharides, while the inner part of the seed, which contains the endosperm and the cotyledons, is rich in fatty oil. If the seeds are taken whole, the inner layer of the testa is only partially digested in the GI tract and they will be excreted in the entire form, and the fatty acids will not be released. The swelling factor should at least be 4 (entire seeds) or 4.5 (powdered drug). Linseed also possesses cholesterol-lowering properties and contains phytoestrogenic lignans.

Plantago Species

Ispaghula, Plantago ovata Forssk. (syn.: Plantago ispaghula Roxb.)†. The various types of psyllium yield useful and commonly used emollients and bulk laxatives that help in maintaining a regular bowel movement.

The dark brown, glossy seeds from *Plantago ovata* (Indian fleawort, blond psyllium, Plantaginaceae) are useful in the treatment of chronic constipation. In cases of simple and chronic constipation and among the elderly, the use of ispaghula husk is reported to be effective. Ispaghula should not be taken within at least half to 1 hour of any other medication, as it may delay their absorption.

The seeds are broadly elliptical in shape, up to 3.5 mm long, and are practically tasteless, becoming mucilaginous when chewed. They can help to maintain or achieve a regular bowel movement and are also useful in IBS. The swelling factor should be greater than 9 for the entire seeds and greater than 40 for the seed husk, which is the most widely used part. The usage is similar to that of psyllium (fleawort, below).

Psyllium, Plantago indica L. (syn.: Plantago psyllium L. and P. arenaria Waldst. & Kit.) and Plantago afra L.†. The brown, shiny, elliptical to ovate seeds (2–3 mm long) are obtained from two species of the plantain family (Plantaginaceae). *Plantago indica* (fleawort, black or dark psyllium and plantain) is used in a similar way and the seeds are narrower and somewhat smaller than ispaghula seeds. An essential characteristic of high-quality material is a high swelling factor.

Wheat bran, Triticum aestivum L. Bran is less useful as a laxative (except when taken as a natural part of the diet, for example in breakfast cereal) since it contains phytic acid, which in high concentrations can complex with, and therefore reduce, the bioavailability of vitamins and minerals taken at the same time. However, in some patients, wheat bran (the husk from the grains of *Triticum aestivum*) is more effective than other swelling agents, and preparations containing it are available for prescribing. These are taken in water.

CHAPTER 18 The Gastrointestinal and Biliary System **193**

Osmotic Laxatives

Osmotic laxatives, such as lactulose or lactose, which are dimeric sugars derived from milk, are a useful and widely used approach to the treatment of long-term constipation. Lactose is split in the GI tract into glucose and galactose, and galactose is not generally resorbed well. Consequently, the bacteria of the colon metabolise this sugar. The resulting acids, including lactic acid and acetic acid, have an osmotic effect, and the bacteria in the colon multiply more rapidly. This results in softening and an increase in the amount of faeces, with a subsequent increase in GI peristalsis.

Stimulant Laxatives

Stimulant laxatives are derived from a variety of unrelated plant species, which only have in common the fact that they contain similar chemical constituents. These are anthraquinones such as emodin (Fig. 18.1) and aloe-emodin, and related anthrones and anthranols. Anthraquinones are commonly found as glycosides in the living plant. Several groups are distinguished, based on the degree of oxidation of the nucleus and whether one or two units make up the core of the molecule. The anthrones are less oxygenated than the anthraquinones and the dianthrones are formed from two anthrone units (Fig. 18.2). Studies using dianthrone glycosides such as sennosides A and B suggest that most of these compounds pass through the upper GI tract without any change; however, they are subsequently metabolised to rhein anthrone in the colon and caecum by the natural flora (mainly bacteria) of the GI tract. Anthranoid drugs act directly on the intestinal mucosa, influencing several pharmacological targets, and the laxative effect is due to increased peristalsis of the colon, reducing transit time and, consequently, the re-absorption of water from the colon. Additionally, the stimulation of active chloride secretion results in an inversion of normal physiological conditions and a subsequent increased excretion of water. Overall, this results in an increase in the faecal volume with an increase in the GI pressure. These actions are based on the well-understood effects of chemically defined constituents; consequently, phytomedicines containing them are usually standardised to specified anthranoid content). While anthranoid-containing extracts are clearly clinically effective, no significant clinical differences in effectiveness between lactulose and senna have been shown.

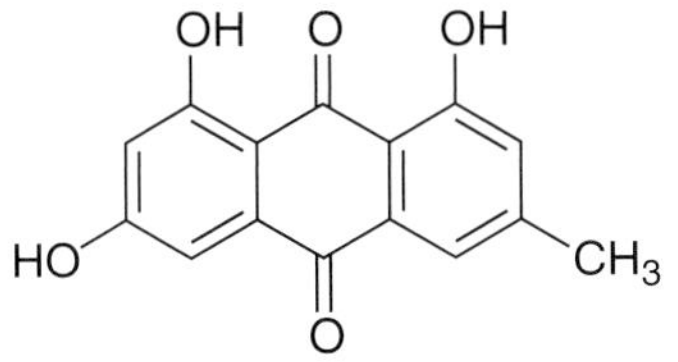

Fig. 18.1 Emodin.

Safety Concerns Related to Anthranoid Drugs

The monomeric aglycones (especially emodin and aloe-emodin) have been shown to have genotoxic and mutagenic effects using bacterial and in vitro systems such as the Ames test, and in mammalian cell lines. The long-term use of anthranoids may result in a (reversible) blackening of the colon (*Pseudomelanosis coli*), which is due to the incorporation of metabolites of the anthranoids and is thought to be associated with an increased risk of colon carcinoma. In practice, few toxic effects have been described, apart from those involving electrolyte loss described earlier. More immediate effects of anthranoid-containing drugs are colic and griping pains due to increased spastic contractions of the smooth musculature of the GI tract. Aloes and senna leaves are particularly prone to producing these. A synthetic derivative, danthrone (also known as dantron; not to be confused with the naturally occurring dianthrone), has been developed and, although effective, it is used only in palliative care due to its carcinogenic potential.

Frangula, *Frangula alnus* Mill. (syn.: *Rhamnus frangula* L.†, Buckthorn, *R. cathartica* L. and Cascara, *Frangula purshiana* (DC.) A.Gray ex J.G.Cooper) (syn.: *R. purshiana* DC.)†

The barks of several species of Rhamnaceae are used for their strong purgative effects. *F. alnus* (glossy buckthorn, frangula) has a milder action than *R. cathartica* (European buckthorn) and the berries are used in veterinary medicine. Cascara, the bark of *F. purshiana* (American buckthorn, known in commerce as Cascara sagrada) is the other main species used medicinally.

F. alnus is a densely foliated, thornless bush or tree, reaching a height of 1–7 m, common in damp environments such as bogs and along streams in North and Central Europe, as well as northern Asia. The cut bark is grey-brown with numerous visible grey-white lenticels. The leaves are broadly elliptical to obovate, about 3.5–5 cm long. The black, pea-sized berries develop from small greenish-white flowers.

Buckthorn (*R. cathartica*) is a thorny shrub with toothed leaves and a reddish-brown bark; the berries are black and globular.

Cascara (*F. purshiana*) is native to the Pacific coast of North America but grows widely elsewhere. It is found in commerce in quilled pieces, often with epiphytes (lichen and moss) attached.

Constituents.

F. alnus: Glucofrangulin A (Fig. 18.3) and B, which are diglucosides differing only in the type of sugar at C6.

R. cathartica: Emodin, aloe-emodin, chrysophanol and rhein glycosides, frangula-emodin, rhamnicoside, alaterin and physcion.

F. purshiana: Cascarosides A (see Fig. 18.3), B, C, D, E and F (which are stereoisomers of aloin and derivatives), with minor glycosides including barbaloin, frangulin, chrysaloin, palmidin A, B and C and the free aglycones.

The anthrone and dianthrone glycosides, which are present in the fresh bark of these species, have emetic effects and may result in colic. In order to oxidise these compounds to anthraquinones with fewer

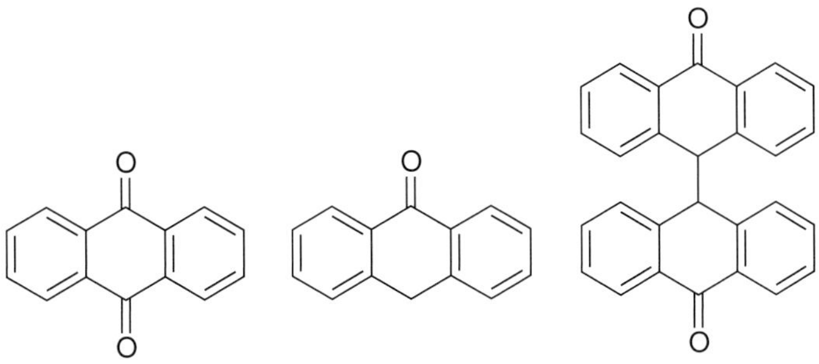

Fig. 18.2 Anthrone derivatives.

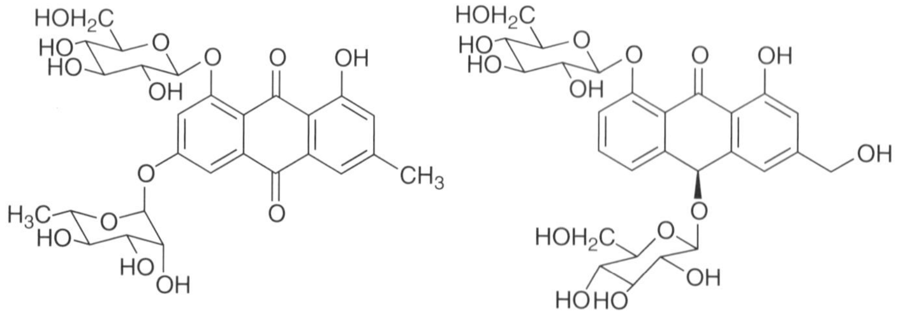

Fig. 18.3 Glucofrangulin A *(left)* and cascaroside A *(right).*

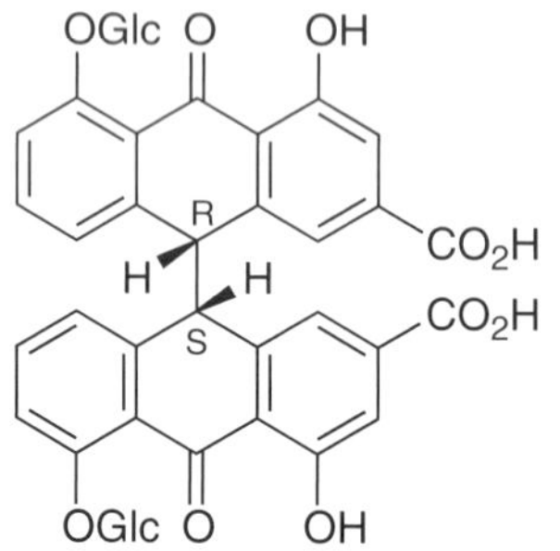

Fig. 18.4 Sennoside B.

undesirable side effects, the drug has either to be kept for a year or it is 'aged artificially' by heating it for several hours to 80–100°C.

Senna, *Cassia senna* L. Leaf and Fruit†

The genus *Cassia* (Fabaceae) is very large, with about 550 species, mostly occurring in warm temperate and tropical climates. The species are not native to Europe and were an important drug of early trading; the name 'senna' is of Arabic origin and was recorded as early as the 12th century. The species was previously split into two species based on their origin: Alexandrian senna (*Cassia senna* L. also known as *C. acutifolia* Delile) and Tinnevelly senna (*C. angustifolia* Vahl). The common names were derived from their original trade sources and are only applied to the fruits (pods). The second origin is considered to be the milder in activity. Both the leaves and the fruits have typical microscopic characteristics, including the highly diagnostic, single-celled warty trichomes and the crystal sheath of calcium oxalate prisms around the fibres, but it is possible to distinguish the two species microscopically.

Constituents.

Leaf: Sennosides A and B (Fig. 18.4), which are based on the aglycones sennidin A and sennidin B; sennosides C and D, which are glycosides of heterodianthrones of aloe-emodin and rhein; palmidin A, rhein anthrone and aloe-emodin glycosides and some free anthraquinones. *C. senna* usually contains greater amounts of the sennosides.

Fruit: Sennosides A and B and a related glycoside sennoside A1. The sennosides, which are dianthrones, differ in their stereochemistry at C_{10} and C_{10}', as well as in their substitution pattern. *C. senna* usually contains greater amounts of the sennosides.

The structure of sennoside B is given in Fig. 18.4. The Eur. Ph. standard is for a glycoside content of not less than 2.5% for the leaf, 3.5% for *C. senna* fruit and 2.2% for *C. angustifolia* fruit, calculated as sennoside B. Flavonoids, tannins and bitter compounds are also present but not defined in the standard. The way in which the plant material is dried has a strong influence on the amount of glycosides remaining and accordingly on the quality of the product.

The other main anthranoid herbal drugs are **aloes** *Aloe vera* (L.) Burm.f.† (syn.: *A. barbadensis* Mill.; and other species) and **rhubarb** (*Rheum* spp.).

INFLAMMATORY GASTROINTESTINAL CONDITIONS: GASTRITIS AND ULCERS

Inflammation of the gastric mucosa, or gastritis, is an acute inflammatory infiltration of the superficial gastric mucosa, predominantly by neutrophils. It is treated with antacids (magnesium and aluminium salts) and emollients (alginate, mucilages), and other phytomedicines such as chamomile and liquorice. These have largely been superseded by the H_2-receptor-blocking agents (cimetidine, ranitidine, etc.) and proton pump inhibitors (omeprazole, lansoprazole). Now that infection with *Helicobacter pylori* is known to be a causal factor in ulceration, antibiotic therapy is the first-line treatment of choice. However, infection is not always the factor involved in chronic gastritis, and gluten intolerance is increasingly implicated as a cause. Symptomatic treatments for mild gastric inflammation contain a mixture of an emollient, to line and soothe the mucosa (e.g. an agar suspension), an antacid, and possibly a carminative such as peppermint or anise oil.

Alginate†

Alginate†, or alginic acid, is an anionic polysaccharide distributed widely in the cell walls of brown algae including *Laminaria* and *Ascophyllum nodosum*. Raw or dried seaweed is washed with acid to remove cross-linking ions that cause the alginate to be insoluble. It is then dissolved in alkali, typically sodium hydroxide, to produce a viscous solution of alginate. The solution is filtered to remove the cell wall debris and leave a clear alginate solution. Alginate binds with water to form a viscous gum and acts as a protective coating over the walls of the stomach and oesophagus.

Chamomile, *Matricaria chamomilla* L.†

German (or Hungarian) chamomile flowers are derived from *M. chamomilla* L. (syn.: *Chamomilla recutita* (L.) Rauschert, *M. recutita* L., Asteraceae, the daisy family). They have a pleasant aromatic odour. The flower heads have a diameter of approximately 10 mm and are composed of many minute flowers (called florets), which are either tongue-shaped ('ligulate florets', found at the margin) or tubular ('disc' florets, found in the disc-like centre). True chamomile has a hollow receptacle (the part of the stalk where the flower parts are attached) and is devoid of the small leaf-like structures (stipules) that are common with the nonmedicinal members of this genus. Chamomile is grown on a large scale, especially in Eastern Europe, Spain, Turkey, Egypt and Argentina, and has been known as a medicinal plant for several thousands of years. It is used internally for spasmodic and inflammatory illnesses of the GI tract.

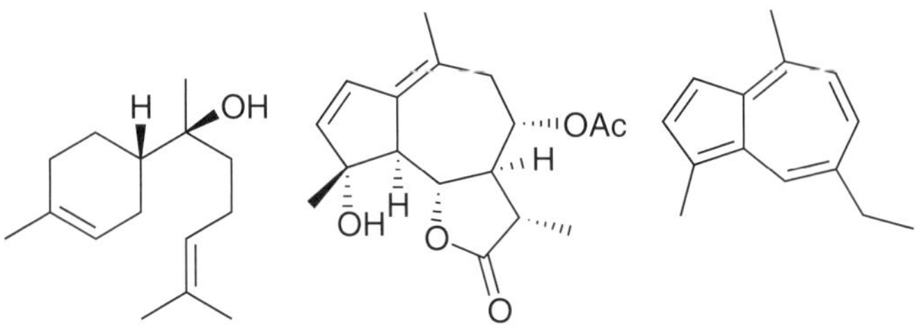

Fig. 18.5 Bisabolol *(left)*, matricin *(middle)* and chamazulene *(right)*.

Constituents. The flower heads are rich in essential oil. Two types of essential oil are recognised: one rich in bisabolol (levomenol) (Fig. 18.5) and the other in bisabolol oxides. Both contain other terpenoid compounds, including guaianolides, such as matricin, which are only found in the crude drug. The characteristic dark blue azulenes (e.g. chamazulene; see Fig. 18.5) are produced during steam distillation and only found in the essential oil. Flavonoids (up to 6%), especially apigenin and apigenin-7*O*-glycoside, caffeic acid derivatives and spiro ethers are also present. The components of the essential oil levomenol (α-bisabolol), its oxides, chamazulene, some unusual spiro ethers and the flavonoids (especially apigenin) are all essential for the therapeutic effects.

Therapeutic uses and available evidence. Chamomile is used in the form of an infusion (tea) due to its mild digestive properties. Anti-inflammatory, spasmolytic, antibacterial and antifungal effects are well established, and chamomile is generally considered to be safe, although allergic reactions may occur as with all plants of the Asteraceae. Chamomile is also used in topical preparations (see Chapter 27) for its antiinflammatory properties.

Note. The flower heads of *Chamaemelum nobile* (L.) All. (syn.: *Anthemis nobilis* L., English chamomile, Roman chamomile†) have a pharmacological profile similar to that of *Matricaria recutita*, and are included in the Eur. Ph. However, there is less scientific and clinical evidence to support their use.

Liquorice, *Glycyrrhiza glabra* L.†

Liquorice (licorice) root is derived from the inner part of the root and underground stem (rhizome) of *G. glabra* (Fabaceae, the legume family). The peeled root is of much higher quality and produced in several European countries. It has a very characteristic taste and smell and is used in confectionery. The sweet taste also makes the identification relatively easy, and adulteration is uncommon.

Liquorice is used to relieve gastric inflammation, specifically in the case of peptic ulcers and duodenal ulcers, but its use as a GI remedy is controversial because of its mineralocorticoid action. Due to the small size of the clinical studies using liquorice extract in GI and ulcerative conditions, no meaningful conclusions can be drawn.

More potent synthetic pharmaceuticals are now available, and it is now rarely used for this purpose. Liquorice and its preparations are contraindicated in cholestatic liver disorders, liver cirrhosis, hypertension, hypokalaemia, severe renal failure and pregnancy. With excessive use, liquorice-containing confectionery may result in similar undesired side effects. Liquorice is also used in respiratory complaints as an expectorant, mucolytic and antitussive agent.

Constituents. The most important bioactive secondary metabolite is glycyrrhizic acid (also known as glycyrrhizin; Fig. 18.6), a water-soluble pentacyclic triterpene saponin that gives the drug its characteristic sweet taste (it is about 50 times sweeter than sucrose). The genin (glycyrrhetinic acid or glycyrrhetin), on the other hand, is not sweet but very bitter. Liquorice also contains numerous flavonoids

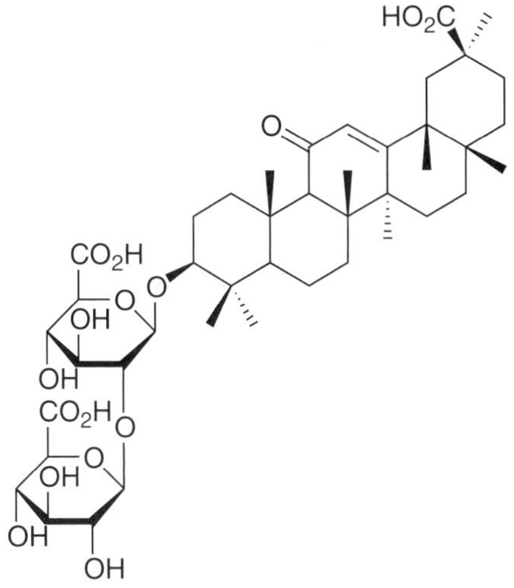

Fig. 18.6 Glycyrrhizic acid.

(chalcones and isoflavonoids), coumarins and polysaccharides, which contribute to the activity.

INFLAMMATORY GASTROINTESTINAL CONDITIONS

These conditions include ulcerative colitis and Crohn's disease, and their aetiology is poorly understood. IBS is characterised by pain in the left iliac fossa, diarrhoea and/or constipation. Symptoms are usually relieved to some extent by defecation or the passage of wind and may respond to the use of bulk laxatives with or without anti-spasmodic (carminative) drugs. Ulcerative colitis is limited to the colon and Crohn's disease may involve any part of the entire GI tract. Inflammatory bowel disease increases the risk of developing colon cancer. Inflammatory cytokines such as tumour necrosis factor (TNF)-α are crucial mediators, and standard treatments include anti-inflammatory agents, immunosuppressants, and TNF blockers. The generally poor treatment outcomes, the high cost and adverse effects limit their therapeutic usefulness.

Tropane alkaloids have been used traditionally. Atropine has been replaced by hyoscine, in the form of the *N*-butyl bromide, which, as a quaternary ion, is poorly absorbed from the GI tract and therefore has fewer antimuscarinic side effects.

Natural remedies include peppermint oil and other essential oil carminatives, and in the case of ulcerative colitis, turmeric (*Curcuma longa* L.) and ispaghula (*Plantago ovata* Forssk.). It is also known that patients self-prescribe marihuana (*Cannabis sativa* L.), but there is no evidence for or against its use.

DYSPEPSIA AND BILIOUSNESS

Dyspepsia and 'biliousness' are closely associated with eating habits and are very common. The symptoms include nausea, pain and cramps, distension, heartburn and the 'inability to digest food', often after rich meals. Traditionally, these conditions were treated either with cholagogues or with bitter stimulants. A cholagogue is an agent that stimulates bile production in the liver or promotes the emptying of the gallbladder and bile ducts. Although clinical evidence is largely lacking, plant-based cholagogues are frequently prescribed based on observational evidence and a long tradition of use, but they should not be used in cases of bile duct obstruction or cholestatic jaundice.

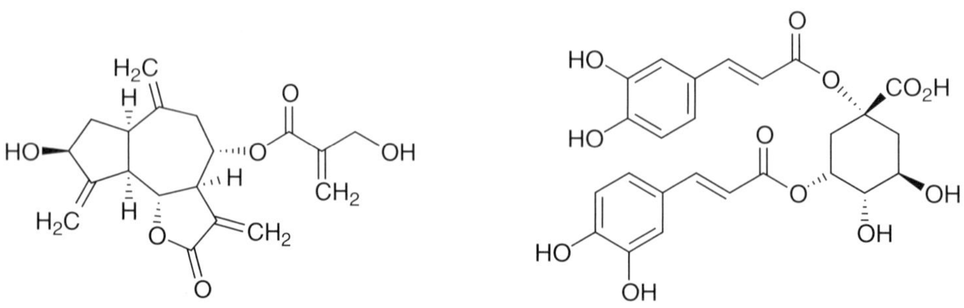

Fig. 18.7 Cynaropicrin *(left)* and cynarin *(right)*.

Bitter stimulants, such as gentian and wormwood, act directly on the mucosa of the upper part of the GI tract and the bitter receptors on the tongue, stimulating the secretion of saliva and gastric juices and influencing the secretion of gastrin. An aperitif containing 'bitters', taken about half an hour before eating, stimulates gastric and biliary secretion; however, it is not known whether these effects are restricted to patients with a reduced secretory reflex, or whether an increase also occurs in healthy people.

Artichoke, *Cynara cardunculus* L. (syn.: *Cynara scolymus* L.)†

This well-known member of the Asteraceae yields the globe artichoke, which is the edible flower head of the plant. The medicinal part is the leaf, which is used to treat indigestion and dyspepsia, and to lower cholesterol levels.

Constituents. The leaf contains the bitter sesquiterpene lactone cynaropicrin, several flavonoids and derivatives of caffeoylquinic acid, including cynarin (Fig. 18.7).

Therapeutic uses and available evidence. In the case of hypercholesterolaemia, there is some evidence for a cholesterol-lowering effect of single-herb artichoke leaf extract, although the effect is modest. Antihepatotoxic effects, cholagogue activity and a reduction of cholesterol and triglyceride levels have been reported, due to the inhibition of cholesterol biosynthesis. Artichoke extracts have been shown to reduce the symptom severity associated with dyspepsia and IBS, and improve parameters such as fat intolerance, bloating, flatulence, constipation, abdominal pain and vomiting,

Gentian, *Gentiana lutea* L.†

The yellow gentian (*G. lutea*, Gentianaceae) is, after ethanol, the most important ingredient of the Alpine beverage *Enzianschnaps*, used as a digestive stimulant, taken after a large meal. Most medicinal products are made using the rapidly dried and nonfermented drug.

The species is rare (but locally abundant) and distributed in the alpine regions of Europe and western Asia. It is a perennial herb up to 1.4 m high with showy yellow flowers. Because of the high risk of over-exploitation (for use as an ornamental and as a medicine), the species is now protected throughout most of its range and attempts are being made to cultivate it. Gentian root in commerce consists of the dried rhizomes and roots of the species. The rhizome is cylindrical and may have a diameter of up to 4 cm, with long roots attached.

Constituents. The compounds responsible for the highly bitter taste are monoterpenoid compounds (Fig. 18.8) such as gentiopicroside—a secoiridoid with a bitter value of 12,000—and amarogentin—with a bitter value of 58,000,000, which is only present in minute amounts. The normally white inner part of the rootstock turns yellow during

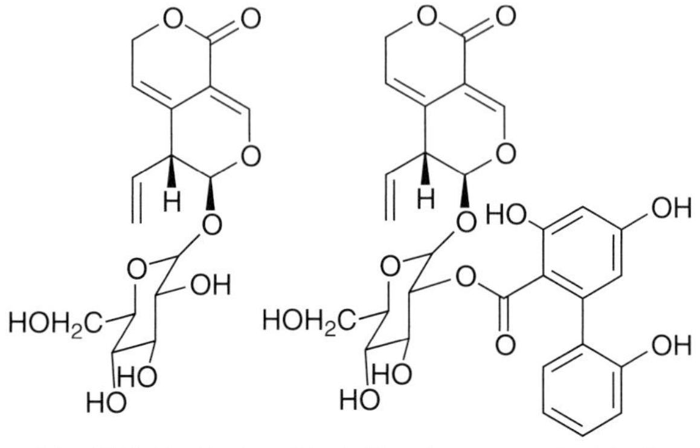

Fig. 18.8 Gentiopicroside *(left)* and amarogentin *(right)*.

fermentation, due to the formation of xanthones, including gentisin. Chemical analysis is carried out following the method of the Eur. Ph., but the 'bitter value' test is also useful. This is a simple and useful measure for establishing the quality of bitter-tasting (botanical) drugs. It is the inverse concentration of the dilution of an extract (or a pure compound), which can still be detected as being bitter to testers with normal bitter taste receptors. In the case of gentian, it should at least be 10,000 (i.e. an extract that has been diluted 10,000 times should still leave a bitter taste).

Therapeutic uses and available evidence. Gentian is indicated for poor appetite, flatulence and bloating, although clinical trial evidence is lacking. Extracts stimulate gastric secretion in cultured rat gastric mucosal cells, and gentiopicroside has been shown to suppress chemically and immunologically induced liver damage in mice.

Wormwood, Absinth, *Artemisia absinthium* L.†

Wormwood is a bitter stimulant derived from the aerial parts of *Artemisia absinthium* (Asteraceae) and is popularly used as a tea. It is a commonly cultivated garden plant. The liqueur was a popular stimulant in many European countries during the latter part of the 19th century and early part of the 20th century and gave rise to the condition known as absinthism, a form of mental disorder, reputed to affect the artist Van Gogh. The plant is still commonly grown in Mediterranean gardens. The leaves and young stems are densely covered with characteristic greyish-white hairs, which give the species its typical appearance.

Several related species are also used as a food (tarragon or estragon, *A. dracunculus* L.) or medicine (*A. annua* L., the source of artemisinin, used to treat malaria and to isolate artemisinin, see Chapter 10 (Antimicrobial Natural Products)).

Constituents. The essential oil contains β-thujone (Fig. 18.9) as the major component, as well as thujyl alcohol, azulenes, bisabolene and others. Sesquiterpene lactones include absinthin, anabsinthin,

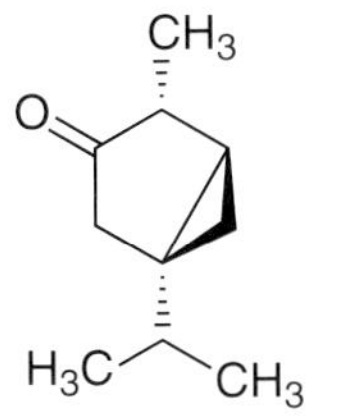

Fig. 18.9 β-Thujone.

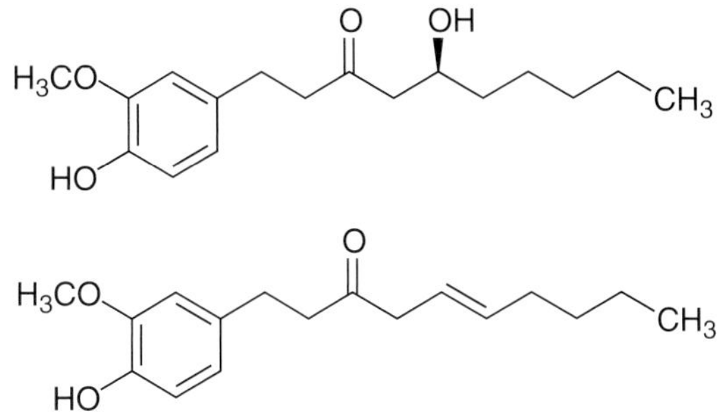

Fig. 18.10 Constituents of fresh and dried ginger.

artemetin, artabsinolides A, B, C and D, artemolin and others. During the process of distillation, the intensively blue chamazulene is formed, which together with the other constituents gives the oil of absinth its characteristic green-blue colour. The sesquiterpene lactone absinthin is responsible for the intensive bitter taste (see section on Gentian for the explanation of bitter value). The essential oil content should be at least 0.2% and the bitter sesquiterpenoids 0.15%–0.4%, to meet Eur. Ph. standards.

Therapeutic uses and available evidence. Wormwood is commonly used as a bitter tonic, a choleretic and formerly as an anthelmintic. Although its use in the form of a tea is considered safe, the essential oil, and the liqueur 'absinthe' distilled from this plant, may be harmful in large doses due to the thujone content, and only used where the thujone has been removed. Most of the evidence is empirical and clinical evidence is limited.

Toxicological risks. Thujone is neurotoxic and hallucinogenic in large doses and can produce epileptic fits and long-lasting psychiatric disturbances. These are considered to be a problem only with the distilled ethanolic beverage (absinthe). Thujone is found in the essential oil of many unrelated species, including sage (*Salvia officinalis*†) and thuja (*Thuja occidentalis*), and is still used medicinally with few ill effects. There is also a dispute as to whether 'absinthism' is anything more than plain alcoholism since thujone levels are not always high enough to cause such severe damage.

NAUSEA AND VOMITING

'Travel sickness' or 'motion sickness' is particularly common in children and is caused by the repetitive stimulation of the labyrinth of the ear. It is most common when travelling by sea, but also happens in cars, aeroplanes and when horse-riding. Vomiting, nausea, dizziness, sweating and vertigo may occur. Prophylactic treatment includes the use of antihistamines (mainly phenothiazines) and cinnarizine, and natural compounds such as the antimuscarinic alkaloid hyoscine, found in the Solanaceae (nightshade family). Morning sickness during pregnancy is also common but few (if any) synthetic drugs are licensed for such a use because of fears of toxicity to the unborn child. Ginger can be a useful antiemetic for this condition, as well as for travel sickness.

Ginger, *Zingiber officinale* Roscoe†

Ginger (Zingiberaceae) is one of the most commonly used culinary spices in the world and has a variety of medicinal uses. The odour and taste are very characteristic, aromatic and pungent. Ginger is cultivated in moist, warm tropical climates throughout south and south-eastern Asia, China, Nigeria and Jamaica. The rhizome is the part used and is available commercially either peeled or unpeeled. African dried ginger is usually unpeeled, and the fresh rhizome, which is widely available for culinary purposes, is always unpeeled. The medicinal use of ginger in Europe has an ancient history and can be traced back to Greek and Roman times. It is mentioned in Ayurvedic and other religious scriptures dating back to 2000 BCE, where it was recognised as an aid to digestion and for cases of rheumatism and inflammation.

Constituents. The rhizome contains 1%–3% essential oil, the major constituents of which are zingiberene and β-bisabolene. The pungent taste is produced by a mixture of phenolic compounds with carbon side chains consisting of seven or more carbon atoms, referred to as gingerols, gingerdiols, gingerdiones, dihydrogingerdiones and shogaols (Fig. 18.10). The shogaols are produced by dehydration and degradation of the gingerols and are formed during drying and extraction. The shogaols are twice as pungent as the gingerols, which accounts for the fact that dried ginger is more pungent than fresh ginger.

Therapeutic uses and available evidence. Uses of ginger are diverse and include as a carminative, antiemetic, spasmolytic, antiflatulent, antitussive, hepatoprotective, antiplatelet aggregation and hypolipidaemic. Many of these actions are substantiated by pharmacological in vivo or in vitro evidence. Particularly important uses are for preventing motion sickness and postoperative nausea, as well as vertigo and morning sickness in pregnancy, and there is some clinical evidence for the efficacy of ginger in these conditions. Ginger consumption has also been reported as beneficial in alleviating the pain and frequency of migraine headaches, and studies on the action in rheumatic conditions have shown a moderately beneficial effect. Antiulcer activity is attributed to the volatile oil, especially the 6-gingesulfonic acid content, and hepatoprotective effects have been noted in cultured hepatocytes, with the gingerols being more potent than the homologous shogaols found in dried ginger. Both groups of compounds are antioxidants and possess free radical scavenging activity. Ginger is well known to produce a warming effect when ingested, and the pungent principles stimulate thermogenic receptors. In Traditional Chinese Medicine medicine, ginger is so highly regarded that it forms an ingredient in about half of all multi-item prescriptions. A distinction is made between the indications for the fresh rhizome (vomiting, coughs, abdominal distension and pyrexia) and the dried or processed rhizome (abdominal pain, lumbago and diarrhoea). This is justifiable since the constituents are present in different proportions in the different preparations. Ginger, both in the fresh and dried form, is generally regarded as safe.

Hyoscine (Scopolamine)†

The alkaloid hyoscine (Fig. 18.11) is usually isolated from *Datura* or *Scopolia* spp., although, as the name suggests, it was originally found in *Hyoscyamus niger* L. It is a popular remedy for motion sickness, given at an oral dose of 400 μg or, more recently, as a transdermal patch containing 2 mg of the alkaloid, which is delivered through the skin over 24 hours. Hyoscine is also used as a premedication, usually in combination with an opiate, to relax the patient and dry up bronchial secretions prior to the administration of halothane anaesthetics.

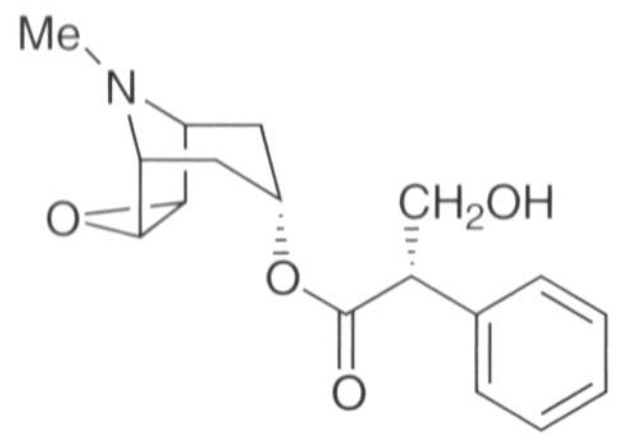

Fig. 18.11 (–)-Hyoscine.

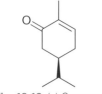

Fig. 18.12 (–)-Carvone.

BLOATING AND FLATULENCE

Flatulence, which is the passage of excessive wind from the body, can be treated with carminatives, which are usually taken with food; they produce a warm sensation when ingested and promote the postprandial elimination of gas. Plant-based carminatives are usually rich in essential oil, such as the fruits ('seeds') of species of the Apiaceae (celery family) and some members of the Lamiaceae (mint family). Many condiments such as cumin and caraway have carminative effects and are used as spices because of their taste *and* their pharmacological effect. The properties of many of these herbs are due to their spasmolytic action, for which some in vitro evidence exists, but the precise mechanism of action is unclear. It seems likely that both the essential oil and other components (e.g. the flavonoids) also contribute to the effect.

Mint Leaves and Oils: *Mentha* Species

Members of the mint family are widely used for their digestive effects and flavouring qualities. They contain similar compounds, but in differing proportions, which results in subtle differences in their taste and properties.

Peppermint, *Mentha × piperita* L.†

Peppermint is a hybrid of *Mentha aquatica* L. and *M. spicata* L., which originated spontaneously and has been known for over 2500 years; the first records are from old Egyptian graves (2600–3200 BCE). Peppermint has a very characteristic, strongly aromatic and penetrating smell and taste. All species of the genus *Mentha* (the mints) have quadrangular (square) stems and decussate, elongated, dentate leaves with a pointed apex, and pinkish-blue flowers up to 5 mm long, and microscopical characteristics include glandular hairs, which are typical of the Lamiaceae. Both the leaves, in the form of a tea, and the oil are used for digestive problems.

Constituents. Peppermint leaf is rich in essential oil (0.5%–4%), the main components being (–)-menthol, menthone, menthyl acetate and menthofuran. The plant also contains the nonvolatile polyphenolics rosmarinic acid and derivatives, flavonoids and triterpenes.

Peppermint oil is derived from the fresh plant by steam distillation and contains approximately 50% (–)-menthol (see Chapter 21).

Therapeutic uses and available evidence. Overall, the evidence is mostly empirical and based on many years of practice. Peppermint is often taken in the form of a tea, which provides a refreshing beverage as well as a mild digestive soothing effect. The oil can be given well diluted with water or as an emulsion (2%, v/v, dispersed in a suitable vehicle) for treating colic and GI cramps in both adults and children, and in the form of enteric-coated capsules for IBS, where it is released directly into the intestine and bowel. The antispasmodic effect of peppermint oil has been well established using a series of in vitro models, the effect being marked by a decline in the number and amplitude of spontaneous contractions, and due at least in part to Ca^{2+}-antagonistic effects.

Peppermint oil has also been shown clinically to enhance gastric emptying.

Japanese Mint, *Mentha arvensis* L.

Japanese mint is rich in menthol (about 80% of the total volatile oil) and is employed as a cheaper substitute for peppermint or for extracting menthol.

Spearmint, *Mentha × spicata* L. (syn.: *M. crispa, M. spicata* var. *crispa*)

Spearmint gives toothpaste, mouthwash and chewing gum their typical taste and smell. It is an important flavouring agent but is of limited medicinal importance. It is easily identifiable from the taste and odour.

Umbelliferous Fruits

The fruits (not 'seeds' as they are commonly known) of several members of the celery family (Apiaceae or Umbelliferae) are used as carminatives as they are rich in essential oil and have an antispasmodic effect. Many of these species are also important as spices. Flower heads are umbels of white or pinkish flowers, which produce the characteristic schizocarp (double) fruits, in which two mericarps are united to form an easily separated fruit.

Caraway, *Carum carvi* L.†

Caraway is the fruit of a mountain herb common in many regions of Europe and Asia.

Constituents. The essential oil (3%–7%) consists mainly of (+)-carvone and (+)-limonene, accounting for 45%–65% and 30%–40%, respectively, of the total oil. Carvone (Fig. 18.12) is considered to be the main component responsible for the spasmolytic action.

Therapeutic uses and available evidence. The fruits are used in cases of dyspepsia, minor GI cramps and flatulence. Little modern clinical evidence is available, but caraway has long been used in products such as infant gripe water. The aqueous extract, and even more so the essential oil, acts as a spasmolytic and has antimicrobial activity.

Fennel, *Foeniculum vulgare* Mill.†

The common fennel is a perennial herb yielding fruit and oil that are used for stomach and abdominal discomfort, as well as a spice in sweets and liqueurs. Other varieties yield the commonly used vegetable fennel. Two pharmaceutically important varieties are distinguished: *Foeniculum vulgare* var. *dulce* (sweet fennel), which is richer in anethole and has a sweet and aromatic taste, and *F. vulgare* var. *vulgare* (bitter fennel), which is rich in fenchone, resulting in a bitter taste. The two varieties are nearly impossible to distinguish microscopically; consequently, taste and smell differentiation, as well as thin-layer chromatography (TLC) analysis, are essential for differentiating the two.

Constituents. All of the aerial parts of fennel are rich in essential oil, with bitter fennel fruit containing 2%–6%, mostly *trans*-anethole (>60% of the oil) and fenchone (>15%) (Fig. 18.13), and with not more than 10% estragole. Sweet fennel contains 1.5%–3% essential oil,

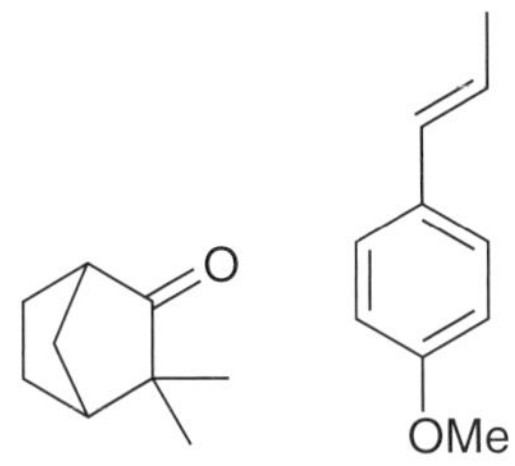

Fig. 18.13 Fenchone *(left)* and anethole *(right)*.

Fig. 18.14 Berberine.

composed of *trans*-anethole (80%–90%) but with very little fenchone (<1%) and less than 5% estragole. Fatty oil and protein are also found in fennel fruit.

Therapeutic uses and available evidence. Fennel is used as a carminative, for indigestion and colic in children, and there is some clinical data in support. It is considered to be safe and is widely used as a spice. Safety concerns have been raised based on the content of the potential carcinogen estragole (methylchavicol; ca 5%–10% of the total essential oil), but no clinical reports for toxicity for fennel have been recorded. The clinical relevance of studies using pure estragole at high doses has been disputed. Fennel oil (the distilled essential oil of both varieties of fennel) is used for the same indications.

Related herbs used for these indications are anise from *Pimpinella anisum* L.†, star anise from *Illicium verum* Hook.f.†, and coriander from *Coriandrum sativum* L.†. The oils of all of these fruits are the subject of monographs in the Eur. Ph.

LIVER DISEASE

Liver damage, cirrhosis and poisoning should only be treated under medical supervision. There is, however, a useful phytomedicine derived from the milk thistle, *Silybum marianum* (L.) Gaertn. (Asteraceae), in the form of an extract known as silymarin. Other medicinal plants as shown below, are widely used for liver disease, although with less clinical evidence in support. Medicinal plants used for 'biliousness' (see section on Dyspepsia and Biliousness) are also used in mild liver disease.

Andrographis, *Andrographis paniculata* (Burm.f.) Nees†

Andrographis is widely used in many Asian systems of medicine to treat jaundice and liver disorders. There are few clinical studies available to support these uses, although numerous in vitro experiments have shown it has liver-protective effects against a variety of hepatotoxins. 14-Deoxyandrographolide, a constituent, desensitises hepatocytes to TNF-α-induced signalling of apoptosis. It appears to be well tolerated, but caution should be exercised when given in conjunction with antithrombotic drugs. In the West, it is more often used as an immune stimulant (see Chapter 21, The Respiratory System, for more detail, including constituents).

Berberis Species and Other Berberine-Containing Drugs

Berberine (Fig. 18.14) is contained in *Berberis* species, for example *B. vulgaris* L., *B. aristata* DC.; in bloodroot, *Sanguinaria canadensis* L.†; goldenseal, *Hydrastis canadensis* L.†; gold thread, *Coptis chinensis* Franch†; and greater celandine, *Chelidonium majus* L.†.

Berberine has antibacterial and amoebicidal properties and is used either as the pure compound or in plant extracts, to treat dysentery and liver disease. Care should be taken when given together with anticancer drugs and with ciclosporin since berberine is known to be a substrate of P-glycoprotein and to affect the expression of cytochrome P (CYP) 450 enzymes.

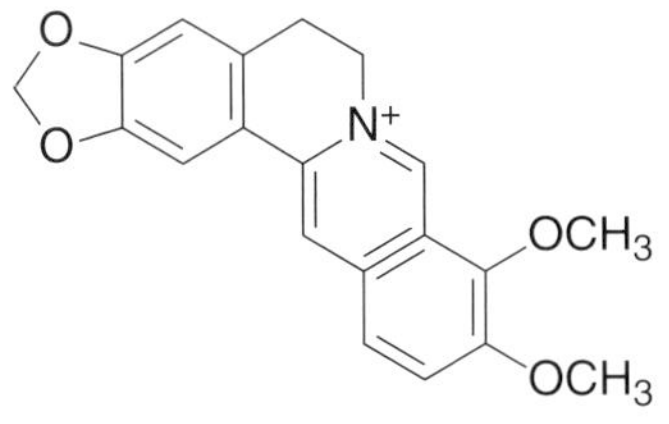

Milk Thistle, *Silybum marianum* (L.) Gaertn.†

The seeds of the milk thistle, *Silybum marianum* (Asteraceae), yield a flavonolignan fraction known as silymarin.

Constituents. The active constituents of the extract silymarin are flavonolignan, mainly silybin (= silibinin), with isosilybin, dihydrosilybin, silydianin, silychristin and others.

Therapeutic uses and available evidence. In many parts of Europe, silymarin is used extensively for liver disease and jaundice. It has been shown to exert an antihepatotoxic effect in animals against a variety of poisons, particularly those of the death cap mushroom *Amanita phalloides*. This fungus contains some of the most potent liver toxins known (the amatoxins and the phallotoxins), both of which cause fatal haemorrhagic necrosis of the liver is used to treat' [patients with chronic hepatitis and cirrhosis] to treat patients with chronic hepatitis and cirrhosis; it is also partially active against hepatitis B virus, is hypolipidaemic and lowers fat deposits in the liver in animals. This extract can be used not only for serious liver disease but also for general biliousness and other digestive disorders. The long-term administration of silymarin (in open studies) significantly increased survival time of patients with alcohol-induced liver cirrhosis. An inhibitory effect of silymarin on the development of metastases has also been reported (both in liver and other cancers), offering opportunities for its use in adjuvant therapy.

Schisandra, *Schisandra chinensis* (Turcz.) Baill.†

Schisandra (Schizandra) berries are the fruit of the magnolia vine and are very important in traditional Chinese medicine where they are used to treat liver disorders such as fatty liver disease, hepatotoxicity caused by immunosuppressive and other drugs, and conditions of general debility. The related species *Schisandra sphenanthera* Rehder & E.H. Wilson is also widely used. See also Chapter 26 (Supportive Therapies for Stress, Ageing, Cancer and Debility).

Constituents. The active constituents are dibenzocyclooctene lignans, known as schisandrins (schizandrins) and gomisins. The nomenclature is confused and, for example, 'schisandrin' is sometimes referred to in the literature as 'schisandrol A', and 'gomisin A' as 'schisandrol B'.

Therapeutic uses and available evidence. A great deal of research has been carried out on the pharmacology of this plant, and liver-protectant effects have been observed in animals, but clinical studies are lacking

Turmeric, *Curcuma longa* L.†

Turmeric is used in Asian medicine to treat liver disorders as well as inflammatory conditions. For details of the herbal drug and its constituents, see Chapter 23 (The Musculoskeletal System). Related species include Javanese turmeric (*Curcuma xanthorrhiza* Roxb.†), which is mostly used for dyspepsia and other GI problems. Turmeric and the curcuminoids are hepatoprotective against liver damage induced by various toxins, including paracetamol (acetaminophen), aflatoxin and cyclophosphamides, and have antispasmodic effects. Turmeric is also hypoglycaemic and hypocholesterolaemic, although clinical studies for liver disease are lacking. The underlying mechanism seems to be linked to the modulation of numerous complex signalling cascades. Turmeric is well tolerated but the bioavailability is poor, and refined extracts of curcumin are normally used, often in combination with pepper to enhance absorption (Ahsan et al 2020).

FURTHER READING

Ahsan, R., Arshad, M., Khushtar, M.A., et al., 2020. A comprehensive review on physiological effects of curcumin. Drug Res. 70, 441–447.

Anhayer, D., Frawley, J., Koch, A.K., et al., 2017. Herbal medicines for gastrointestinal disorders in children and adolescents: a systematic review. Pediatrics 139 (6), e20170062.

Chua, L.S., 2014. Review on liver inflammation and antiinflammatory activity of *Andrographis paniculata* for hepatoprotection. Phytother. Res. 28 (11), 1589–1598.

EMA, 2013. Assessment report on *Glycyrrhiza glabra* L. and/or *Glycyrrhiza inflata* Bat. and/or *Glycyrrhiza uralensis* Fisch., radix. Eur. Med. Agency. Available at: http://www.ema.europa.eu/docs/en_GB/document_library/Herbal_-_HMPC_assessment_report/2012/08/WC500131285.pdf.

EMA, 2013. Community herbal monograph on *Plantago ovata* Forssk., seminis tegumentum. Eur. Med. Agency. Available at: http://www.ema.europa.eu/docs/en_GB/document_library/Herbal_-_Community_herbal_monograph/2013/07/WC500146508.pdf.

Hosseinzadeh, H., Nassiri-Asl, M., 2015. Pharmacological effects of *Glycyrrhiza* species and its bioactive constituents: update and review. Phytother. Res. 29 (12), 1868–1886.

McKay, D.L., Blumberg, J.B., 2006. A review of the bioactivity and potential health benefits of chamomile tea (*Matricaria recutita* L.). Phytother. Res. 20, 519–530.

McKay, D.L., Blumberg, J.B., 2006. A review of the bioactivity and potential health benefits of peppermint tea (*Mentha piperita* L.). Phytother. Res. 20, 619–633.

Nikkhah Bodagh, M., Maleki, I., Hekmatdoost, A., 2018. Ginger in gastrointestinal disorders: a systematic review of clinical trials. Food Sci. Nutr. 7 (1), 96–108.

Obolskiy, D., Pischel, I., Feistel, B., Glotov, N., Heinrich, M., 2011. *Artemisia dracunculus* L. (tarragon): a critical review of its traditional use, chemical composition, pharmacology and safety. J. Agric. Food Chem. 59, 11367–11384.

Panahi, Y., Kianpour, P., Mohtashami, R., et al., 2018. Efficacy of artichoke leaf extract in non-alcoholic fatty liver disease: a pilot double blind randomized controlled trial. Phytother. Res. 32 (7), 1382–1387.

Samadi, M., Moradinazar, M., Khosravy, T., et al., 2022. A systematic review and meta-analysis of pre-clinical and clinical studies on the efficacy of ginger for the treatment of fatty live disease. Phytother. Res. 36 (3), 1182–1193. https://doi.org/10.1002/ptr.7390.

Soleimani, V., Delghandi, P.S., Moallem, S.A., Karimi, G., 2019. Safety and toxicity of silymarin, the major constituent of milk thistle extract: an updated review. Phytother. Res. 33 (6), 1629–1638.

Zhou, M., Deng, Y., Liu, L., et al., 2021. The pharmacological activity of berberine, a review for liver protection. Eur. J. Pharmacol. 890, 173655.

Zhu, P., Li, J., Fu, X., Yu, Z., 2019. Schisandra fruits for the management of drug-induced liver injury in China: a review. Phytomedicine 59, 152760.

The Cardiovascular System

Cardiovascular (CV) disorders are responsible for a major reduction in healthy life years, many years of poor chronic health and multiple deaths. They are a consequence of lifestyle and diet as well as being linked to genetic predisposition. Serious conditions such as heart failure must be treated only by a qualified physician, but some forms of CV disease respond well to changes in diet, taking more exercise, phytotherapy and the use of nutritional supplements.

Cardiology has benefited greatly from the introduction of semisynthetic drugs based on natural products, including aspirin, an antiplatelet agent derived from salicin, and warfarin, an anticoagulant derived from dicoumarol. Others have been developed using a natural product as a template. For example, verapamil, a calcium channel antagonist used to treat hypertension and angina, is based on the opium alkaloid papaverine; nifedipine, a calcium channel antagonist, and amiodarone, an antiarrhythmic, were both developed from khellin, the active constituent of khella (*Visnaga daucoides* Gaertn., syn.: *Ammi visnaga* (L.) Lam.). Cocaine from the coca plant (*Erythroxylum coca* Lam.) has cardioactive as well as central nervous system effects and was the starting material for the development of the antiarrhythmics procaine and lignocaine, which are more effective and without the unwanted stimulant activity.

Conditions suitable for supportive herbal treatment include chronic venous insufficiency (CVI), thrombosis and atherosclerosis. Hypertension and cardiac arrhythmias are usually treated with prescription drugs, although mild forms may benefit from phytomedicines. Diuretics are widely used as antihypertensives, but herbal diuretics are not sufficiently potent to reduce blood pressure. They are often incorporated into remedies for female urinary tract complaints (see Chapter 24) or to reduce bloating (mild water retention, for example premenstrual).

HEART FAILURE AND ARRHYTHMIAS

These conditions were formerly treated with cardiac glycosides (cardenolides and bufadienolides) such as digoxin, isolated from the foxglove. Other species such as lily of the valley (*Convallaria majalis* L.), which contains convallatoxin (a mixture of cardenolides), and squill (*Drimia maritima* (L.) Stearn), which contains the bufadienolides scillaren A and proscillaridin, and ouabain, isolated from *Strophanthus* spp., were formerly used. The cardiac glycosides have a positive inotropic effect, meaning that they increase the force of the contractions of the heart. They are emetic and toxic in large doses and have a cumulative effect and are therefore unsuitable for use in the form of herbal extracts. Single isolated compounds for which the pharmacokinetics can be monitored, such as digoxin, are used but have largely been superseded by safer drugs.

Arrhythmias are mainly treated with synthetic drugs, although alkaloids including quinidine (from *Cinchona* spp.; Fig. 19.1), ajmaline, from *Rauvolfia* spp., and sparteine, from broom (*Cytisus scoparius* (L.) Link), have been used historically.

There are, however, other herbal drugs that have beneficial effects upon the heart, the most important of which are hawthorn (*Crataegus* spp.) and motherwort (*Leonurus cardiaca* L.), which will be discussed later.

Foxglove (Digitalis) Leaf, *Digitalis purpurea* L.†

The very common purple foxglove (*Digitalis purpurea*) and its close relative the woolly foxglove (*D. lanata* Ehrh., Plantaginaceae) yield cardiac glycosides. They are indigenous to Europe and cultivated elsewhere. They do not have a long history of herbal use because of their toxicity, although in 1785, based on reports from a local herbalist in Shropshire, the famous surgeon William Withering described their use for 'dropsy' (a historic term for congestive heart failure), and this was the first time an effective treatment for this condition had been found. The leaves are the source of the drug and are usually gathered in the second year of growth.

Constituents

Both species contain cardenolides, which are glycosides of the steroidal aglycones digitoxigenin, gitoxigenin and gitaloxigenin. There are very many cardiac glycosides, but the most important is digoxin (Fig. 19.2) and to a much lesser extent digitoxin, and the purpurea glycosides A and B. *D. lanata* contains higher concentrations of glycosides, including digoxin and lanatosides, and is the main source of digoxin for the pharmaceutical industry.

Therapeutic Uses and Available Evidence

Digoxin increases the force of myocardial contractility and reduces conductivity within the atrioventricular node. It is used primarily in the treatment of supraventricular tachycardia and heart failure and is given as a once-daily dosage in the range 62.5–250 micrograms. Digitalis glycosides increase the force of the contractions of the heart without increasing the oxygen consumption and slow the heart rate when atrial fibrillation is present. Due to their cumulative effect, the glycosides can easily give rise

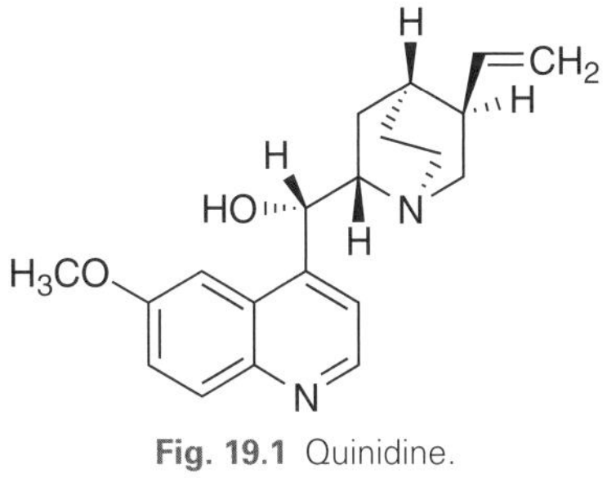

Fig. 19.1 Quinidine.

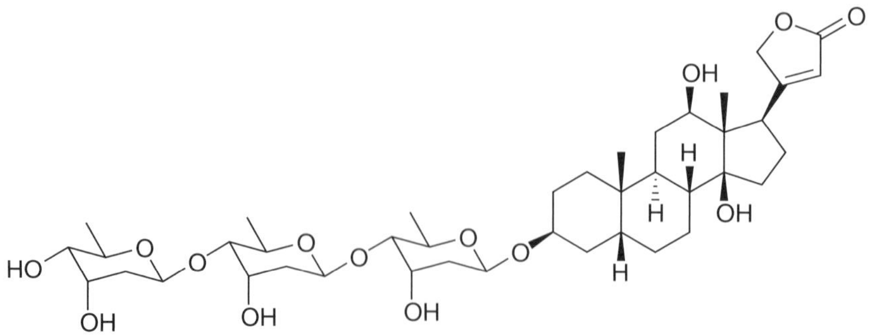

Fig. 19.2 Digoxin.

to toxic symptoms, such as nausea, vomiting and anorexia, especially in the elderly, thus blood levels should be monitored.

Hawthorn, *Crataegus* spp.†

Hawthorn (sometimes known as mayflower or whitethorn) is a common plant found in hedgerows and gardens throughout Europe and elsewhere. The flowers, leaves and berries of at least three species and their hybrids are used: mainly *Crataegus laevigata* (Poir.) DC., *C. monogyna* Jacq., (Rosaceae) as well as *C. rhipidophylla* Gand. (syn.: *C. oxyacantha* L.). These are hairless, thorny, deciduous shrubs with 3–5 lobed leaves, bearing white, dense clusters of flowers, followed by deep red fruits containing one seed (in *C. monogyna*) or two seeds (in *C. laevigata*). The flowers appear in early summer and the berries or 'haws' in early autumn. Jams and wines are often made from the fruit.

Constituents

The main constituents of the leaf are flavonoids, including vitexin, vitexin-4-rhamnoside, quercetin and quercetin-3-galactoside, hyperoside, rutin, vicentin and orientin; the fruit contains flavonoids, procyanidins, catechins and epicatechin dimers, as well as phenolic acids such as chlorogenic and caffeic acids. Amines such as phenethylamine and its methoxy derivative, as well as dopamine, acetylcholine and tyramine, have also been isolated. Hawthorn preparations are often standardised to contain 4–30 mg of flavonoids, calculated as hyperoside, or 30–160 mg of procyanidins, calculated as epicatechin. The leaf and flower are assayed for flavonoid content, whereas the berries are assayed for anthocyanin content.

Therapeutic Uses and Available Evidence

Hawthorn is used as a cardiac tonic, hypotensive, coronary and peripheral vasodilator, antiatherosclerotic and antiarrhythmic. Animal studies have shown beneficial effects on coronary blood flow, blood pressure and heart rate, as well as improved circulation to the extremities. Hawthorn extract inhibits myocardial Na^+, K^+-ATPase and exerts a positive inotropic effect and relaxes the coronary artery; it also repolarises the potassium current in the ventricular muscle and prolongs the refractory period, thus exerting an antiarrhythmic effect.

Positive outcomes from clinical trials using hawthorn extracts have been reported but there are inconsistencies in terms of the clinical criteria used (sample size, preparation, dosage, among others). The usual recommended dose of standardised extract is 160–900 mg daily. Few side effects have been observed, although nausea and headache have been reported infrequently.

Motherwort, *Leonurus cardiaca* L.†

Motherwort, *Leonurus cardiaca*, is a perennial herb indigenous to central Europe but now established in temperate regions throughout the world. The aerial parts are used for cardiovascular and gynaecological disorders in many traditional systems of medicine. Other species of *Leonurus* (Lamiaceae) are used in Chinese medicine for similar indications.

Constituents

The active ingredients include the labdane and clerodane diterpenes (e.g. forskolin, leocardin iridoids (e.g. harpagide, leonuride, ajugoside), alkaloids (e.g. leonurine, stachydrine), phenylethanoid glycosides (e.g. verbascoside, lavandulifolioside)), flavonoids (e.g. hyperoside, rutin and quercetin glycosides), triterpenes (e.g. ursolic acid) and many others.

Therapeutic Uses and Available Evidence

There is pharmacological evidence for antiarrhythmic effects of motherwort extracts, and some clinical evidence for antihypertensive and sedative activity. Long treatment is necessary for results to show, but motherwort appears to be safe and may prove a useful adjunctive treatment for mild heart disease.

VENOUS INSUFFICIENCY AND CIRCULATORY DISORDERS

Improvements in circulatory disorders can be elicited via different pharmacological effects, particularly those involving antiinflammatory and antioxidant activity. Plant drugs with these actions are important in the treatment of haemorrhoids, varicose veins, impaired visual acuity and even in memory enhancement, when blood flow to the brain may be affected. They usually contain saponins with antiinflammatory activity, or anthocyanidins and other antioxidants. The most important are bilberry, butcher's broom, horse chestnut, ginkgo and garlic.

Bilberry, *Vaccinium myrtillus* L.†

The bilberry, also known as the huckleberry or blueberry (*Vaccinium myrtillus*, Ericaceae), grows on acid soil in hilly and mountainous regions of Europe, Asia and North America. It is cultivated extensively for its delicious fruit, which ripen from July to September. The soft blue-black berries, about 0.5–1 cm in diameter, have a persistent calyx ring at the apex and contain numerous small oval seeds. Both the ripe fruit and the leaves are used medicinally. Some other members of the genus are used for similar indications.

Constituents

The fruit contains anthocyanosides (Fig. 19.3), mainly galactosides and glucosides of cyanidin, delphinidin and malvidin, together with vitamin C and volatile flavour components, such as *trans*-2-hexenal

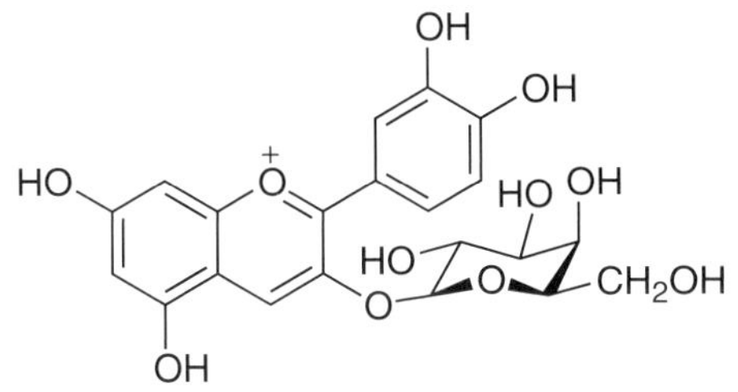

Fig. 19.3 Cyanidin-3-*O*-galactoside.

and ethyl-2- and -3-methylbutyrates. Unlike other *Vaccinium* spp., bilberry does not contain arbutin or other hydroquinone derivatives.

Therapeutic Uses and Available Evidence

The berries were traditionally used as an antidiabetic, and an astringent and antiseptic for diarrhoea. However, they are now more important as general health foods and agents to improve blood circulation in conditions such as vision disorders including retinopathy caused by diabetes or hypertension, as well as for other forms of venous insufficiency. The anthocyanosides are mainly responsible for these effects, due to their antioxidant and free radical scavenging properties, particularly in the case of the ophthalmic and vascular systems. They have antiplatelet effects and inhibit some proteolytic enzymes. Extracts are also antiinflammatory, antiulcer and antiatherosclerotic and reduce fluid retention. The usual daily dose of a standardised anthocyanoside extract of bilberry is 480 mg, taken in divided doses. Few side effects have been observed, as would be expected of a widely consumed food substance.

Butcher's Broom, *Ruscus aculeatus* L.†

Butcher's broom (*Ruscus aculeatus*, Asparagaceae) is an evergreen shrub native to Europe, and is found in dry woods and among rocks. It is often cultivated for its tough, spiky twigs and 'leaves', which can be preserved and used for decoration. The true leaves are reduced to small scales and the stems flattened at the ends into oval 'cladodes' that resemble leaves, each bearing a small white flower in the centre, followed by a round scarlet berry, and ending in a sharp spine. The rhizome or whole plant can be used.

Constituents

The active compounds are saponin glycosides, including ruscine and ruscoside, aculeosides A and B, which are based on ruscogenin (1β-hydroxydiosgenin) and neoruscogenin.

Therapeutic Uses and Available Evidence

Butcher's broom has antiinflammatory effects and is used mainly for venous insufficiency, especially varicose veins and haemorrhoids. The ruscogenin derivatives have been shown to reduce vascular permeability and improve symptoms of retinopathy and lipid profiles of diabetic patients.

The extract is either taken internally as a decoction or, more often, applied topically in the form of an ointment (or a suppository in the case of haemorrhoids). The saponins inhibit elastase activity in vitro and for this reason extracts are widely used in cosmetic preparations. When applied topically, few side effects have been observed, apart from occasional irritation.

Ginkgo, *Ginkgo biloba* L.†

Ginkgo is used in CNS disorders (see Chapter 22 for further detail) but also in cases of peripheral arterial occlusive disease and other circulatory disorders. Although probably less potent than some synthetic drugs, it has the advantage of being well tolerated. Ginkgo improves blood circulation and can alleviate some of the symptoms of tinnitus, intermittent claudication and altitude sickness. Ginkgo extracts have complex effects on isolated blood vessels. The ginkgolides are specific platelet-activating factor (PAF) antagonists and inhibit effects produced by PAF, including platelet aggregation and cerebral ischaemia. The usual dose is 120–160 mg of extract daily.

Horse Chestnut, *Aesculus hippocastanum* L.†

Aesculus hippocastanum (Sapindaceae) is native to Western Asia but cultivated and naturalised in most temperate regions. It is a large tree, bearing large sticky leaf buds, which open in early spring. The leaves are composed of 5–7 large oval leaflets; the flowers have a candle-like appearance and are white or pink in colour. The fruits are spiny capsules, each with two to four compartments containing the well-known large shiny brown seeds or 'conkers'. The seeds, and occasionally the bark, are used medicinally.

Constituents

Both seeds and bark contain a complex mixture of saponins based on protoescigenin and barringtogenol-C, which is known as 'aescin' (or 'escin'), although this term refers more properly to the isomeric compound aescin (Fig. 19.4). More than 30 saponins have been identified, including α- and β-escin, together with escins Ia, Ib, IIa, IIb, IIIa, etc. Sterols and other triterpenes such as friedelin, taraxerol and spinasterol are present, as well as coumarins (e.g. esculin = aesculin) and fraxin, flavonoids and anthocyanidins.

Therapeutic Uses and Available Evidence

Extracts of horse chestnut, or, more usually, extracts standardised to the aescin content, are used particularly for conditions involving CVI, bruising and sports injuries. They can be taken internally or applied topically. Oral horse chestnut seed extracts standardised to aescin have been found to be safe and efficacious for treating patients with CVI-related signs and symptoms (leg pain, pruritus (itching) and oedema (swelling)). It is also indicated for preventing thrombosis during long flights and may be beneficial in the treatment of cerebral oedema. Venotonic effects, and an improvement in capillary resistance, have been noted in healthy volunteers. Aescin has been shown to reduce oedema, decrease capillary permeability and increase venous tone, and horse chestnut extract to contract both veins and arteries in vitro, with veins being the more sensitive. It is widely used in cosmetics. The usual dose of extract daily is 600 mg, which corresponds to about 100 mg of escin. Extracts are well tolerated at therapeutic doses, but higher amounts can cause gastrointestinal upset with internal use, and occasional irritation with external application.

Red Root Sage, *Salvia miltiorrhiza* Bunge†

The root and rhizome of *Salvia miltiorrhiza* (Lamiaceae), also known as Danshen, are widely used in traditional Chinese medicine to treat many types of cardiovascular diseases, including ischaemic and circulatory disorders such as angina, after stroke, and atherosclerosis. The root has a characteristic bright red colour due to the tanshinone content.

Constituents

The main active constituents are diterpene quinones, known as tanshinones. Tanshinone I, tanshinone II, and cryptotanshinone are the major constituents, although nearly 40 variants of the basic tanshinone structures have been found in the roots. The total tanshinone content of the roots is about 1%, with tanshinone I and II and cryptotanshinone being the major components.

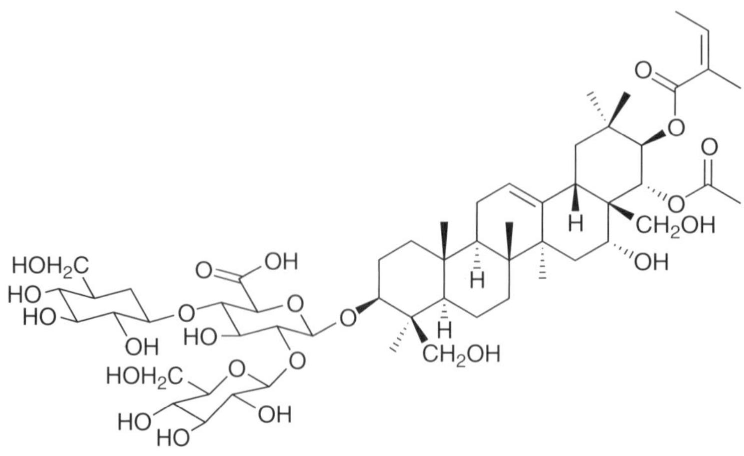

Fig. 19.4 Aescin.

Therapeutic Uses and Available Evidence

Animal studies have shown many relevant effects, such as protecting heart muscle from ischaemia and improving microcirculation. The isolated tanshinones have been shown to reduce fever and inflammation, inhibit platelet aggregation, dilate the blood vessels and aid urinary excretion of toxins. *S. miltiorrhiza* has a mild vasodilatory effect but does not increase cardiac output. Clinical studies carried out in China have shown benefit to patients with heart and circulatory diseases, including ischaemic stroke and acute myocardial infarction, and to improve glycaemic control in diabetes, *S. miltiorrhiza* seems to be safe and well tolerated, but there is potential for drug interactions, especially with other cardiovascular drugs.

Red Vine Leaf, *Vitis vinifera* L.

Certain varieties of grape vine (*Vitis vinifera*, Vitaceae, a plant that needs no description) produce red leaves that are used in the treatment of CVI and in particular, varicose veins. The definition of the herbal drug covers not only the species and plant part but also the use of a specific coloured variety.

Constituents

Vine leaves contain a wide range of polyphenols including quercetin-3-O-beta-D-glucuronide and isoquercitrin (the main flavonoids), anthocyanins, oligomeric proanthocyanidins, catechin, epicatechin monomers and dimers, gallic acid, astilbin and *trans*-resveratrol, along with organic acids, mainly malic and oxalic acid. The dried leaves should contain at least 4% of total polyphenols and 0.2% of anthocyanins.

Therapeutic Uses and Available Evidence

Positive effects in terms of improving the symptoms of CVI (tired, heavy and swollen legs or pain and tension in the legs) and reducing leg oedema compared to placebo were shown for ethanolic and aqueous wine leaf extracts and for a proprietary extract (AS 195). Red vine leaf extracts are also used to improve the microcirculation and aid wound healing. In vitro studies indicate that they have antioxidant and antiinflammatory properties, and that they inhibit platelet aggregation and hyaluronidase, and reduce oedema, possibly by reducing capillary permeability. Preclinical in vivo experiments demonstrated antiinflammatory and capillary wall thickening effects.

Red vine leaf extract can be applied topically and taken internally, and is well tolerated, although minor gastrointestinal effects have been reported. Commercial products are usually standardised to 90% polyphenols and 5% astilbin, with a daily dose of 360 mg red vine leaf extract being the recommended internal dose.

ANTIPLATELET AND ANTIATHEROSCLEROTIC DRUGS

These conditions are closely related in that atherosclerosis predisposes to thrombus formation, and can result in peripheral arterial disease, myocardial infarction and stroke. As well as improving diet and taking regular exercise, preventative drugs can be taken, many of which are natural products of some kind. Antiplatelet drugs are used prophylactically to decrease platelet aggregation and inhibit thrombosis. Aspirin has antiplatelet effects at doses that are lower (75–300 mg daily) than for pain relief (300 mg to 1 g, up to four times daily), but newer antiplatelet drugs such as clopidogrel, and more recently, ticagrelor and prasugrel, are used increasingly.

Many items of diet also have antiplatelet effects, for example, the flavonoids and anthocyanidins, as well as garlic, which is used also for its antiatherosclerotic effects. These foods form part of the 'Mediterranean diet', other elements of which include olive oil, which contains monounsaturated fatty acids, which also lower blood cholesterol levels, and red wine, which contains anthocyanidins (see bilberry, mentioned earlier). High-fibre foods, and phytomedicines used as bulk laxatives (such as ispaghula and psyllium husk), lower plasma lipid levels and can be used as adjuncts to a low-fat diet.

Diabetes and atherosclerosis may be a consequence of obesity, in a generalised inflammatory condition known as metabolic syndrome. Herbs and supplements may be used to address these complications, and some (such as fenugreek and garlic, mentioned later) may improve several parameters of cardiovascular risk. Others (gymnema, karela) address hyperglycaemic control

Garlic, *Allium sativum* L.†

The garlic bulb (*Allium sativum*, Amaryllidaceae) is composed of a number of small bulbs or 'cloves', covered with papery, creamy-white bracts. Garlic is cultivated worldwide and is used in many forms of cooking. The drug in commerce is the powder prepared from the cut, dried or freeze-dried bulb.

Constituents

Garlic contains a large number of sulfur compounds, which are responsible for the flavour and odour of garlic, as well as the medicinal effects. The main compound in the fresh plant is alliin, which on crushing undergoes enzymatic hydrolysis by alliinase to produce allicin (*S*-allyl-2-propenthiosulfinate; Fig. 19.5). This in turn forms a wide range of compounds, such as allylmethyltrisulfide, diallyldisulfide, ajoene and others, many of which are volatile. Sulfur-containing peptides such as

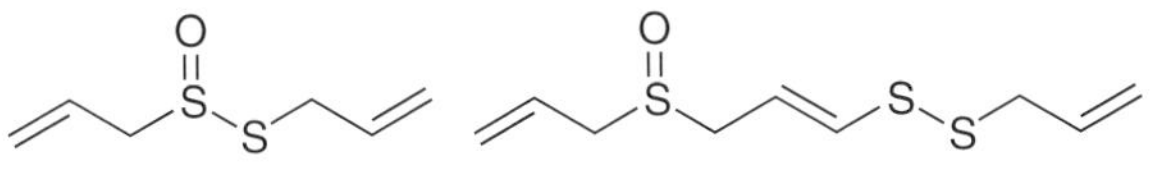

Fig. 19.5 Allicin (left) and ajoene (right).

glutamyl-S-methylcysteine, glutamyl-S-methylcysteine sulfoxide and others are also present.

Therapeutic Uses and Available Evidence

Different types of garlic preparations are available, such as quantified, allicin-rich extracts, aged garlic extracts (particularly in the Far East) and capsules containing the oil (older products). All have different compositions, but it is recognised that the sulfur-containing compounds must be present for the therapeutic effect. Deodorised products, except for those containing the precursor allicin, are ineffective.

Meta-analyses and systematic reviews of clinical studies have concluded that garlic has numerous beneficial effects in reducing risk factors associated with atherosclerosis, such as peripheral arterial occlusive disease. S-Allylcysteine inhibits nuclear factor kappa B (NF-κB) synthesis and low-density lipoprotein (LDL) oxidation, which are both implicated in atherosclerosis. Allicin is also antioxidant, and garlic extracts protect endothelial cells from oxidised LDL damage. It is known that ajoene (see Fig. 19.5) is a potent antithrombotic agent, as is 2-vinyl-4H-1,3-dithiin to a lesser extent. Other health benefits attributed to garlic are antibacterial, antiviral and antifungal effects, and chemopreventative activity against carcinogenesis in various experimental models. Diallylsulfide is thought to inhibit carcinogen activation via cytochrome P450-mediated oxidative metabolism, and epidemiological evidence suggests that a diet rich in garlic reduces the incidence of cancer.

Garlic has few side effects, but due to the antiplatelet effects, care should be taken if given in combination with other cardiovascular drugs due to additive effects.

Fenugreek, *Trigonella foenum-graecum* L.

Fenugreek is the dried, ripe seeds of *Trigonella foenum-graecum* (Fabaceae), an aromatic annual plant that grows up to 60 cm high. It is indigenous to China, India, Indonesia and the Mediterranean region and cultivated worldwide. The seeds are oblong-rhomboidal in shape and can be up to 5 mm long; they are yellowish-brown to reddish-brown in colour, and taste slightly bitter. Fenugreek seeds and leaf have a wide culinary use.

Constituents

The seeds contain pyridine-type alkaloids, including trigonelline and choline; steroidal saponins based on diosgenin, yamogenin, tigogenin and others; fenugreekine (a sapogenin-peptide ester); furostanol glycosides trigofoenosides A–G; sterols; and flavonoids, including orientin, isoorientin and isovitexin). There is a high mucilage content and a small concentration of essential oil.

Therapeutic Uses and Available Evidence

Fenugreek has a long history of traditional use, as an appetite stimulant, aphrodisiac, to enhance lactation, and as a hypocholesterolaemic and hypoglycaemic agent. Hypoglycaemic activity has been documented for trigonelline, and the steroidal saponins have cholesterol-lowering effects in preclinical studies.

The hypoglycaemic and hypocholesterolaemic effects of fenugreek are supported by clinical evidence. Fasting and postprandial blood glucose concentrations, glycosylated haemoglobin, total cholesterol, triglyceride and LDL concentrations have been shown to be reduced, and the total lipid profile improved, with fenugreek preparations.

Fenugreek may cause gastrointestinal disturbances and allergic reactions; cross-reactivity may occur in individuals with peanut or chickpea allergy.

Black Seed, *Nigella sativa* L.

The seeds and seed-oil of *Nigella sativa* (Ranunculaceae), also known as black cumin, are widely used in food and very highly regarded in traditional medicine systems of the Middle East and Asia, including Ayurveda, Siddha, Unani and Tibb, where it is a prophetic medicine.

They are used to treat a wide variety of ailments, inflammatory conditions including arthritis, and cardiovascular disorders including hypertension and diabetes, asthma, bronchitis and respiratory complains, dysentery, worms and skin conditions.

Constituents

The major active constituent of the seeds and oil is thymoquinone (Fig. 19.6), with lesser amounts of thymol, thymodihydroquinone, carvacrol and p-cymene. The seeds also contain alkaloids including the nigellamines, nigellicine, nigellidine and others, saponins based on α-hederin, and flavonoids, which contribute to the overall therapeutic effects of black seed.

Therapeutic Uses and Available Evidence

Nigella has demonstrated antiinflammatory, antidiabetic, antilipidemic and antihypertensive effects in many preclinical studies. Clinical trials have been carried out on the oil and extracts of the seed to establish the cardiovascular effects, and meta-analyses have shown that seed extracts and oil produce significant improvements in glycaemic control, lipid profiles, and biomarkers of inflammatory and oxidative stress.

The antiasthmatic properties of seed extract and oil have also been assessed in clinical studies, with positive outcomes reported, including in children. However, many of the trials do not use well-characterised products, and further studies are needed. The antiinflammatory effects of nigella in lung conditions are attracting interest as an adjunctive treatment in SARS-related diseases including COVID-19. Thymoquinone has well-documented pharmacological properties including neuroprotective, anticancer, radioprotective and other effects, and is widely studied due to its multiple mechanisms of action.

ANTIDIABETIC HERBS

Generally, the herbs used for diabetes are those mentioned earlier, which have general benefits in related metabolic diseases, but several are used for their hypoglycaemic benefits.

Gymnema, *Gymnema sylvestre* (Retz.) R. Br. ex Sm.

Gymnema sylvestre (Apocynaceae) grows wild in India, Sri Lanka and tropical Africa. It is a large woody climber with small yellow flowers. The leaves, which are ovate and hairy on both surfaces, have a slightly bitter taste, and if chewed this is followed by a remarkable temporary loss of sensitivity to the taste of sugar and other sweeteners. This unusual property has no relation to the hypoglycaemic effects, although may have originally been the rationale for its traditional use.

Constituents

The leaves and root contain saponins known collectively as 'gymnemic acid', which consists of a mixture of gymnemic acids, gymnemasins, gymnasiades, gymnemosides and their aglycones. Gurmarin, a

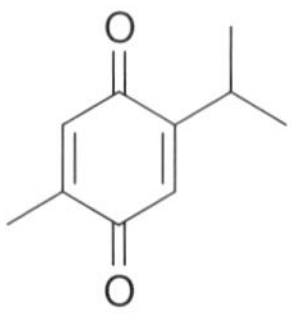

Fig. 19.6 Thymoquinone.

polypeptide, is responsible for the desensitisation of the palate to sweet tastes.

Therapeutic Uses and Available Evidence

The herb is a traditional treatment for diabetes in India. The anti-hyperglycaemic properties are due to the gymnemic acids and other saponins. In preclinical studies gymnema increased plasma insulin concentrations, and/or lowered serum total cholesterol or triglycerides. Systematic reviews of clinical studies have shown modest improvements in glycaemic control and reducing lipid levels in patients with type 2 diabetes.

Gymnema is well tolerated, but care should be taken when used in conjunction with other antidiabetic agents.

Karela, *Momordica charantia* L.

The bitter gourd or bitter melon, karela (*Momordica charantia*, Cucurbitaceae), is grown throughout India, China, Africa, the Caribbean and parts of America. It is a slender, climbing shrub with kidney-shaped, lobed leaves. The fruit resembles a cucumber with numerous ridges or warts and soft spines. It has an intensely bitter taste. Both the leaves and fruit are used medicinally.

The plant is widely used in the treatment of diabetes. The fruit is eaten as a vegetable; the leaf may be made into a type of 'bush tea', called 'cerassie'.

Constituents

The species contains triterpene (cucurbitane-type) glycosides called momordicosides A–L and the goyaglycosides A–H, as well as momordicin, momordicinin and cucurbitanes I, II and III and goyasaponins I, II and III. Proteins and lectins present include α-, β- and γ-momorcharins and momordins a and b.

Therapeutic Uses and Available Evidence

Both the fruit and the leaf have hypoglycaemic effects. There is substantial evidence demonstrating hypoglycaemic effects for karela extracts in preclinical studies, and also in patients with diabetes, although trials are of variable quality.

Karela has also been used to treat asthma, skin infections and hypertension. Contraceptive and teratogenic effects have been described in animals, so karela should be avoided by pregnant women until further information is available; cooking the vegetable may denature some of the toxins.

FURTHER READING

Angeloni, S., Spinozzi, E., Maggi, F., et al., 2021. Phytochemical profile and biological activities of crude and purified *Leonurus cardiaca* extracts. Plants (Basel) 10 (2), 195.

Azhdari, M., Zilaee, M., Karandish, M., et al., 2020. Red vine leaf extract (AS 195) can improve some signs and symptoms of chronic venous insufficiency, a systematic review. Phytother. Res. 34 (10), 2577–2585. https://doi.org/10.1002/ptr.6705.

Chan, S.W., Chu, T.T.W., Choi, S.W., et al., 2021. Effect of short-term bilberry supplementation on glycemic control, cardiovascular disease risk factors and antioxidant status in Chinese patients. Phytother. Res. 35 (6), 3236–3245.

Devangan, S., Varghese, B., Johny, E., et al., 2021. The effect of supplementation with *Gymnema sylvestre* on glycaemic control in type 2 diabetes patients: a systematic review and meta-analysis Phytother. Res. 34 (12), 6802–6812.

Gallelli, L., 2019. Escin: a review of its anti-edematous, anti-inflammatory, and venotonic properties. Drug Des. Devel. Ther. 13, 3425–3437. https://doi.org/10.2147/DDDT.S207720.

Gong, J., Fang, K., Dong, H., Wang, D., Hu, M., Lu, F., 2016. Effect of fenugreek on hyperglycaemia and hyperlipidemia in diabetes and prediabetes: a meta-analysis. J. Ethnopharmacol. 194, 260.

Hallajzadeh, J., Milajerdi, A., Mobini, M., et al., 2020. Effects of *Nigella sativa* on glycemic control, lipid profiles, and biomarkers of oxidative stress: a systematic review and meta-analysis of randomized controlled trials. Phytother. Res. 34 (10), 2586–2608.

Heshmat-Ghahdarijani, K., Mashayekhiasl, N., Amerizadeh, A., et al., 2020. Effect of fenugreek consumption on serum lipid profile: a systematic review and meta-analysis. Phytother. Res. 34 (9), 2230–2245.

Holubarsch, C.J.F., Colucci, W.S., Eha, J., 2018. Benefit-risk assessment of *Crataegus* extract WS 1442: an evidence-based review. Am. J. Cardiovasc. Drugs 18, 25–36. https://doi.org/10.1007/s40256-017-0249-9.

Imaizumi, V.M., Laurindo, L.F., Manzan, B., et al., 2022. Garlic: a systematic review of the effects on cardiovascular diseases. Crit. Rev. Food Sci. Nutr. 23, 1–23.

Islam, M.N., Hossain, K.S., Sarker, P.P., et al., 2021. Revisiting the pharmacological potentials of *Nigella sativa* seed: a promising option for COVID-19 prevention and cure. Phytother. Res. 35 (3), 1329–1344.

Jia, Q., Zhu, R., Tian, Y., et al., 2019. *Salvia miltiorrhiza* in diabetes: a review of its pharmacology, phytochemistry, and safety. Phytomedicine 58, 152871.

Kohandel, Z., Farkhondeh, T., Aschner, M., et al., 2021. Antinflammatory effects of thymoquinoe and its protective effects against several diseases. Biomed. Pharmacother. 138, 111492.

Kooti, W., Hasanzadeh-Noohi, Z., Sharafi-Ahvazi, N., et al., 2016. Phytochemistry and pharmacology, and therapeutic uses of black seed (*Nigella sativa*). Chinese J. Nat. Med. 14 (10), 732–745.

Kosehira, M., Machida, N., Kitaichi, N., 2020. A twelve-week long intake of Bilberry extract (*Vaccinium myrtillus* L.) improved objective findings of ciliary eye muscle contraction of the eye: a randomized, double blind, placebo-controlled parallel-group comparison trial. Nutrients 12 (3), 600.

Liu, L.M., Wang, Y., Zhang, T., Wang, S., 2021. Advances in the chemical constituents and chemical analysis of *Ginkgo biloba* leaf, extract and phytopharmaceuticals. J. Pharm. Biomed. Anal. 193, 113704.

Masullo, M., Pizza, C., Piacente, S., 2016. Ruscus genus: a rich source of bioactive steroidal saponins. Planta Med. 82 (18), 1513–1524.

Monjotin, N., Tenca, G., 2022. Lymphotonic activity of *Ruscus* extract, hesperidin methyl chalcone and vitamin C in human lymphatic smooth muscle cells. Microvasc. Res. 139, 104274. https://doi.org/10.1016/j.mvr.2021.104274.

Orhan, I.E., 2018. Phytochemical and pharmacological activity profile of *Crataegus oxyacantha* L. (Hawthorn) – a cardiotonic herb. Curr. Med. Chem. 25 (37), 4854–4865.

Peter, E.L., Kasali, F.M., Deyno, S., et al., 2019. *Momordica charantia* L. lowers elevated glycaemia in type 2 diabetes mellitus patients: a systematic review and meta-analysis. J. Ethnopharmacol. 231, 311–324.

Peter, E.L., Nagendrappa, P.B., Kaligirwa, A., et al., 2021. The safety and efficacy of *Momordica charantia* L. in animal models of type 2 diabetes: a systematic review and meta-analysis. Phytother. Res. 35 (2), 637–656.

Quesada, I., de Paola, M., Torres-Palazzolo, C., et al., 2020. Effect of garlic's active constituents in inflammation, obesity and cardiovascular disease. Curr. Hypertens. Rep. 22 (1), 6.

Ribeiro, M., Alvarenga, L., Cardozo, L.F.M.F., 2021. From the distinctive smell to therapeutic effects: garlic for cardiovascular, hepatic, gut, diabetes and chronic kidney disease. Clin. Nutr. 40 (7), 4807–4819.

Rodrigues, J.P.B., Fernandes, A., Dias, M.I., 2021. Phenolic compounds and bioactive properties of *Ruscus aculeatus* L. (Asparaginaceae): the pharmacology of an underexploited subshrub. Molecules 26 (7), 1882.

Saadat, S., Aslani, M.R., Ghorani, V., et al., 2021. The effects on *Nigella sativa* respiratory, allergic and immunologic disorders, evidence from experimental and clinical studies, a comprehensive and updated review. Phytother. Res. 35 (6), 2968–2996.

Shang, A., Cao, S.-Y., Xu, X.-Y., et al., 2019. Bioactive compounds and biological functions of garlic (*Allium sativum* L.). Foods 8 (7), 246. https://doi.org/10.3390/foods8070246.

Wang, X., Yang, Y., Liu, X., Gao, X., 2020. Pharmacological properties of tanshinones, the natural products from *Salvia miltiorrhiza*. Adv. Pharmacol. 87, 43–70.

Wojtyniak, J., Szymanski, M., Matlawska, I., 2013. *Leonurus cardiaca* L. (motherwort): a review of its phytochemistry and pharmacology. Phytother. Res. 27 (8), 1115–1120.

Wu, M., Liu, L.T., Xing, Y.W., Yang, S.J., Li, H., Cao, Y., 2020. Roles and mechanisms of hawthorn and its extracts on atherosclerosis: a review. Front. Pharmacol. 11, 118.

20

Weight-Loss Supplements

These very popular products are widely available, claiming to act in various ways, for example, by suppressing the appetite or inhibiting fat and/or carbohydrate absorption, as with fibre supplementation, by 'speeding up' metabolism, and/or by inducing thermogenesis and increasing lipolysis. There is a lack of good clinical evidence for their efficacy in relation to these claims. Many of these supplements are also taken for the purpose of improving athletic performance and increasing stamina, and users may take several products at the same time, which raises safety concerns.

Some of the most common ingredients of weight-loss supplements contain caffeine, which acts as a stimulant and appetite suppressant. These include **guarana** (see Chapter 22), **green tea** (see Chapter 26) and **green coffee bean** extracts. **Hoodia** is an appetite suppressant, and **bitter orange peel**, **chilli peppers**, **garcinia** and **kelp** are considered to increase metabolism. Multi ingredient products are common. Many other supplements are advertised as beneficial during weight-loss regimens, but few are clinically proven, and some, such as the stimulant **ephedra** (see Chapter 21), are responsible for cases of poisoning and other adverse effects. For review, see Watanabe *et al.* (2020).

BITTER ORANGE, *CITRUS × AURANTIUM* L. (RUTACEAE) †

Bitter orange peel extract is widely used in weight-loss products.

Constituents

Bitter orange peel contains *p*-synephrine (Fig. 20.1) as the main active compound. There are also citrus flavonoids, such as naringenin, and essential oil components.

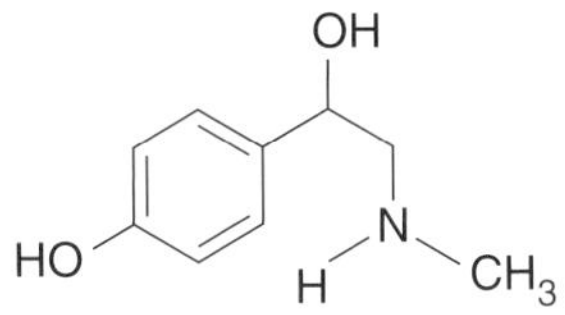

Therapeutic Uses and Available Evidence

There are few clinical studies showing efficacy for bitter orange extracts or *p*-synephrine, but animal studies have shown thermogenic effects. Concerns have been expressed about the use of products containing *C. aurantium* extract; however, there is some confusion between *p*-synephrine and *m*-synephrine (phenylephrine), a stimulant used as a nasal decongestant. Based on current knowledge, the use of bitter orange extracts and *p*-synephrine appears to be safe at doses recommended, and a clinical study assessing the cardiovascular effects of bitter orange extract (equivalent to 49 mg *p*-synephrine) found no significant changes in heart rates, systolic blood pressure or blood chemistry at any time point, nor were any adverse effects reported (Shara *et al.* 2016).

CHILLI PEPPERS, *CAPSICUM FRUTESCENS* L. AND OTHERS (SOLANACEAE)†

Chilli peppers are eaten everywhere and used widely in medicine, including for weight loss.

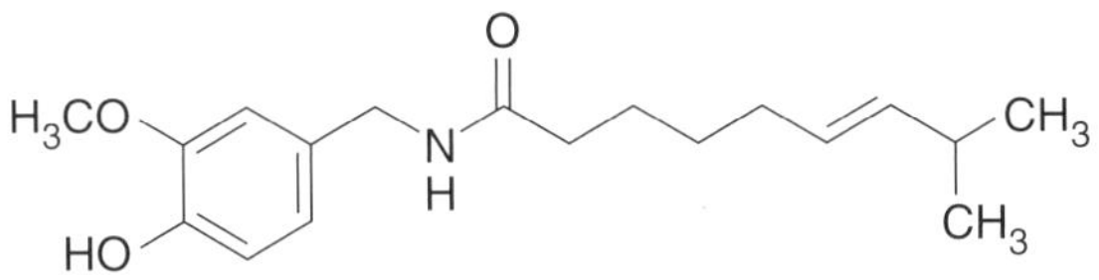

Fig. 20.1 *p*-Synephrine.

Fig. 20.2 Capsaicin.

Constituents

The extract known as 'capsaicin' contains pungent substances, capsaicinoids, based on capsaicin (Fig. 20.2), and non pungent analogues called capsinoids, and many other compounds.

Therapeutic Uses and Available Evidence

Capsaicinoids are thermogenic and human studies have shown them to increase satiety and fullness, preventing overeating. The capsinoids are also of interest for weight loss and appear to be without safety concerns (Avila *et al.* 2021).

GREEN COFFEE BEAN, *COFFEA ARABICA* L. AND OTHER VARIETIES (RUBIACEAE)

Extracts of unripe coffee beans are common ingredients of weight-loss products.

Constituents

Green coffee beans contain caffeine and high concentrations of chlorogenic acid derivatives.

Therapeutic Uses and Available Evidence

Systematic reviews suggest that green coffee extract can improve lipid profiles and reduce body weight, but the contribution of caffeine to this effect is not known, and studies were generally of poor methodological quality. Caffeine-containing herbs may cause serious central nervous system and cardiovascular adverse reactions (e.g. ischaemic stroke, cardiac arrest) if used with conventional medicines and/or herbals with similar effects, e.g. bitter orange, ephedra.

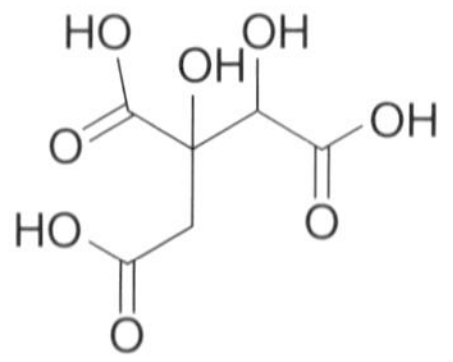

Fig. 20.3 Hydroxycitric acid.

HOODIA, *HOODIA GORDONII* (MASSON) SWEET EX DECNE. AND RELATED SPECIES (APOCYNACEAE)

The stem of the hoodia plant is traditionally used as an appetite suppressant by bushmen in the Kalahari Desert. It is becoming endangered due to overharvesting, and there is thought to be considerable illegal trade and adulteration of hoodia products.

Constituents

Steroidal (pregnane) glycosides, based on hoodigogenin and calogenin. A mixture of glycosides, known as P57, is the main appetite-suppressant component.

Therapeutic Uses and Available Evidence

Human clinical studies have confirmed appetite suppression by a P57-enriched extract of hoodia, although side effects, such as nausea, flatulence, and increases in blood pressure and heart rate, are associated with consumption of the high doses required to achieve a clinical effect (Smith and Krygsman 2014).

GARCINIA, *GARCINIA GUMMI-GUTTA* (L.) N. ROBSON (CLUSIACEAE)

The extract of the rind of the fruit of *G. gummi-gutta* (formerly *G. cambogia* (Gaertn.) Desr.) and its major constituent hydroxycitric acid are widely used in weight-loss products. The fruit is also used as a flavouring in food.

Constituents

Plant acids, mainly hydroxycitric acid (Fig. 20.3), and also ascorbic acid.

Therapeutic Uses and Available Evidence

The evidence is conflicting: garcinia extracts are reported to exhibit antiobesity activity by regulating serotonin levels related to satiety,

increasing fat oxidation and decreasing de novo lipogenesis; however, clinical studies have not shown effects persisting beyond 12 weeks of intervention. Liver toxicity has been reported, and a possible interaction with serotonin re-uptake inhibiting drugs (Semwal *et al.* 2015).

KELP, BLADDERWRACK *FUCUS VESICULOSUS* L., *FUCUS SERRATUS* L., *ASCOPHYLLUM NODOSUM* (L.) LE JOLIS (FUCACEAE)†

The thallus (whole plant) of these seaweeds is used to aid weight loss and as a source of iodine to support thyroid function, which may also help weight loss.

Constituents

Polysaccharides, the fucoidans, alginic acid and laminarin, with minerals, mainly iodine.

Therapeutic Uses and Available Evidence

There is little clinical evidence for the use of kelp for weight loss, although it does alter glucose homeostasis in humans. Anti-obesity effects have been described for fucoidan, with reduced triglyceride, cholesterol and low-density lipoprotein levels. High doses should be avoided due to the iodine content, which is very variable (Kim *et al.* 2014).

FURTHER READING

Avila, D.L., Nunes, N.A.M., Almeida, P.H.R.F., Gomes, J.A.S., Rosa, C.O.B., Alvarez-Leite, J.I., 2021. Signaling targets related to anti-obesity effects of capsaicin: a scoping review. Adv. Nutr. 12 (6), 2232–2243.

Kim, M.J., Jeon, J., Lee, J.S., 2014. Fucoidan prevents high-fat diet-induced obesity in animals by suppression of fat accumulation. Phytother. Res. 28 (1), 137–143.

Semwal, R.B., Semwal, D.K., Vermaak, I., Viljoen, A., 2015. A comprehensive scientific overview of *Garcinia cambogia*. Fitoterapia 102, 134–148.

Shara, M., Stohs, S.J., Mukattash, T.L., 2016. Cardiovascular safety of oral p-synephrine (bitter orange) in healthy subjects: a randomized placebo-controlled cross-over clinical trial. Phytother. Res. 30 (5), 842–847.

Smith, C., Krygsman, A., 2014. *Hoodia gordonii*: to eat, or not to eat. J. Ethnopharmacol. 155, 987–991.

Watanabe, M., Risi, R., Masi, D., Caputi, A., Balena, A., Rossini, G., et al., 2020. Current evidence to propose different food supplements for weight loss: a comprehensive review. Nutrients 12 (9), 2873.

21

The Respiratory System

Minor common disorders of the respiratory system can generally be treated successfully using herbal medicines which may also be helpful as a supportive measure in more serious diseases, such as bronchitis, emphysema and pneumonia, alongside antibiotic therapy if appropriate.

The global pandemic caused by the coronavirus SARS-CoV-2 has resulted in a dramatic increase in the demand for herbal medicines for use in the treatment of COVID-19-related symptoms. An epidemic of SARS (not COVID), in 2003, was treated with traditional Chinese herbal medicines, including *Houttuynia cordata* and *Isatis tinctoria* in addition to corticosteroids, resulting in a reduction of fever and lowered rate of mortality. The potential for natural products as leads for development of novel treatments for COVID-19 is being investigated, although the clinical evidence for the treatment of COVID-19 is limited as yet.

Upper respiratory tract infections such as coughs, colds and sore throats are common reasons for visiting a healthcare professional but are very suitable for self-medication, including with herbal medicines. For colds and flu-like viral infections, in addition to analgesics and anti-inflammatories, decongestants (menthol, eucalyptus), bronchiolytics and expectorants (ipecacuanha, thyme, senega), demulcents (mallow), antibacterials and antivirals (linden and elder flowers, elderberries, pelargonium) and immune system modulators (echinacea, astragalus, andrographis) are popular and effective. Traditionally, garlic and echinacea have been used in combination for allergic and infective rhinitis.

Asthma is becoming more prevalent for many reasons and is usually treated prophylactically with inhaled steroids, and symptomatically with bronchodilators, many of which are either of natural origin (e.g. theophylline and ephedrine) or were developed from natural products.

Antimuscarinic drugs (e.g. atropine), which have bronchodilator effects and also dry secretions, have largely been superseded by derivatives such as ipratropium. Cough suppressants and expectorants are very popular, although there is limited clinical evidence for their effectiveness. The most important antitussives are codeine and other derivatives obtained from the opium poppy, and expectorants include ipecacuanha and senega.

ANTIALLERGICS

Many flavonoids have antiallergic properties, although not as potent as, for example, cetirizine, desloratadine or chlorphenamine.

Khella, *Visnaga daucoides* Gaertn. (syn.: *Ammi visnaga* (L.) Lam.)

Also known as the 'toothpick plant', as the woody pedicels have been used for this purpose, khella (Apiaceae) is a herbaceous annual reaching 1.5 m in height, with divided filiform leaves and typically umbelliferous flowers. The herbal drug is derived from the fruits, which are very small, broadly ovoid and usually found as separate greyish-brown mericarps. It has a long history of use in the Middle East, especially

Egypt, as an antispasmodic in renal colic, for asthma and as a coronary vasodilator for angina.

Constituents

The active constituents are furanocoumarins, the most important being khellin (Fig. 21.1), together with visnagin, visnadin and khellol glucoside.

Therapeutic Uses and Available Evidence

Khellin, visnadin and visnagin are vasodilators, with calcium-channel-blocking and spasmolytic activity. Khellin was the starting material for the development of several important semisynthetic derivatives such as sodium cromoglycate, which is widely used as a prophylactic treatment for asthma, hay fever and other allergic conditions, in the form of an inhaler or eyedrops, or orally for allergic digestive disorders. Nifedipine (a calcium channel antagonist and vasodilator) used in heart disease, and amiodarone, a cardiac antiarrhythmic, were also developed using khellin as a lead compound.

Butterbur, *Petasites hybridus* (L.) G. Gaertn., B. Mey. & Scherb.

Petasites hybridus (syn.: *P. vulgaris, Tussilago petasites*, Asteraceae) is a downy perennial, common in damp places throughout Europe, with large heart-shaped leaves and lilac-pink brush-like flowers in early spring before the leaves appear. The root and herb are used.

Constituents

Butterbur contains sesquiterpene lactones (eremophinolides), including a series of petasins and isopetasins, neopetasin, petasalbin, furanopetasin, petasinolides A and B, and flavonoids including isoquercetin glycosides. All parts of the plant contain unsaturated, toxic pyrrolizidine alkaloids (PAs; senecionine, integerrimine, senkirkine, petasitine and neopetasitine), usually with higher concentrations in the root.

Therapeutic Uses and Available Evidence

Butterbur is used for allergic and respiratory problems and there is evidence to support this use, although it cannot be recommended due to safety concerns. A proprietary PA-free CO_2 extract of *P. hybridus* prepared from the leaves, and standardised to 8 mg total petasins, is approved in some European countries for the symptomatic treatment of allergic rhinitis (hay fever) and related symptoms.

BRONCHODILATORS AND DECONGESTANTS

Ephedra, *Ephedra* spp.†

Ephedra, also known as Ma Huang (*Ephedra sinica* Stapf and other species of the Ephedraceae) is an ancient Chinese medicine, which is now used worldwide. It was the original source of ephedrine, a useful decongestant and bronchodilator, which is used to treat nasal

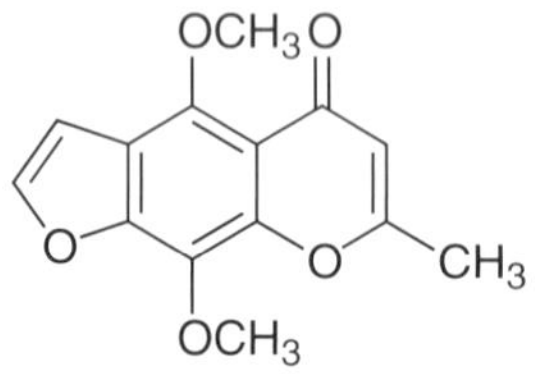

Fig. 21.1 Khellin.

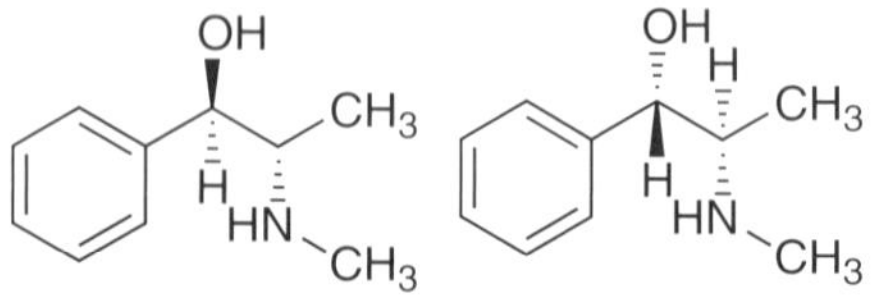

Fig. 21.2 Ephedrine *(left)* and pseudoephedrine *(right).*

congestion in the form of nasal drops. Pseudoephedrine is now used more widely for respiratory congestion as it has fewer central nervous system (CNS) stimulatory properties. The drought-tolerant plant has slender green stems, which are jointed in branches of about 20 tufts about 15 cm long, and terminate in a sharp, recurved point. The leaves are reduced to sheaths surrounding the stems.

Constituents

The main active constituents are the alkaloids, up to about 3% of the stem, but widely varying; the major alkaloid is (–)-ephedrine (Fig. 21.2), with (+)-pseudoephedrine, norephedrine, norpseudoephedrine, ephedroxane, *N*-methylephedrine, maokonine, transtorine and the ephedradines A–D.

Therapeutic Uses and Available Evidence

For at least 5000 years *Ephedra* has been used in China for asthma and hay fever, as a bronchodilator, sympathomimetic and CNS and cardiac stimulant. Herbalists also use it to treat enuresis, allergies, narcolepsy and other disorders, and antiinflammatory activity has been observed in extracts. Ephedrine is used in the form of elixirs and nasal drops, and in the emergency treatment of some types of bradycardias.

Toxicological Risks

Ephedra herb has been abused as a slimming aid, and as an ergogenic agent in sports and athletics, but this is risky. Hypertension and other cardiovascular events, and exacerbation of hepatitis, have been noted with high doses. The absorption of ephedrine and pseudoephedrine is slower after ingestion of the herbal drug than for the isolated alkaloids. The ephedradines, mahuannins and maokonine, are mildly hypotensive, but the herb and the isolated alkaloids should be avoided by hypertensive patients and in cases of thyrotoxicosis, narrow-angle glaucoma and urinary retention.

Theophylline†

The xanthine theophylline (Fig. 21. 3) is found in cocoa (*Theobroma cacao* L.), coffee (*Coffea* spp.) and tea (*Camellia sinensis* (L.) Kuntze) but is almost invariably used as the isolated compound. It is indicated in reversible airways obstruction, particularly in acute asthma. There is a narrow margin between therapeutic and toxic doses, and the half-life is highly variable between patients, especially smokers or with concurrent administration of other drugs.

Side effects include tachycardia and palpitations, nausea and other gastrointestinal upsets, which can be reduced by using sustained-release preparations.

Inhalations

Essential-oil-containing herbal drugs and their volatile constituents are used as chest rubs, steam inhalations and baths, and in nasal sprays and pastilles or lozenges, for their decongestant properties. They are particularly useful for infants, children, asthmatics and pregnant women for whom systemic decongestants may not be appropriate. Oils distilled

from the aerial parts of the pine family (e.g. the common Pumilio (Alpine) pine (*Pinus mugo* Turra), the European larch (*Larix decidua* Mill.) and the fir tree (*Abies* spp.)) and the Australian Myrtaceae (e.g. eucalyptus and tea-tree oil) are used frequently.

Camphor†

Camphor (Fig. 21. 4), a pure compound, is extracted from the Asian camphor tree (*Cinnamomum camphora* (L.) J. Presl, Lauraceae). It is often combined with the essential-oil-containing drugs as an aromatic stimulant and decongestant. Camphor has antiseptic, antiinflammatory, secretolytic and decongestant effects. It was formerly taken internally for colds, diarrhoea and other complaints, in small doses, but it is now only used externally.

Toxicological Risks

Camphor can be used safely if the dose of camphor is less than 11% of the formulation and if it is applied on an unbroken skin, e.g. for inhaling as a vapour rub. Overdose causes vomiting, convulsions and palpitations, and can be fatal.

Eucalyptus Oil, *Eucalyptus* spp.†

The blue gum tree, *Eucalyptus globulus* Labill. (Myrtaceae), and related species yield a highly characteristic oil that is widely used as a decongestant, insect repellent, antiseptic and solvent. The leaves are scimitar-shaped, 10–15 cm long and about 3 cm wide, short-stalked and rounded at the base, with numerous transparent oil glands.

Constituents

The oil contains 1,8-cineole (eucalyptol; Fig. 21.5) as the major component, with terpineol, α-pinene, *p*-cymene and small amounts of ledol, aromadendrene and viridiflorol, aldehydes, ketones and alcohols.

Therapeutic Uses and Available Evidence

The leaf and oil are traditional Australian Aboriginal remedies for coughs, colds and bronchitis. The oil may be taken internally in small doses, as an ingredient of cough mixtures, sweets and pastilles, or applied externally in the form of a liniment, ointment or vapour rub or bath additive for inhalation. The leaf extract and oil have antiseptic effects against a variety of bacteria and yeasts, and are used in pharmaceutical products such as dentifrices and cosmetics. The oil is insect repellent, insecticidal and larvicidal and widely used in skin products for these purposes.

Menthol and Eucalyptus Inhalation BP for steam inhalation is used as a decongestant.

Eucalyptus oil is irritant when undiluted and, although safe as an inhalation, should not be taken internally as fatalities have been reported.

Menthol†

Menthol is a monoterpene (see Fig. 21.5) extracted from essential oils of *Mentha* spp. (especially *M. arvensis* L.) or synthesised. It is an effective decongestant used in nasal sprays and inhalers, and an antiinflammatory and cooling agent in skin inflammation and sunburn when applied topically.

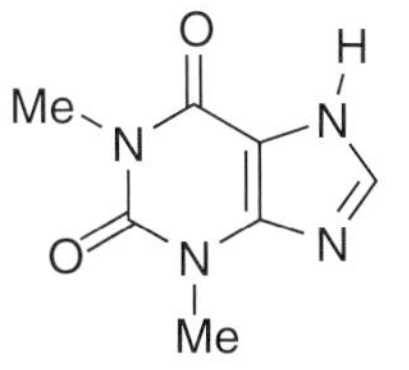

Fig. 21.3 Theophylline.

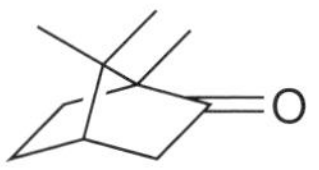

Fig. 21.4 Camphor.

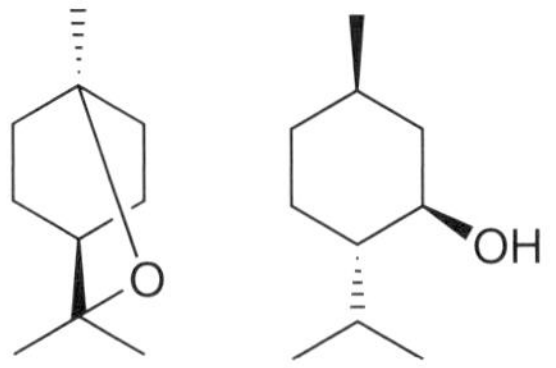

Fig. 21.5 1,8-Cineole *(left)* and (−)-menthol *(right)*.

EXPECTORANTS AND MUCOLYTICS

The purpose of these is to reduce the viscosity of mucus in the respiratory tract to enable expectoration. They are included in cough mixtures which, although efficacy is often difficult to demonstrate, are very popular. Expectorants are usually used in conjunction with decongestants, demulcents, analgesics and, occasionally, antibiotics.

Balm of Gilead (Poplar Buds), *Populus* spp.

Poplar buds (from various *Populus* spp., including *P. × candicans* Aiton (syn.: *P. × gileadensis* Rouleau), *P. balsamifera* L. and *P. nigra* L., Salicaceae) are collected in the spring before they open. The buds of all species are similar, being about 2 cm long and 0.5 cm wide, with narrow, brown, overlapping scales; the inner scales are sticky and resinous. The bark of these species is also used.

Constituents

All species contain the phenolic glycosides salicin (salicyl alcohol glucoside), populin (benzoyl salicin) and an essential oil composed of α-caryophyllene, with cineole, bisabolene and farnesene. Flavonoids (pinocembrin and pinobanksin) and lignans based on isolariciresinol are also present.

Therapeutic Uses and Available Evidence

Balm of Gilead is an ingredient of herbal cough mixtures, and ointments used for rheumatic and other muscular pains. Little evidence is available for efficacy, but there is a long history of traditional use

Thyme and Wild Thyme, *Thymus vulgaris* L. and *Thymus serpyllum* L.†

Thymus vulgaris (garden or common thyme) and *T. serpyllum* (wild thyme, mother of thyme or serpyllum, Lamiaceae) are indigenous to Europe, especially the Mediterranean region, and are cultivated extensively.

They are bushy or prostrate shrubs with small, elliptical, shortly stalked leaves, which are up to about 6 mm long and 0.5–2 mm broad, with entire recurved margins. Wild thyme leaves are a little broader and the margins are not recurved, with long trichomes at the base.

Constituents

The essential oil has the major constituent thymol, with lesser amounts of carvacrol, 1,8-cineole, borneol, thymol methyl ether and α-pinene. The flavonoids (apigenin, luteolin, thymonin, etc.) and the polyphenolic acids (labiatic, rosmarinic and caffeic) contribute to the antiinflammatory and antimicrobial effects.

Therapeutic Uses and Available Evidence

Thyme, and oil of thyme, are antitussive, expectorant and spasmolytic, and, as such, are used for coughs, bronchitis, sinusitis, whooping cough and similar respiratory complaints. The activity is mainly due to thymol, which is expectorant and antiseptic; thymol, carvacrol and the flavonoid fraction are spasmolytic. Thymol (see Chapter 27, Fig. 27.3) is a popular ingredient of mouthwashes and dentifrices because of its antiseptic and deodorant properties. The oil may be taken internally in small doses of up to 0.3 mL, unless for use in a mouthwash, which is not intended to be swallowed in significant amounts. Thymol is irritant and toxic in high doses, and should be used with care.

Senega, *Polygala senega* L.†

Senega (snake root, rattlesnake root, *Polygala senega*, Polygalaceae) is native to the United States, whereas in Chinese medicine, senega may also refer to *P. tenuifolia* Willd.; both species are used for similar purposes. The root is light yellowish-grey with a knotty crown from which slender stems arise, bearing the remains of rudimentary leaves and buds at the base.

Constituents

The active constituents are triterpenoid saponins, the mixture generally known as 'senegin', and are based on the aglycones presenegenin, senegenin, hydroxysenegin, polygalacic acid and senegnic acid. They include the E- and Z-senegins II, III and IV; E- and Z-senegasaponins a, b and c; and others.

Therapeutic Uses and Available Evidence

Senega is used primarily for chronic bronchitis, catarrh, asthma and croup. The saponins are the active constituents; they have immunomodulating activity, and are antiinflammatory and antiseptic.

Ivy, *Hedera helix* L.†

Ivy is a saponin-containing expectorant herb. It is a common climbing plant, found in Europe, northern and eastern Asia and introduced into America. *Hedera helix* (Araliaceae) leaves are dark green and leathery, shiny, with 3–4 triangular lobes. The berries are small, purplish-black and globular, with the calyx ring visible at the apex. Both leaves and berries are used in herbal preparations.

Constituents

The active constituents are saponins based on oleanolic acid, bayogenin and hederagenin, including the hederosaponins (hederacosides) B, C and D, and α- and β-hederin; the polyyne falcarinol and the flavonoids.

Therapeutic Uses and Available Evidence

Ivy extracts are used in preparations for bronchitis and catarrh. The saponins and sapogenins are expectorant and antifungal and there is some evidence of efficacy. These preparations are safe and well tolerated, with adverse events being mainly gastrointestinal disorders. Ivy constituents have been well researched, and several modes of action postulated. In addition to their mucolytic activity, the saponins act on G protein-linked β_2-adrenergic receptors of epithelial lung cells, resulting in an indirect β_2-sympathomimetic and bronchodilator effect. Ivy can be irritant and allergenic due to the saponin and falcarinol content.

Tolu Balsam, *Myroxylon balsamum* (L.) Harms†

The resin, which is collected from incisions in the bark and sapwood of *Myroxylon balsamum* (Fabaceae), is a light brown, fragrant, balsamic resin, softening when warm and becoming brittle when cold. It has a pleasant, sweetish, aromatic, vanilla-like odour.

Constituents

The main constituents of the balsam are cinnamic and benzoic acids, their esters such as benzyl benzoate and cinnamyl cinnamate, and esters with resin alcohols, including coniferyl and hydroconiferyl benzoates.

Therapeutic Uses and Available Evidence

Balsam of tolu is expectorant, stimulant and antiseptic. It is used in cough mixtures and pastilles, and as a lozenge base. Although there is no clinical evidence, many balsams are used for similar purposes. Balsam of tolu is an ingredient in Friar's balsam, which is used as a steam inhalation and also as a protectant in skin formulations. The antimicrobial activity is due to the benzyl benzoate and benzyl cinnamate content.

Tolu balsam, like many other balsam resins, can cause allergic reactions.

Ipecacuanha, *Carapichea ipecacuanha* (Brot.) L. Andersson†

'Ipecac' is obtained from the root and rhizome of *Carapichea ipecacuanha* (better known under its synonym *Cephaelis ipecacuanha* A. Rich, Rubiaceae). *C. ipecacuanha* root is twisted and reddish brown, with a characteristic ringed appearance. It is native to tropical central and south America and cultivated in southern Asia.

Constituents

Ipecac root contains about 2%–3% isoquinoline alkaloids as the active constituents. The most important are emetine (Fig. 21.6) and cephaeline, with psychotrine and others.

Therapeutic Uses and Available Evidence

Ipecac extract is included in cough preparations because of its expectorant activity. It is a rapidly acting emetic and has been employed to induce vomiting in cases of poisoning or drug overdose, but this use has been superseded by more effective and less drastic measures. The alkaloids are amoebicidal, but the emetic activity means that they are rarely used for this purpose.

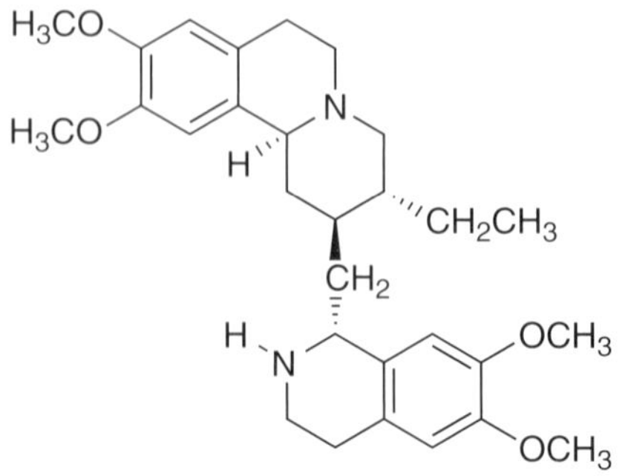

COUGH SUPPRESSANTS

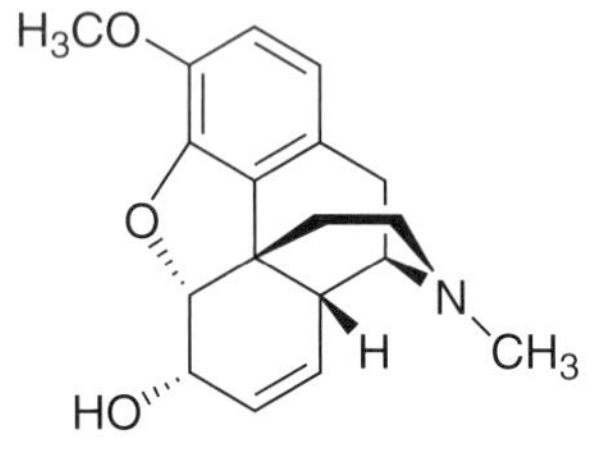

Cough is a reflex action and a symptom of other diseases such as asthma and colds due to 'nasal drip'. It is also an adverse reaction to some classes of drugs. Cough suppressants may be useful in some

Fig. 21.6 Emetine.

Fig. 21.7 Codeine.

instances, but they are not recommended for children who are highly susceptible to respiratory depression caused by opiates. Codeine and semisynthetic opiates such as dextromethorphan are the most common antitussives.

Codeine†

Codeine (Fig. 21.7) from the opium poppy (*Papaver somniferum* L.) is occasionally used to treat cough, formulated as a linctus or pastille, but in much lower doses than for diarrhoea and pain (see chapters 18 and 22). The dose for treating diarrhoea or pain is much higher. Although used widely, its efficacy is not supported by clinical research. Codeine is sedating and constipating and in large doses causes respiratory depression. As it is liable to abuse, codeine is available only on prescription in many countries.

HERBAL MEDICINES USED IN COLDS AND INFLUENZA—DEMULCENTS AND EMOLLIENTS

Medicinal plants used to treat colds and flu have antiviral, anti-inflammatory, demulcent or immunomodulating effects, and many have several of these properties. They are often used in combination, as herbal teas, for the supportive therapy of respiratory disease, and are usually pleasant. Herbs rich in mucilage are also used for respiratory conditions, for example, the lichen 'Icelandic Moss' from *Cetraria islandica* (L.) Ach. (Parmeliaceae).

Coltsfoot, *Tussilago farfara* L.

Coltsfoot (Asteraceae) is a common wild plant in Britain and Europe, growing in damp places. The bright yellow flowers appear in early spring before the leaves. The leaves are hoof-shaped, with angular teeth on the margins, green above and coated with matted, long white hairs on the lower surface. Both the leaves and flowers have been used medicinally.

Constituents

The main active constituent is a mucilage composed of acidic polysaccharides, together with flavonoids, triterpenes and sterols. Pyrrolizidine alkaloids, including senkirkine, tussilagine and isotussilagine, may be present in variable amounts, usually minor (about 0.015%) or absent, depending on source.

Therapeutic Uses and Available Evidence

Coltsfoot is used for irritating or spasmodic coughs, whooping cough, bronchitis, laryngitis and asthma. The polysaccharides are antiinflammatory, immunostimulant and demulcent, and the flavonoids have antiinflammatory and antispasmodic action. The pyrrolizidine alkaloids cause hepatotoxicity in rats fed daily on high doses, but not on low-dose regimens, and appear not to cause damage to human chromosomes in vitro. However, until further evidence is available, coltsfoot is not suitable for self-medication.

Elderflower and Elderberry (Fruit), *Sambucus nigra* L.†

Sambucus nigra (Viburnaceae), the black or European elder, is one of the most popular herbal medicines for the treatment of upper respiratory viral infections. Elder is a common European hedge tree or shrub. The flowers appear in May as small, creamy-white, flat-topped umbel-like clusters and are followed by small, shiny, purplish-black berries. Most parts of the plant are used, but most commonly the flowers and berries, which are used to make refreshing drinks and country-style wines, and cordials which are taken medicinally for their reputed antioxidant and antiviral properties. Related species such as (e.g. Danewort, *S. ebulus* L.) are also used but are more toxic.

Constituents

Flowers. The active constituents are triterpenes, including ursolic and oleanolic acid derivatives; flavonoids, mainly quercetin and chlorogenic acid derivatives, with naringenin as the major compound; and a small amount of essential oil.

Fruit. The berries contain cyanidin-3-*O*-sambubuioside, cyanidin-3-osambubioside-5-*O*-glucoside and their coumaroyl derivatives; other constituents include flavonol glycosides of rutin, kaempferol, and isorhamnetin and caffeoylquinic acid derivatives.

Therapeutic Uses and Available Evidence

Elder flowers are used as an infusion or herbal tea, and a mixture with peppermint is a traditional remedy for colds and influenza. They induce perspiration, which is thought to be beneficial in such cases. In vitro activity has been shown against several strains of influenza virus. The usual dose is about 3 g of flowers infused with 150 mL of hot water but is not critical. Elder flowers are nontoxic, and no side effects have been reported.

Elderberries

A reduction in the duration of flu symptoms and for other viral infections has been reported for elderberry preparations, and there is preclinical evidence supporting their potential use and safety for the adjunctive treatment of coronavirus. The effects are attributed to an increase in inflammatory cytokine production as well as a direct antiviral action.

The berries should not be eaten raw as they contain lectins, which can cause gastrointestinal disturbances, but which are destroyed by heat.

Linden Flowers, *Tilia* spp.†

Linden flowers (also called 'lime flowers' though not related to lime fruit) are from *Tilia rubra* DC., *T. cordata* Mill., *T.* × *europaea* L. and their hybrids (Tiliaceae), ornamental trees native to Europe. The pedicel bears three to six yellowish-white, five-petalled, fragrant flowers on stalks half-joined to an oblong bract.

Constituents

The flowers contain low levels of essential oil (containing linalool, germacrene, geraniol, 1,8-cineole, 2-phenyl ethanol and others); flavonoids (hesperidin, quercetin, astragalin, tiliroside); a mucilage of arabinose, galactose and rhamnose polysaccharides; polyphenolics such as chlorogenic and caffeic acids; and GABA (γ-aminobenzoic acid).

Therapeutic Uses and Available Evidence

Linden flowers are used for feverish colds, catarrh, coughs and influenza. They are used as herbal teas to induce diaphoresis (perspiration), as with elder flowers. The polysaccharides are soothing and adhere to epithelial tissue, producing a demulcent effect. The other main use of the flowers is for nervous disorders; the extract is thought to act as an agonist for the peripheral benzodiazepine receptor. Mild sedative effects have been shown in mice. Linden flowers are nontoxic and no side effects have been reported.

Mallow Flower and Leaves, *Malva sylvestris* L.†

The common mallow (*Malva sylvestris*, Malvaceae) is a wild plant indigenous to southern Europe but naturalised worldwide. The leaves are downy, with 5–7 lobes, and prominent veins on the under surface. The flowers are mauve, with darker veins; both are used medicinally.

Constituents

The main constituents are mucilages, sulfated flavonol glycosides such as gossypin-3-sulfate, hypolaetinglucoside-3'-sulfate and others, and anthocyanins (malvin, the diglucoside of malvidin, and delphinidin).

Therapeutic Uses and Available Evidence

Mallow is a demulcent. An infusion is used for colds and coughs, and the mucilage from the leaves is antiinflammatory with anticomplement activity. Little clinical evidence is available but there is a long tradition of historical use. No adverse effects are known.

Marshmallow Leaf and Root, *Althea officinalis* L.†

Both the leaves and the rootstock of the marshmallow (Malvaceae) are used as a demulcent, expectorant and emollient. The plant is a downy perennial reaching up to 2 m in height with leaves broadly ovate or cordate, 10–20 cm long and about 10 cm wide, with three to seven rounded lobes, palmate veins and a crenate margin. The flowers are pink, five-petalled, and up to 3 cm in diameter. The root is fibrous, cream-white when peeled, and deeply furrowed longitudinally.

Constituents

Both rootstock and leaves are rich in mucilage, consisting of polysaccharides composed of L-rhamnose, D-galactose, D-galacturonic acid and D-glucuronic acid and others. It also contains common flavonoids, especially derivatives of kaempferol and quercetin.

Therapeutic Uses and Available Evidence

Both the leaves and root are used internally for coughs and bronchial complaints and for gastric and urinary inflammation including cystitis. They may be applied externally as a soothing poultice and to aid wound healing. The mucilages have demonstrated biological activity, including the stimulation of phagocytosis in vitro, and antimicrobial and antiinflammatory activities. Polysaccharides isolated from the roots have been found to have antitussive activity. The most common use of extracts of marshmallow root is in the making of confectionery.

GENERAL HERBAL MEDICINES USED IN COLDS AND INFLUENZA—ANTIINFECTIVE AGENTS

Pelargonium, *Pelargonium sidoides* DC. and *P. reniforme* (Andrews) Curtis†

The tubers, stems and root of two southern African species of *Pelargonium*, *P. sidoides* and *P. reniforme* (Geraniaceae) have been used for centuries to treat a range of infectious conditions. The herbal medicine prepared from them is widely known as 'Umckaloabo', a fusion of two Zulu terms, 'Umkuhlune' = coughing and fever, and 'Uhlabo' = chest pains.

Constituents

The main active components are hydrolysable tannins, (+)-catechin, gallic acid and methyl gallate, including a unique series of *O*-galloyl-*C*-glucosylflavones. Flavonoids including myricetin and quercetin-3-*O*-beta-D-glucoside, coumarins including scopoletin and umckalin, are present in both species. A series of benzopyranones has been isolated from *P. sidoides*. Pelargoniins (a type of ellagitannin) and a diterpene, reniformin, have been identified in *P. reniforme*.

Therapeutic Uses and Available Evidence

In several European countries, a standardised extract of *P. sidoides* (EPs 7630, known as Umckaloabo, and Kaloba) is registered for the indication 'acute bronchitis', and as an adjunctive treatment for chronic obstructive pulmonary disease (COPD). Systematic reviews assessing the efficacy of *P. sidoides* preparations in acute respiratory infections provide some evidence that EPs 7630 may be effective in alleviating symptoms in adults and children, but concerns about the quality of some studies remain. The extract is safe and well tolerated. EPs 7630 has been shown in vitro to interfere with the replication of respiratory viruses including seasonal influenza A, respiratory syncytial virus, coronavirus and coxsackie virus. There is some clinical evidence for the efficacy of EPs 7630 in other viral respiratory infections, with preliminary data on human coronavirus.

Other contributory mechanisms include the modulation of immunological responses through an increase in monocyte-related, and a decrease in neutrophil-related, chemokines; and by increasing the frequency of ciliary beats, thus helping to remove pathogens. Extracts of *Pelargonium* species inhibit the adherence of bacteria mucous membrane.

EPs 7630 extract is given to athletes to help strengthen their immune systems, which can be compromised by extreme exercise, and to protect against colds. Athletes submitted to intense physical activity found the extract increased the production of immunoglobulin A in saliva, and decreased levels of interleukin-15 and interleukin-6 in serum, suggesting a modulation of the immune response associated with the upper airway mucosa.

IMMUNOSTIMULANTS

Immune stimulation is usually measured using parameters such as an increase in numbers of circulating immune cells, or enhanced phagocytosis after inoculation with a pathogen. It is notoriously difficult to substantiate claims for the prevention of disease, since very large clinical studies are needed for statistical validity, and these are difficult and expensive to perform. Echinacea, astragalus and andrographis are widely used for the treatment of upper respiratory diseases, with evidence to support some of their claims.

Echinacea, *Echinacea pallida* (Nutt.) Nutt., *E. purpurea* (L.) Moench and *E. angustifolia* DC.†

Members of the genus *Echinacea* (Asteraceae) are widely distributed in North America and have a long tradition of use, both by the Indigenous peoples and the settlers, who developed the first commercial preparations during the 19th century. Both aerial parts and secondary roots are used, and juice of *E. purpurea*, expressed from the fresh herb, is also used. The three species are used as immunostimulants to treat and prevent colds and other respiratory infections. The complex situation regarding species, part of plant used and method of production makes clinical efficacy difficult to assess. Echinacea is often combined with garlic, for the treatment of colds and allergic rhinitis.

Constituents

The alkylamides are considered to be the most relevant immune modulating compounds, although polysaccharides and caffeic acid derivative are also present, and contribute to the overall therapeutic effect. The alkylamides are a complex mixture of unsaturated fatty acid derivatives with a diene, diyne or tetraene structure linked via an esteramide bond to a (2)-methylpropane or (2)-methylbutane residue. They are found throughout the plant in all three species. The caffeic acid derivatives, including echinacoside (Fig. 21.8) (*E. pallida* root) and cichoric acid (*E. purpurea* aerial parts) are found in many medicinal plants and can serve as quality markers.

Therapeutic Uses and Available Evidence

Echinacea preparations are used to relieve the symptoms of the common cold and influenza-type infections. Meta-analyses show that *Echinacea* preparations appear to be efficacious both therapeutically (reducing symptoms and duration) and in terms of prophylaxis against the common cold, and are safe. However, *Echinacea* preparations tested in clinical trials differ greatly. A mechanism of action has been postulated, suggesting that the alkylamides bind to the cannabinoid-2- (CB2) receptor to exert antiinflammatory and immune-modulatory effects. Alkylamides inhibit LPS-induced inflammation and exert modulatory effects on cytokine expression, but these effects are not exclusively related to CB2 binding.

Echinacea appears to be safe, although allergic reactions have been reported. The risk of drug interactions is low.

Astragalus, *Astragalus mongholicus* Bunge†

Astragalus mongholicus (syn.: *Astragalus membranaceus* (Fisch.) ex Bunge, Fabaceae) is a herbaceous perennial native to north-eastern China, central Mongolia and Siberia. The root is known in Chinese medicine as Huang qi. The use of *Astragalus* root, as a general tonic, dates back to the legendary Chinese emperor Shen-Nong. The root consists of a long cylindrical tap root, which is internally yellowish in colour, with the rootlets removed.

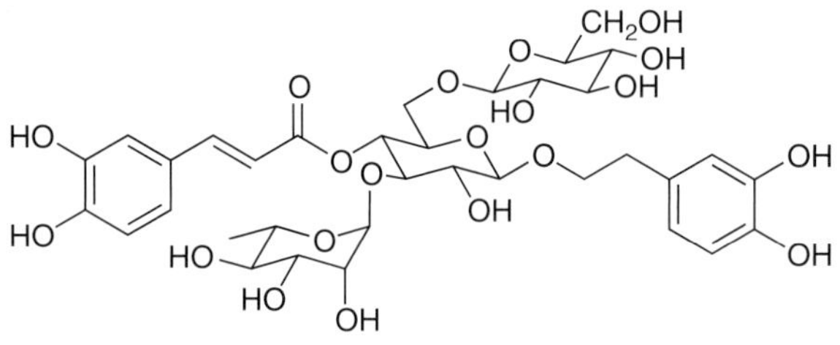

Fig. 21.8 Echinacoside.

Constituents

Triterpenoid saponins, the astragalosides I–VIII, and their acetyl derivatives, agroastragalosides I–IV, astramembranins I and II and others; isoflavones including formononetin and kumatakenin, and polysaccharides known as astrogalactoglucans.

Therapeutic Uses and Available Evidence

Overall, there is anecdotal evidence that astragalus alone and in combination may help in the treatment of the common cold or for impaired immunity. Clinical studies, supported by data from over 1000 patients in China, support the use of astragalus as an immunostimulant for use in colds and upper respiratory infections. It is also used prophylactically. Antiinflammatory effects have been shown to be modulated via inflammatory mediators and the MAPK signalling pathway, resulting in the inactivation of NF-κB, and immunomodulation has been demonstrated in a wide range of in vitro and in vivo models.

In general, astragalus is well tolerated, and there is little data showing toxicity. Some authorities recommend avoiding in autoimmune diseases, but drug interactions with immunosuppressant drugs such as ciclosporin and tacrolimus have not been reported.

Andrographis, *Andrographis paniculata* (Burm. f.) Wall†

Andrographis paniculata (Acanthaceae), also known as 'green chiretta', is an erect annual herb found in many regions of Asia. It is extremely bitter in taste and has been referred to as the 'king of bitters'. It is important in Ayurveda where it is known as 'kalmegh' and in Thai and other Asian traditional medical systems.

Constituents

The main actives are diterpenes, andrographolide and its analogues, neoandrographolide, isoandrographolide and many others. Flavonoids and polyphenols such as 7-*O*-methylwogonin, apigenin, onysilin and 3,4-dicaffeoylquinic acid are present; an alkaloid, andrographine and sesquiterpene lactones, paniculides A, B and C, have been isolated from the root.

Therapeutic Uses and Available Evidence

Andrographis and its preparations are used to treat a range of respiratory tract infections. *A. paniculata* (both alone or plus usual care) has been shown to improve overall symptoms of acute respiratory tract infections when compared to placebo, usual care, and other herbal therapies, with no major adverse events recorded.

Andrographis is a promising drug used to treat viral infection, although there is insufficient evidence to decide whether this includes coronavirus infections specifically, but the Thai government has allowed its trial use in state hospitals based on the pharmacological profile extracts and andrographolide.

Andrographolide has been shown to have immunostimulatory activity, shown by an increase in proliferation of lymphocytes and production of interleukin-2, and anti-inflammatory activity has been demonstrated by an inhibition of NF-κB, nitric oxide, PGE2, IL-1β, IL-6, LTB4, TXB2 and histamine.

Based on systematic reviews, the herbal extract alone (or in combination with *Eleutherococcus*) may be an appropriate treatment for uncomplicated acute upper respiratory tract infection, having significant drying effect on the nasal secretions of cold sufferers, with a very low level of serious adverse events with an overall good safety profile.

FURTHER READING

Auyeung, K.K., Han, Q.-B., Ko, J.K., 2016. *Astragalus membranaceus*: a review of its protection against inflammation and gastrointestinal cancers. Am. J. Chin. Med. 44, 1–22.

Blosa, M., Uricher, J., Nebel, S., Zahner, C., Butterweck, V., Drewe, J., 2021. Treatment of early allergic and late inflammatory symptoms of allergic rhinitis with *Petasites hybridus* leaf extract (Ze 339): results of a noninterventional observational study in Switzerland. Pharmaceuticals 14, 180. https://doi.org/10.3390/ph14030180.

Brendler, T., Al-Harrasi, A., Bauer, R., Gafner, S., Hardy, M.L., Heinrich, M., et al., 2021. Botanical drugs and supplements affecting the immune response in the time of COVID-19: implications for research and clinical practice. Phytother. Res. 35 (6), 3013–3031. https://doi.org/10.1002/ptr.7008.

Chen, Z., Liu, L.J., Gao, C., Vong, C.T., Yao, P., Yang, Y., et al., 2020. Astragali Radix (Huangqi): a promising edible immunomodulatory herbal medicine. J. Ethnopharmacol. 258, 112895. https://doi.org/10.1016/j.jep.2020.112895.

David, S., Cunningham, R., 2019. Echinacea for the prevention and treatment of upper respiratory tract infections: a systematic review and meta-analysis. Complement. Ther. Med. 44, 18–26. https://doi.org/10.1016/j.ctim.2019.03.011.

EFSA (EFSA Panel on Food Additives and Nutrient Sources), 2013. Scientific opinion on safety evaluation of *Ephedra* species in food. EFSA J. 11 (11), 3467. https://doi.org/10.2903/j.efsa.2013.3467.

EMA (European Medicines Agency), 2018. Assessment Report on *Pelargonium sidoides* DC and/or *Pelargonium reniforme* Curt., Radix. Committee on Herbal Medicinal Products (HMPC). EMA/HMPC/444251/2015.

Fazio, S., Pouso, J., Dolinsky, D., Fernandez, A., Hernandez, M., Clavier, G., et al., 2009. Tolerance, safety and efficacy of *Hedera helix* extract in inflammatory bronchial diseases under clinical practice conditions: a prospective, open, multicentre postmarketing study in 9657 patients. Phytomedicine 16, 17–24.

Ferreira-Santos, P., Badim, H., Salvador, Â.C., Silvestre, A.J., Santos, S.A., Rocha, S.M., et al., 2021. Chemical characterization of *Sambucus nigra* L. flowers aqueous extract and its biological implications. Biomolecules 11, 1222.

Harnetta, J., Oakes, K., Carè, J., Leache, M., Brown, D., Brown, D., Cramer, H., et al., 2020. The effects of *Sambucus nigra* berry on acute respiratory viral infections: a rapid review of clinical studies. Adv. Integrat. Med. 7, 240–246.

Hu, X.Y., Wu, R.H., Logue, M., Blondel, C., Lai, L.Y.W., Stuart, B., et al., 2017. *Andrographis paniculata* (Chuān Xīn LiáÂn) for symptomatic relief of acute respiratory tract infections in adults and children: a systematic review and meta-analysis. PLoS One 12 (8), e0181780. https://doi.org/10.1371/journal.pone.0181780.

Jabbari, M., Daneshfard, B., Emtiazy, M., Khiveh, A., Hashempur, M.H., 2017. Biological effects and clinical applications of dwarf elder (*Sambucus ebulus* L.). Rev. J. Evid. Based Complementary Altern. Med. 22 (4), 996–1001.

Jia, W., Gao, W., 2003. Is traditional Chinese medicine useful in the treatment of SARS? Phytother. Res. 17, 840–841.

Keck, T., Strobl, A., Weinhaeusel, A., Funk, P., Michaelis, M., 2021. Pelargonium extract EPs 7630 in the treatment of human corona virus-associated acute respiratory tract infections – a secondary subgroup-analysis of an open-label, uncontrolled clinical trial. Front. Pharmacol. 12, 666546. https://doi.org/10.3389/fphar.2021.666546.

Koncz, D., Tóth, B., Roza, O., Csupor, D., 2021. A systematic review of the European Rapid Alert System for Food and Feed: tendencies in illegal food supplements for weight loss. Front. Pharmacol. 11, 611361. https://doi.org/10.3389/fphar.2020.611361.

Lang, C., Röttger-Lüer, P., Staiger, C., 2015. A valuable option for the treatment of respiratory diseases: review on the clinical evidence of the ivy leaves dry extract EA 575®. Planta Med. 81, 968–974.

Luna Jr., L.A., Bachi, A.L., Novacs c Brito, R.R., Eid, R.G., Suguri, V.M., Oliveira, P.W., et al., 2011. Immune responses induced by *Pelargonium sidoides* extract in serum and nasal mucosa of athletes after exhaustive exercise: modulation of secretory IgA, IL-6 and IL-15. Phytomedicine 18, 303–308.

Marchese, A., Orhan, I.E., Daglia, M., Barbieri, R., Di Lorenzo, A., Nabavi, S.F., et al., 2016. Antibacterial and antifungal activities of thymol: a brief review of the literature. Food Chem. 210, 402–414. https://doi.org/10.1016/j.foodchem.2016.04.111.

Merarchi, M., Dudha, N., Das, B.C., Garg, M., 2021. Natural products and phytochemicals as potential anti-SARS-CoV-2 drugs. Phytother. Res. 35 (10), 5384–5396.

Mikulic-Petkovsek, M., Samoticha, J., Eler, K., Stampar, F., Veberic, R., 2015. Traditional elderflower beverages: a rich source of phenolic compounds with high antioxidant activity. J. Agric. Food Chem. 63, 1477–1487.

Perić, A., Kovačević, S.V., Barać, A., Gaćeša, D., Perić, A.V., Vojvodić, D., 2020. Effects of *Pelargonium sidoides* extract on chemokine levels in nasal secretions of patients with non-purulent acute rhinosinusitis. J. Drug Assess. 9 (1), 145–150. https://doi.org/10.1080/21556660.2020.1838176.

Porter, R.S., Bode, R.F., 2017. A review of the antiviral properties of black elder (*Sambucus nigra* L.) products. Phytother. Res. 31, 533–554. https://doi.org/10.1002/ptr.5782.

Sa-Ngiamsuntorn, K., Suksatu, A., Pewklian, P., Thongsri, P., Kanjanasirirat, P., Manopwisedjaroen, S., et al., 2021. Anti-SARS-CoV-2 activity of *Andrographis paniculata* extract and its major component andrographolide in human lung epithelial cells and cytotoxicity evaluation in major organ cell representatives. J. Nat. Prod. 84, 1261–1270.

Sierocinski, E., Holzinger, F., Chenot, J.F., 2021. Ivy leaf (*Hedera helix*) for acute upper respiratory tract infections: an updated systematic review. Eur. J. Clin. Pharmacol. 77, 1113–1122. https://doi.org/10.1007/s00228-021-03090-4.

Silveira, D., Prieto-Garcia, J.M., Boylan, F., Estrada, O., Fonseca-Bazzo, Y.M., Jamal, C.M., et al., 2020. COVID-19: is there evidence for the use of herbal medicines as adjuvant symptomatic therapy? Front. Pharmacol. 11, 1479. https://doi.org/10.3389/fphar.2020.581840.

Song, W.J., Chung, K.F., 2020. Pharmacotherapeutic options for chronic refractory cough. Exp. Opin. Pharmacother. 21, 1345–1358.

Stolz, D., Barandun, J., Borer, H., Bridevaux, P.O., Brun, P., Brutsche, M., et al., 2018. Diagnosis, prevention and treatment of stable COPD and acute exacerbations of COPD: the Swiss Recommendations. Respiration 96 (4), 382–398. https://doi.org/10.1159/000490551.

Tiboc Schnell, C.N., Filip, G.A., Decea, N., Moldovan, R., Opris, R., Man, S.C., et al., 2021. The impact of *Sambucus nigra* L. extract on inflammation, oxidative stress and tissue remodeling in a rat model of lipopolysaccharide-induced subacute rhinosinusitis. Inflammopharmacology 29 (3), 753–769. https://doi.org/10.1007/s10787-021-00805-y.

Timmer, A., Günther, J., Motschall, E., Rücker, G., Antes, G., Kern, W.V., 2013. *Pelargonium sidoides* extract for treating acute respiratory tract infections. Cochrane Database Syst. Rev. 10, CD006323.

WHO, 2021. Key Technical Issues of Herbal Medicines with Reference to Interaction with Other Medicines. World Health Organization, Geneva.

Willcox, M., Simpson, C., Wilding, S., Stuart, B., Soilemezi, D., Whitehead, A., et al., 2021. *Pelargonium sidoides* root extract for the treatment of acute cough due to lower respiratory tract infection in adults: a feasibility double-blind, placebo-controlled randomised trial. BMC Complement Med. Therap. 21, 48. https://doi.org/10.1186/s12906-021-03206-4.

Worakunphanich, W., Thavorncharoensap, M., Youngkong, S., Thadanipon, K., Thakkinstian, A., 2021. Safety of *Andrographis paniculata*: a systematic review and meta-analysis. Pharmacoepidemiol. Drug Saf. 30, 727–739.

Zhang, B.M., Wang, Z.B., Xin, P., Wang, Q.H., Bu, H., Kuang, H.X., 2018. Phytochemistry and pharmacology of genus *Ephedra*. Chin. J. Nat. Med. 16 (11), 811–828.

22

The Central Nervous System

Drugs acting on the central nervous system (CNS) include the centrally acting (mainly opioid) analgesics, antiepileptics, anti-Parkinson agents, and for treating psychiatric and mood disorders, anxiety and insomnia. Plant-derived drugs are important in these, although not usually for self-medication. They are also of historical interest; for example, the antipsychotic drug reserpine, isolated from *Rauvolfia* species, revolutionised the treatment of schizophrenia and enabled many patients to avoid hospitalisation before the introduction of the phenothiazines (such as chlorpromazine) and the newer atypical antipsychotics (olanzapine, quetiapine and risperidone). Unfortunately, reserpine depletes neurotransmitter concentrations in the brain (it is used as a pharmacological tool in neuroscience for this purpose) and can cause severe depression. There are no currently useful antipsychotics obtained from plants, and most antiepileptics are synthetic, with the exception of cannabidiol (CBD), from *Cannabis sativa*, which is licensed for the treatment of some severe forms of childhood epilepsy and is discussed later.

Phytotherapy can however provide useful support for milder conditions. The prevalence of depression and anxiety in the general population is around one in six people, and around 40% of people with mental health problems will have symptoms of both anxiety and depression. Sleep disturbances, such as insomnia and early morning awakening, are characteristic of depression and anxiety, although they can also occur independently. Around one-third of adults will experience insomnia at some time, and most do not seek treatment from a physician. In such cases, phytotherapy may help to re-establish a regular pattern of sleep.

Migraine is a common disorder and can be severely debilitating. Opioid analgesics may be used, and the synthetic 5-HT$_1$ (5-hydroxytryptamine) antagonists (sumatriptan, rizatriptan, zolmitriptan and others) are highly effective in acute migraine, and ergotamine is a potent drug which is used as a last resort in severe attacks of migraine. Prophylaxis is usually with β-blockers such as propranolol, although low-dose anticonvulsants and antidepressants may be effective. Feverfew and butterbur have been traditionally used to prevent migraine attacks and are discussed later.

In dementia and Alzheimer disease, natural compounds play a role in symptomatic treatment. Galantamine (from the snowdrop, *Galanthus nivalis*) and derivatives of physostigmine (e.g. rivastigmine) are cholinesterase inhibitors. Some plant extracts, such as sage and rosemary, have reputedly similar, but milder, effects in memory improvement. *Ginkgo biloba* has cognition-enhancing properties and is used in mild forms of dementia.

HYPNOTICS AND SEDATIVES

Plant species used as herbal sedatives and/or hypnotics are not as potent as synthetic drugs (with the exception of tropane and opium alkaloids) but, as with synthetic hypnotics, are generally intended for short-term use.

Hops, *Humulus lupulus* L.†

Humulus lupulus (Cannabaceae), often referred to by its common name of hops, has been used traditionally for insomnia, neuralgia and excitability. It is cultivated in many temperate countries for fermenting into beers and vinegars. The parts of the plant used medicinally are the female flower heads (composed of overlapping bracts, which enclose the ovary) known as strobiles, and the detached resinous glandular trichomes, known as lupulin. Hops have a highly characteristic odour and bitter taste.

Constituents

The main active constituents of hops are the bitter principles found in the oleoresin. These include the α-acid humulone and the β-acid lupulone, and their degradation products, such as 2-methyl-3-buten-2-ol (Fig. 22.1). Other constituents include flavonoids, chalcones, tannins and volatile oils.

Therapeutic Uses and Available Evidence

Modern indications for hops include sleep disturbances and restlessness. Sedative and hypnotic activities have been documented in vivo (mice) for extract of hops, and clinical studies provide some evidence of the hypnotic effects of hops given in combination with valerian. Hops are nontoxic, as their use in beer would suggest. Cheers!

Lemon Balm, *Melissa officinalis* L.†

The leaves of *Melissa officinalis* (syn.: melissa, balm and 'sweet balm', Lamiaceae) are used traditionally for its sedative effects, as well as for gastrointestinal disorders. The extract has antiviral properties when applied externally.

Constituents

The volatile oil of melissa contains mainly monoterpenes, particularly aldehydes (e.g. citronellal, geranial and neral) and sesquiterpenes (e.g. β-caryophyllene). Flavonoids, including quercetin, apigenin and kaempferol, and polyphenols (e.g. hydroxycinnamic acid derivatives) are also present in the herb. Melissa, as specified in the European Pharmacopoeia (Eur. Ph.), contains not less than 4.0% of total hydroxycinnamic derivatives, expressed as rosmarinic acid, in the dried herb.

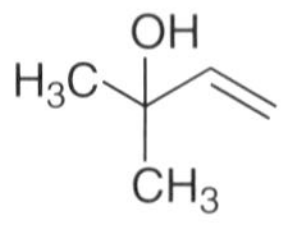

Fig. 22.1 2-Methyl-3-buten-2-ol.

Therapeutic Uses and Available Evidence

Sedative and antispasmodic effects have been documented for melissa extracts using in vivo studies (mice, rats). It is used for nervous or sleeping disorders and functional gastrointestinal complaints. There has been little investigation of the sedative effects of melissa alone in individuals with sleeping disorders, but clinical trials of melissa in combination with other herbal sedatives (e.g. valerian and hops) have provided some supportive evidence. Lemon balm is usually taken in the form of a herbal tea. Melissa extracts are also applied topically in cases of herpes simplex resulting from Herpes simplex virus type 1 (HSV-1) infection (see Antimicrobial Natural Products).

Lemon balm is regarded as nontoxic, although it should not be taken excessively due to its reputed antithyroid activity.

Kava, *Piper methysticum* G. Forst.

Piper methysticum G. Forst (Piperaceae), known by the common names kava-kava or kawa, has been used in the Pacific Islands, notably Fiji, for hundreds of years. It is a small shrub with heart-shaped leaves and thick, woody roots and rhizomes, which are ground or chewed to release the actives. These are then fermented to make the ceremonial drink kava, which induces a relaxed sociable state, and is given to visiting dignitaries.

Kava is used medicinally for its tranquillising properties and kava phytomedicines, based on a solvent extract, were popular until hepatotoxic effects associated with kava use led to a widespread prohibition of kava products in the early 2000s. This was later revoked but damage to the reputation and sales of kava remains.

Constituents

The main constituents of kava are the kavalactones (also known as kavapyrones), including kavain, dihydrokavain, methysticin, yangonin and desmethoxyyangonin.

Therapeutic Uses and Available Evidence

Preclinical studies indicate that kava extracts potentiate gamma-aminobutyric acid type A (GABA$_A$) receptor activity, and their efficacy in relieving anxiety and depression is supported by data from randomised controlled trials. There are conflicting views as to whether poor-quality kava raw material is involved in the reported toxicity, whether there are toxic constituents or metabolites, and if there is a pharmacogenomic component to the toxicity.

Passionflower, *Passiflora incarnata* L.†

Passionflower (*Passiflora incarnata*, Passifloraceae), also known as passiflora and maypop, is a vine native to South America, but now grown worldwide. The flower shows a distinctive shape of a cross and the name passion refers to Christian connotations rather than romantic. The herb, consisting of the dried leaf and flower, is used medicinally. The edible passion fruit is from *P. edulis* Sims.

Constituents

The main active constituents include the flavonoids, particularly chrysin and related compounds such as schaftoside, isoschaftoside, orientin, homoorientin, vitexin, isovitexin, kaempferol, luteolin, quercetin, rutin, saponaretin and saponarin. Alkaloids of the harman type

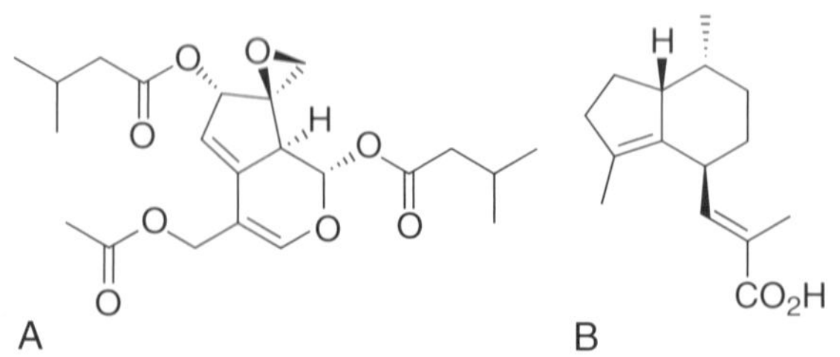

Fig. 22.2 A) Valtrate and B) Valerenic acid.

are present in low concentrations (the presence of harmine, harmaline, harmol and harmalol has been disputed) as well as β-carbolines. Passiflora Eur. Ph. contains not less than 1.5% of total flavonoids, expressed as vitexin.

P. edulis contains similar classes of compounds and cycloartane triterpenoids, such as the cyclopassifloic acids and cyclopassiflosides.

Therapeutic Uses and Available Evidence

The historical uses of passionflower herb include treatment of insomnia, hysteria, nervous tachycardia and neuralgia. Modern uses include restlessness and insomnia due to nervous tension. In the UK, products authorised under the Traditional Herbal Medicinal Products Directive (THMPD) containing passionflower are indicated for the temporary relief of symptoms associated with stress, such as mild anxiety, based on traditional use only.

Preclinical studies have shown sedative and anxiolytic activity for extracts and certain constituents. Modulation of the GABA system is involved in the anxiolytic effects and sedative properties are attributed at least in part to the flavonoid, particularly chrysin, content. There are few clinical studies of passiflora, and systematic reviews have reported that there is insufficient evidence to draw definitive conclusions regarding its effects in anxiety. Generally, passiflora is well tolerated with few side effects; however, there are isolated case reports of nausea and tachycardia.

Valerian, *Valeriana officinalis* L.†

Valeriana officinalis (Caprifoliaceae), commonly known as valerian, all-heal, and many other names, is among the most well documented of all medicinal plants, particularly in northern Europe. It is widely cultivated. Related species of *Valeriana* are used in Asia for similar indications; valerian has a long history of traditional use in the treatment of conditions involving nervous excitability and insomnia. The herbal drug comprises the root and rhizome, which are yellowish-grey to pale greyish-brown. It has a characteristic smell which is usually described as unpleasant.

Constituents

The main components are the volatile oil and the iridoid valepotriate constituents. The volatile oil contains monoterpenes and sesquiterpenes, such as β-bisabolene, caryophyllene, valeranone, valerianol, valerenol, valerenal, valerenic acid and derivatives (Fig. 22.2). The valepotriate compounds include valtrate, didrovaltrate and isovaltrate. The valepotriates readily decompose on storage and processing, to form mainly baldrinal and homobaldrinal, which are also unstable. Valerian also contains alkaloids, including valerianine and valerine, and amino acids such as arginine, GABA, glutamine and tyrosine.

Therapeutic Uses and Available Evidence

In Europe, valerian preparations (tablets, tinctures) have been approved for the temporary relief of symptoms of mild anxiety and to aid sleep, generally based on traditional use evidence. In vivo studies (in mice) have demonstrated CNS-depressant activity for the volatile oil, the valepotriates and the valepotriate degradation products, particularly valerenal and valerenic acid, leading to increased concentrations of the inhibitory neurotransmitter GABA in the brain by inhibiting its catabolism, inhibiting uptake and/or by inducing GABA release. Increased GABA concentrations are associated with decreased CNS activity, which may at least partly explain the sedative effects.

Clinical trials have tested the effects of valerian preparations on subjective (e.g. sleep quality) and objective (e.g. sleep structure) sleep parameters, and on measures of stress. Some, but not all, of these studies provide evidence to support the traditional uses of valerian. Several preparations contain valerian root in combination with other herbs reputed to have hypnotic and/or sedative effects, such as hops (*Humulus lupulus*) and Melissa (*Melissa officinalis*).

Valerian preparations should not be taken before driving a car or operating machinery if drowsiness is experienced; also, the effect may be enhanced by alcohol consumption. There are isolated reports of hepatotoxicity associated with valerian-containing products, although causality has not been established, and gastrointestinal symptoms.

ANTIDEPRESSANTS

Saffron, *Crocus sativus* L.

Crocus sativus (Iridaceae), is a perennial herb indigenous to southwestern Asia and southern Europe and is cultivated in many other countries, particularly Iran, China and India. The flower produces drooping red stigmas, which, when dried, are used medicinally. Saffron has a range of traditional uses, including the treatment of abdominal pain and fever. Clinical research has explored the effects of saffron in depression, Alzheimer disease and other conditions. Saffron is used widely as a culinary spice and colouring agent.

Saffron is extremely expensive, due to the labour required for its collection: around 150,000 flowers are individually picked to produce 1 kg of the herb. The high price means it is a common target for adulteration, with other plant materials, synthetic dyes and fibres. Adulterants include petals from safflower (*Carthamus tinctorius* L.) and calendula (*Calendula officinalis* L.); powdered turmeric rhizomes *Curcuma longa* L.); and dye extracted from buddleia flowers (*Buddleja officinalis* Maxim.). 'Old' saffron material is also sometimes used as a 'bulking agent'.

Constituents

The major constituents are carotenoids, including crocins (e.g. crocin, a glucoside) and crocetin, safranal (a monoterpene), and picrocrocins (e.g. picrocrocin, a monoterpene glucoside); the vitamins riboflavin and thiamine are also present.

Therapeutic Uses and Available Evidence

The crocins, crocetin and safranal have antiinflammatory, immunomodulatory, antioxidant and antiplatelet effects and are thought to contribute to the antidepressant effect of saffron. Preclinical studies have shown serotonergic activity and anxiolytic effects.

A systematic review of trials involving patients diagnosed with major depressive disorder found that *C. sativus* was more effective than placebo and as effective as conventional antidepressant medicines when administered at doses of 30 mg/day for up to 8 weeks.

Although saffron is used in food, the quantity used is very small compared to the therapeutic dose, and investigation of its safety profile when used as a medicine is required. Saffron elicits toxic effects at daily doses of 5 g or higher (the stigmas from about 750 flowers), but the cost means that such doses are unlikely to be ingested, and for the same reason, its wider medicinal use may be limited.

St John's Wort, *Hypericum perforatum* L.†

The common name St John's wort is used for most species of the genus *Hypericum* (Hypericaceae). In Western countries, it usually refers to *Hypericum perforatum*, a herbaceous perennial plant native to Europe and Asia, though other species are used medicinally elsewhere. Herbal products containing St John's wort have been among the top-selling herbal preparations in recent years. The dried herb consists of the flowering tops, including leaves, unopened buds and flowers. It is commonly used to treat depression and anxiety.

Constituents

St John's wort contains a series of naphthodianthrones, which include hypericin and pseudohypericin, and prenylated phloroglucinols, such as hyperforin and adhyperforin. Initially, hypericin was considered to be the antidepressant constituent of St John's wort, although evidence has now emerged that hyperforin (Fig. 22.3) is also a major contributor to the antidepressant activity. St John's wort also contains other biologically active constituents, such as flavonoids, and an essential oil composed mainly of β-caryophyllene, caryophyllene oxide spathulenol, tetradecanol, viridiflorol, α- and β-pinene, and α- and β-selinene.

Therapeutic Uses and Available Evidence

St John's wort extracts inhibit synaptosomal uptake of the neurotransmitters, serotonin (5-HT), dopamine and noradrenaline (norepinephrine) and GABA, and may have dopaminergic activity and effects on cortisol, which may influence concentrations of relevant neurotransmitters. Evidence from randomised controlled trials indicates that St John's wort extracts are more effective than placebo, and as effective as certain conventional antidepressants, in the treatment of major depression. Generally, a few weeks' treatment

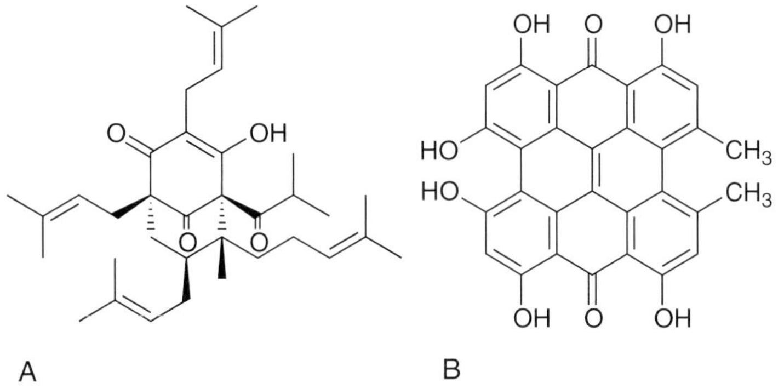

Fig. 22.3 A) Hyperforin and B) Hypericin.

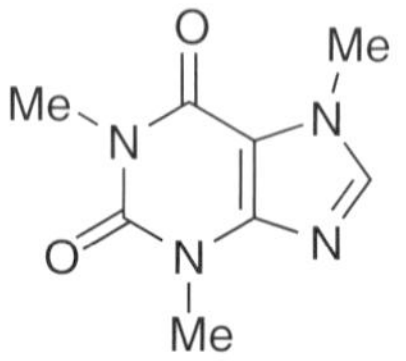

Fig. 22.4 Caffeine.

Fig. 22.5 Cocaine.

is required before marked improvement is seen and St John's wort is generally well tolerated when used at recommended doses for up to 12 weeks. Clinical trials of St John's wort indicate that it has a more favourable short-term safety profile than that of some conventional antidepressants. Adverse effects reported are usually mild, and include gastrointestinal symptoms, dizziness, confusion and tiredness and, rarely, photosensitivity (due to the hypericin content). However, constituents of St John's wort induce both cytochrome P450 drug-metabolising enzymes and P-glycoprotein (a drug transporter), and can interact with prescribed medicines including anticonvulsants, ciclosporin, digoxin, HIV protease inhibitors, oral contraceptives, selective serotonin reuptake inhibitors, tacrolimus, theophylline, triptans and warfarin. Patients taking these medicines with St John's wort should seek medical advice: in most cases, St John's wort treatment should be stopped, and dose adjustment of the prescribed medicines concerned may be necessary. Women taking St John's wort concurrently with an oral contraceptive should use additional contraceptive measures and it should not be used during pregnancy and lactation.

STIMULANTS

CNS stimulants are now rarely employed therapeutically, with the exception of caffeine, although they were historically used in the treatment of barbiturate poisoning (e.g. picrotoxin) or as a tonic (strychnine). Cola nut extract is used in many herbal tonics and, of course, soft drinks. Guarana is an ingredient of some 'energy' drinks and 'healthy' nutritional products. Both cola nut and guarana contain caffeine as the active constituent. Cocaine is rarely used medicinally, but its recreational use causes major health and other problems.

Caffeine†

Caffeine is a methylxanthine derivative found in tea, coffee and cocoa (Fig. 22.4). It is a mild stimulant, and is added to many analgesic preparations to enhance activity; there is some evidence from clinical trials to support this, though the mechanism is not well understood. High doses of caffeine may lead to gastric irritation, insomnia, a feeling of anxiety, diuresis, muscle tremors and tachycardia, among other symptoms, and can induce withdrawal syndrome following prolonged use.

Cola Nut, *Cola* spp.†

Cola, or kola nut (*Cola nitida* (Vent.) Schott & Endl., *Cola acuminata* (P. Beauv.) Schott & Endl., Malvaceae), is native to West Africa and extensively cultivated in the tropics, particularly Nigeria, Brazil and Indonesia. The seed is found in commerce as the dried, fleshy cotyledons, without the testa. They are red-brown in colour, convex on one side and flattened on the other, up to 5 cm long and about 2.5 cm in diameter. *C. acuminata* is generally smaller.

Cola contains the xanthine derivative caffeine (see Fig. 22.4), with traces of theobromine and theophylline. Tannins and phenolics, including catechin, epicatechin, kolatin, kolatein, kolanin, and amines, including dimethylamine, methylamine, ethylamine and isopentylamine, are also present, together with thiamine and other B vitamins.

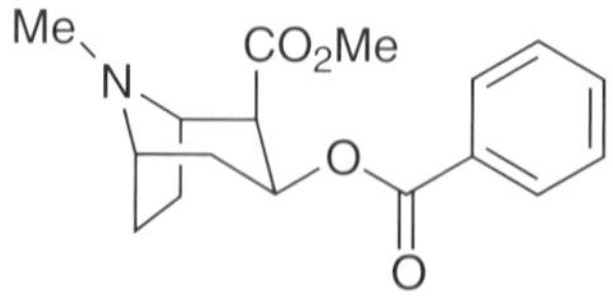

Caffeine is a mild stimulant and has diuretic properties; cola extracts are also astringent and antidiarrhoeal due to the tannin content. Cola extracts are an ingredient of many tonics for depression and tiredness, and to stimulate the appetite. Cola extract is safe, apart from any effects due to high doses of caffeine (see earlier).

Guarana, *Paullinia cupana* Kunth†

Guarana (Sapindaceae) is a vine indigenous to the Amazonian rainforest. The seeds are ground to a paste and used in cereal bars, or extracted and made into a stimulant drink. The effects are similar to those of cola (see earlier). The main active constituent is caffeine, which was formerly known as guaranine, and other methylxanthines; it also contains tannins. The stimulant properties of guarana are well-documented in preclinical studies and, to a lesser extent, clinical trials.

Cocaine†

Cocaine (Fig. 22.5) is a tropane alkaloid extracted from the leaf of coca, *Erythroxylum coca* Lam. and *E. novogranatense* (D. Morris) Hieron. (Erythroxylaceae). These shrubs grow at high altitudes in the South American Andes. The leaf was—and still is—traditionally chewed (along with lime to assist buccal absorption) to alleviate symptoms of altitude sickness and fatigue. Cocaine is rarely used medicinally, except as a local anaesthetic in eye surgery, and the supply and use of cocaine are strictly regulated in most countries.

Analgesics

Several types of analgesics are recognised: those that act via the CNS (the opioids), which will be discussed briefly here, the cannabinoids from *Cannabis sativa*, and the nonopiate and nonsteroidal anti-inflammatory drugs, such as the salicylates, which are covered in Chapter 23. It is very common for the two types to be used in combination, for example, aspirin with codeine. The opioid analgesics and their derivatives have never been surpassed as painkillers in efficacy or patient acceptability despite their disadvantages. They are obtained from the opium poppy (*Papaver somniferum*) and the most important are still the alkaloids morphine and codeine. Numerous derivatives, such as oxycodone, dihydrocodeine, fentanyl, buprenorphine and etorphine, have been developed that have different therapeutic and pharmacokinetic profiles, or can be administered via a different route (buccal tablets such as those containing buprenorphine, or transdermal patches, such as with fentanyl). Several of these are so potent that they have led to epidemics of addiction and deaths by overdose in many parts of the world.

Opium, *Papaver somniferum* L.†

The opium poppy (*Papaver somniferum*, Papaveraceae) is an annual that is native to Asia but cultivated widely for food (the seed and seed oil), for medicinal purposes, and as a garden ornamental. It has been used for centuries as a painkiller, sedative, cough suppressant and antidiarrhoeal, and features in many ancient medical texts, myths, legends and histories. The flowers vary in colour but are usually pale lilac with a purple base spot. The fruits, or capsules, are subspherical, depressed at the top with the radiating stigma in the centre, below which are the small valves through which the small, greyish, kidney-shaped seeds are dispersed. The latex, which exudes from the unripe capsule when scored, dries to form a tarry resin, raw opium. Originally, for pharmaceutical use, it was treated to form 'prepared opium', but the whole dried capsule (known as 'poppy straw') is more commonly used commercially to extract the alkaloids. The supply and use of these products are strictly regulated in most countries.

Poppy seeds are very widely used in cooking, especially breads and crackers, and to produce oil. These products may contain traces of opium alkaloids, but they are present in such small amounts that no pharmacological effects have been observed.

Constituents

Alkaloids represent about 10% of the dried latex or raw opium. The major alkaloid is morphine (Fig. 22.6), with codeine and thebaine and lesser amounts of many others including narceine, narcotine, papaverine, salutaridine, oripavine and sanguinarine.

Therapeutic Uses and Available Evidence

Opium has potent narcotic and analgesic properties. The total alkaloidal extract is known as 'papaveretum' and was formerly used for pre-operative analgesia and severe pain. Pain management now requires precise doses and sophisticated formulations for safety and efficacy, and only isolated opium alkaloids are used. Morphine is a very potent analgesic, used for severe pain in the short term (e.g. kidney stone), or for terminal illness, and is the starting material for the production of diamorphine (heroin). Codeine is less potent than morphine, although it is a very useful analgesic for moderate to severe pain, for example for migraine, dental and gynaecological pain. All the opioid analgesics have side effects, which include nausea, constipation and drowsiness; they cause respiratory depression and have a potential for dependence, which varies according to their capacity to induce euphoria. A withdrawal syndrome is common after prolonged administration, and especially after long-term addiction.

MIGRAINE

The aetiology of migraine is not fully known and various pharmacological approaches are used in its treatment. Analgesics, particularly codeine, can be used to relieve an attack, although their capacity to induce nausea can cause problems, and salicylates can cause stomach discomfort. The newer synthetic drugs sumatriptan, naratriptan and others are highly effective in acute attacks, and β-blockers and pizotifen taken regularly are used to prevent recurrences. If all else fails, ergotamine can be used in limited doses for acute attacks. Butterbur and feverfew have been investigated for migraine prophylaxis and are described later.

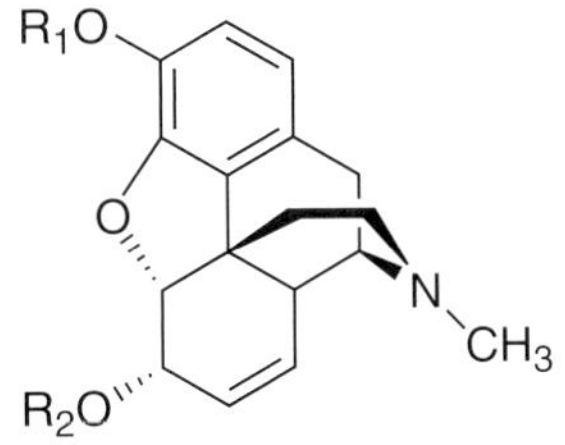

Ergotamine†

Ergotamine is an alkaloid extracted from ergot (*Claviceps purpurea*), a parasitic fungus that grows on cereals, usually rye. It can be used to treat severe migraine that cannot be controlled with other drugs, but it can cause severe adverse reactions and there are restrictions as to the maximum daily and weekly doses.

Feverfew, *Tanacetum parthenium* (L.) Sch. Bip.†

Feverfew (syn.: *Chrysanthemum parthenium* (L.) Bernh., Asteraceae) is a perennial reaching 60 cm, with a downy erect stem. It is a common garden plant and is a popular medicinal plant in many parts of the world, to treat rheumatism and menstrual problems. The aerial parts are used. The leaves are yellowish-green, alternate, stalked, ovate and pinnately divided with an entire or crenate margin. The flowers, which appear in June to August, are up to about 2 cm in diameter and arranged in corymbs of up to 30 heads, with white ray florets and yellow disc florets and downy involucral bracts.

Constituents

The sesquiterpene lactones are the active constituents, the major one being parthenolide (Fig. 22.7), with numerous others reported from the species (e.g. santamarine). It also contains small amounts of essential oil (0.02% to 0.07%), with α-pinene and derivatives, camphor and others.

Therapeutic Uses and Available Evidence

The main use of feverfew today is as a prophylactic and treatment for migraine. The fresh leaves may be eaten, usually with other foods to disguise the nauseous taste, or a standardised extract taken daily to prevent migraine attacks. Although some clinical studies have shown efficacy, others have not, and further work is needed to identify which extracts may be effective.

Feverfew extracts inhibit secretion of serotonin from platelet granules and proteins from polymorphonuclear leukocytes (PMNs). Since serotonin is implicated in the aetiology of migraine and PMN secretion is increased in rheumatoid arthritis, these findings substantiate the use of feverfew to some extent. Parthenolide is a potent inhibitor of NF-κB, and the sesquiterpene lactones as a class inhibit prostaglandin production and arachidonic acid release. This explains the antiplatelet and antifebrile actions to some extent, but feverfew extract with the parthenolide removed also has antiinflammatory activity. Feverfew may produce side effects such as dermatitis, and soreness or ulceration of the mouth. Contact dermatitis has been described in workers handling material from this species, caused by exposure to the allergenic sesquiterpene lactones.

Butterbur, *Petasites hybridus* (L.) G. Gaertn., B. Mey. & Schreb.

Butterbur is used in seasonal allergic rhinitis but has also been investigated clinically for its effects in migraine prophylaxis.

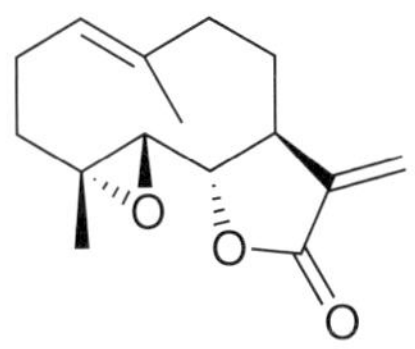

Fig. 22.6 Morphine (R$_1$ = R$_2$ = H) and codeine (R$_1$ = CH$_3$, R$_2$ = H).

Fig. 22.7 Parthenolide.

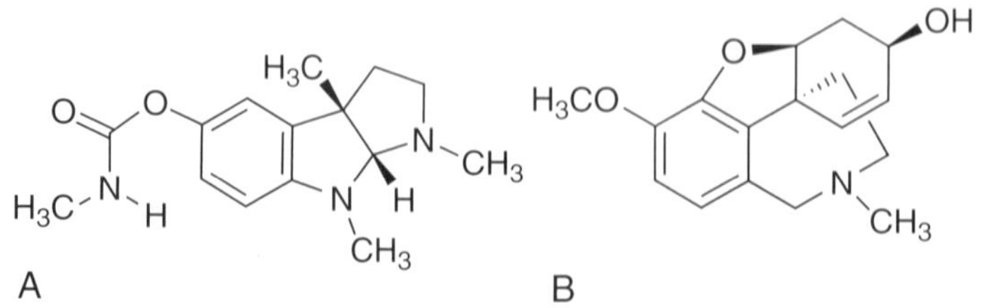

Fig. 22.8 A) Physostigmine and B) Galantamine.

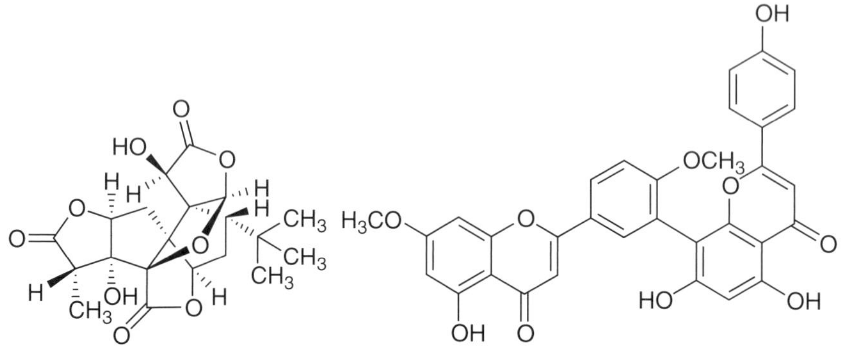

Fig. 22.9 A) Ginkgolide A and B) Ginkegetin.

Therapeutic Uses and Available Evidence

Butterbur and some of its constituents show antiinflammatory effects in preclinical studies, but clinical investigation is limited. However, its use in migraine prophylaxis cannot be recommended due to safety concerns regarding its pyrrolizidine alkaloid content.

DRUGS USED FOR COGNITIVE ENHANCEMENT AND IN DEMENTIA

There are few effective treatments for improving memory, especially in dementia. Acetylcholinesterase-inhibiting drugs are available to treat Alzheimer disease with varying degrees of success. Rivastigmine is a reversible, noncompetitive inhibitor of acetylcholinesterase. It is a semisynthetic derivative of physostigmine, an alkaloid found in the Calabar bean (*Physostigma venenosum* Balf.); a highly poisonous plant indigenous to West Africa. Galantamine (= galanthamine), an alkaloid extracted from the snowdrop (*G. nivalis* L.), was introduced around 2001 (Fig. 22.8). These drugs appear to slow down progression of the disease for a limited period, but do not cure it, and have side effects making them unacceptable to many patients.

Ginkgo, *Ginkgo biloba* L.†

Ginkgo, the maidenhair tree (Ginkgoaceae), is an ancient 'fossil' tree indigenous to China and Japan and cultivated elsewhere. It is very hardy and is reputed to be the only species to have survived a nuclear explosion. The leaves are glabrous and bilobed, each lobe being triangular with fan-like, prominent, radiate veins. The leaves are used medicinally.

Constituents

Ginkgo contains two major classes of actives, both of which contribute to the activity: ginkgolides A, B and C, and bilobalide, which are diterpene lactones; and the biflavone glycosides, such as ginkgetin, isoginkgetin and bilobetin (Fig. 22.9). Ginkgolic acids are present in the fruit, but normally only in very minor amounts in the leaf.

Therapeutic Uses and Available Evidence

Ginkgo has been investigated clinically for its effects in a range of conditions including tinnitus, peripheral arterial occlusive disease, chronic venous insufficiency, acute ischaemic stroke, visual disorders and antidepressant-related sexual dysfunction. It is perhaps best known for its use in cognitive impairment, reducing or preventing memory deterioration due to ageing and milder forms of dementia. Its effects are the result of improving blood circulation to the brain and its antiinflammatory and antioxidant properties. The effects of ginkgo include modulation of neurotransmitter uptake and receptor changes during ageing, cerebral ischaemia and neuronal injury. Inhibition of nitric oxide may also be involved.

Many clinical trials have assessed the effects of ginkgo extracts (most commonly the standardised *G. biloba* leaf extract EGb-761) in patients with cognitive impairment, including Alzheimer disease and other forms of dementia, although not all are of high methodological quality. Reviews limited to higher-quality studies found that ginkgo was more effective than placebo in patients with dementia, and there are conflicting results as to whether ginkgo has beneficial effects on cognitive function in cognitively intact individuals.

Ginkgo has been reported to cause dermatitis and gastrointestinal disturbances in large doses, although rarely. Allergic reactions in sensitive individuals are more likely to be due to ingestion of the fruits due to the ginkgolic acids, which usually are absent from leaf extracts and ginkgo products, or present only in very small amounts. There are isolated reports of bleeding associated with use of ginkgo either alone or when used concurrently with antiplatelet and anticoagulant agents, and nonsteroidal antiinflammatory drugs.

ANTIEPILEPTICS

Herbal drugs are used in traditional medicine to treat epilepsy, but with little evidence and reportedly weak effects. The exception is cannabis, or more specifically CBD, one of the most significant new antiepileptic drugs to be licensed recently.

CANNABIDIOL

CBD (Fig. 22.10) is the main nonpsychoactive cannabinoid in marijuana, *Cannabis sativa* L. (Cannabaceae). In contrast to the well-known Δ^9-tetrahydrocannabinol (THC), which causes euphoria by activation of cannabinoid CB_1 receptors, CBD has very low affinity for both CB_1 and CB_2 receptors and has little abuse potential. CBD exerts multiple pharmacological effects including anticonvulsive, analgesic, antiinflammatory and behavioural effects via several mechanisms, including modulation of the endocannabinoid system and transient receptor potential (TRP) channels, activation of peroxisome proliferator-activated receptor γ (PPARγ) and 5-HT_{1A} receptors, GPR55 antagonism and inhibition of adenosine reuptake. Although CBD has become one of the most widely selling supplements globally, its effects on drug-resistant seizures in children with severe early-onset epilepsy are of greater importance. High-quality randomised clinical trials (RCT) have shown that the addition of CBD to conventional antiepileptic regimens resulted in a greater reduction in frequency of seizures than placebo, in patients with Dravet or Lennox–Gastaut syndromes, and these and other robust studies have led to the approval of CBD (Epidiolex, a 99% pure CBD extract) for the treatment of these rare forms of epilepsy in patients of 2 years and older.

Other Central Nervous System Effects

Most CBD sales are related to products with nonspecific health indications, but the possible benefits of CBD in mood and psychotic disorders, anxiety and depression, has been well reviewed, but the evidence remains promising but inconclusive. Clinical studies assessing CBD (alone, and not with THC, as in an extract) for pain relief are limited. Most are of poor methodology and conclusions cannot be drawn, but a high-quality RCT in patients with multiple sclerosis, spinal cord injury, brachial plexus damage and limb amputation found a significant improvement of pain control in the CBD group.

Safety of Cannabidiol

Doses up to 600 mg are reportedly well tolerated. RCTs in epileptic patients have found adverse events are slightly higher in patients treated with CBD than placebo. Adverse events were drowsiness, decreased appetite and diarrhoea.

CBD inhibits CYP2C and CYP3A4 enzymes which can lead to a pharmacokinetic interaction with the antiepileptic drug clobazam, resulting in increased sedation, which can be resolved with a reduction of the clobazam dose. This interaction is considered beneficial, and part of the therapeutic effect of CBD as an adjunct to conventional antiepileptic drug treatment.

Almost all the available safety data are derived from the use of Epidiolex, and not to nonapproved CBD products freely available in the market, which may cause adverse events due to the variable quality, contamination or adulteration.

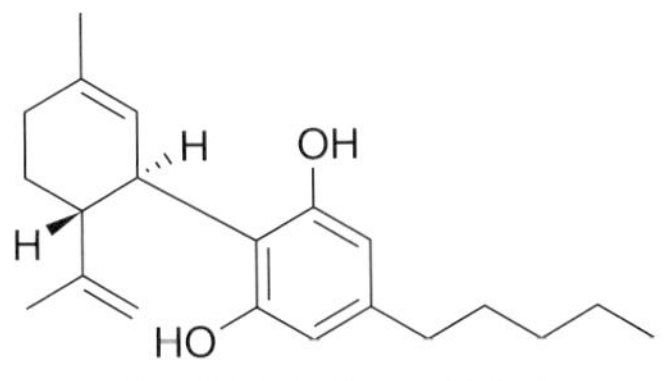

Fig. 22.10 Cannabidiol.

FURTHER READING

Arzimanoglou, A., Brandl, U., Cross, J.H., Gil-Nagel, A., Lagae, L., Landmark, C.J., et al., 2020. Epilepsy and cannabidiol: a guide to treatment. Epileptic Disord. 22 (1), 1–14. https://doi.org/10.1684/epd.2020.1141.

Bauer, I., 2019. Travel medicine, coca and cocaine: demystifying and rehabilitating *Erythroxylum*—a comprehensive review. Trop. Dis. Travel Med. Vaccines 5, 20. https://doi.org/10.1186/s40794-019-0095-7.

Borrás, S., Martínez-Solís, I., Ríos, J.L., 2021. Medicinal plants for insomnia related to anxiety: an updated review. Planta Med. 87 (10–11), 738–753. https://doi.org/10.1055/a-1510-9826.

Das, G., Shin, H.-S., Tundis, R., Gonçalves, S., Tantengco, O., Campos, M.G., et al., 2021. Plant species of sub-family Valerianaceae—a review on its effect on the central nervous system. Plants (Basel). 10 (5), 846. https://doi.org/10.3390/plants10050846.

Ghazizadeh, J., Sadigh-Eteghad, S., Marx, W., Fakhari, A., Hamedeyazdan, S., Torbati, M., et al., 2021. The effects of lemon balm (*Melissa officinalis* L.) on depression and anxiety in clinical trials: a systematic review and meta-analysis. Phytother. Res. 35 (12), 6690–6705. https://doi.org/10.1002/ptr.7252.

Guadagna, S., Barattini, D.F., Rosu, S., Ferini-Strambi, L., 2020. Plant extracts for sleep disturbances: a systematic review. Evid. Based Complement. Alternat. Med. 2020, 3792390. https://doi.org/10.1155/2020/3792390.

Heinrich, M., Teoh, H.L., 2004. Galanthamine from snowdrop—the development of a modern drug against Alzheimer's disease from local Caucasian knowledge. J. Ethnopharmacol. 92, 147–162.

Kaur, J., Famta, P., Famta, M., Mehta, M., Satija, S., Sharma, N., et al., 2021. Potential anti-epileptic phytoconstituents: an updated review. J. Ethnopharmacol. 268, 113565. https://doi.org/10.1016/j.jep.2020.113565.

Lelli, D., Cortese, L., Pedone, C., 2021. Use of plant-derived natural products in sleep disturbances. Adv. Exp. Med. Biol. 1308, 217–224. https://doi.org/10.1007/978-3-030-64872-5_15.

Metz, C.N., Pavlov, V.A., 2021. Treating disorders across the lifespan by modulating cholinergic signaling with galantamine. J. Neurochem. 58 (6), 1359–1380. https://doi.org/10.1111/jnc.15243.

Miroddi, M., Calapai, G., Navarra, M., Minciullo, P.L., Gangemi, S., 2013. *Passiflora incarnata* L: ethnopharmacology, clinical application, safety and evaluation of clinical trials. J. Ethnopharmacol. 150 (3), 791–804.

Moragrega, I., Ríos, J.L., 2021. Medicinal plants in the treatment of depression: evidence from preclinical studies. Planta Med. 87 (9), 656–685. https://doi.org/10.1055/a-1338-1011.

Nielsen, S., Germanos, R., Weier, M., Pollard, J., Degenhardt, L., Hall, W., et al., 2018. The use of cannabis and cannabinoids in treating symptoms of multiple sclerosis: a systematic review of reviews. Curr. Neurol. Neurosci. Rep. 18, 8.

Nowak, A., Kojder, K., Zielonka-Brzezicka, J., Wróbel, J., Bosiacki, M., Fabiańska, M., et al., 2021. The use of *Ginkgo biloba* L. as a neuroprotective agent in the Alzheimer's disease. Front. Pharmacol. 12, 775034. https://doi.org/10.3389/fphar.2021.775034.

Premoli, M., Aria, F., Bonini, S.A., Maccarinelli, G., Gianoncelli, A., Pina, S.D., et al., 2019. Cannabidiol: recent advances and new insights for neuropsychiatric disorders treatment. Life Sci. 224, 120–127.

Presley, C.C., Lindsley, C.W., 2018. DARK classics in chemical neuroscience: opium, a historical perspective. ACS Chem. Neurosci. 9 (10), 2503–2518. https://doi.org/10.1021/acschemneuro.8b00459.

Rajapakse, T., Davenport, W.J., 2019. Phytomedicines in the treatment of migraine. CNS Drugs 33 (5), 399–415. https://doi.org/10.1007/s40263-018-0597-2.

Schimpl, F.C., da Silva, J.F., de Carvalho Gonçalves, J.F., Mazzafera, P., 2013. Guarana: revisiting a highly caffeinated plant from the Amazon. J. Ethnopharmacol. 150 (1), 14–31.

Shakeri, A., Sahebkar, A., Javadi, B., 2016. *Melissa officinalis* L.—a review of its traditional uses, phytochemistry and pharmacology. J. Ethnopharmacol. 188, 204–228. https://doi.org/10.1016/j.jep.2016.05.010.

Song, Y.N., Wang, Y., Zheng, Y.H., Liu, T.L., Zhang, C., 2021. Crocins: a comprehensive review of structural characteristics, pharmacokinetics and therapeutic effects. Fitoterapia 153, 104969. https://doi.org/10.1016/j.fitote.2021.104969.

Thomsen, M., Schmidt, M., 2021. Health policy versus kava (*Piper methysticum*): anxiolytic efficacy may be instrumental in restoring the reputation of a major South Pacific crop. J. Ethnopharmacol. 268, 113582. https://doi.org/10.1016/j.jep.2020.113582.

White, C.M., 2019. A review of human studies assessing cannabidiol's (CBD) therapeutic actions and potential. J. Clin. Pharmacol. 9, 923–934.

Wider, B., Pittler, M.H., Ernst, E., 2015. Feverfew for preventing migraine. Cochrane Database Syst. Rev. 4, CD002286. https://doi.org/10.1002/14651858.CD002286.pub3.

Williamson, E.M., Liu, X., Izzo, A.A., 2020. Trends in use, pharmacology, and clinical applications of emerging herbal nutraceuticals. Br. J. Pharmacol. 177 (6), 1227–1240. https://doi.org/10.1111/bph.14943.

Xing, B., Li, S., Yang, J., Lin, D., Feng, Y., Lu, J., et al., 2021. Phytochemistry, pharmacology, and potential clinical applications of saffron: a review. J. Ethnopharmacol. 281, 114555. https://doi.org/10.1016/j.jep.2021.114555.

Yang, G., Wang, Y., Sun, J., Zhang, K., Liu, J., 2016. *Ginkgo biloba* for mild cognitive impairment and Alzheimer's disease: a systematic review and meta-analysis of randomized controlled trials. Curr. Top. Med. Chem. 16 (5), 520–528.

23

The Musculoskeletal System

Acute inflammatory disorders are not normally treated with phytomedicines, but for chronic inflammatory conditions, they may offer a gentle, long-term solution. Analgesic and antiinflammatory drugs such as paracetamol, aspirin and ibuprofen are used for such conditions, but side effects can limit their acceptability. Nonsteroidal antiinflammatory drugs (NSAIDs) act mainly via inhibition of cyclo-oxygenase (COX) enzymes, also known as prostaglandin synthases (PGS). At present three are known, COX-1, COX-2 and COX-3 (a splice variant of COX-1, sometimes referred to as COX-1b). Inhibition of COX-1 (e.g. with aspirin, ibuprofen and diclofenac) reduces levels of the gastroprotective prostaglandins, leading to inflammation of the gastrointestinal lining and even ulceration and bleeding. COX-2, however, is only induced in response to proinflammatory cytokines and is not found in normal tissue (unlike COX-1). It is associated particularly with oedema and the nociceptive and pyretic effects of inflammation. Treatment with inhibitors of COX-2 does not produce such severe gastrointestinal side effects, but there are concerns about their cardiovascular safety. Other targets for treating inflammatory diseases include 5-lipoxygenase (LOX), nuclear factor kappa B (NF-κB) (which is activated in rheumatoid arthritis and other chronic inflammatory conditions) and certain cytokines that inhibit the activity of tumour necrosis factor-α (TNF-α). Chronic expression of nitric oxide (NO) is also associated with various inflammatory conditions, including arthritis.

DRUGS USED IN ARTHRITIS, RHEUMATISM AND MUSCLE PAIN

The classic NSAID, aspirin, was originally developed as a result of studies on salicin, obtained from willow bark (see below and—for historical aspects—Chapter 2). Although at first the effects of salicin were only linked to the hydrolysed product salicylic acid, it is now known that plant antiinflammatory agents tend to have fewer gastrointestinal side effects than salicylates in general. There are also several combination herbal products on the market, for which little clinical data are available, but which are very popular and seem to produce few side effects.

Bromelains (Ananase)[†]

Bromelain is a mixture of proteolytic enzymes extracted from the fruits and and stem of the pineapple (*Ananas comosus* (L.) Merr.) and other species of bromeliads (Bromeliaceae). The active constituents are protease-inhibiting enzymes. Bromelain is used clinically to treat bruising, arthritis, joint stiffness and pain, and to improve healing postoperatively, including after dental procedures. It is antiinflammatory in animal studies and may be an effective alternative to NSAIDs, as shown in several clinical trials, and has been proposed for the treatment of osteoarthritis, dysmenorrhoea and sports injuries.

Some evidence exists for the efficacy of bromelain in treating postoperative oedema and pain after tooth extraction. While bromelain is claimed to be useful in the treatment and prevention of osteoarthritis, the clinical evidence remains preliminary. Bromelain is generally well tolerated, but side effects include minor gastrointestinal upsets.

Devil's Claw, *Harpagophytum procumbens* (Burch.) DC. ex Meisn.[†]

Devil's claw (Pedaliaceae) is named from the claw-like appearance of the fruit. The storage roots are collected in the savannahs of southern Africa (mainly the Kalahari Desert) and, while still fresh, cut into small pieces and dried. The main exporters are South Africa and Namibia. Devil's claw was used traditionally as a tonic for 'illnesses of the blood', fever, kidney and bladder problems, during pregnancy and as an obstetric remedy for induction or acceleration of labour, as well as for expelling the retained placenta. *H. zeyheri* Decne. is also used medicinally.

Constituents

The most important actives are the bitter iridoids, harpagide and harpagoside (Fig. 23.1), with 8-O-p-coumaroylharpagide, procumbide, 6'-O-p-coumaroylprocumbide, pagide and procumboside; the triterpenoids oleanolic and ursolic acids; β-sitosterol; and a glycoside harproside. Other compounds present include phenylethyl glycosides, such as verbascoside and isoacteoside, polyphenolic acids (caffeic, cinnamic and chlorogenic acids) and flavonoids, such as luteolin and kaempferol.

Therapeutic Uses and Available Evidence

In Europe, a tea made from the powdered root has been used traditionally for the treatment of dyspeptic disorders such as indigestion and lack of appetite. This effect is due to the presence of bitter glycosides, the iridoids. The antiinflammatory effects are now of much more significance, and clinical research, using chemically well-characterised extracts, for the treatment of rheumatic conditions and lower back pain has demonstrated the superiority of these to placebo in patients with osteoarthritis, non-radicular back pain and other chronic and acute pain, and their therapeutic equivalence to conventional forms of treatment. Devil's claw is generally well tolerated and appears to be a suitable alternative to NSAIDs, which often have gastrointestinal side effects.

The mechanism of action is not fully known: fractions containing the highest concentration of harpagoside inhibited COX-1 and COX-2 activity and greatly inhibited NO production, whereas the fraction containing mainly the other iridoids increased COX-2 and did not alter NO and COX-1 activities. Harpagoside suppresses the lipopolysaccharide (LPS)-induced production of inflammatory

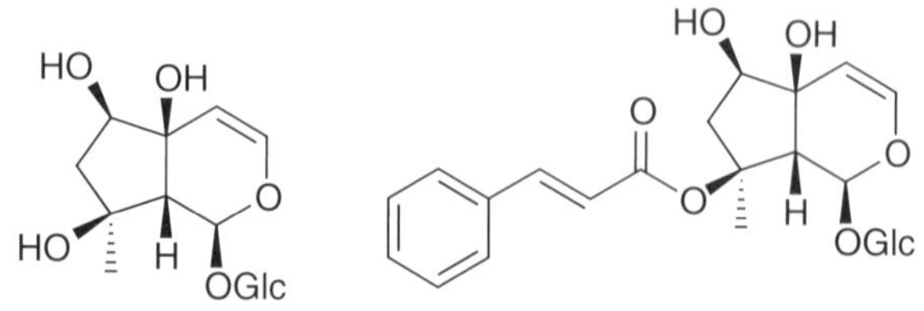

Fig. 23.1 Harpagide *(left)* and harpagoside *(right)*.

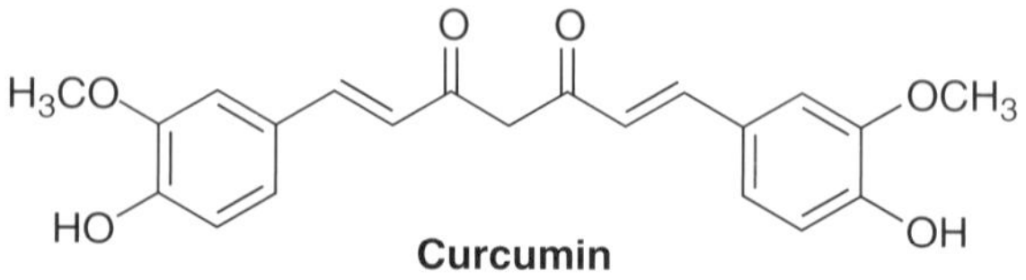

Fig. 23.2 Curcumin.

cytokines (IL-1β, IL-6 and TNF-α) and is probably the main active constituent, but other components modulate the synthesis of inflammatory mediators.

Extracts are generally well tolerated but should not be used for patients with gastric or duodenal ulceration. The aqueous extract possesses a spasmogenic action on rat uterine muscles, lending credence to the popular obstetric uses but suggesting that it should be avoided in pregnant women. Side effects include minor gastrointestinal upsets. Devil's claw products are used in veterinary medicine, especially in horses and dogs.

Rosehip, *Rosa canina* L.[†]

Rosehips of the wild or dog rose (*Rosa canina* L., Rosaceae) are botanically 'pseudofruits', composed of fruits (achenes) enclosed in a fleshy receptacle. The trichomes found inside rose hips are irritant and are often removed before powdering the fruit. There are several types of rosehip preparation available: rosehip and seed (the ripe pseudofruits, including the seed); rosehip (the ripe seed receptacle, freed from seed and attached trichomes); and rosehip seed (the ripe, dried seed). The whole pseudofruit, i.e. rosehip with seed, is most commonly used and widely investigated.

Constituents

Antiinflammatory constituents isolated from rosehip extracts include the triterpene acids, oleanolic, betulinic and ursolic acids; oleic, linoleic and alpha-linolenic acids; and a series of galactolipids, which are thought to be a major contributor to the effects.

Therapeutic Uses and Available Evidence

Traditionally, rose hips were used as a source of vitamin C and were made into syrups for that purpose, but modern use is now focused on their antiinflammatory effects. Several clinical trials have suggested that patients with rheumatoid arthritis may benefit from additional treatment with rose hip. Extracts of rosehips have displayed potent antiinflammatory and antinociceptive activities in several in vivo experimental models, but the mechanism of action and the contribution of the different active constituents are still not fully known.

Turmeric, *Curcuma longa* L.[†]

The rhizomes of turmeric (syn. *C. domestica* Val., Zingiberaceae) are widely traded as a ready-prepared and ground, dark yellow powder with a characteristic taste and odour. Turmeric is used in religious ceremonies by Hindus and Buddhists. It is important in Asian, and increasingly, global cuisine and as a food colouring agent. Javanese turmeric (*Curcuma xanthorrhiza* Roxb.[†]) is mostly used for gastrointestinal discomfort.

Turmeric preparations are promoted with a wide range of claims, but evidence is accumulating to support its efficacy in a wide variety of inflammatory, liver and digestive disorders.

Constituents

The curcuminoids, a mixture known as curcumin (Fig. 23.2), consisting of analogous phenolic diarylheptanoids including curcumin, monodemethoxycurcumin and bisdemethoxycurcumin, are the bright yellow compounds responsible for many of the effects. There is an essential oil (about 3%–5%), containing about 60% sesquiterpene ketones (turmerones), including ar-turmerone, α-atlantone, zingiberene, with borneol, α-phellandrene, eugenol and others; and polysaccharide fractions containing such as glycans, the ukonans A–D.

Therapeutic Uses and Available Evidence

The main indications for turmeric are linked to its antiinflammatory and antihepatotoxic effects. It is widely used as an antiinflammatory, digestive aid, antiseptic and general tonic. It is given internally and applied externally to wounds and insect bites. The efficacy of curcumin and its regulation of multiple targets, as well as its safety, mean that turmeric has received considerable interest as a potential agent for the prevention and/or treatment of arthritis, skin disease, allergies, inflammatory bowel disease, Alzheimer's disease, prostate inflammation, renal disease, diabetes and many others. Curcumin has been studied as an anticancer agent and inhibits inducible NO synthase (iNOS) via a mechanism involving the proinflammatory transcription factor NF-κB.

The use of turmeric as an adjunctive cancer treatment, in combination with antineoplastic agents, is under current investigation. Curcumin inhibits drug transporters involved in the development of drug resistance, and a review of its effects in combination with cisplatin suggests this may constitute a new cancer therapeutic approach.

Clinical evidence is urgently needed for many indications. Turmeric is well tolerated, but its poor bioavailability limits its therapeutic usefulness. Preparations which combine turmeric with piperine, or as liposomes or microencapsulated formulations, show enhanced absorption, but improved methods for novel delivery are required to utilise turmeric to its full extent.

Willow Bark, *Salix* spp.[†]

Salix spp., including *S. purpurea* L., *S. × fragilis* L., *S. daphnoides* Vill. and *S. alba* L. (Salicaceae), are trees and shrubs common in alpine ecosystems, flooded areas and along the margins of streams. Willow bark is a European phytomedicine with a long tradition of use for chronic forms of pain, rheumatic diseases, fever and headache. As is well known, the constituent salicin served as a lead for the development of aspirin (acetylsalicylic acid).

Constituents

Phenolic glycosides, including salicin (Fig. 23.3), phenolic acids, tannins (mainly dimeric and polymeric procyanidins) and flavonoids, are the most prominent groups of compounds. The most common willow bark dry extract has a salicin content of 15%–18%.

Very few pharmacological studies of individual compounds from willow bark (and their metabolites) have been conducted. The extract, however, exerts effects on several proinflammatory targets, including both isoforms of COX, and willow bark water extract STW 33-1 has been shown to produce a significant inhibition of TNF-α and NF-κB in activated monocytes.

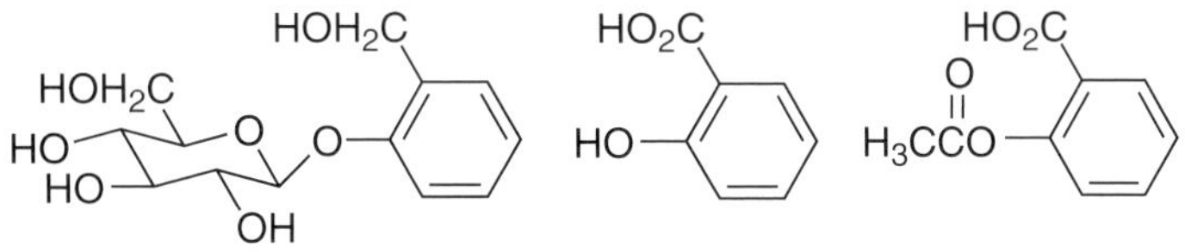

Fig. 23.3 Salicin *(left)*, salicylic acid *(middle)*, Acetylsalicylic acid (Aspirin) *(right)*.

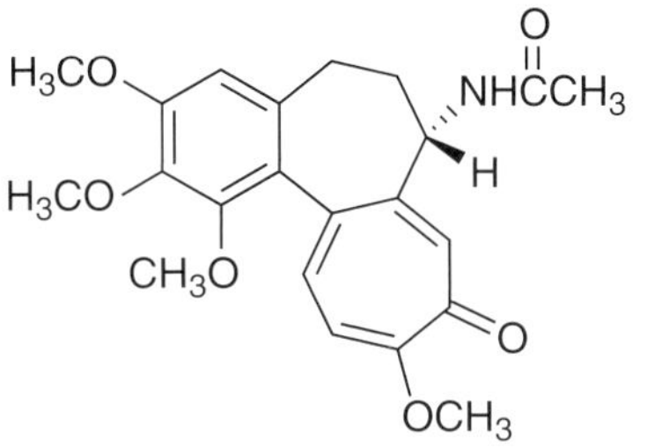

Fig. 23.4 Colchicine.

Therapeutic Uses and Available Evidence

The effectiveness of an extract of willow bark (which is licensed as a medicine in Germany) has been shown to be superior to a placebo for osteoarthritis and lower back pain, and with fewer side effects than, for example, aspirin. However, further, more stringent clinical and mechanistic studies are needed. In very high doses, the side effects of salicylates may be encountered, although these are rarely seen at therapeutic levels of the extract. In general, the effective dose contains lower amounts of salicylate than would be expected by calculation, and a form of synergy is thought to be operating within the extract. High-quality products (willow bark powder or aqueous or hydroalcoholic extracts) used at the usual therapeutic levels are not associated with serious adverse events.

GOUT

Gout is a very painful, localised inflammation of the joints (particularly those of the thumb and big toe) caused by hyperuricaemia and the formation of needle-like crystals of uric acid in the joint. For prevention, the xanthine oxidase inhibitor allopurinol is the drug of choice, but an alternative is sulfinpyrazone, which increases the excretion of uric acid. Prophylactic treatment should never be initiated during an acute attack as it may prolong it. Acute gout is treated with indometacin or other NSAIDs (but not aspirin), but, if inappropriate, colchicine can be used.

Colchicine[†]

Colchicine (Fig. 23.4) is an alkaloid extracted from the corms and flowers of *Colchicum autumnale* L., the autumn crocus or meadow saffron (Colchicaceae, formerly Liliaceae). The plant grows from bulbs in meadows throughout Europe and North Africa, typically appearing during the autumn, with the fruit developing over winter and dispersing prior to the first mowing of the meadows. The leaves and the fruit appear during spring.

Colchicine is used in the acute phase of gout particularly when NSAIDs are either ineffective or contraindicated. Doses of colchicine may need to be reduced if administered concurrently with CYP3A4/P--glycoprotein inhibitors such as diltiazem and verapamil.

Low-dose colchicine (0.5–1 mg) is now being evaluated as a treatment for severe inflammatory pulmonary and cardiovascular inflammation in COVID-19 patients, based on its interaction with several inflammatory pathways and antiviral effects. In large doses, colchicine is cardiotoxic, and this may limit its use, but it is also effective in low doses in patients with recent myocardial infarction, to reduce inflammation and prevent further ischaemic cardiovascular events.

Colchicine is occasionally also used as prophylaxis for familial Mediterranean fever. It is an important tool for biochemical research, as an inhibitor of the separation of the chromosomes during mitosis (e.g. to produce polyploid organisms). Colchicine is a fascinating drug but definitely not a herbal medicine. It is highly toxic and causes gastrointestinal upsets such as nausea, vomiting, abdominal pain and diarrhoea even at therapeutic doses.

TOPICAL ANTIINFLAMMATORY AGENTS

Most topical antirheumatics are rubefacients and redden the skin by increasing blood flow. They are used for localised pain or when systemic drugs are not appropriate. Many contain salicylates, and capsaicin is used for severe pain (e.g. with shingles). They should not be used in children, pregnant or breastfeeding women or with occlusive dressings. Arnica is also very popular, despite little clinical evidence to support its use.

Arnica, *Arnica montana* L.[†]

Arnica (Asteraceae) is widely used in many European countries, but as *A. montana* is protected, other species are used as substitutes. Extracts and tinctures of the flowerheads are applied topically, for bruising, sprains and swellings, usually in the form of a cream or gel.

Constituents

Arnica species are rich in sesquiterpene lactones of the pseudoguianolide type. The most abundant in *A. montana* are helenalin (Fig. 23.5), and 11α,13-dihydrohelenalin. Flavonoids, including quercetin and kaempferol derivatives, coumarins and an essential oil are also present.

Therapeutic Uses and Available Evidence

Extracts of arnica and the pure sesquiterpene lactone helenalin have been shown to exert antiinflammatory effects in vivo in animal models, although few clinical studies have been carried out, and those published have shown equivocal results. Helenalin has well-documented effects on several transcription factors, including NF-κB and nuclear factor of activated T-cells (NFAT). Arnica preparations suppress matrix metalloproteinase-1 (MMP1) and MMP13 mRNA levels in chondrocytes at low concentrations, possibly due to inhibition of DNA binding of the transcription factors activator protein-1 (AP-1) and NF-κB. The cytotoxicity of the sesquiterpene lactones is well documented, and allergic reactions may occur. In phytotherapy, arnica is always used externally and the sesquiterpene lactones have been shown to be absorbed through the skin producing a localised effect, although highly diluted arnica preparations are taken internally in homoeopathy.

Capsaicin[†]

Capsaicin, 8-methyl-*N*-vanillyl-trans-6-nonenamide, is the pungent oleo-resin of the fruit of the chilli pepper (*Capsicum frutescens* L., and some varieties of *C. annuum* L., Solanaceae), also known as capsicum, cayenne, or hot chilli. Green and red (or bell) peppers and paprika are produced by milder varieties. The plant is indigenous to tropical America and Africa but widely cultivated. Related capsaicinoids such as dihydrocapsaicin, nordihydrocapsaicin and homodihydrocapsaicin are present in the resin. These are esters of vanillyl amine with C_8–C_{13} fatty acids.

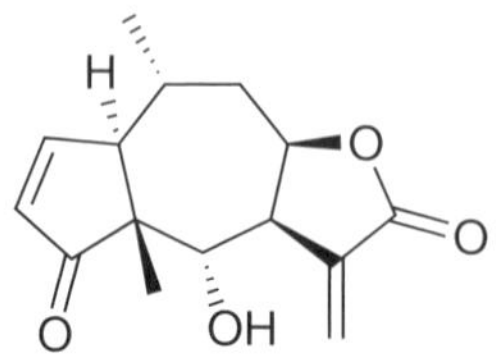

Fig. 23.5 Helenalin.

Therapeutic Uses and Available Evidence

Capsaicin acts on vanilloid receptors and is a well-known transient receptor potential vanilloid subtype 1 (TRPV1) agonist, causing inflammation, but it also desensitises sensory nerve endings to pain stimulation by depleting the neuropeptide substance P from local C-type nerve fibres. It is used as a local analgesic in the treatment of postherpetic neuralgia, diabetic neuropathy, osteoarthritis and for pruritus and in the management of intractable neuropathic pain. Capsaicin has long been used in cough and cold remedies, and since the vanilloid 1 (TRPV1) receptor is a sensor of airway irritation and initiator of the cough reflex, there is a rationale for that usage.

For external use, capsaicin is normally formulated as a cream containing 0.025%, 0.075% or 0.75%, or applied via a transdermal patch. Capsaicin produces severe irritation and should not be applied near the eyes, mucous membranes or broken skin. It should be avoided in children and pregnant or breastfeeding women.

Wintergreen Oil, *Gaultheria procumbens* L., *Betula lenta* L.

Wintergreen oil is now most often obtained from *Betula lenta* (Betulaceae) rather than *Gaultheria procumbens* (Ericaceae), although both have similar compositions and the characteristic odour of methyl salicylate.

Constituents

The oil is mainly methyl salicylate (about 98%), which is produced by enzymatic hydrolysis of phenolic glycosides during maceration and steam distillation.

Therapeutic Uses and Available Evidence

Methyl salicylate is antiinflammatory and antirheumatic. Oil of wintergreen is used mainly in the form of an ointment or liniment for rheumatism, sprains, sciatica, neuralgia, muscular pain and, highly diluted, in mouthwashes. It can cause irritation and should not be applied near the eyes, mucous membranes or on broken skin, and should be avoided in children and pregnant or breastfeeding women. It is also used in insecticidal products.

MUSCLE CRAMP

Quinine[†]

Quinine is isolated from the bark of *Cinchona* spp. Quinine salts can be effective in reducing the incidence of muscle cramps but should be avoided for routine use because of their cardiac toxicity. For further information on quinine, including the structure, see Chapter 10 (Antiinfective Agents).

FURTHER READING

Ahsan, R., Arshad, M., Khushtar, M., Ahmad, M.A., Muazzam, M., Akhter, M.S., et al., 2020. A comprehensive review on physiological effects of curcumin. Drug Res. 70, 441–447.

Axmann, S., Hummel, K., Nöbauer, K., Razzazi-Fazeli, E., Zitterl-Eglseer, K., 2019. Pharmacokinetics of harpagoside in horses after intragastric administration of a Devil's Claw (*Harpagophytum procumbens*) extract. J. Vet. Pharmacol. Ther. 42, 37–44.

Dai, W., Yan, W., Leng, X., Chen, J., Hu, X., Ao, Y., 2021. Effectiveness of *Curcuma longa* extract versus placebo for the treatment of knee osteoarthritis: a systematic review and meta-analysis of randomized controlled trials. Phytother. Res. 35 (11), 5921–5935.

de Souza, G.M., Fernandes, I.A., Dos Santos, C., Falci, S., 2019. Is bromelain effective in controlling the inflammatory parameters of pain, edema, and trismus after lower third molar surgery? A systematic review and meta-analysis. Phytother. Res. 33, 473–481.

Drogosz, J., Janecka, A., 2019. Helenalin – a sesquiterpene lactone with multidirectional activity. Curr. Drug Targets 20, 444–452.

Gruenwald, J., Uebelhack, R., Moré, M.I., 2019. *Rosa canina* – rose hip pharmacological ingredients and molecular mechanics counteracting osteoarthritis – a systematic review. Phytomedicine 60, 152958.

He, J., Li, X., Wang, Z., Bennett, S., Chen, K., Xiao, Z., et al., 2019. Therapeutic anabolic and anticatabolic benefits of natural Chinese medicines for the treatment of osteoporosis. Front. Pharmacol. 10, 1344.

Hussain, Y., Islam, L., Khan, H., Filosa, R., Aschner, M., Javed, S., 2021. Curcumin-cisplatin chemotherapy: a novel strategy in promoting chemotherapy efficacy and reducing side effects. Phytother. Res. 35 (12), 6514–6529. https://doi.org/10.1002/ptr.7225.

Kunnumakkara, A.B., Bordoloi, D., Padmavathi, G., Monisha, J., Roy, N.K., Prasad, S., et al., 2017. Curcumin, the golden nutraceutical: multitargeting for multiple chronic diseases. Br. J. Pharmacol. 174, 1325–1348.

Menghini, L., Recinella, L., Leone, S., Chiavaroli, A., Cicala, C., Brunetti, L., et al., 2019. Devil's Claw (*Harpagophytum procumbens*) and chronic inflammatory diseases: a concise overview on preclinical and clinical data. Phytother. Res. 33, 2152–2162.

Moran, M.M., Szallasi, M.M., 2018. Targeting nociceptive transient receptor potential channels to treat chronic pain: current state of the field. Br. J. Pharmacol. 175 (12), 2185–2203.

Oketch-Rabah, H.A., Marles, R.J., Jordan, S.A., Dog, T.L., 2019. United States pharmacopeia safety review of willow bark. Planta Med. 85, 1192–1202.

Pascart, T., Lioté, F., 2019. Gout: state of the art after a decade of developments. Rheumatology 58, 27–44.

Tardif, J.C., Kouz, S., Waters, D.D., Bertrand, O.F., Diaz, R., Maggioni, A.P., et al., 2019. Efficacy and safety of low-dose colchicine after myocardial infarction. N. Engl. J. Med. 381 (26), 2479–2505.

Tawfeek, N., Mahmoud, M.F., Hamdan, D.I., Sobeh, M., Farrag, N., Wink, M., et al., 2021. Phytochemistry, pharmacology and medicinal uses of plants of the genus *Salix*: an updated review. Front. Pharmacol. 12, 593856.

Wang, Z., Singh, A., Jones, G., Winzenberg, T., Ding, C., Chopra, A., et al., 2021. Efficacy and safety of turmeric extracts for the treatment of knee osteoarthritis: a systematic review and meta-analysis of randomised controlled trials. Curr. Rheumatol. Rep. 23 (2), 11.

24

Female Hormonal and Reproductive Conditions

Herbal medicines are commonly taken by women seeking a more natural or gentle treatment for menopause and dysmenorrhoea, and to facilitate conception, childbirth and lactation. Many preparations used for these conditions contain herbs with oestrogenic effects and are known as phytoestrogens, whereas other herbs are considered to have the capacity to regulate hormone levels without necessarily being oestrogenic.

MENOPAUSAL SYMPTOMS

Herbal medicines are widely used to manage menopause, including not only the acute symptoms such as hot flushes and night sweats but also associated anxiety, memory impairment, fatigue and insomnia. Herbal products formulated for the menopause often include herbs specifically for these central nervous system (CNS) symptoms, such as melissa, valerian, ginkgo, passiflora and St John's wort. Herb used for more specific menopausal symptoms include sage, black cohosh, evening primrose oil and agnus castus as well as herbs and supplements containing phytoestrogenic compounds, such as red clover, fenugreek, soya, linseed, rhubarb, liquorice, alfalfa, fennel and anise.

PHYTOESTROGENS

These compounds act as mild oestrogens or, in certain circumstances, as antioestrogens (by binding to oestrogen receptors and preventing occupation by natural oestrogens). They have a wide range of other effects, including chemopreventive activity. Many pulses (which are legumes) contain phytoestrogens, as do linseed and hops. The main chemical types of phytoestrogen are the isoflavones, coumestans, lignans and stilbenoids; some species of palm even contain similar hormones (e.g. estriol) to those found in the human body. The common occurrence of these substances has implications for men as well as for women, in that the incidence of benign prostatic hyperplasia in men, and menopausal symptoms in women, is lower in societies that consume significant amounts of foods containing these substances in their normal diet. No significant associations between phytoestrogen intake and breast cancer risk have been found, and soya phytoestrogen intake may have a beneficial effect on tumour recurrence. As most studies have not involved women with breast cancer and are of short duration, it would be wise for patients with hormone-dependent cancers to avoid taking these phytomedicines. Very many classes of compounds have oestrogenic effects to different extents and under different physiological conditions; the most important are discussed in the following sections.

Red Clover, *Trifolium pratense* L.

Red (or pink) clover (Fabaceae) is widely distributed throughout Europe, naturalised in North America and found in many other parts of the world. The flower heads are ovoid, red or pinkish purple, about 2–3 cm in diameter, composed of numerous individual, keeled flowers. The leaflets are trefoil, often with a whitish crescent in the centre. Both the leaves and isolated isoflavones are used medicinally.

Constituents

The major actives are phytoestrogens of two types: the isoflavones genistein (Fig. 24.1), afrormosin, biochanin A, daidzein, formononetin, pratensein, calycosin, pseudobaptigenin, orobol, irilone and trifoside, as well as their glycoside conjugates; and coumestans coumestrol and medicagol (see Fig. 24.1).

Therapeutic Uses and Available Evidence

Red clover was traditionally used for skin complaints such as psoriasis and eczema, and as an expectorant in coughs and bronchial conditions. However, it has recently been used more as a source of isoflavones, for a natural method of hormone replacement therapy. The isoflavones are oestrogenic in animals, and biochanin A inhibits metabolic activation of the carcinogen benzo[a]pyrene in a mammalian cell culture, suggesting chemopreventive properties. Red clover extracts also inhibit cytochrome P450 3A4 in vitro, which supports such a use.

Systematic reviews and meta-analyses of randomised trials of red clover extracts for treating hot flushes in menopausal women show conflicting results, but as with other phytoestrogen supplements, there is some indication that high concentrations may reduce the incidence and severity of hot flushes.

Red clover is generally considered safe, although there has not been a comprehensive investigation of its safety profile.

Soya, *Glycine max* (L.) Merr.

Soya (Fabaceae) is a low-growing, typically leguminous crop plant, producing white or yellow beans. It is an important item in the diet of people from many countries and is used in many ways. For example, 'soya milk' is used as a substitute for animal milk in allergic people (especially babies) and by vegetarians and can be made into yoghurt. The protein is used as a meat substitute and to make tofu and is fermented into condiments such as soy sauce. The fresh (edamame) beans and bean sprouts are eaten raw in salads and used in stir-fry dishes; the flour can be made into bread and cakes.

Constituents

Soya contains phytoestrogens of two chemical types: isoflavones including genistein, daidzein and their derivatives, ononin, isoformononetin and others; and coumestans such as coumestrol (especially in the sprouts). There is a fixed oil composed mainly of linoleic and linolenic acids, as well as phytosterols including β-sitosterol and stigmasterol.

Therapeutic Uses and Available Evidence

Preparations containing an isoflavone fraction of soya are used medicinally. The available epidemiological evidence suggests that a diet high in soya can reduce menopausal symptoms and prostate enlargement, but systematic reviews have concluded there is no definitive evidence that phytoestrogen 'supplements', including soy extracts, reduce the frequency or severity of hot flushes and night sweats in peri- or postmenopausal women.

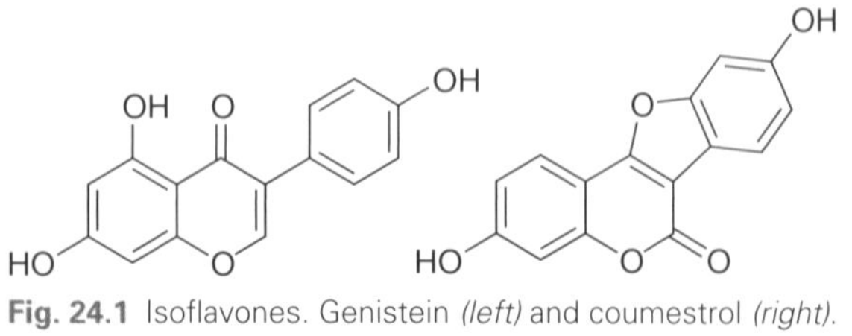

Fig. 24.1 Isoflavones. Genistein *(left)* and coumestrol *(right)*.

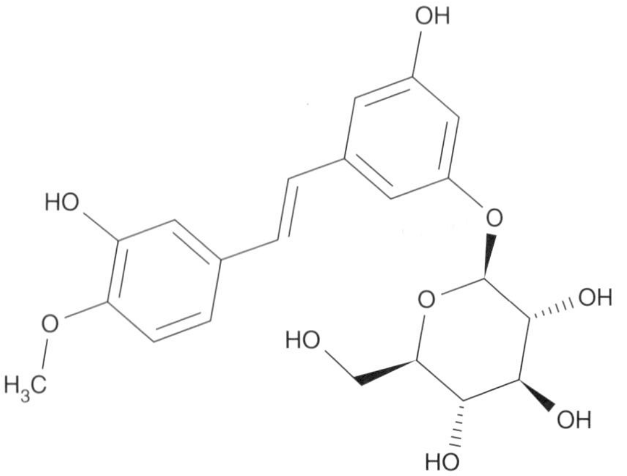

Fig. 24.2 Rhaponticin.

Dietary inclusion of whole soya foods appears to produce a reduction in some clinical risk factors for osteoporosis. Cardiovascular disease and lipid profiles in menopausal women are reportedly improved by consumption of whole soya foods, although further research is necessary. At present it appears that they are beneficial with few adverse effects. A systematic review of soy, red clover and isoflavones for menopausal symptoms in women with breast cancer concluded that better evidence confirming safety is required before use of higher doses (>100 mg daily) of isoflavones can be recommended. Soya is considered to be nontoxic.

Rhubarb, *Rheum rhaponticum* L.

Rhubarbs, *Rheum* spp. (Polygonaceae), are cultivated worldwide for medicinal and food use. The most popular are garden rhubarb (*Rheum rhabarbarum* L.), rhapontic or Siberian rhubarb (*R. rhaponticum* L.) and Chinese rhubarb (*R. officinale* Baill.) The young petioles (leaf stalks) are used as food, but the leaves are toxic due to their high oxalate content. The roots are used medicinally for a variety of indications, depending on their different active constituents.

Constituents

The anthraquinone constituents, which include aloe-emodin and chrysophanol (see Chapter 18), are responsible for the laxative and several other properties, particularly in *R. officinale,* but rhapontic rhubarb contains higher concentrations of stilbenoids which have oestrogenic effects. These include piceatannol and resveratrol glycosides as well as galloyl derivatives, rhapontigenin *O*-glucoside (rhaponticin, Fig. 24.2) and desoxyrhapontigenin *O*-glucoside (desoxyrhaponticin), pterostilbene glycosides and resveratrol dimers.

Therapeutic Uses and Available Evidence

Rhubarb has anticancer, antiparasitic, digestive, both laxative *and* antidiarrhoeal, as well as oestrogenic effects, depending on the nature and composition on the extract. It is widely used in Chinese medicine. A special root extract of *R. rhaponticum* (ERr 731), consisting mainly of rhaponticin (see Fig. 24.2) and desoxyrhaponticin, is used for treating menopausal symptoms. Extracts and isolated compounds show a strong binding affinity to oestrogen receptors, and clinical studies, especially with ERr 731, have demonstrated efficacy in alleviating menopausal symptoms. Details of these and other properties of rhubarb can be found in the Further Reading section.

Pomegranate, *Punica granatum* L.

Pomegranate (Lythraceae) originated from the Mediterranean region but is now grown widely in Asia, the Middle East and the Americas for their fruits, which are used in sauces, juices, liqueurs and foods. The deciduous trees are up to 6 m tall, and the popular red fruit needs little description. Pomegranates have long been symbolic in religious texts, ancient mythology, traditional medicine and folklore, and particularly in association with female fertility. The bark of the trunk and root is a traditional vermifuge, used to treat tapeworm, and as an insecticide.

Constituents

Fruit and seed. The juice is rich in vitamin C and polyphenols such as anthocyanins, flavonoids and ellagitannins, which include punicalin, punicalagin, tellimagrandins and granatins. The fruit peel contains similar compounds and lignans such as isolariciresinol and pomegralignan. The seeds contain phytoestrogens including genistein, daidzein and coumestrol.

Stem and root bark. Alkaloids are present in the bark and include pelletierine, pseudopelletierine and their derivatives.

Therapeutic Uses and Available Evidence

Pomegranate juice and extracts have demonstrated a wide range of beneficial properties such as antimicrobial, chemopreventive, antioxidant and antiinflammatory effects, and as such, they are popular ingredients of foods and drinks marketed to promote general health. The fruit's ubiquitous use does not detract from the considerable evidence available on the properties of pomegranate and its potential therapeutic benefits.

The traditional use of pomegranate fruit extracts in female conditions, and particularly in infertility, has been investigated in cases of polycystic ovary syndrome (PCOS). Preclinical studies have shown that pomegranate extracts are oestrogenic and inflammatory, and in a study of PCOS-induced rats, pomegranate fruit extract was found to increase serum oestrogen levels and reduce symptoms. A small randomised clinical trial (RCT) on 23 women with PCOS found that pomegranate fruit extract improved the serum levels of sex hormones (testosterone reduction) and their lipid profile. However, no information is available on actual pregnancy outcomes.

HORMONE-REGULATING HERBS

These act via mechanisms other than, or in addition to, phytoestrogenic effects, one of which may be via dopamine modulation and prolactin and other hormone release. They are not well investigated in human studies.

Black Cohosh, *Actaea racemosa* L.†

Black cohosh (syn.: *Cimicifuga racemosa* (L.) Nutt., Ranunculaceae) is also known as 'squawroot' because of its traditional use for female complaints. In North America, where the species originates, it was also used to treat snakebite, hence another synonym, 'black snakeroot'. It has also been used for a variety of disparate disorders, including

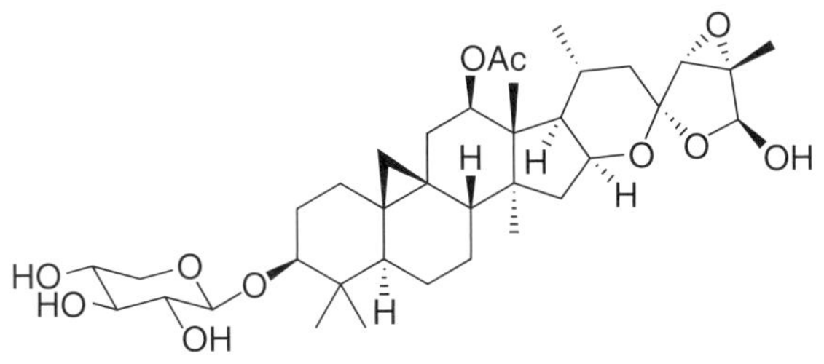

Fig. 24.3 Actein.

rheumatism, sciatica, chorea and tinnitus. The parts used medicinally are the rhizomes and roots. There are substantial issues with the quality of black cohosh raw material in the supply chain: adulteration with other *Actaea* species in particular is a significant problem.

Constituents

The active components of black cohosh are the triterpene glycosides, such as actein (Fig. 24.3), 27-deoxyactein and several cimicifugosides; the flavonoids may contribute to the activity.

Therapeutic Uses and Available Evidence

Hormonal and antiinflammatory effects have been described for black cohosh. Reductions in serum luteinising hormone concentrations have been documented for methanolic and lipophilic extracts in preclinical studies, but there are conflicting data on the oestrogenic activity of the herb.

Evidence from well-designed Randomised Clinical Trials does not consistently show significant beneficial effects of black cohosh preparations in peri- or postmenopausal women. No significant differences were found between black cohosh and placebo in the frequency of hot flushes or menopausal symptom scores. Epidemiological studies and clinical trials indicate that black cohosh use is not associated with an increased risk of breast cancer, although these studies are of short duration.

Black cohosh has been associated with hepatotoxic reactions, ranging from abnormal liver function test values to severe hepatitis requiring liver transplantation. Regulatory action was taken in several countries, usually requiring label warnings to be added regarding the association with liver adverse reactions. There is a view that poor-quality black cohosh material in the supply chain is an explanation for at least some of the cases observed, many of which do not adequately describe the type of black cohosh product used.

Adverse effects reported include skin reactions, gastrointestinal disturbances and lowering of blood pressure with high doses. Black cohosh should be avoided during pregnancy and lactation because of insufficient data.

Chasteberry, *Vitex agnus-castus* L.†

Vitex agnus-castus (Lamiaceae) is also known by the common names 'chasteberry' and 'chaste tree', or simply as 'agnus castus'. It has a history of traditional use for menstrual problems, including pre-menstrual symptoms and dysmenorrhoea, and for menopausal complaints. It was considered historically to reduce the libido, especially in men, hence the names 'chasteberry', 'agnus castus' (which means 'chaste lamb') and 'monk's pepper'. *V. agnus-castus* is native to the Mediterranean. It is a shrub or small tree, 1–6 m in height. The berries are reddish-black and around 2–4 mm in diameter, and the parts are used medicinally.

Constituents

Agnus castus contains the diterpene constituents (e.g. rotundifuran), flavonoids, mainly vitexin, casticin, kaempferol and quercetagetin, as well as iridoids.

Therapeutic Uses and Available Evidence

Extracts of agnus castus and isolated diterpene constituents display dopamine receptor-binding activity and associated inhibition of prolactin synthesis and release. Modern uses of agnus castus include menstrual cycle disorders, premenstrual syndrome (PMS) and cyclical mastalgia (breast pain).

There is some evidence from RCTs to support the effects of agnus castus in relieving breast pain in women with mastalgia and PMS as well as premenstrual dysphoria, and in lowering prolactin concentrations in hyperprolactinaemia including in mastalgia. It does not reportedly affect concentrations in women with normal basal prolactin concentrations.

Evidence from RCTs is lacking for agnus castus in menopausal symptoms, but preclinical evidence suggests this area warrants investigation. Although generally considered safe, agnus castus is not recommended during pregnancy, and should not be used during lactation as it may suppress milk production; its effects upon neonates are not known.

Sage, *Salvia officinalis* L.†

Sage is a well-known culinary herb and used as traditional medicine for its antiinflammatory and antiseptic properties, for example as a gargle for sore throats and laryngitis. However, a more recent use is in the treatment of menopausal hot flushes and excessive perspiration.

Therapeutic Uses and Available Evidence

The diterpene constituents are the main actives for menopausal symptoms, via a mechanism of action involving binding to Gamma Amino Butyric Acid/γ-Amino Butyric Acid (GABA) receptors in the brain, and oestrogenic effects. Its effects in the treatment of excessive sweating have been approved by the Commission E.

Evening *Primrose Oil*†

Eveningeflu primrose is used for many inflammatory disorders, due to its high polyunsaturated fatty acid content, in dermatology (see Chapter 27) and for PMS and menopausal disorders. The use in PMS is not well supported by clinical studies, but recent trials have found it useful in alleviating psychological symptoms in menopausal women.

POSTMENOPAUSAL OSTEOPOROSIS

Osteoporosis is a common disorder affecting mainly elderly people and especially women, where it is exacerbated by a steep decline in oestrogen after the menopause. Most conventional treatments rely either upon oestrogen replacement, or selective oestrogen receptor modulation (SERM) in women, or the use of drugs that prevent the breakdown of bone tissue, such as the bisphosphonates. A good diet is important for maintaining bone health, and several studies have shown that consumption of fruit and vegetables can enhance bone growth. Although there are few herbal treatments for osteoporosis, traditional Chinese medicine (TCM) offers some examples of potentially useful treatments, namely, kudzu, *Pueraria* species and *Epimedium* (see Chapter 25). *Epimedium* contains the osteogenic and phytoestrogenic prenylated flavonoid icariin (Fig. 25.2), and kudzu contains the isoflavone puerarin (Fig. 24.4).

Kudzu, *Pueraria* Spp.†

The kudzu vines (*Pueraria montana* var. *lobata* (Willd.) Sanjappa & Pradeep (syn.: *P. lobata* (Willd.) Ohwi), *P. montana* var. *chinensis*

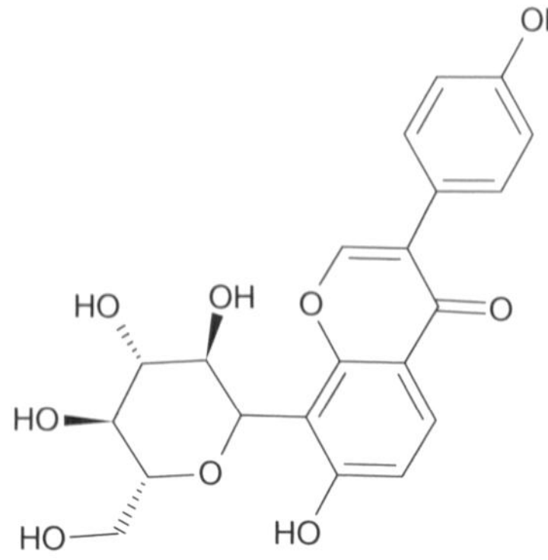

Fig. 24.4 Puerarin.

(Ohwi) Sanjappa & Pradeep (syn.: *P. thomsonii* Benth.) and *P. candollei* var. *mirifica* (Airy Shaw & Suvat.) Niyomdham) today are invasive species found in many warmer and humid regions, especially in the southern states of America and on some Oceanian islands. In addition to its other activities, kudzu root has recently been advocated as a treatment for alcoholism, with limited clinical evidence to support this use, as well as for cerebrovascular and neurological degenerative conditions. It is phytoestrogenic and used as a hormone-replacement therapy.

Constituents

The root contains isoflavones including puerarin, daidzein, genistein and their derivatives.

Therapeutic Uses and Available Evidence

Puerarin, the major active constituent, is thought to be responsible for most of the therapeutic effects. Several animal models have shown osteogenic properties for puerarin, mediated via various complementary mechanisms promoting osteogenesis and inhibition of Receptor activator of Nuclear Kappa B Ligand (RANKL)-induced osteoclastogenesis, but clinical studies for the use of kudzu in osteoporosis are lacking.

INFERTILITY

The inability to achieve a successful pregnancy affects 15%–17% of couples globally, with about 50% related to female factors. Traditional herbal medicines have long been used to treat female infertility, although few clinical studies are available to support this. Popular herbs for infertility include agnus castus, pomegranate and phytoestrogenic herbs such as red clover, often as part of a wholistic regime with a dietary component. The intention is to 'improve' a woman's reproductive health in general or treat underlying causes such as PCOS or endometriosis.

PREGNANCY AND CHILDBIRTH

Taking (any) medicine during pregnancy is generally not advisable as safety to the mother and foetus cannot be guaranteed. Raspberry leaf is included here because it has a widespread folklore use in facilitating childbirth, and it is often recommended that it be taken during pregnancy for this purpose, despite a lack of evidence as to its efficacy.

Ergometrine†

Ergometrine (Fig. 24.5) is an alkaloid extracted from ergot (*Claviceps purpurea* (Fr.) Tul.), a parasitic fungus growing on cereals, usually rye.

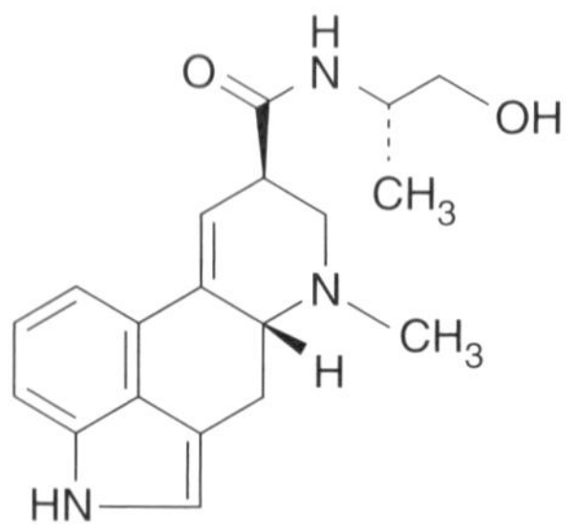

Fig. 24.5 Ergometrine.

It contracts the uterus and is sometimes used to manage the third stage of labour (in conjunction with oxytocin), and to control postpartum haemorrhage if the placenta has not been completely expelled. It must be used only under expert care and is contraindicated in pregnancy due to its abortifacient effects.

Raspberry Leaf, *Rubus idaeus* L.

Raspberry leaf (*Rubus idaeus*, Rosaceae) 'tea' has been used for centuries to facilitate childbirth, and it is usually recommended that it be drunk freely before and during confinement for maximum benefit. The raspberry shrub is well known and is cultivated in many temperate countries for the fruit.

Constituents

The leaves contain tannins and flavonoids, mainly glycosides of kaempferol and quercetin, including rutin, uncharacterised polypeptides.

Therapeutic Uses and Available Evidence

Small clinical observational studies in Australia have given conflicting results regarding a shortening of labour and reduction in medical intervention, but untoward effects apart from anecdotal reports of diarrhoea and strong Braxton Hicks contractions have been reported. Uterine relaxant effects have been demonstrated in animals, and raspberry leaf appears to affect only the pregnant uterus in both rats and humans, with no activity on the nonpregnant uterus. Recent reviews have concluded that in the absence of good clinical data, raspberry leaf cannot be recommended in pregnancy, although it has shown no evidence of causing harm.

LACTATION

Herbs and special diets have long been used traditionally to improve milk flow after childbirth. These herbs are known as 'galactogogues', and among them the most frequently cited are the phytoestrogenic herbs anise, *Pimpinella anisum* L., and fennel, *Foeniculum vulgare* Mill. fruits, which contain anethole, and fenugreek, *Trigonella foenumgraecum* L., with ginger, *Zingiber officinale* Roscoe; turmeric, *Curcuma longa* L.; and shatavari, *Asparagus racemosus* Willd. also being popular. There is little clinical evidence to support this use, but the long tradition suggests they are well accepted and generally safe.

URINARY TRACT INFECTION

Acute or serious urinary tract infections (UTIs), including cystitis, may need antibiotic therapy, but for milder or chronic symptoms, herbal medicines are often used. This applies more commonly to women, although the treatment is the same for men. The most important are bearberry and cranberry. Bearberry is used for acute cystitis over a short period, whereas cranberry juice and extracts are more usually taken long term to prevent recurrent episodes.

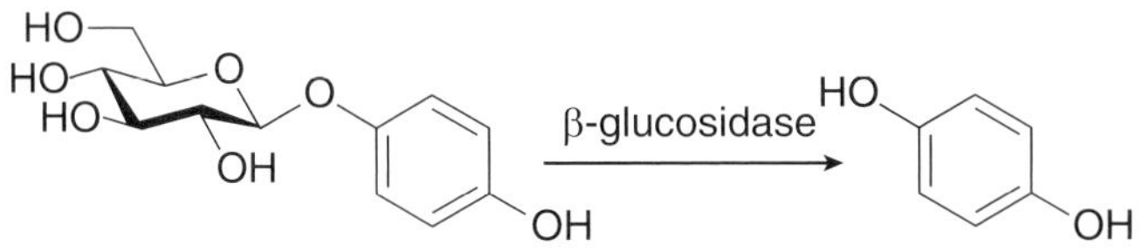

Fig. 24.6 Hydrolysis of arbutin.

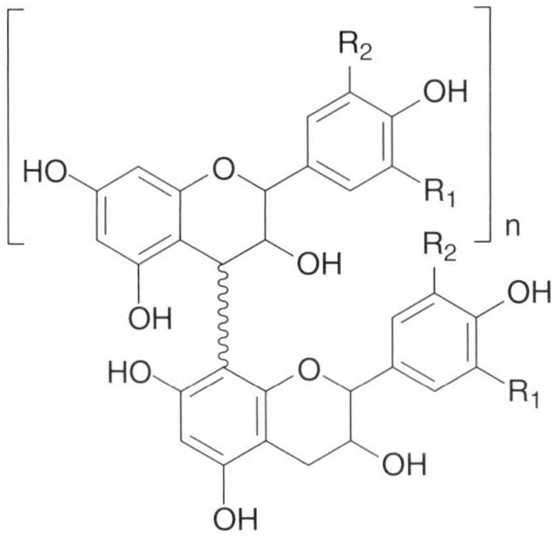

Fig. 24.7 Proanthocyanidins.

Bearberry, *Arctostaphylos uva-ursi* (L.) Spreng.†

The leaves of the shrub *Arctostaphylos uva-ursi* (Ericaceae), widely known as uva-ursi or bearberry, are used to treat cystitis and urethritis, although the efficacy is not supported by evidence from RCTs.

Constituents

The hydroquinone glycoside arbutin, which is hydrolysed in vivo by the enzyme β-glucosidase to give the diphenol, hydroquinone (Fig. 24.6), is the major constituent. Other constituents include terpenoids such as α- and β-amyrin, flavonoids and tannins.

Therapeutic Uses and Available Evidence

Hydroquinone is a potent phenolic antiseptic that is very active against many bacteria, in particular those that are liable to cause UTIs such as *Escherichia coli* and *Pseudomonas aeruginosa*. Uva-ursi preparations require that the urine be alkaline for it to have antiseptic properties and, as such, acidic foods including cranberry juice (see the following section) should be avoided during treatment. Hydroquinone is a very reactive and biologically active compound and is cytotoxic and mutagenic, causing changes to bladder epithelial cells. Short-term use of the herb does not seem to pose any problems, but high doses and prolonged usage should be avoided, and it should not be used during pregnancy or for renal disorders.

Cranberry Juice, *Vaccinium macrocarpon* Aiton

The juice of the berries of *Vaccinium macrocarpon* and related species (Ericaceae), or a freeze-dried extract, are very popular remedies for UTIs. Originally from North America, they are now used widely elsewhere for the same purpose. They are incorporated into foods and beverages for their general health benefits, based mainly on antioxidant properties.

Constituents

Flavonoid polymers, the proanthocyanidins (PACs), are mainly responsible for the antibacterial activity. These PACs are exceptionally complex and vary in the number of flavonoid units, the way these are connected, and the functional groups present on each unit (Fig. 24.7). They are highly polar and soluble in water, ethanol and methanol.

Therapeutic Uses and Available Evidence

Many clinical trials in a range of UTIs have been reported and the best evidence for efficacy found for the *prevention* of recurrent UTIs.

Cranberry juice and proanthocyanidins have been shown to affect the binding of *E. coli*, which is a major causative agent of UTIs, to uroepithelial cells, inhibiting the adherence of this bacterium and allowing its clearance. Cranberry juice has a high sugar and acid content, and extracts of cranberry are often used instead. Registered products containing extracts standardised to PAC content have been subjected to rigorous clinical studies and have shown positive results. Concerns that cranberry juice interacts with warfarin are now considered unfounded, as is a possible increase in the risk of kidney stone formation.

FURTHER READING

Akbaribazm, M., Goodarzi, N., Rahimi, M., 2021. Female infertility and herbal medicine: an overview of the new findings. Food Sci. Nutr. 9 (10), 5869–5882. https://doi.org/10.1002/fsn3.2523.

Bernstein, N., Akram, M., Yaniv-Bachrach, Z., Daniya, M., 2021. Is it safe to consume traditional medicinal plants during pregnancy? Phytother. Res. 35, 1908–1924.

Echeverria, V., Echeverria, F., Barreto, G.E., et al., 2021. Estrogenic plants: to prevent neurodegeneration and memory loss and other symptoms in women after menopause. Front. Pharmacol. 12, 644103. https://doi.org/10.3389/fphar.2021.644103.

Hudek Turković, A., Gunjača, M., Marjanović, M., et al., 2022. Proteome changes in human bladder T24 cells induced by hydroquinone derived from *Arctostaphylos uva-ursi* herbal preparation. J. Ethnopharmacol. 289, 115092.

Kenda, M., Glavač, N.K., Nagy, M., Dolenc, M.S., 2021. Herbal products used in menopause and for gynecological disorders. Molecules 26 (24), 7421. https://doi.org/10.3390/molecules26247421.

Kolodziejczyk-Czepas, J., Liudvytska, O., 2020. *Rheum rhaponticum* and *Rheum rhabarbarum*: a review of phytochemistry, biological activities and therapeutic potential. Phytochem. Rev. 20 (3), 589–607.

Liabsuetrakul, T., Choobun, T., Peeyananjarassri, K., Islam, Q.M., 2018. Prophylactic use of ergot alkaloids in the third stage of labour. Cochrane Database Syst. Rev. 6 (6), CD005456. https://doi.org/10.1002/14651858.CD005456.pub3.

Lim, T.K., 2012. *Punica granatum*. In: Edible Medicinal and Non-Medicinal Plants, pp. 136–194. Springer, Dordrecht, Netherlands. https://doi.org/10.1007/978-94-007-5653_10.

Liu, H., Zhu, R., Wang, L., et al., 2018. Radix Salviae miltiorrhizae improves bone microstructure and strength through Wnt/β-catenin and osteoprotegerin/receptor activator for nuclear factor-κB ligand/cathepsin K signaling in ovariectomized rats. Phytother. Res. 32, 2487–2500.

Madden, E., McLachlan, C., Oketch-Rabah, H., Calderón, A.I., 2021. Safety of cranberry: evaluation of evidence of kidney stone formation and botanical drug-interactions. Planta Med. 87 (10–11), 803–817. https://doi.org/10.1055/a-1497-6241.

Rahte, S., Evans, R., Eugster, P., et al., 2013. *Salvia officinalis* for hot flushes: towards determination of mechanism of activity and active principles. Planta Med. 79 (9), 753–760.

Safdari, F., Motaghi Dastenaei, B., Kheiri, S., Karimiankakolaki, Z., 2021. Effect of evening primrose oil on postmenopausal psychological symptoms: a triple-blind randomized clinical trial. J. Menopausal Med. 2, 58–65. https://doi.org/10.6118/jmm.21010.

Słupski, W., Jawień, P., Nowak, B., 2021. Botanicals in postmenopausal osteoporosis. Nutrients 13 (5), 1609. https://doi.org/10.3390/nu13051609.

Vandecasteele, K., Ost, P., Oosterlinck, W., 2012. Evaluation of the efficacy and safety of *Salvia officinalis* in controlling hot flashes in prostate cancer patients treated with androgen deprivation. Phytother. Res. 26 (2), 208–213. https://doi.org/10.1002/ptr.3528.

Wu, S., Li, T., 2017. Diverse phytochemicals and bioactivities in the ancient fruit and modern functional food pomegranate (*Punica granatum*). Molecules 22 (10), 1606.

Xia, J.Y., Yang, C., Xu, D.F., et al., 2021. Consumption of cranberry as adjuvant therapy for urinary tract infections in susceptible populations: a systematic review and meta-analysis with trial sequential analysis. PLoS One 16 (9), e0256992.

Zhang, Z., Lam, T.M., Zuo, Z., 2013. Radix puerariae: an overview of its chemistry, pharmacology, pharmacokinetics and clinical use. J. Clin. Pharmacol. 53 (8), 787–811.

25

The Male Reproductive System

Disorders of prostate gland occur frequently in older men and should be investigated to eliminate the possibility of prostate cancer. However, after diagnosis, benign conditions are often suitable for self-treatment with herbal medicines.

BENIGN PROSTATIC HYPERPLASIA

Benign prostatic hyperplasia (BPH) is so common that it can almost be considered a normal part of male ageing. The symptoms are increased frequency and difficulty in urinating, due to enlargement of the prostate gland surrounding the ureter, which restrict the flow of urine. Severe and acute cases may require surgery and drug treatment. α-Blockers relax smooth muscle in BPH and improve urinary flow, but they have side effects including drowsiness, dizziness and dry mouth. 5α-reductase inhibitors prevent the conversion of testosterone to the more potent androgen dihydrotestosterone, reducing prostate size and improving urine flow. Herbal medicines may be helpful in BPH, although complete reversal of the enlargement of the prostate is not possible.

Nettle, *Urtica dioica* L. (Urticaceae)†

Urtica dioica, the stinging nettle, grows to approximately 60–120 cm in height, with serrated leaves and stinging hairs on both the leaf and stem. The root and herb are used medicinally, as teas and extracts, and the young leaves are used in food (after denaturing the sting by boiling).

Constituents

Root. Several classes of compounds are thought to be responsible for the therapeutic effect. The main constituents are lignans, including pinoresinol, secoisolariciresinol, dehydrodiconiferyl alcohol and neo-olivil; triterpenes based on oleanolic and ursolic acids; and lectins, a mixture known as *U. dioica* agglutinin, composed of at least six isolectins.

Leaf. The leaf and stem contain flavonoids, mainly isorhamnetin, kaempferol and quercetin glycosides and glycoprotein, with indoles such as histamine and serotonin, betaine, acetylcholine, caffeic, chlorogenic and caffeoyl malic acids.

Therapeutic Uses and Available Evidence

Nettle root extracts are used for symptomatic relief of BPH. In vitro and in vivo (in mice) studies measuring sex hormone-binding globulin to human prostate membranes, and proliferation of prostatic epithelial and stromal cells, suggest beneficial effects on BPH tissue. Compounds from the roots are reported to be aromatase inhibitors. There is evidence from some clinical trials to support the use of nettle root extracts in BPH.

Nettle herb extracts and teas inhibit the proinflammatory transcription factor (nuclear factor kappa B (NF-κB)); partially inhibit cyclooxygenase and lipoxygenase; and inhibit tumour necrosis factor and interleukin-1β secretion stimulated by lipopolysaccharide.

Nettle preparations are generally considered safe, and few adverse events have been reported in clinical trials. The stinging sensation and dermatitis from contact with nettle plants are, of course, well known and thought to be due to both chemical and mechanical irritation.

Pumpkin, *Cucurbita pepo* L. (Cucurbitaceae)

Pumpkins are widely grown and well known for their food use.

Constituents

Pumpkin seeds are a rich source of lycopene, which is thought to benefit prostate health. They have a high essential fatty acid content, the most important being linoleic acid, palmitic acid, stearic acid, oleic acid and phytosterols including sitosterol and stigmasterol, as well as tocopherol (vitamin E).

Therapeutic Uses and Available Evidence

Pumpkin seed oil has been found to reduce testosterone-induced prostatic hyperplasia in rats, by a mechanism thought to involve 5α-reductase inhibition.

Several randomised controlled trials (RCTs) have shown that long-term administration of products containing pumpkin seed extract or oil can relieve the symptoms of BPH. It is often used in conjunction with saw palmetto (see later). Pumpkin seeds and oil are extremely safe, with adverse events only rarely reported.

Pygeum Bark, *Prunus africana* (Hook. f.) Kalkman (Rosaceae)†

The African prune (also known as *Pygeum africanum*, Hook. f.), is a tropical evergreen tree indigenous to central and southern Africa. The whole or fragmented dried bark of the stems and branches is used medicinally. The use of pygeum bark is becoming more widespread throughout Europe and the United States, and the tree is in danger of becoming scarce due to over harvesting of the bark.

Constituents

The bark contains sterols and pentacyclic triterpenes, including abietic, oleanolic, ursolic and crataegolic acids, *N*-butylbenzene sulfonamide and esters of ferulic acid.

Therapeutic Uses and Available Evidence

Traditionally used for micturition problems and now for BPH, pygeum extract has antiproliferative and apoptotic effects on proliferative prostate fibroblasts and myofibroblasts but not on smooth muscle cells. Other *Prunus* species have recently been investigated in preclinical studies for their effects in testosterone-induced BPH. Systematic reviews of RCTs have concluded the extract may be useful for men with

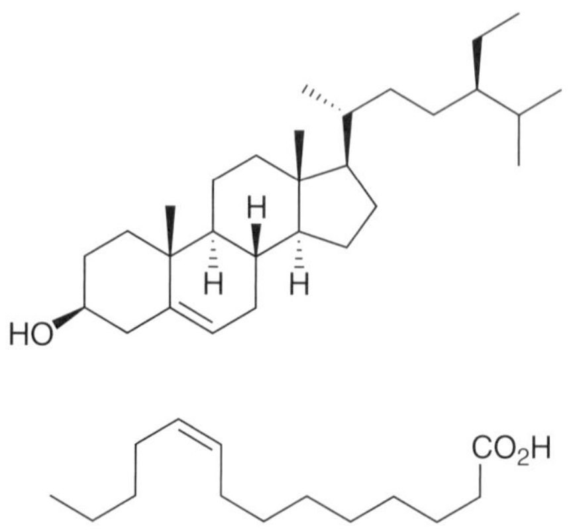

Fig. 25.1 β-Sitosterol *(top)* and myristoleic acid *(bottom)*.

lower urinary tract symptoms consistent with BPH, although further work is needed. Acute and chronic toxicity and mutagenicity tests have shown no adverse effects, and the extract appears to be well tolerated in men when administered over long periods. Pygeum is often used in combination with nettle.

Saw Palmetto, *Serenoa repens* (W. Bartram) Small (Arecaceae)†

Serenoa repens (*S. serrulata* (Michx.) Hook. f. ex B.D. Jacks., *Sabal serrulata* (Michx.) Schult. f.) or saw palmetto is a small 'fan' palm that produces abundant berries with a diameter of 1–2 cm, which are used traditionally for cystitis and male hormone disorders, including prostatic enlargement. Most commercial saw palmetto comes from the United States.

Constituents

The major constituents include the fatty acids capric, caprylic, lauric, oleic, myristoleic, palmitic, linoleic and linolenic acids; monoacyl glycerides; phytosterols such as β-sitosterol, campesterol, stigmasterol, lupeol and cycloartenol (Fig. 25.1); long-chain alcohols (farnesol, phytol and polyprenolic alcohols) and flavonoids. A series of immunostimulant, high-molecular-weight polysaccharides containing galactose, arabinose, mannose, rhamnose and glucuronic acid has been isolated. There are substantial variations in the quality of saw palmetto products, which influence efficacy.

Therapeutic Uses and Available Evidence

Liposterolic and ethanolic extracts of saw palmetto inhibit 5α-reductase (the enzyme that catalyses the conversion of testosterone to 5α-dihydrotestosterone in the prostate) in vitro; other studies have described beneficial effects in animal models of BPH. Spasmolytic activity has been documented in vivo (rats) for an ethanolic extract of saw palmetto. In vitro growth arrest of prostate cancer LNCaP, DU145, and PC3 cells and in vivo oestrogenic and antiinflammatory activities have been reported, which may be due to the high content of β-sitosterol.

The results of clinical studies are less conclusive. Systematic reviews of RCTs of saw palmetto extracts have failed to show efficacy. Adverse events were mild and did not occur any more frequently than with a placebo.

PROSTATITIS AND CHRONIC PELVIC PAIN SYNDROME

Chronic prostatitis or chronic pelvic pain syndrome (CPPS) is characterised by pain in the pelvic, perineal and penile areas, the lower abdomen and during urination or ejaculation. It is often diagnosed by biopsy during investigations for prostate cancer. The underlying mechanisms are unknown but hidden urinary tract infections and inflammation are common causes. Drug treatment is usually with antibiotics and antiinflammatories and in this context, herbal medicines for long-term CPPS management can be useful and include cranberry extract to inhibit urinary infection (see Chapter 24), turmeric as an antiinflammatory, together with the herbs described above for BHP.

ERECTILE DYSFUNCTION

Failure to produce a satisfactory or sustainable erection may be due to psychogenic, vascular, neurogenic or endocrine disorders (such as diabetes), drug treatment (such as with antihypertensives and antidepressants), but often with no identifiable cause. Erectile dysfunction (ED) is extremely common and can be very distressing but, in many cases, can be treated successfully with 5-phosphodiesterase (5-PD) inhibiting drugs such as sildenafil (Viagra).

Several herbal products claim to treat ED. There is no good clinical evidence of efficacy for any of these, although some have pharmacological activities in common with sildenafil.

Damiana, *Turnera diffusa* Willd. ex Schult. (Passifloraceae)

Damiana grows in tropical and subtropical areas of Central and South America. The leaves are used as a tonic and to treat male sexual dysfunction, and in some areas they are smoked to produce relaxation. They have been included in 'legal highs', but there is little clinical evidence available for any of these uses.

Constituents

Damiana contains traces of cyanogenetic glycosides and the hydroquinone glycoside arbutin, together with an essential oil composed of pinenes, thymol and others.

Therapeutic Uses and Available Evidence

No clinical evidence is available for the use of damiana in humans, but a study in rats has found that the extract can enhance recovery in 'sexually exhausted' rats, via the nitric oxide pathway.

Epimedium, Horny Goat Weed, *Epimedium brevicornu* Maxim, *E. sagittatum* (Siebold & Zucch.) Maxim (Berberidaceae) and Related Species

Epimedium herb is widely used in traditional Chinese medicine for a variety of disorders and is increasingly used to treat ED. The properties were apparently discovered after noticing that when goats ate it, they were eager to mate. Epimediums are sprawling perennial herbs, with cordate leaves and white, cream, pink, yellow or lavender flowers. Although native to Asia and the Mediterranean region, they are widely cultivated.

Constituents

The main constituents of the herb are prenylated flavonoids, the most important being icariin (Fig. 25.2) and its analogues and metabolites, epimedins A, B and C and the saggitatosides, together with other flavonoids.

Therapeutic Uses and Available Evidence

Icariin has phosphodiesterase type 5 inhibitory effects (the mechanism of action of sildenafil) and may also have neurotrophic effects, supporting its use in ED. A small double-blind clinical trial found that a

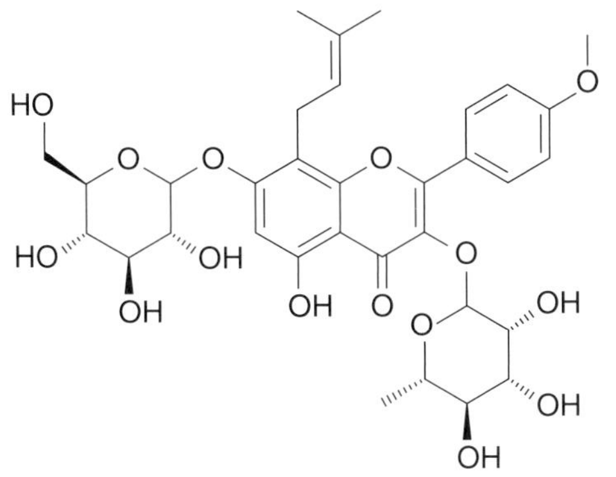

Fig. 25.2 Icariin.

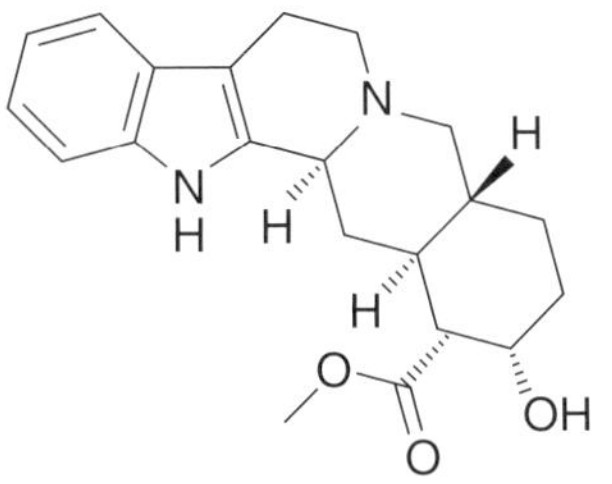

Fig. 25.3 Yohimbine.

daily dose of an epimedium-containing herbal product enhanced sexual satisfaction.

Epimedium is used to treat and prevent osteoporosis in both men and women, where it may exert its effects through the induction of bone morphogenetic protein-2 and NO synthesis, subsequently regulating gene expression and contributing to the induction of osteoblast proliferation and differentiation.

Yohimbe, *Pausinystalia johimbe* (K. Schum) Pierre ex Beille (Rubiaceae)

Yohimbe bark occurs as flat or slightly quilled pieces, often covered with lichen. It is a very popular supplement used to treat sexual dysfunction, but has been linked to reports of toxicity, including priapism, hypertension and even heart attack, and is on the US Food and Drug Administration's list of dangerous supplements. There are many contraindications and potential drug interactions, so its use cannot be recommended.

Constituents

The bioactive constituents are indole alkaloids, the major being yohimbine, together with coryantheine, α- and β-yohimbane and pseudoyohimbine.

Therapeutic Uses and Available Evidence

Yohimbine[†] (Fig. 25.3) is an α-2 adrenergic blocker and coryantheine is an α-1 adrenergic blocker, both of which may contribute to activity, so yohimbe bark may be more effective than yohimbine alone. Priapism has been reported after taking the bark extract as well as from yohimbine.

MALE FERTILITY AND LIBIDO ENHANCERS

Many herbal and nutritional products used for men's sexual health are the same as those used by athletes for their anabolic or testosterone-boosting properties. The most prominent include *Tribulus terrestris* (caltrops), *Eurycoma longifolia* (tongkat ali), *Lepidium meyenii* (maca), *Mucuna pruriens* (mucuna), *Trigonella foenum-graceum* (fenugreek), *Withania somnifera* (ashwaghanda) and *Nigella sativa* (black seed).

Of these, only mucuna, fenugreek and black seed have shown moderate effects in improving testosterone levels and improving seminal parameters in patients with oligozoospermia. Further details on these and other herbal medicines used for these conditions can be found in the papers cited in the Further Reading list.

FURTHER READING

Anand Ganapathy, A., Hari Priya, V.M., Kumaran, A., 2021. Medicinal plants as a potential source of phosphodiesterase-5 inhibitors: a review. J. Ethnopharmacol. 267, 113536. https://doi.org/10.1016/j.jep.2020.113536.

Brunetti, P., Lo Faro, A.F., Tini, A., Busardò, F.P., Carlier, J., 2020. Pharmacology of herbal sexual enhancers: a review of psychiatric and neurological adverse effects. Pharmaceuticals 13 (10), 309. https://doi.org/10.3390/ph13100309.

Csikós, E., Horváth, A., Ács, K., Papp, N., Balázs, V.L., Dolenc, M.S., et al., 2021. Treatment of benign prostatic hyperplasia by natural drugs. Molecules 26 (23), 7141. https://doi.org/10.3390/molecules26237141.

Hu, M., Wazir, J., Ullah, R., Wang, W., Cui, X., Tang, M., et al., 2019. Phytotherapy and physical therapy in the management of chronic prostatitis-chronic pelvic pain syndrome. Int. Urol. Nephrol. 51 (7), 1081–1088.

Jena, A.K., Vasisht, K., Sharma, N., Kaur, R., Dhingra, M.S., Karan, M., 2016. Amelioration of testosterone induced benign prostatic hyperplasia by *Prunus* species. J. Ethnopharmacol. 190, 33–45.

Rehman, S.U., Choe, K., Yoo, H.H., 2016. Review on a traditional herbal medicine, *Eurycoma longifolia* Jack (Tongkat Ali): its traditional uses, chemistry, evidence-based pharmacology and toxicology. Molecules 21 (3), 331.

Santos, H.O., Howell, S., Teixeira, F.J., 2019. Beyond tribulus (*Tribulus terrestris* L.): the effects of phytotherapics on testosterone, sperm and prostate parameters. J. Ethnopharmacol. 235, 392–405.

Thu, H.E., Mohamed, I.N., Hussain, Z., Jayusman, P.A., Shuid, A.N., 2017. *Eurycoma longifolia* as a potential adoptogen of male sexual health: a systematic review on clinical studies. Chin. J. Nat. Med. 15 (1), 71–80.

26

Supportive Therapies for Stress, Ageing, Cancer and Debility

Many people use preventative medicines as a way of maintaining and improving their health, and this approach is an essential element of most Asian traditional medicine systems. Substances used in this way have been collected together here as they are typically used for general health and well-being, to prevent degenerative conditions, including ageing and some forms of cancer, and for numerous other health and medical conditions. Most of the herbs mentioned here originated in China, India and other parts of Asia. In traditional Chinese medicine (TCM), they are used to treat 'empty' diseases, to restore 'qi' energy and tonify the organs, having a balancing effect on yin and yang rather than affecting only one. These traditional medicines are believed to strengthen the immune system, improve memory and alertness, enhance sexual performance, promote healing and/or stimulate appetite. In Western countries, the Chinese herbs ginseng, ginkgo, astragalus, schisandra, baical skullcap and tea, as well as reishi mushroom, are used in this way. In Ayurveda, some rejuvenating and tonic herbs are called 'rasayanas', and these are considered to have a beneficial effect, balancing the tridosha (see Chapter 16). In Asian medicine, ashwagandha and *Centella asiatica* (gotu kola) are very widely used as tonics and/or for other purposes. Many of these herbs contain saponins or steroidal compounds of some kind, and these may act in a similar way to corticosteroids or enhance the effect of naturally occurring steroid hormones in the body. This type of drug is known as an adaptogen and is considered to be a substance that helps the body to deal with or adapt to stress or other adverse conditions.

This is a fast-growing area of phytotherapy, but use of these herbal drugs is often based on very limited scientific evidence.

CANCER CHEMOPREVENTION

During the 1960s and 1970s, L.W. Wattenberg's work at the University of Minnesota, United States, showed that various compounds, especially from fruits and vegetables (indoles and isothiocyanates), could inhibit chemically induced tumours in laboratory animals. Termed 'chemoprophylaxis of carcinogenesis', this was of obvious benefit to maintenance of human health and had enormous dietary significance. After intensive studies using retinoids (vitamin A-related natural products), the term 'cancer chemoprevention' was first used and the area has now developed into a well-defined discipline.

Cancer chemoprevention is 'the prevention of cancer in human populations by ingestion of chemical agents that prevent carcinogenesis'. (N.B. It is distinct from cancer prevention (e.g. through cessation of cigarette smoking) and cancer chemotherapy (the use of cytotoxic drugs after cancer diagnosis)). Large epidemiological studies have demonstrated that dietary factors may reduce the incidence of cancers. For example, inverse associations have been found between the incidence of lung cancer among people who smoke and consume carotene-rich foods, as well as for vitamin C intake and oesophageal and stomach cancers, selenium and various cancers, and vitamin E and lung cancer. Epidemiological studies can identify potential leads for chemopreventive agents, which can then be tested in laboratory experiments. Almost 600 'chemopreventive' agents are known; they are usually classified as inhibitors of carcinogen formation (ascorbic acid, tocopherols, phenols); inhibitors of initiation (phenols, flavones); and inhibitors of postinitiation events (β-carotene, retinoids, terpenes). Many are constituents of food or beverages (e.g. tea) and are sometimes called 'functional foods' or 'nutraceuticals'.

Chemopreventive agents may work in synergy, with several components contributing to the overall effect, which may be the case with plant drugs. This approach has great promise, with both natural products and synthetics being potentially useful. Dietary campaigns by government bodies, the American Cancer Society and other scientific organisations recommend that 5–7 servings of vegetables be consumed daily to function as a source of cancer chemopreventive agents. However, it is not reasonable to assume that consuming chemopreventive agents will safeguard humans from known carcinogenic risks, such as smoking. As knowledge of chemopreventive agents increases, they will play a more important role in cancer prevention. Chemoprevention and its mechanisms are discussed in Chapter 9.

CANCER SUPPORT

Many patients with cancer use various therapies to help their recovery, and dietary measures are often advocated. These usually involve increasing vegetable and whole grain and reducing or omitting meat intake. Herbal medicines and nutritional supplements are also popular, as an attempt to improve general health before or during cancer treatment, to enhance well-being and to counteract the adverse effects of chemotherapy or radiotherapy. The concurrent use of herbal and conventional medicines has led to concerns of clinical interactions with prescribed drugs. For example, the dangers of co-administration of St John's wort with many drugs, including some anticancer drugs, such as irinotecan, are now recognised and patients are made aware of them. Other herbal medicines are of less concern with respect to drug interactions, but each situation should be assessed. In China, TCM is routinely used as a supporting or adjunctive therapy in patients with cancer, and lingzhi mushroom (*Ganoderma lucidum*) is particularly widely used. Beneficial interactions between herbs and drugs may also occur, but this approach should be practised only by clinical specialists, usually in integrated TCM hospitals or similar environments.

TONICS, STIMULANTS, ADAPTOGENS AND SUPPORTIVE THERAPIES

Açai Berry, *Euterpe oleracea* Mart.

The fruits of the palm *Euterpe oleracea* (açai, Arecaceae) are claimed to have a range of health-promoting and therapeutic benefits due to their reportedly high content of antioxidants. Açai has a history of use as a medicinal plant and as a staple food in many parts of Brazil. Traditionally, it has been used to treat fevers, skin complications, digestive disorders and parasitic infections. In recent years, açai berry has been advertised widely, for example, via the Internet.

Constituents

Açai has a relatively high content of polyphenols. Most notable are anthocyanins and flavonoids, as well as fatty acids. Small amounts of lignans have also been reported.

Therapeutic Uses and Available Evidence

Açai berries have become very popular despite a lack of definitive scientific evidence to support their uses. The high content of polyphenols has been linked with several activities, including antioxidant, antiinflammatory, antiproliferative and cardioprotective properties, following preclinical studies. Clinical data are mostly limited to small studies involving healthy volunteers; one small study explored the antiinflammatory effects of an açai beverage in patients with metabolic syndrome, and another reported açai improves exercise tolerance in athletes.

Ashwagandha, *Withania somnifera* (L.) Dunal†

Ashwagandha, also known as winter cherry (Solanaceae) and 'Indian ginseng', is a woody shrub native to the Middle East, Africa and parts of Asia, growing in stony and semiarid regions; it is cultivated widely. The leaves are elliptical with an acute apex and the flowers campanulate and greenish yellow, developing into red berries enclosed in a papery membrane. The dried root is used medicinally. Ashwagandha has been used in Ayurvedic medicine for more than 4000 years, as an adaptogen, sedative and tonic for debility. It is used to enhance fertility in both men and women and as an aphrodisiac. Ashwagandha is also widely used for inflammation, colds, asthma and many other disorders. The name 'ashwagandha' comes from the Sanskrit *ashva* (meaning 'horse') and *gandha* (meaning 'smell') and refers to the odour of the root.

Constituents

The root contains steroidal lactones (the withanolides A–Y), withaferin A (Fig. 26.1), withasomniferols A–C and others, phytosterols (e.g. the sitoindosides) and the alkaloids anahygrine, cuscohygrine, ashwagandhine, ashwagandhinine, withasomnine, withaninine, somniferine and others.

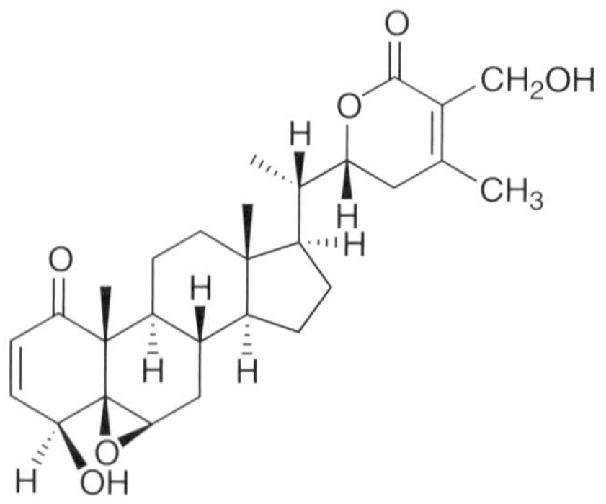

Therapeutic Uses and Available Evidence

Ashwagandha root extracts have adaptogenic, antistress, antioxidant, immunomodulatory and sedative properties. Many of these pharmacological effects have been substantiated in animal studies. The extract is also reported to be anxiolytic, acting via the (γ-amino butyric acid [GABA]) GABAergic system. Numerous other actions have been documented in preclinical studies, including antimicrobial, antiinflammatory, antitumour, neuroprotective, cardioprotective and antidiabetic activities.

There is an increasing amount of clinical research on ashwagandha across a range of therapeutic areas. Some trials involving patients with sleep disorders, diabetes mellitus, cognitive dysfunction, anxiety or male infertility have reported beneficial effects, but systematic reviews

Fig. 26.1 Withaferin A.

of these studies conclude that definitive evidence from well-designed clinical trials to support the pharmacological effects of ashwagandha remains limited. Few adverse events occurred in clinical trials involving patients who received ashwagandha, but comprehensive data on the safety profile of ashwagandha are required. High doses can cause gastrointestinal irritation, and there are isolated reports of hepatotoxic reactions, although causality has not been established.

Centella, *Centella asiatica* (L.) Urb.†

Centella herb is described in Chapter 27 (Topical Phytotherapy). In addition to its wound-healing effects, the plant is considered a 'rasayana' in Ayurvedic medicine (a therapy that helps maintain and promote health) and is used in TCM and other Asian systems. It is believed to enhance the immune system and is considered to have a rejuvenating, neurological 'tonic' with a mild sedative effect. The immunomodulating effects of the herb have been shown in vitro and in vivo in mice. Preclinical studies in rodents have shown that asiatic acid (a triterpene) and certain other constituents of centella have benefits on memory and learning and that centella extract protects against certain types of neurodegeneration. Several bioactive constituents of centella cross the blood–brain barrier in animal models, and the mechanisms for the neuroprotective effects may involve antioxidant activity and protection of mitochondrial function. Other reported effects for the herb or its constituents include antiinflammatory, antiepileptic, antimicrobial and antiulcer activity and spasmolytic effects.

Despite the popular use of centella in traditional medicine systems, there is a lack of robust clinical research, and the pharmacological effects reported from preclinical studies mostly are unsubstantiated in humans. A systematic review of five randomised controlled trials exploring the effects of centella on cognitive function found no effects on any cognitive function domain, but some trials found that centella may improve working memory. Six other trials, which assessed centella given in combination with other (mainly herbal) ingredients, also found no effect on overall cognitive function.

Centella is taken orally, usually in the form of an extract. Clinical trials of a standardised water extract of the aerial parts have used doses of 250, 500 and 750 mg daily (equivalent to 22.5, 25.0 and 37.5 mg pentacyclic triterpenes, respectively).

Ginseng, *Panax ginseng* C.A. Mey.,† *Eleutherococcus senticosus* (Rupr. & Maxim.) Maxim.† (syn.: *Acanthopanax senticosus* (Rupr. & Maxim.) Harms) and Related 'Ginseng' Species

Ginseng root in commerce is obtained from *Panax ginseng* (Korean or Chinese ginseng, Araliaceae) and other species. American ginseng is from *P. quinquefolius* L., but Siberian ginseng, *Eleutherococcus senticosus* (Araliaceae), is from a different (but related) genus.

P. ginseng is native to China and cultivated widely elsewhere. The root is spindle shaped, ringed, and divided into two or three equal branches. Red Korean ginseng (from *P. ginseng*) is approximately 8 years old; it is matured and roasted and is the most highly regarded form. Adulteration and substandard material are common in the trade, and proper authentication is essential. Adulteration with other species of the same genus or with unrelated species (including sawdust) and/or the admixing of other plant parts of *P. ginseng* are just some of the many examples of adulteration. Sadly, there seems to be no limit to the ingenuity of adulterating a high-value botanical drug such as *P. ginseng* (root), and this clearly impacts both on the patients' experience with the use of products and the results of bioscientific research on the species.

Constituents

All types contain saponin glycosides (the ginsenosides Ra, Rb, Rg$_1$, Rg$_2$, Rs, etc.; Fig. 26.2). The ginsenosides are sometimes referred to as the panaxosides, but this nomenclature uses the suffixes A–F, which do not correspond to those of the ginsenosides.

In Siberian ginseng (*E. senticosus*), the saponins (eleutherosides A–F) are chemically different but have similar properties. Glycans (panaxans) also occur in *P. ginseng*. The actual composition of ginseng extracts depends upon the species and method of preparation.

Therapeutic Uses and Available Evidence

Ginseng is taken as a tonic for numerous purposes, including debility, insomnia, natural and premature ageing, to increase alertness and improve sexual inadequacy, for diabetes, and as an adaptogen to relieve stress and improve stamina and concentration. These effects may be due to changes in cholinergic activity and also neuroprotection, as well as through antioxidant activity. The adaptogenic effect may be due to the elevation of serum concentrations of corticosteroids and the reduction of catecholamines, which results in homeostasis. Ginsenoside Rb$_1$ acts as a central nervous system (CNS) sedative, and Rg$_1$ has antifatigue and stimulant properties. In animals, an extract increases the capacity of skeletal muscle to oxidise free fatty acids in preference to glucose to produce cellular energy, which would support the antifatigue activity seen in conventional exhaustion tests. Ginseng also has a traditional use in diabetes, and the glycans (panaxans A–E) are hypoglycaemic in mice. Other documented effects include immunomodulatory activity, potentiation of analgesia and anticancer effects (by ginsenosides R$_{s3}$ and R$_{s4}$).

There is a substantial body of clinical research on ginseng, particularly *P. ginseng*, but few studies are of high methodological

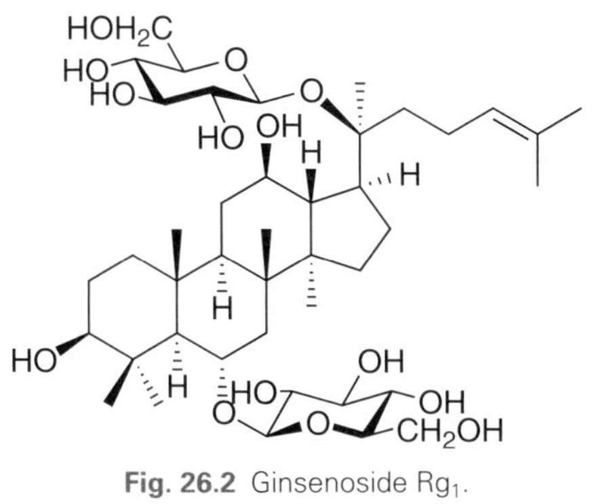

quality and clinical trials vary with respect to doses and populations studied. It has been recognised that modified extracts, such as hydrolysed dammarane saponin extracts, may provide a more targeted approach.

Eleutherococcus has also been tested in clinical trials for cognitive function and physical and mental endurance, but, again, more rigorous clinical trials are required to confirm these findings.

The dose of ginseng used is very variable depending on the age of the patient and the length of the course of treatment. Ginseng is taken widely, and side effects are relatively well documented; they include oestrogenic effects, hypertension and irritability.

Lingzhi or Reishi Mushroom, *Ganoderma* spp.†

Ganoderma lucidum (Curtis Fr.) P. Karst., *G. japonicum* (Fr. Lloyd) and other species of mushroom (Ganodermataceae) grow on tree stumps (mainly conifers) in China, Japan and North America. This mushroom is now cultivated for commerce. In China, the fungus is known as lingzhi and, in Japan, as reishi. The fruiting body takes several forms, including a rare, branched or 'antler' type, in addition to the more usual mushroom shape. The colour varies from red, through orange and brown, to black, with the red and antlered varieties being more highly prized. The cap is circular, kidney- or fan-shaped, leathery, with a smooth or rippled upper surface, and an undersurface that shows the spore tubes. Lingzhi is a very important Chinese medicine; it has been immortalised in Oriental paintings and was used frequently by Taoist monks.

Constituents

The mature fruiting body of the fungus contains a series of triterpenes, mainly lanostanes, such as the ganoderic acids A–Z, ganoderals A and B, ganoderiols A and B, epoxyganoderiols A–C, ganolucidic acids A–E, lucidones A–C and lucidenic acids A–M. Polysaccharides, mainly glucans and arabinoxyoglucans, and peptidoglycans (known as ganoderans A–C) are also present.

Therapeutic Uses and Available Evidence

Lingzhi is used as an adaptogen and general tonic, in the hope of prolonging life, retarding ageing and generally improving well-being and mental faculties. The most common indication for use is to enhance the immune system, and preclinical studies support this, as well as antioxidant, lipid-lowering and antiinflammatory activities. The active principles are considered to be the triterpenes and polysaccharides. Extracts inhibit angiotensin-converting enzyme and produce hypotensive effects, and animal studies have provided evidence of hypoglycaemic effects.

Clinical evidence to support the use of ganoderma preparations is limited, including when reishi is used as an adjunctive treatment to chemotherapy and radiation in cancer patients to support immune system resistance.

The dose of the dried fruiting body of the fungus is 6–12 g daily, or the equivalent in extract. Lingzhi is well tolerated, although transient side effects of gastrointestinal disturbance and rashes in sensitive individuals have been reported. Animal studies have shown no toxic effects after intake of long-term high doses. However, comprehensive data on the safety profile of lingzhi are lacking, and, as with other immune modulators, lingzhi should probably be avoided in people with autoimmune disease.

Rosenroot, *Rhodiola rosea* L.

Also known as *Sedum rosea* (L.) Scop., golden root and Aaron's rod, *Rhodiola rosea* (Crassulaceae) grows in cold regions of the world, including much of the Arctic, mountainous regions of Central Asia

Fig. 26.2 Ginsenoside Rg$_1$.

and Europe, and the Rocky Mountains. It is a dioecious perennial reaching 5–35 cm in height.

Constituents

The main active constituents of the root and rhizome are monoterpene alcohols and their glycosides, such as salidroside (previously known as rhodioloside or rhodosin), rhodioniside, rhodiolin, rosin, rosavin, rosarin and rosiridin. These compounds are thought to be responsible for the adaptogenic properties of *Rhodiola*. Other phenolic constituents such as caffeic acid, chlorogenic acid and flavonoids (catechins and proanthocyanidins) are present. Geraniol and other essential oil constituents, such as geranyl formate, geranyl acetate, benzyl alcohol and phenylethyl alcohol, give the root its rose-like odour.

Therapeutic Uses and Available Evidence

Rhodiola has a long history of use in traditional medicine, particularly in TCM; it is used as a 'brain tonic' and stimulant, to reduce fatigue and improve stamina, and to prevent stress. Their adaptogenic effects, including neuroprotective, cardioprotective, antifatigue, antidepressive, anxiolytic and CNS-stimulating activities, have been shown in preclinical studies, and several mechanisms of action that may contribute to the reported effects have been identified, including interactions with the Hypothalamic-pituitary-adrenal (HPA) system (reducing cortisol levels) and defence mechanism proteins (e.g. some heat shock proteins). Unregulated products are often of poor quality, and an additional problem relates to the use (often interchangeably) of different *Rhodiola* species in Chinese medicine. According to the Chinese Pharmacopoeia 2010, only *R. crenulata* can be used medicinally, and, consequently, this species also enters the trade. Of course, this problem is linked both to poor pharmacognostic authentication and to a lack of knowledge along the value chains of the botanical drugs.

Due to the low quality of clinical trials, evidence for *Rhodiola* preparations is usually inconclusive, and systematic reviews of clinical trials of *Rhodiola* in physical and mental fatigue, and ischaemic heart disease, have either drawn cautiously positive conclusions or concluded there is insufficient evidence to assess efficacy. Few adverse events associated with *Rhodiola* have been reported, but a comprehensive investigation of its safety profile is lacking.

Schisandra, *Schisandra chinensis* (Turcz.) Baill.†

The magnolia vine (*Schisandra chinensis*, Schisandraceae) is also known as gomishi in Japan and as bei-wuweizi in China. It is a monoecious liana, native to Northern China, Korea, Japan and eastern Russia, usually found climbing round tree trunks. The leaves are elliptical, and the flowers are cream with a pleasant odour. The fresh berries are scarlet, small and ovoid, hanging in clusters and are the main botanical drug used. When dry, they are wrinkled, dark reddish brown, containing a sticky pulp and a yellow kidney-shaped seed. *Schisandra sphenanthera* Rehder & E.H. Wilson (nan-wuweizi) is also widely used for similar purposes.

Constituents

The active constituents are lignans, including schizandrin A (= deoxyschisandrin or wuweizu A), schizandrin B (= wuweizu B or γ-schizandrin B; Fig. 26.3), schizandrol A (= schizandrin), schizandrol B (= gomisin A), schisandrin C, schisantherin A (= gomisin C), schisantherin B (= gomisin B), gomisins H, K, L, M, N, schizanhenol, wuweizu C, schisantherin C and others.

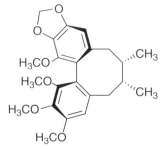

Fig. 26.3 Schisandrin B.

Therapeutic Uses and Available Evidence

Schisandra has been used in China since ancient times to prolong life and increase energy ('qi') and act as a general and sexual tonic, especially for men. It is also used to reduce sweating, detoxify the liver, enhance kidney function and suppress cough in lung disease. Many pharmacological studies support the use of schisandra: for example, the adaptogenic and antifatigue properties have been tested in racehorses in which a beneficial effect on physical recovery and a general improvement in performance were observed. Schizanhenol and schizandrin B protect against peroxidative damage associated with ageing and ischaemia in the rat brain. Schisandra is used for liver disease (see Chapter 18), including that induced by chemotherapy and immunosuppressive drugs. Deoxyschisandrin, gomisin A, B and C increase liver cytochrome P450 enzymes, which supports the detoxifying and anticancer properties attributed to the plant. Antitumour-promoting and antiinflammatory properties have also been shown in skin, and the lignans are known to be platelet-activating factor antagonists.

Clinical evidence to support the uses of schisandra as a general supportive therapy is limited. Randomised, placebo-controlled trials involving small numbers of adults have reported beneficial effects on muscle strength following 12 weeks' treatment with schisandra extract and improvements in perimenopausal and postmenopausal symptoms. Daily doses of powdered berry are usually 1.5–6 g, or sometimes higher.

Few toxicity studies have been carried out, and comprehensive investigation of the safety profile of schisandra is required; until then, schisandra should be avoided during pregnancy (possible uterine stimulation) and epilepsy. Schisandra has been associated with an increase in gastric acidity and may cause allergy in susceptible individuals.

Skullcap, *Scutellaria baicalensis* Georgi.†

Scutellaria baicalensis (huang qin, Lamiaceae) is sometimes known as baical skullcap to differentiate it from American skullcap (*S. lateriflora* L.). It grows in northern China, Siberia and Manchuria (a large region in northeast Asia). The leaves are opposite, lanceolate and sessile with an acute apex. The flowers are blue, with a helmet-shaped upper lip (hence the name). The root is the part used medicinally.

Constituents

The root contains flavonoids, including baicalin, baicalein, wogonin, chrysin, oroxylin A, skullcapflavones I and II and others (Fig. 26.4).

Therapeutic Uses and Available Evidence

Skullcap is used for a wide variety of ailments, particularly fevers, infections, jaundice, thirst and nosebleeds, and as an antidote and sedative. It is important in TCM and is an ingredient in numerous TCM formulae.

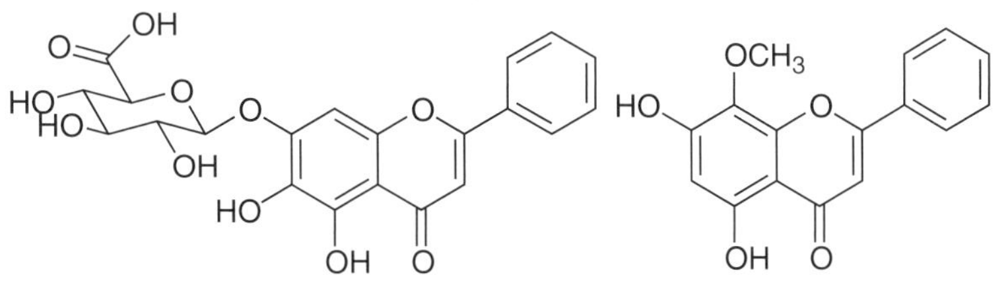

Fig. 26.4 Baicalin (left) and wogonin (right).

Preclinical studies with skullcap extracts and its isolated constituents provide evidence for antioxidant, immunomodulatory, antitumour, antibacterial, antiviral, hepatoprotective and other effects. Baicalin is antiinflammatory and antiallergic; it inhibits the generation of inflammatory cytokines and is synergistic with β-lactam antibiotics against methicillin-resistant *Staphylococcus aureus* in vitro. Extracts of *S. baicalensis* inhibit lipid peroxidation in rat liver, and wogonin suppresses production of hepatitis B virus surface antigen. The flavones interact with the benzodiazepine-binding site of the GABA$_A$ receptor, with wogonin and baicalein being the most potent; this supports the sedative use. Baicalein is antigenotoxic in vitro and inhibits adhesion molecule expression induced by thrombin and cell proliferation of several types of cells. Wogonin inhibits nitric oxide production in activated C6 rat glial cells, acting via nuclear factor (NF)-κB inhibition and thus suppressing cell death. Many other mechanistic studies support the antiinflammatory and other uses of skullcap, but despite this, and the extensive traditional use, clinical evidence from well-designed trials is lacking. Pharmacokinetic and tolerability studies involving single doses (100–800 mg) of baicalein in healthy volunteers found it to be well tolerated, although adverse events occurred more frequently with baicalein than with placebo, most commonly elevated high-sensitivity C-reactive protein and high triglyceride concentrations. A comprehensive investigation of the safety profile of baical skullcap is still required.

Green Tea, *Camellia sinensis* (L.) Kuntze.†

Tea (*Camellia sinensis*, Theaceae) is cultivated in China, India, Sri Lanka, Kenya, Indonesia and elsewhere. Green tea is produced in China and Japan; it is not processed and thus differs from black tea, which is fermented and produced in India, Sri Lanka and Kenya. Oolong tea is partially fermented. The leaf buds and very young leaves are used to prepare the beverage and extracts for medicinal use.

Constituents

Tea contains caffeine and much smaller amounts of other xanthines, such as theophylline and theobromine. The polyphenols are the antioxidant constituents: in green tea, these are mainly (−)-epigallocatechin (Fig. 26.5), together with theogallin, trigalloyl glucose; in black tea, they have been oxidised to form the 'tea pigments', the theaflavins, thearubigins and theaflavic acids.

Therapeutic Uses and Available Evidence

Tea is a stimulant, diuretic, astringent and antioxidant. Green tea is used medicinally more frequently than black tea. The stimulant and diuretic properties are due to the caffeine content and the astringency and antioxidant effects to the polyphenols. Tea is also antimicrobial and anticariogenic and is reputed to help weight loss. Tea is useful in diarrhoea and, in China, is used for many types of dysentery.

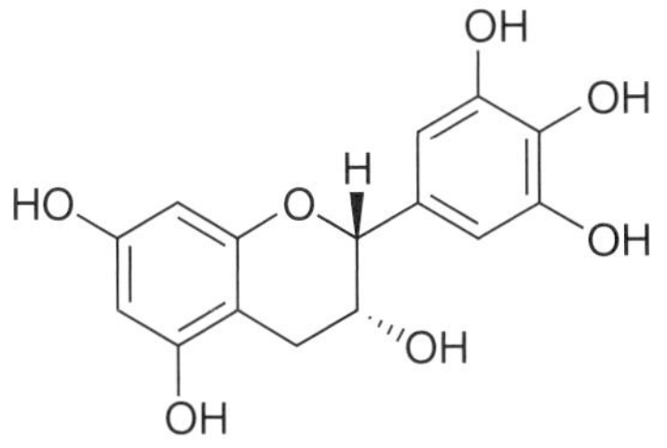

Fig. 26.5 (−)-Epigallocatechin.

The polyphenols in green tea have cancer chemopreventive properties due to their antioxidant capacity. Antiinflammatory and antitumour effects have been described and attributed to inhibition of the transcription factor NF-κB.

Black tea consumption has been associated with a lower risk of death from ischaemic heart disease and has been shown to reverse endothelial dysfunction in coronary heart disease. Habitual consumption of green tea has been associated with a lower incidence of cancer, and black tea is believed to have similar health benefits, which are ascribed to the tea pigments. Cochrane reviews of randomised trials and observational studies have concluded that there is insufficient and conflicting evidence for green tea in cancer prevention or for achieving or maintaining weight loss in overweight or obese adults but that consumption of green or black tea is associated with a reduced risk of cardiovascular disease. Recent systematic reviews have reported that green or black tea consumption for 4–24 weeks does not significantly affect blood pressure or blood lipid profile in adults and that green tea does not affect serum concentrations of adiponectin (a hormone that may help protect against the development of diabetes mellitus and atherosclerosis). Consumption of three to five cups of tea daily was not associated with safety concerns.

Tea is drunk in nearly every country in the world for its refreshing and mildly stimulating effects. There is no recommended dose for tea, and consumption varies widely. Tea as a beverage is nontoxic in the usual amounts ingested, although it can cause gastrointestinal upsets and nervous irritability, due to the caffeine content. There is now some concern about the safety of concentrated preparations or excessive consumption of green tea. Cases of hepatotoxicity have been associated with consumption of high doses of green tea-containing dietary supplements (10–29 mg/kg/d p.o.). Symptoms resolved following cessation of green tea, but re-injury occurred in some people who reused the same preparations, suggesting a causative effect of the green tea. A comprehensive review undertaken by a United States Pharmacopoeia expert panel concluded that there was a clear association between ingestion of green tea extracts and the occurrence of severe hepatotoxicity; the review also concluded that the hepatotoxic effect is rare and that specific constituents of green tea, particularly (−)-epigallocatechin-3-O-gallate (EGCG) and other catechins, are likely to be involved.

TABLE 26.1   Examples of 'Superfoods' and Their Important Constituents

Food	Important Constituents
Avocado	Phosphorus, potassium, magnesium, calcium; vitamins A, C, K, folate; fibre
Beans and other low-fat legumes	Folate, potassium, magnesium, iron, protein, fibre
Beetroot	Iron, magnesium; folate; antioxidants (betacyanin)
Blueberries and other coloured berries, such as raspberries and blackberries	Blueberries: anthocyanins; vitamins C and K; fibre
Broccoli and other cruciferous vegetables, including Brussels sprouts, cauliflower, cabbage, or kale	Broccoli: vitamins A, C, K; folate; fibre; sulforaphane and isothiocyanates
Chocolate (dark)	Cocoa: iron, magnesium, manganese, phosphorous, zinc; antioxidants (catechins, procyanidins)
Dragon fruit, Pitaya fruit	Fibre; vitamins C and E; lycopene
Kiwi fruit (green)	Fibre
Oatmeal	Fibre
Olive oil	Unsaturated fats
Pomegranate	Vitamins A, C, E; iron
Quinoa	Essential amino acids; vitamins; minerals; protein
Spinach	Iron (but is poorly absorbed); lutein, zeaxanthin
Spirulina	Magnesium, manganese, phosphorus; B vitamins, including B_{12}; essential fatty acids, e.g. gamma-linolenic acid
Tomatoes	Lycopene
Walnuts	Omega-3 fatty acids; fats (help absorb vitamins A, D, E and K)

SUPERFOODS

'Superfoods' is a contemporary term used to describe foods that are believed to be, or promoted as being, beneficial to health; in many instances, this is driven by marketing strategies.

Foods that have in recent years been hailed as superfoods include those that contain fibre, plant proteins and/or high concentrations of antioxidant compounds, such as vitamins A, C and E, and omega-3 fatty acids. Many of the so-called superfoods are fruits or vegetables or otherwise originate from plants; some are animal products or animal by-products (e.g. salmon, eggs, yoghurt). Table 26.1 lists some popular 'superfoods' and their important constituents.

Many of these foods are, of course, used as ('super') ingredients in naturally derived health and nutrition products and supplements, as well as in drinks, and beauty, personal care and hygiene products. The total global superfoods market across all categories (foods and drinks, health products, personal care, pet care) is substantial and is predicted to continue to grow.

Where intended for oral use, superfoods are often formulated as powders, often in combination with other superfoods and herbal substances, for adding to blended drinks, food recipes and meals; others are components of single- or multiingredient tablets and capsules marketed for daily use.

Many health claims have been made in association with these foods and marketed products, from supporting well-being, boosting energy, regulating metabolism and strengthening immunity, to lowering blood pressure, lowering cholesterol, improving exercise performance, and preventing dementia and cancer. Although superfoods are promoted as being beneficial to health, most of the evidence relating to health claims associated with their consumption is inconclusive. In addition, there is evidence that some may be harmful.

The European Food Safety Authority (EFSA) has issued guidance on the types of studies required to substantiate health claims relating to antioxidants, as well as for claims relating to physical performance, gut health and immunity, appetite and weight management and others.

Recently, the EFSA determined that daily consumption of approximately 200 g of the flesh of green kiwifruit (described as *Actinidia deliciosa* var. Hayward) maintains normal defecation without causing diarrhoea.

There is a large body of literature on the phytochemistry and pharmacological properties of many of the so-called superfoods and their bioactive constituents, and an increasing number of clinical trials and epidemiological studies exploring their effects in humans (for reviews of evidence for selected foods, see Further Reading). Much of this literature emphasises that comprehensive clinical investigations are still required to understand the clinical pharmacology, efficacy and safety profile of these foods and their constituent phytochemicals, as well as possible synergistic interactions with those found in other foods.

Rather than looking to a few 'superfoods' for their health benefits, it is probably more appropriate to adhere to a 'superdiet' that is balanced and healthy and rich in fruits, vegetables and wholegrain foods. It is also important to consider that research with superfoods often uses extracts, rather than the food in its natural state, and so there may be differences in composition and, ultimately, biologic effects.

FURTHER READING

Amirpoor, A., Zavar, R., Amerizadeh, A., Asgary, S., Moradi, S., Farzaei, M.H., et al., 2021. Effect of beetroot consumption on serum lipid profile: a systematic review and meta-analysis. Curr. Probl. Cardiol. 47, 100887.

Arring, N.M., Millstine, D., Marks, L.A., Nail, L.M., 2018. Ginseng as a treatment for fatigue: a systematic review. J. Altern. Complement. Med. 24, 624–633.

Barnes, J., Anderson, L.A., Phillipson, J.D., 2007. Rhodiola. In: Herbal Medicines. Pharmaceutical Press, London, pp. 500–505.

Bejar, E., Upton, R., Cardellina, J.H., 2017. Adulteration of Rhodiola (*Rhodiola rosea*) rizome and root and extracts. Botanical Adulterants Bull. 1–8 2017.

Bhuyan, D.J., Alsherbiny, M.A., Perera, S., Low, M., Basu, A., Devi, O.A., et al., 2019. The odyssey of bioactive compounds in avocado (*Persea americana*) and their health benefits. Antioxidants 8 (10), 426.

Bishop, K.S., Kao, C.H., Xu, Y., Glucina, M.P., Paterson, R.R., Ferguson, L.R., 2015. From 2000 years of *Ganoderma lucidum* to recent developments in nutraceuticals. Phytochemistry 114, 56–65.

Biswas, D., Mandal, S., Chatterjee Saha, S., Tudu, C.K., Nandy, S., Batiha, G.E., et al., 2021. Ethnobotany, phytochemistry, pharmacology, and toxicity of *Centella asiatica* (L.) Urban: a comprehensive review. Phytother. Res. 35, 6624–6654.

Bjelakovic, G., Nikolova, D., Gluud, L.L., Simonetti, R.G., Gluud, C., 2012. Antioxidant supplements for prevention of mortality in healthy participants and patients with various diseases. Cochrane Database Syst. Rev. 3, CD007176.

Björnsson, H.K., Björnsson, E.S., Avula, B., Khan, I.A., Jonasson, J.G., Ghabril, M., et al., 2020. Ashwagandha-induced liver injury: a case series from Iceland and the US drug-induced liver injury network. Liver Int. 40 (4), 825–829.

Booker, A., Zhai, L.X., Gkouva, C., Li, S.Y., Heinrich, M., 2016. From traditional resource to global commodities: a comparison of *Rhodiola* species using NMR spectroscopy-metabolomics and HPTLC. Front. Pharmacol. 7, 254.

Chan, S.W., Tomlinson, B., Chan, P., Lam, C.W.K., 2021. The beneficial effects of *Ganoderma lucidum* on cardiovascular and metabolic disease risk. Pharm. Biol. 59, 1161–1171.

Chang, S.K., Alasalvar, C., Shahidi, F., 2019. Superfruits: phytochemicals, antioxidant efficacies, and health effects—a comprehensive review. Crit. Rev. Food Sci. Nutr. 59, 1580–1604.

Cho, Y.H., Lee, S.Y., Lee, C.H., Park, J.H., So, Y.S., 2021. Effect of *Schisandra chinensis* Baillon extracts and regular low-intensity exercise on muscle strength and mass in older adults: a randomized, double-blind, placebo-controlled trial. Am. J. Clin. Nutr. 113, 1440–1446.

Dong, R., Li, L., Gao, H., Lou, K., Luo, H., Hao, S., et al., 2021. Safety, tolerability, pharmacokinetics, and food effect of baicalein tablets in healthy Chinese subjects: a single-center, randomized, double-blind, placebo-controlled, single-dose phase I study. J. Ethnopharmacol. 274, 114052.

EFSA Panel on Dietetic Products, Nutrition and Allergies (EFSA NDA Panel), Turck, D., Bresson, J.L., Burlingame, B., Dean, T., Fairweather-Tait, S., et al., 2018. Guidance for the scientific requirements for health claims related to antioxidants, oxidative damage and cardiovascular health. EFSA J. 16 (1), e05136.

EFSA Panel on Nutrition, Novel Foods and Food Allergens (NDA), Turck, D., Castenmiller, J., De Henauw, S., Hirsch-Ernst, K.I., Kearney, J., et al., 2021. Green kiwifruit (lat. *Actinidia deliciosa* var. Hayward) and maintenance of normal defecation: evaluation of a health claim pursuant to Article 13(5) of Regulation (EC) no 1924/2006. EFSA J. 19, e06641.

Filippini, T., Malavolti, M., Borrelli, F., Izzo, A.A., Fairweather-Tait, S.J., Horneber, M., et al., 2020. Green tea (*Camellia sinensis*) for the prevention of cancer. Cochrane Database Syst. Rev. 3, CD005004.

Gerontakos, S., Taylor, A., Avdeeva, A.Y., Shikova, V.A., Pozharitskaya, O.N., Casteleijn, D., et al., 2021. Findings of Russian literature on the clinical application of *Eleutherococcus senticosus* (Rupr. & Maxim.): a narrative review. J. Ethnopharmacol. 278, 114274.

Haghighatdoost, F., Nobakht, M.G.,B.F., Hariri, M., 2017. Effect of green tea on plasma adiponectin levels: a systematic review and meta-analysis of randomized controlled clinical trials. J. Am. Coll. Nutr. 36, 541–548.

Heinrich, M., Dhanji, T., Casselman, I., 2011. Açaí (*Euterpe oleracea* Mart.)—a phytochemical and pharmacological assessment of the species' health claims. Phytochem. Lett. 4 (1), 10–21.

Ichim, M.C., de Boer, H.J., 2021. A review of authenticity and authentication of commercial ginseng herbal medicines and food supplements. Front. Pharmacol. 11, 612071.

Igho-Osagie, E., Cara, K., Wang, D., Yao, Q., Penkert, L.P., Cassidy, A., et al., 2020. Short-term tea consumption is not associated with a reduction in blood lipids or pressure: a systematic review and meta-analysis of randomized controlled trials. J. Nutr. 150, 3269–3279.

Ishaque, S., Shamseer, L., Bukutu, C., Vohra, S., 2012. *Rhodiola rosea* for physical and mental fatigue: a systematic review. BMC Complement. Altern. Med. 12, 70.

Jia, A., Zhang, Y., Gao, H., Zhang, Z., Zhang, Y., Wang, Z., et al., 2021. A review of *Acanthopanax senticosus* (Rupr and Maxim.) Harms: from ethnopharmacological use to modern application. J. Ethnopharmacol. 268, 113586.

Jin, X., Ruiz Beguerie, J., Sze, D.M., Chan, G.C., 2016. *Ganoderma lucidum* (Reishi mushroom) for cancer treatment. Cochrane Database Syst. Rev. 4, CD007731.

Joshi, M., Prabhakar, B., 2020. Phytoconstituents and pharmaco-therapeutic benefits of pitaya: a wonder fruit. J. Food Biochem. 44, e13260.

Jurgens, T.M., Whelan, A.M., Killian, L., Doucette, S., Kirk, S., Foy, E., 2012. Green tea for weight loss and weight maintenance in overweight or obese adults. Cochrane Database Syst. Rev. 12, CD008650.

Klupp, N.L., Chang, D., Hawke, F., Kiat, H., Cao, H., Grant, S.J., et al., 2015. *Ganoderma lucidum* mushroom for the treatment of cardiovascular risk factors. Cochrane Database Syst. Rev. 2, CD007259.

Latocha, P., 2017. The nutritional and health benefits of kiwiberry (*Actinidia arguta*)—a review. Plant Foods Hum. Nutr. 72, 325–334.

Le, T.N., Chiu, C.H., Hsieh, P.C., 2020. Bioactive compounds and bioactivities of *Brassica oleracea* L. var. Italica sprouts and microgreens: an updated overview from a nutraceutical perspective. Plants 9, 946.

Li, X., Chen, W., Xu, Y., Liang, Z., Hu, H., Wang, S., et al., 2021. Quality evaluation of randomized controlled trials of *Rhodiola* species: a systematic review. Evid. Based Complement. Alternat. Med. 2021, 9989546.

Liu, J., Xu, D., Chen, S., Yuan, F., Mao, L., Gao, Y., 2021. Superfruits in China: bioactive phytochemicals and their potential health benefits—a review. Food Sci. Nutr. 9, 6892–6902.

Mazzanti, G., Di Sotto, A., Vitalone, A., 2015. Hepatotoxicity of green tea: an update. Arch. Toxicol. 89 (8), 1175–1191.

Melini, V., Melini, F., 2021. Functional components and anti-nutritional factors in gluten-free grains: a focus on quinoa seeds. Foods 10 (2), 351.

Oketch-Rabah, H.A., Roe, A.L., Rider, C.V., Bonkovsky, H.L., Giancaspro, G.I., Navarro, V., et al., 2020. United States Pharmacopeia (USP) comprehensive review of the hepatotoxicity of green tea extracts. Toxicol Rep. 7, 386–402.

Park, J., Han, S., Park, H., 2020. Effect of *Schisandra chinensis* extract supplementation on quadriceps muscle strength and fatigue in adult women: a randomized, double-blind, placebo-controlled trial. Int. J. Environ. Res. Public Health 17, 2475.

Park, J.Y., Kim, K.H., 2016. A randomized, double-blind, placebo-controlled trial of *Schisandra chinensis* for menopausal symptoms. Climacteric 19, 574–580.

Puttarak, P., Dilokthornsakul, P., Saokaew, S., Dhippayom, T., Kongkaew, C., Sruamsiri, R., et al., 2017. Effects of *Centella asiatica* (L.) Urb. on cognitive function and mood related outcomes: a systematic review and meta-analysis. Sci. Rep. 7, 10646.

Ru, W., Wang, D., Xu, Y., He, X., Sun, Y.E., Qian, L., et al., 2015. Chemical constituents and bioactivities of *Panax ginseng* (C. A. Mey.). Drug Discov. Ther. 9 (1), 23–32.

Samec, D., Urlic, B., Salopek-Sondi, B., 2019. Kale (*Brassica oleracea* var. *acephala*) as a superfood: review of the scientific evidence behind the statement. Crit. Rev. Food Sci. Nutr. 59, 2411–2422.

Shergis, J.L., Zhang, A.L., Zhou, W., Xue, C.C., 2013. *Panax ginseng* in randomised controlled trials: a systematic review. Phytother. Res. 27 (7), 949–965.

Shu, L., Cheung, K.L., Khor, T.O., Chen, C., Kong, A.N., 2010. Phytochemicals: cancer chemoprevention and suppression of tumor onset and metastasis. Cancer Metastasis Rev. 29, 483–502.

Smith, I., Williamson, E.M., Putnam, S.E., Farrimond, J., Whalley, B.J., 2014. Effects and mechanisms of ginseng and ginsenosides on cognition. Nutr. Rev. 72 (5), 319–333.

Song, M.-Y., Wang, J.-H., Eom, T., Kim, H., 2015. *Schisandra chinensis* fruit modulates the gut microbiota composition in association with metabolic markers in obese women: a randomized, double-blind placebo-controlled study. Nutr. Res. 35 (8), 655–663.

Sorrenti, V., Castagna, D.A., Fortinguerra, S., Buriani, A., Scapagnini, G., Willcox, D.C., 2021. Spirulina microalgae and brain health: a scoping review of experimental and clinical evidence. Mar. Drugs 19 (6), 293.

Sun, B., Wu, L., Wu, Y., Zhang, C., Qin, L., Hayashi, M., et al., 2020. Therapeutic potential of *Centella asiatica* and its triterpenes: a review. Front. Pharmacol. 11, 568032.

Tandon, N., Yadav, S.S., 2020. Safety and clinical effectiveness of *Withania somnifera* (Linn.) Dunal root in human ailments. J. Ethnopharmacol. 255, 112768.

Torbati, F.A., Ramezani, M., Dehghan, R., Amiri, M.S., Moghadam, A.T., Shakour, N., et al., 2021. Ethnobotany, phytochemistry and pharmacological features of *Centella asiatica*: a comprehensive review. Adv. Exp. Med. Biol. 1308, 451–499.

van den Driessche, J.J., Plat, J., Mensink, R.P., 2018. Effects of superfoods on risk factors of metabolic syndrome: a systematic review of human intervention trials. Food Funct. 9, 1944–1966.

Wang, Z.-L., Wang, S., Kuang, Y., Hu, Z.-M., Qiao, X., Ye, M., 2018. A comprehensive review on phytochemistry, pharmacology, and flavonoid biosynthesis of *Scutellaria baicalensis*. Pharm. Biol. 56, 465–484.

Williamson, E.M., Liu, X., Izzo, A.A., 2020. Trends in use, pharmacology, and clinical applications of emerging herbal nutraceuticals. Br. J. Pharmacol. 177 (6), 1227–1240. https://doi.org/10.1111/bph.14943.

Wong, J.H., Barron, A.M., Abdullah, J.M., 2021. Mitoprotective effects of *Centella asiatica* (L.) Urb.: anti-inflammatory and neuroprotective opportunities in neurodegenerative disease. Front. Pharmacol. 12, 687935.

Yang, K., Qiu, J., Huang, Z., Yu, Z., Wang, W., Hu, H., et al., 2022. A comprehensive review of ethnopharmacology, phytochemistry, pharmacology, and pharmacokinetics of *Schisandra chinensis* (Turcz.) Baill. and *Schisandra sphenanthera* Rehd. et Wils. J. Ethnopharmacol. 284, 114759.

Yao, R., Heinrich, M., Weckerle, C.S., 2018. The genus *Lycium* as food and medicine: a botanical, ethnobotanical and historical review. J. Ethnopharmacol. 212, 50–66.

Yu, L., Qin, Y., Wang, Q., Zhang, L., Liu, Y., Wang, T., et al., 2014. The efficacy and safety of Chinese herbal medicine, Rhodiola formulation in treating ischemic heart disease: a systematic review and meta-analysis of randomized controlled trials. Complement. Ther. Med. 22 (4), 814–825.

Zhao, T., Tang, H., Xie, L., Zheng, Y., Ma, Z., Sun, Q., et al., 2019. *Scutellaria baicalensis* Georgi. (Lamiaceae): a review of its traditional uses, botany, phytochemistry, pharmacology and toxicology. J. Pharm. Pharmacol. 71, 1353–1369.

27

Topical Phytotherapy: Skin, Hair, Eye, Ear, Nose and Throat

Inflammatory and infectious skin diseases have a high prevalence everywhere, and inflammation of the eye, ear, nose and throat (ENT) is often treated with similar herbal extracts, formulated according to use. Antiinfective phytochemicals are covered separately in Chapter 10, but local applications are considered here.

In the areas of dry and itchy skin, inflammation and wound healing, medicinal plants and natural extracts and oils have an important role to play.

DRY AND ITCHY SKIN CONDITIONS, DERMATITIS AND ECZEMA

Dry and scaly skin conditions can arise from many causes. Diagnosis should be carried out initially by a medical practitioner to exclude infection, infestation or serious disorders. Emollient preparations, based on peanut (arachis) oil or oat extracts, are usually the first line of treatment. These conditions also affect the ear, but the main use of eardrops containing oils, such as almond, arachis and olive, is to soften wax prior and facilitate removal.

Almond Oil†

Almond oil is obtained from the seed of *Prunus amygdalus* Batsch. (Rosaceae). It is a fixed oil (i.e. a nonvolatile oil), also known as sweet almond oil, and consists of triglycerides, mainly triolein and trilinolein, together with fatty acids, including palmitic, lauric, myristic and oleic acids.

Arachis Oil†

Arachis oil (also known as groundnut or peanut oil) is expressed from *Arachis hypogaea* L. (Fabaceae). It is a fixed oil consisting mainly of glycerides of oleic and linoleic acids. It is an ingredient of emollient creams and bath oils. Peanuts are dangerously allergenic to some individuals, and the oil should be avoided in these patients as a precaution.

Olive Oil†

Olive oil is expressed from the fruits of *Olea europaea* L. (Oleaceae). Virgin (or cold-expressed) olive oil has a greenish tinge and is used as a food; refined oil is yellowish. Both have a characteristic odour. Olive oil is a fixed oil containing glycerides of oleic acid (about 70%–80%), with smaller amounts of linoleic, palmitic and stearic acid glycerides.

Oats

Oats (*Avena sativa* L., Poaceae) are a widely distributed cereal crop. The seeds, with the husks removed, are crushed to form a coarse powder, which is creamy white in colour. They are widely used in foods, and the health benefits are widely recognised. Oat tinctures are taken internally for their reputed sedative activity, which remains unproven. Colloidal oatmeal, a powder of finely ground oats, has a long traditional use as a skin emollient, and is widely used in dermatological applications for eczema.

Constituents

Oats contain proteins (prolamines known as avenin, avenalin and gliadin), polyphenols known as avenanthramides, starch and soluble polysaccharides (mainly β-glucans and arabinogalactans), saponin glycosides including avenacosides A and B as well as soyasaponin I. The fatty oil is composed of phytosterols including cholesterol, β-sitosterol and Δ^5-avenasterol, avenoleic, oleic, ricinoleic and linoleic acids as well as vitamin E.

Therapeutic Uses and Available Evidence

Colloidal oats are used in bath preparations for eczema and itchy or dry skin, and oat extracts are recommended for regular use over a long period. The avenanthramides demonstrate potent antiinflammatory and antiirritant effects, although the clinical properties derive from a variety of chemical constituents. The starches and beta-glucans are responsible for the protective and water-holding functions of oats, and the presence of phenolics confers antioxidant and antiinflammatory activities. Some of the oat phenols are also strong ultraviolet absorbers, and the saponins confer a cleansing effect.

INFLAMMATORY SKIN CONDITIONS

Allergic reactions, psoriasis, burns, bruising and general inflammation of skin are common. Severe cases are treated with corticosteroids under medical supervision, as well as emollient preparations, many of which are soothing and antiinflammatory herbal products.

Aloe Vera

'Aloe vera' is the gel obtained from the centre of the fleshy leaves of *Aloe vera* (L.) Burm. f. and other species of *Aloe* (Asphodelaceae) and is differentiated from the anthraquinone-rich exudate or 'aloes', which is used as a purgative. It is a common practice to cut the leaf to use the fresh gel for burns and other inflammatory skin conditions. Aloe vera is added to skin cosmetics, postradiotherapy inflammation, 'after sun' preparations and numerous other products.

Constituents

The gel contains polysaccharides consisting mainly of glucomannans, glycoproteins such as aloctins, enzymes such as carboxypeptidases and variable amounts of anthraquinone glycosides.

Therapeutic Uses and Available Evidence

Aloe vera gel is used mainly as extracted, in a stabilised and a preserved formula. For dermatological preparations, there is some evidence for antibacterial, antiinflammatory, emollient and moisturising effects.

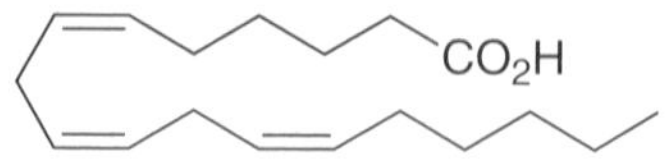

Fig. 27.1 γ-Linolenic acid.

The polysaccharides are important as soothing and immunostimulating agents. Some of the glycoproteins have similar effects, while the anthraquinone derivatives are antibacterial. Taken internally, the gel has been reported to be effective in the treatment of stomach and aphthous (mouth) ulcers. Aloe vera gel is helpful in the treatment of burns and to aid wound healing. In ultraviolet (UV)-induced erythema, aloe vera gel displayed some antiinflammatory effects, supporting its use as an after-sun treatment and postradiotherapy emollient.

Evening Primrose Oil†

Evening primroses, *Oenothera biennis* L. and other spp. (Onagraceae) are common ornamentals that were originally used medicinally by indigenous North American people. The plant is a hairy perennial with alternate, lanceolate leaves and large, yellow, four-petalled flowers that develop into long, elongated fruit capsules containing the seeds from which the fixed oil is extracted.

Constituents

The seed oil contains ~70% *cis*-linoleic acid and ~9% *cis*-γ-linolenic acid (Fig. 27.1).

Therapeutic Uses and Available Evidence

The therapeutic benefits are ascribed mainly to the γ-linolenic acid content, taken internally and applied externally. Supplementation with omega-6 essential fatty acids (omega-6 EFAs) may be helpful in the treatment of atopic dermatitis since patients with atopic dermatitis have imbalances in EFA levels. EFAs play a vital role in skin structure and physiology, and their deficiency replicates the symptoms of atopic dermatitis.

Studies of EFA supplementation in atopic dermatitis have produced conflicting results. Evening primrose oil may have a beneficial effect on itching, crusting, oedema and redness after several weeks, although the evidence of efficacy is equivocal. Evening primrose oil is usually taken in conjunction with vitamin E to prevent oxidation.

Note: The seed oil of *Borago officinalis* L. (borage, Boraginaceae), or starflower oil, is used in a similar way to evening primrose oil, but contains two to three times more γ-linolenic acid.

Marigold, *Calendula officinalis* L.†

Calendula officinalis (or 'pot' marigold) is one of the best-known medicinal plants of Europe. Its origin is unclear, but it has been cultivated for many centuries. Its wide use as an ornamental has increased the botanical variability of the species. The flower heads are large, with a diameter of up to 5 cm, and yellow-orange. Some varieties have both ligulate (tongue-shaped) and radiate florets, others have only the ligulate type. The European Pharmacopoeia (Eur. Ph.) requires that flower heads only containing ligulate florets should be used.

Constituents

Marigold flowers contain saponins based on oleanolic acid, including calendasaponins A, B, C and D, triterpene pentacyclic alcohols such as faradol, arnidiol, erythrodiol, calenduladiol, heliantriols A1, B0, B1 and B2, taraxasterol and lupeol; flavonoids, including hyperoside and rutin; and sesquiterpene and ionone glycosides such as officinosides A, B, C and D, loliolide and arvoside A.

Therapeutic Uses and Available Evidence

Inflammatory skin conditions, including dermatitis, abrasions, wound healing and after radiotherapy. The antiinflammatory properties are due in part to the lipophilic triterpene alcohols, notably the esters of faradiol, shown using in vivo models. Marigold extracts prevent ultraviolet B (UVB) irradiation-induced growth-stimulating hormone (GSH) depletion in mice and increase gelatinase activity, which may be beneficial for skin healing and pro-collagen synthesis. Oral and topical administration improved healing of excision wounds in rats and reduced the time needed for re-epithelisation, stimulating proliferation and migration of fibroblasts. Detailed studies are lacking, but the use of *Calendula* in radiotherapy-induced inflammation is of increasing research interest.

Chamomile, *Matricaria chamomilla* L.†

Chamomile is used internally as an antiinflammatory for gastric conditions and as a calming herbal tea (see Chapter 18 for details of the flowers and constituents), and extracts and the oil are often incorporated into soothing and antiinflammatory skin preparations, including for children. As with *Calendula*, a potential use after radiotherapy has been identified for a gel containing chamomile extracts.

ORAL AND THROAT IRRITATION

These can be treated topically with antiinflammatory and antiseptic products, such as mouthwashes and gels, and are incorporated into artificial saliva products, used for relieving dry mouth, which are composed of either animal mucins or hydroxymethyl cellulose derivatives.

Many different essential oils are used as oral antiseptics, deodorisers and antiinflammatory agents, including mint, clove, eucalyptus and lemon oils, as well as isolated constituents such as menthol and thymol.

Clove, *Syzygium aromaticum* (L.) Merr. & L.M. Perry†

Cloves are obtained from the flower buds of *Syzygium aromaticum* (syn.: *Eugenia caryophyllata* Thunb., Myrtaceae), which are collected prior to opening. The buds are brown, about 1–1.5 cm long, and have a very characteristic shape. On pressing a clove with the fingernail, oil should be exuded. Cloves are used as a culinary spice.

Constituents

The buds are very rich in essential oil (15%–20%), consisting mainly of eugenol (Fig. 27.2), usually 85%–90%, with minor constituents including acetyl eugenol, α- and β-caryophyllene and methyl salicylate. Tannins, such as eugeniin, casuarictin, tellimagrandin I, and flavonoids, are found in the plant material but not in the oil.

Therapeutic Uses and Available Evidence

Clove oil is used for the symptomatic relief of toothache and is a constituent of many dental preparations. It has deodorising, antiseptic, antispasmodic and antiinflammatory properties, due mainly to the eugenol content. Clove extracts are used in cosmetics and perfumery.

Thymol†

Thymol (Fig. 27.3) was originally extracted from thyme (*Thymus* spp.) and is present in many oils, including ajowan, but is now more easily synthesised chemically. It has antiseptic, deodorising and antiinflammatory properties and is widely used in skin and dental products (e.g. compound thymol glycerine). Thymol causes irritation in high concentrations when applied externally and should not be swallowed

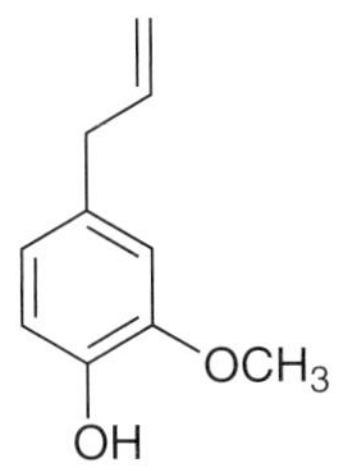

Fig. 27.2 Eugenol.

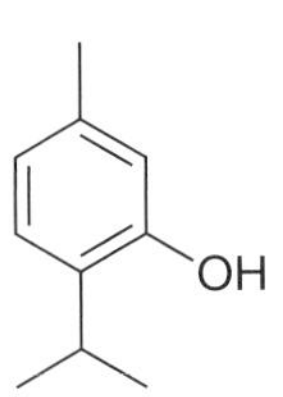

Fig. 27.3 Thymol.

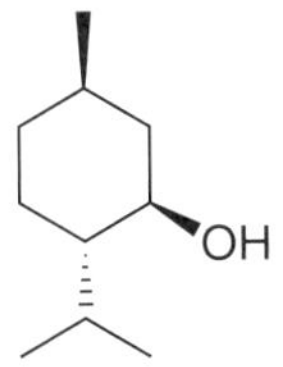

Fig. 27.4 (−)-Menthol.

in significant amounts. Normal doses associated with the herb do not normally cause problems.

Peppermint Oil, *Mentha × piperita* L.†

Peppermint oil has antiseptic, deodorising and antiinflammatory properties and is widely used in dental products as a deodoriser. Other species of mint, such as spearmint, are also used for the same purpose. Menthol is used in antiinflammatory skin products, especially for sunburn, due to its cooling effect.

Constituents

The major constituents are menthol (30%–55%) and menthone (14%–32%), with isomenthone (2%–10%), menthofuran (1%–9%), menthyl acetate (3%–5%), 1,8-cineole (6%–14%), limonene (1%–5%), pulegone (not more than 4.0%) and carvone (not more than 1.0%). Menthol (Fig. 27.4) can cause irritation in high concentrations.

Tea Tree and Tea Tree Oil, *Melaleuca alternifolia* Cheel†

The oil distilled from the leaves and stems of the tea tree has a long traditional usage amongst indigenous peoples of North Australia and New South Wales. The oil is used topically as an antimicrobial for skin infections, to reduce bruising and for insect bites. Tea tree oil products are now popular throughout Europe and the United States, and include soaps, shampoos, creams, lotions and gels. The leaves and twigs undergo distillation to produce the oil, which is pale yellow to colourless.

Constituents

The major component is terpinen-4-ol (Fig. 27.5), which may be present at concentrations as high as 30%. Some varieties are rich in 1,8-cineole, which is present in *Eucalyptus* oil, but the best-quality tea tree oils are low in 1,8-cineole and high in terpinen-4-ol. Other monoterpenes present include γ- and α-terpineol, α- and β-pinene, limonene and cymene; and the sesquiterpenes cubebol, cubenol and δ-cadinene. The composition of the oil also depends on the method of distillation.

Therapeutic Uses and Available Evidence

Tea tree oil is now used worldwide in the form of skin creams for pimples and acne, pessaries for vaginal thrush, as an inhalation for respiratory disorders and in pastilles for sore throats. It is also popular as a lotion for the treatment of lice, mite infestations, dandruff and other hair and scalp disorders. The oil has broad-spectrum antimicrobial activity against *Staphylococcus aureus*, *Escherichia coli* and various pathogenic fungi and yeasts, including *Candida albicans*, and may be useful as an antiseptic. To date, there is no evidence for the induction of bacterial resistance after repeated low-dose applications of tea tree oil.

The most active constituents include terpinen-4-ol, γ-terpinene, α-terpineol and linalool which demonstrate broad-spectrum activity towards Gram-negative bacteria. Clinical trials have supported many of the uses of tea tree oil, although most of the studies are rather small. Undiluted essential oils can cause skin irritation and tea tree oil should be used with care.

The related manuka tree (*Leptospermum scoparium* J.R. Forst & G. Forst) is sometimes referred to as 'New Zealand tea tree' and is used for similar purposes. Honey made from this plant (Manuka honey) is widely promoted as an antibacterial agent.

Lemon Balm, *Melissa officinalis* L.†

Lemon balm has a long history of use as an antimicrobial and carminative as well as a mild sedative. See Chapter 22 (The Central Nervous System) for details and constituents. Topical formulations containing extracts of *Melissa officinalis* are marketed for herpes simplex virus skin lesions, with clinical data and in vitro studies in support. The antiviral properties are mainly due to the polyphenolic acids.

Witch Hazel, *Hamamelis virginiana* L.†

Witch hazel (*Hamamelis virginiana*, Hamamelidaceae) is indigenous to North America and Canada. The leaves are broadly oval, up to 15 cm long, 7 cm broad, the margin dentate or crenate, the apex acute and the base asymmetrically cordate. The distilled extract, known simply as 'witch hazel', is used as an astringent in skin and eye inflammation.

Constituents

The leaves and bark contain tannins, composed mainly of gallotannins with some condensed catechins and proanthocyanins. These include 'hamamelitannin', which is a mixture of related tannins, including galloylhamameloses and flavonoids.

Therapeutic Uses and Available Evidence

Witch hazel is widely used for the treatment of haemorrhoids, bruises, skin irritation, spots and blemishes, and soothing ophthalmic preparations. Hamamelitannin inhibits tumour necrosis factor (TNF)-mediated endothelial cell death without altering TNF-induced upregulation of endothelial adhesiveness, which may explain the antihaemorrhagic use. The proanthocyanidins, gallotannins and gallates are highly active as free radical scavengers, and protective effects on fibroblast cells against hydrogen peroxide-induced damage have been reported.

Clinical studies have demonstrated the efficacy of topically applied witch hazel in inflammatory conditions, including UV-irradiated burning and atopic dermatitis. Witch hazel is used in after-shave lotions and in cosmetic preparations. The evidence for its use is mostly based on empirical evidence and very little systematic data are available. Rarely, allergic contact dermatitis has been reported.

Eyebright, *Euphrasia officinalis* L.

Euphrasia spp. (Scrophulariaceae) have a long history of use in eye inflammation, as the name would suggest, and are used in soothing skin preparations, especially for the area around the eye. They are found in meadows and grassy vegetation throughout Europe and temperate Asia. The leaves are opposite near the base and alternate above, about 1 cm long, lanceolate and dentate; the axillary flowers are two-lipped, small and white, often tinged with purple or with a yellow spot.

Constituents

Eyebright contains iridoid glycosides, such as aucubin, geniposide, catalpol, luproside, eurostoside, euphroside, veronicoside, verproside and others; lignans including coniferyl glucosides and eukovoside; and tannins and polyphenolic acids, including gallic, caffeic and ferulic acids.

Therapeutic Uses and Available Evidence

Euphrasia is a traditional remedy for inflammatory disorders of the eye. Although few clinical studies have been carried out, and the overall evidence is weak, they are popular and do not raise safety concerns.

Psoriasis

There are many forms of psoriasis, with different symptom manifestations, degrees of severity and involvement with other autoimmune diseases such as arthritis. Severe forms are treated by specialist dermatologists with immune suppressants, cytotoxic agents and vitamin D derivatives. Milder symptoms are traditionally treated with herbal medicine agents, such as oats, *Centella*, aloe vera (see earlier), turmeric, Oregon grape (*Mahonia aquifolium*), which contains berberine, and *Cestrum diurnum*, which contains vitamin D analogues. Cannabis also has antiinflammatory effects in preclinical models of psoriasis, but at present there are no effective herbal therapies for this condition. Traditional Chinese medicine is widely used for inflammatory skin disorders, including eczema and psoriasis, but usually on an individual basis, therefore making it difficult to evaluate.

WOUND HEALING

Centella asiatica (L.) Urb.†

Centella asiatica (Apiaceae), also known as gotu kola, Indian pennywort, Brahmi and Mandukaparani, is an important medicinal plant throughout the world. The leaves of this small plant are kidney-shaped (reniform), long-stalked with rounded apices. The pinkish to red flowers are borne in small, rounded umbels. It is a native of tropical and subtropical Asia and generally grows along streams, ditches and in low wet areas. As a consequence, this makes the species prone to exposure to sewage, so there is a risk of high levels of bacterial and other contaminations (including heavy metals). In Sri Lanka and other countries, it is an element of the local cuisine, used as a vegetable or in salads.

Constituents

The triterpenes are generally considered to be the major active metabolites. They are mainly pentacyclic triterpenic acids of the ursane or oleanane types, and their glycosides, and include asiatic acid, the asiaticosides, madecassic acid, madecassoside, brahmoside, brahmic acid, brahminoside, thankuniside, the centellasaponins and others. There are differences depending on the geographical origin of the plant. Flavonoids

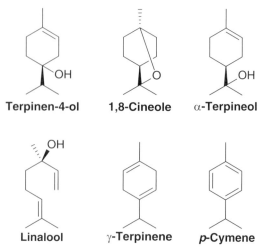

Fig. 27.5 Monoterpenes in tea tree oil.

and a small amount of essential oil, with α-humulene, β-caryophyllene and bicyclogermacrene as the main constituents, are present.

Therapeutic Uses and Available Evidence

A wide range of pharmacological uses have been reported, including as a general tonic (see Chapter 26). Extracts are widely used in treating skin conditions, including wound healing, inflammation, psoriasis, keloid and prevention of stretch marks during pregnancy. They are applied topically, and preparations are taken internally for mental disorders, to improve memory, for atherosclerosis and to improve venous insufficiency.

Despite the lack of clinical studies, pharmacological studies support the use of *Centella* in skin conditions. Extracts have been shown to significantly increase the wound-breaking strength in a rat incision wound model, improving the rate of epithelisation and wound contraction. *Centella* has been suggested as a topical antipsoriatic agent, and extracts have been shown to inhibit keratinocyte replication.

TOPICAL INSECTICIDAL AGENTS

Control of insects is a huge problem due to their potential for transmitting disease, spoiling foods and devastating crops, and causing skin infestations in animals and humans. Agricultural methods and eradicating insect disease vectors—such as the *Anopheles* mosquito which transmits malaria, and *Aedes* species which carry the Zika and Dengue fever viruses—are obviously different from those involved in treating humans, although similar insecticidal compounds are used if they meet safety requirements.

Before the advent of synthetic pesticides, all insecticides were derived from natural products, mainly terpenoids such as essential oils (e.g. tea tree, lavender, citronella, eucalyptus, which are still widely used, including as insect repellents), neem, pyrethrum, and quassia. Delphinium and veratrum alkaloids were formerly used, but they are highly toxic and can be absorbed through the skin. Pyrethroids are extremely important insecticidal agents, both in their natural form and as the starting material for the semisynthetic pyrethroids. They are also used medicinally to treat infestations with lice and scabies.

HEAD LICE

Infestations with head lice, *Pediculus humanus capitis* (Anoplura: Pediculidae), are a common problem throughout the world, and particularly amongst children where they are easily transmitted.

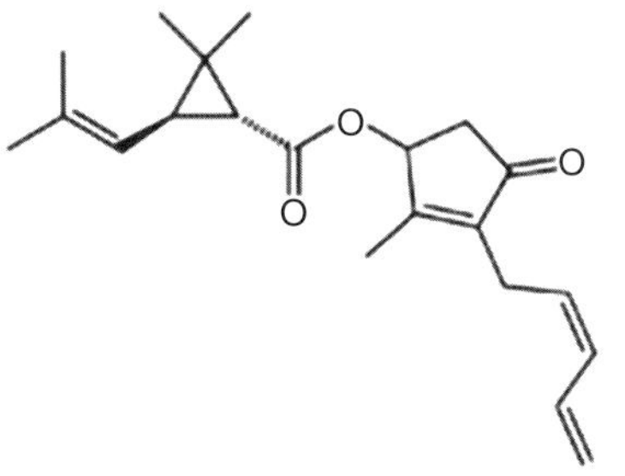

Fig. 27.6 Pyrethrin I.

Fig. 27.7 Azadirachtin.

The adult stages of the louse are actually easy to kill—they do not survive long away from the body and can be suffocated with occlusive treatments such as dimeticone and mineral oil. The eggs (nits) are the main problem; they have a waterproof covering, and most insecticides only act once the louse has hatched. This means that either multiple treatments or persistent insecticides must be used; however, the use of persistent compounds facilitates the development of resistance: as concentrations fall, lice can survive more easily and acquire resistance. This has occurred with permethrin (see the following section). Body lice are more robust and can survive for much longer periods away from the body; they also transmit disease, whereas head lice are considered to be mainly a social problem. The following natural products are of historical importance and are still used.

Pyrethrum (Insect) Flowers, *Chrysanthemum* spp.

Tanacetum cinerariifolium Sch.Bip. and *T. coccineum* (**Willd.**) **Grierson (Asteraceae), formerly classified as *Pyrethrum* or *Chrysanthemum* spp., are known as insect flowers.** They are indigenous to the Balkans but widely cultivated elsewhere. The unopened flower heads are about 7 cm in diameter, with creamy-white ligulate and yellow tubular florets.

Constituents

All species contain pyrethrins, which are esters of chrysanthemic and pyrethric acids and are the actives. They are known as pyrethrins I (Fig. 27.6) and II, cinerins I and II and jasmolins I and II.

Therapeutic Uses and Available Evidence

The natural pyrethrins are used to treat lice and scabies infestations and to kill other types of insects (houseflies etc.) which are not necessarily causes of skin infestation. Pyrethrin I (see Fig. 27.6) is the most potent of the naturally occurring compounds, although all have a knock-down effect on insects. The natural products have been used to develop semisynthetic derivatives such as permethrin, phenothrin, tetramethrin, cypermethrin and decamethrin, which can be more potent and offer more chemical stability. All of these have been shown to have clinical efficacy, but the semisynthetic compounds are more likely to lead to resistance arising because of their persistence. Pyrethrum is mostly considered to be harmless to humans and animals, and may be used as a spray, lotion, powder or fumigant. Pyrethroids are much less toxic to humans than synthetic insecticides, but care should be taken as they can cause irritation or allergic reactions.

Quassia Wood, *Picrasma excelsa* Planch and *Quassia amara* L.

Picrasma excelsa and *Quassia amara* (Simaroubaceae), known as quassia or bitter wood, and Japanese quassia (*P. ailanthoides* Planch.) occur in commerce as logs, chips or shredded. They have a wide folklore use

as insecticides, but extracts must be used immediately after preparation as they are unstable, which limits their usefulness.

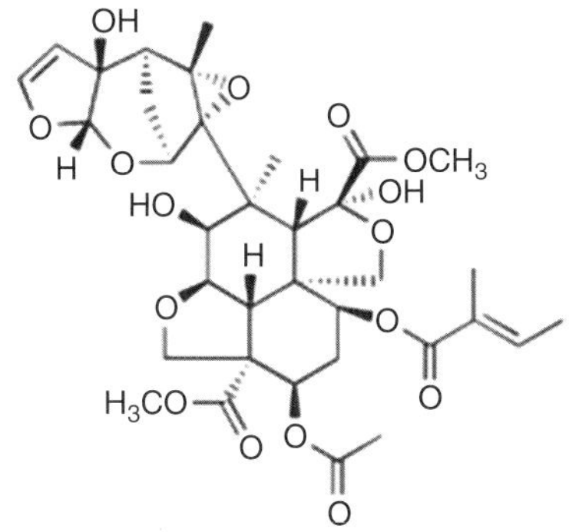

Constituents

The wood contains quassinoids such as quassin, isoquassin (= picrasmin) and others, depending on the species. *P. excelsa* and *Q. amara* also contain carboline alkaloids, and *P. ailanthoides* contains a series of picrasidine alkaloids.

Therapeutic Uses and Available Evidence

Quassia is an insecticide, anthelmintic, febrifuge and antimalarial, although efficacy in malaria is unproven. It has been used as a fresh infusion to treat head lice, although little evidence for efficacy is available. The quassinoids are insecticidal, cytotoxic and amoebicidal both in vitro and in vivo. Quassia is used to flavour bitter alcoholic and soft drinks and to stimulate the appetite. It is nontoxic when applied externally, and safe in small doses when ingested.

Neem, *Azadirachta indica* A. Juss.

The neem tree (Meliaceae) is a vitally important medicinal plant in Asia, where it is used to treat a wide spectrum of diseases, especially skin conditions. There is a strong tradition in India of neem use as a personal insecticide and to control infestations in crops. All parts of the plant are used, and lotions and shampoos containing seed oil and extracts are marketed as head lice treatments. These are very popular, and although their efficacy has not been conclusively proven in clinical trials, there is evidence to show their usefulness.

Constituents

Neem contains limonoids such as the azadirachtin (Fig. 27.7) and nimbin derivatives as the active constituents, together with flavonoids, tannins and coumarins.

Therapeutic Uses and Available Evidence

Neem seed extracts have shown activity against head lice and their eggs, and when used topically they are considered safe. Neem extracts are also used internally in some traditional medicine systems, but there are concerns about their safety.

Essential Oils

Many essential oils and their components have pediculicidal (and other insecticidal) effects. Tea tree and its component terpenen-4-ol are particularly effective. Some mono- and sesquiterpenes are more potent at killing lice than eggs, and vice versa, so a mixture (as is found naturally in an essential oil) may be more clinically effective than an isolated terpene. Essential oils also have the advantage of penetrating the egg covering and killing the developing louse. Despite the long history of use and the wide application in this area, there are few good clinical trials showing efficacy. Many essential oils are known allergens and they are also readily absorbed through the skin, but their use in moderate concentrations on the hair does not seem to pose any great risk.

FURTHER READING

Burgess, I.F., 2011. Head lice. BMJ Clin. Evid. 2011, 1703.

Bylka, W., Znajdek-Awizeń, P., Studzińska-Sroka, E., Dańczak-Pazdrowska, A., Brzezińska, M., 2014. *Centella asiatica* in dermatology: an overview. Phytother. Res. 28 (8), 1117–1124.

Capone, K., Kirchner, F., Klein, S.L., Tierney, N.K., 2020. Effects of colloidal oatmeal topical dermatitis cream on skin microbiome and skin barrier properties. J. Drugs Dermatol. 19 (5), 524–531.

Dabholkar, N., Rapalli, V.K., Singhvi, G., 2020. Potential herbal constituents for psoriasis treatment as protective and effective therapy. Phytother. Res. 35 (5), 2429–2444.

Dagley, N., Dagli, R., Mahmoud, R.S., Baroudi, K., 2015. Essential oils, their therapeutic properties, and implications in dentistry: a review. Int. Soc. Prev. Community Dent. 5 (6), 335–340.

Ferreira, E.B., Ciol, M.A., de Meneses, A.G., Bontempo, P.S.M., Hoffman, J.M., Reis, P.E.D.D., 2020. Chamomile gel versus urea cream to prevent radiation dermatitis in head and neck cancer patients: results from a preliminary clinical trial. Integr. Cancer Ther. 19, 153473542092174.

Liang, J., Cui, L., Li, J., Guan, S., Zhang, K., Li, J., 2021. Aloe vera: a medicinal plant used in skin wound healing. Tiss. Eng. Part B Rev. 27 (5), 455–474.

Liska, D.J., Kern, H.J., Maki, K.C., 2016. Cranberries and urinary tract infections: how can the same evidence lead to conflicting advice? Adv. Nutr. 7 (3), 498–506.

Marchese, A., Orhan, I.E., Daglia, M., Barbieri, R., Di Lorenzo, A., Nabavi, S.F., et al., 2016. Antibacterial and antifungal activities of thymol: a brief review of the literature. Food Chem. 210, 402–414.

Natella, F., Guantario, B., Ambra, R., Ranaldi, G., Intorre, F., Burki, C., et al., 2021. Human metabolites of Hamafortin™ (*Hamamelis virginiana* L. extract) modulates fibroblast extracellular matrix components in response to UVA radiation. Front. Pharmacol. 12, 747638.

Nicolaus, C., Junghanns, S., Hartmann, A., Murillo, R., Ganzera, M., Merfort, I., 2017. In vitro studies to evaluate the wound healing properties of *Calendula officinalis* extracts. J. Ethnopharmacol. 196, 94–103.

Paudel, D., Dhungana, B., Caffe, M., Krishnan, P., 2021. A review of the health beneficial properties of oats. Foods 10 (11), 2591.

Sanchez, M., Gonzalez-Burgos, E., Iglesias, I., Gómez-Serranillos, M.P., 2020. Pharmacological update properties of *Aloe vera* and its major active constituents. Molecules 25 (6), 1324.

Shakeri, A., Sahebkar, A., Javadi, B., 2016. *Melissa officinalis* L. – a review of its traditional uses, phytochemistry and pharmacology. J. Ethnopharmacol. 188, 204–228.

Singh, V., Roy, M., Garg, N., Kumar, A., Arora, S., Malik, D.S., 2021. An insight into the dermatological applications of neem: a review on traditional and modern aspect. Recent Adv. Antiinfect. Drug Discov. 16 (2), 94–121.

Williamson, E.M., 2007. The medicinal use of essential oils and their components for treating lice and mite infestations. Nat. Prod. Comm. 2 (12), 1303–1310.

Youn, B.H., Kim, Y.S., Yoo, S., Hur, M.H., 2021. Antimicrobial and hand hygiene effects of tea tree essential oil disinfectant: a randomized control trial. Int. J. Clin. Pract. 75 (8), e14206.

Naming Herbal Drugs: Pharmaceutical (Latinised), Common English and Accepted Botanical Names (Binomials) and Synonyms

Quality control of herbal products is based upon authentication of the starting material. This plant material may be referred to in different terms, and these may change at different stages during the long and complex supply chain leading from the agricultural environment to the product taken by the patient or consumer. This is further complicated by language issues, trading terms, local names, medical perspectives and official national nomenclature, and the reassigning of species by taxonomists.

The binomial system is the basis of identification and authentication. In the case of medicinal plants, it is even more important to be accurate as patient safety depends upon it. There are excellent online resources available to check the current names in use for medicinal plants (Kew's Medicinal Plant Names Service; https://mpns.science.kew.org) and for plants in general (www.worldfloraonline.org). For more detail and explanation of this essential topic, which ascertains reproducibility of research, see Allkin and Patmore (2022).

To harmonise definitions of herbal drugs, pharmaceutical names may be applied: these are Latin translations derived from the plant organ and all, or part, of a species name. When used in the context of a pharmacopoeial monograph (but not otherwise), pharmaceutical names include a statement that defines very precisely the species and part of the plant to which the monograph refers but may not reflect the current accepted botanical name (binomial). Although Latinised, pharmaceutical names are not italicised by convention, as is the binomial scientific name, and the two should not be confused. The pharmaceutical name is a literal translation: for Cinnamon, i.e. 'bark of cinnamon', 'Cinnamomum' becomes 'Cinnamomi' cortex; for St John's wort, 'Hypericum' aerial parts, or herb, becomes 'Hyperici' herba and so on.

Some pharmaceutical names in pharmacopoeial monographs have more than one species listed. This is because their uses and constituents are similar enough to allow them to comply with the same standards. Usually, these are related species within the same genus (hawthorn may be *Crataegus monogyna* Jacq. or *C. laevigata* (Poir.) DC., or a mixture of both, and devil's claw may be *Harpagophytum procumbens* (Burch.) DC. ex Meisn. or *H. zeyheri* Decne., or both). Rarely, a preparation can be obtained from botanically unrelated species; for example, anise oil Ph. Eur. can be obtained from either aniseed or star anise: despite having very different nonvolatile components, the essential oil from these two species is very similar. Some names specify the use of a particular variety (bitter fennel and sweet fennel, for example), because chemical differences within the same species mean they need separate monograph standards. If a plant (e.g. marshmallow, echinacea) has several different organs used medicinally, such as leaf and root, these herbal drugs will have separate monographs. Differently processed herbal drugs from the same plant organ

also usually have separate monographs (e.g. bilberry fruit, fresh and dried; peony, processed and untreated).

Table A.1 gives examples of the pharmaceutical names for more than 150 important herbs that are official in the Ph. Eur., many of which are further discussed in this book. Important former names—not always true synonyms—areoccasionally included to explain the discrepancy between the monograph title and accepted binomial (e.g. evodia fruit, poria). The list is not by any means restricted to European herbs and reflects the increasing global importance of traditional medicines of China, Asia, the Americas, the Middle East and elsewhere. All Ph. Eur. monographs are incorporated into the British Pharmacopoeia; these are given English titles. Pharmaceutical names are also used in the Chinese Pharmacopoeia and other official texts. The list has several purposes:

- It shows the range of herbal species used medicinally and which are considered sufficiently important within pharmacy and medicine to warrant standards for quality being officially published. Monographs require a great deal of collaborative work between regulatory authorities, independent scientists and commercial companies that produce herbal products and who provide information and expertise at no cost. The preparation of pharmacopoeial monographs is time consuming and expensive, requiring laboratory investigation and validation of analytical methods, and batch data and samples to establish reasonable and achievable standards for quality. Thus inclusion in this list is indicative of significant interest and trade in a medicinal plant. The list is not exhaustive, and new monographs are continually added to the Ph. Eur. at the request of member states.

- The current accepted botanical name (binomial), the pharmaceutical name and the part of the plant used medicinally can be checked in Table A.1 to facilitate literature searching. English names may be used for some herbal drugs; these do not always include the plant organ (part).

- Herbal drugs included in the list have, by definition, published standards and validated methods for assessing quality. These are as simple and robust as possible, as it is mandatory for manufacturers comply with them. Chemical reference standards—pure compounds for use in pharmacopoeial tests—can be purchased from the relevant regulatory authority.

- If a plant is not subject to a monograph, the list in Table A.1 can also be used to identify related species that are included, and these can be used as a starting point for developing analytical methods. Pharmacopoeial monographs are harmonised as much as possible, in that the same systems (HPTLC, HPLC, GC, etc.—see chemical analysis chapter 7) are used for related drugs or those containing similar classes of compounds.

TABLE A.1   Herbal Drug Names and Definitions Focusing on Botanical Drugs Available on European Markets

Latin Pharmaceutical Name	English Monograph Name	Accepted Botanical Name of Species	Part of Plant Used
Abelmoschi corolla	Abelmoschus flower	*Abelmoschus manihot* (L.) Medik	Flower
Absinthii herba	Wormwood	*Artemisia absinthium* L.	Herb
Acanthopanacis gracilistyli cortex	Acanthopanax bark	*Eleutherococcus nodiflorus* (Dunn) S.Y. Hu (syn.: *Acanthopanax gracilistylus* W.W. Sm.)	Root bark
Agni casti fructus	Agnus castus fruit	*Vitex agnus-castus* L.	Fruit
Agrimonia herba	Agrimony	*Agrimonia eupatoria* L.	Herb
Akebiae caulis	Akebia stem	*Akebia quinata* (Houtt.) Decne; *A. trifoliata* (Thunb.) Koidz.	Stem
Alchemillae herba	Alchemilla	*Alchemilla vulgaris* L.	Herb
Allii sativi bulbi pulvis	Garlic powder	*Allium sativum* L.	Bulb
Aloe barbadensis	Barbados/Curaçao aloes	*Aloe barbadensis* Mill.	Dried leaf juice
Aloe capensis	Cape aloes	*Aloe ferox* Mill.	Dried leaf juice
Althaeae folium	Marshmallow leaf	*Althaea officinalis* L.	Leaf
Althaeae radix	Marshmallow root		Root
Andrographidis herba	Andrographis herb	*Andrographis paniculata* (Burm.f.) Nees.	Herb
Angelicae archangelicae radix	Angelica archangelica root	*Angelica archangelica* L.	Root
Angelicae dahuricae radix	Angelica dahurica root	*Angelica dahurica* (Hoffm.) Benth. & Hook. f. ex Franch. & Sav.	Root
Anisi fructus	Aniseed	*Pimpinella anisum* L.	Fruit
Anisi stellati fructus	Star anise	*Illicium verum* Hook. f.	Fruit
Arnicae flos	Arnica flower	*Arnica montana* L.	Flower
Astragali mongholici radix	Astragalus mongholicus root	*Astragalus mongholicus* Bunge	Root
Atractylodis lancea rhizoma	Atractylodes lancea rhizome	*Atractylodes lancea* (Thunb.) DC.	Rhizome
Atractylodis macrocephalae rhizoma	Largehead atractylodes rhizome	*Atractylodes macrocephala* Koidz.	Rhizome
Aucklandiae radix	Aucklandia root	*Saussurea costus* (Falc.) Lipsch. (syn.: *Aucklandia lappa* Decne. et al.)	Root
Aurantii amari epicarpium et mesocarpium	Bitter orange peel	*Citrus aurantium* L., ssp. *aurantium* (syn.: *C. aurantium* var. *amara* Engl.)	Epicarp and mesocarp
Ballotae nigrae herba	Black horehound	*Ballota nigra* L.	
Balsamum peruvianum	Peru balsam	*Myroxylon balsamum* (L.) Harms var. *pereirae* (Royle) Harms	Exudate
Balsamum tolutanum	Tolu balsam	*Myroxylon balsamum* (L.) Harms var. *balsamum*	Oleoresin
Belladonnae folium	Belladonna leaf	*Atropa belladonna* L.	Leaf
Benzoe sumatranus	Sumatra benzoin	*Styrax benzoin* Dryand.	Resin
Benzoe tonkinensis	Siam benzoin	*Styrax tonkinensis* (Pierre) Craib ex Hartwich	Resin
Betulae folium	Birch leaf	*Betula pendula* Roth. *B. pubescens* Ehrh.	Leaf
Bistortae rhizoma	Bistort rhizome	*Persicaria bistorta* (L.) Samp. (syn.: *Polygonum bistorta* L.)	Rhizome
Boldi folium	Boldo leaf	*Peumus boldus* Molina	Leaf
Bupleuri radix	Bupleurum root	*Bupleurum chinense* DC. *B. scorzonerifolium* Willd.	Root
Calendulae flos	Calendula flower	*Calendula officinalis* L.	Flower petals
Capsici fructus	Capsicum	*Capsicum annuum* L. var. *minimum*, *C. frutescens* L.	Fruit
Carthami flos	Safflower flower	*Carthamus tinctorius* L.	Flower
Carvi fructus	Caraway	*Carum carvi* L.	Fruit
Caryophylli flos	Clove	*Syzygium aromaticum* (L.) Merr. & L.M. Perry (syn.: *Eugenia caryophyllata* Thunb.).	Flower bud
Centaurii herba	Centaury	*Centaurium erythraea* Rafn. s.l. et al.	Herb
Centellae asiaticae herba	Centella	*Centella asiatica* (L.) Urb.	Herb
Chamomilla romanae flos	Chamomile flowers	*Chamaemelum nobile* (L.) All. (syn.: *Anthemis nobilis* L.)	Flowerhead
Chelidonii herba	Greater celandine	*Chelidonium majus* L.	Herb
Cimicifugae rhizoma	Black cohosh	*Actaea racemosa* L. (syn.: *Cimicifuga racemosa* (L.) Nutt.)	Rhizome
Cinchonae cortex	Cinchona bark	*Cinchona pubescens* Vahl, *C. calisaya* Wedd., *C. ledgeriana* Moens ex Trimen	Bark
Cinnamomi cortex	Cinnamon	*Cinnamomum verum* J. Presl. (*C. zeylanicum* Blume)	Peeled inner bark
Codonopsis radix	Codonopsis root	*Codonopsis pilosula* (Franch.) Nannf.	Root
Coicis semen	Coix seed	*Coix lacryma-jobi* L.	Ripe seed

Continued

TABLE A.1   Herbal Drug Names and Definitions Focusing on Botanical Drugs Available on European Markets—cont'd

Latin Pharmaceutical Name	English Monograph Name	Accepted Botanical Name of Species	Part of Plant Used
Colae semen	Cola	*Cola nitida* (Vent.) Schott & Endl., *C. acuminata* (P. Beauv.) Schott & Endl.	Seed
Coptidis rhizoma	Chinese goldthread rhizome	*Coptis chinensis* Franch. and others	Rhizome
Coriandri fructus	Coriander	*Coriandrum sativum* L.	Fruit, 'seed'
Crataegi folii cum flore	Hawthorn leaf and flower	*Crataegus monogyna* Jacq., *C. laevigata* (Poir.) DC.	Leaf and flower; fruit
Crataegi fructus	Hawthorn berries		
Curcumae longae rhizoma	Turmeric rhizome	*Curcuma longa* L.	Rhizome
Curcumae zanthorrhizae rhizoma	Javanese turmeric	*Curcuma zanthorrhiza* Roxb.	Rhizome
Cynarae folium	Artichoke leaf	*Cynara cardunculus* L. (syn.: *C. scolymus* L.)	Leaf
Digitalis purpureae folium	Digitalis leaf	*Digitalis purpurea* L.	Leaf
Echinaceae angustifoliae radix	Narrow-leaved coneflower root	*Echinacea angustifolia* DC.	Root
Echinaceae pallidae radix	Pale coneflower root	*Echinacea pallida* (Nutt.) Nutt.	Root
Echinaceae purpureae herba	Purple coneflower herb	*Echinacea purpurea* (L.) Moench	Herb
Echinaceae purpureae radix	Purple coneflower root		Root
Ecliptae herba	Eclipta herb	*Eclipta prostrata* (L.) L.	Herb
Eleutherococcus radix	Siberian ginseng	*Eleutherococcus senticosus* (Rupr. & Maxim.) Maxim.	Root
Ephedrae herba	Ephedra herb	*Ephedra sinica* Stapf, and others	Herb
Eucalypti aetheroleum	Eucalyptus oil	*Eucalyptus globulus* Labill. and others	Essential oil
Eucommiae cortex	Eucommia bark	*Eucommia ulmoides* Oliv.	Bark
Evodia fructus	Evodia fruit	*Tetradium ruticarpum* (A. Juss.) T.G. Hartley (formerly *Evodia ruticarpa*)	Fruit
Foeniculi amari fructus	Bitter fennel	*Foeniculum vulgare* Mill. subsp. *vulgare* var. *vulgare*	Fruit
Foeniculi dulcis fructus	Sweet fennel	*F. vulgare* Mill subsp. *vulgare* var. *dulce*	
Fucus vel Ascophyllum	Kelp, bladderwrack	*Fucus vesiculosus* L., *F. serratus* L., *Ascophyllum nodosum* Le Jolis	Thallus
Ganoderma lucidum	Ganoderma	*Ganoderma lucidum* (Curtis) P. Karst.	Fruiting body
Gastrodiae rhizoma	Gastrodia rhizome	*Gastrodia elata* Blume	Root
Frangulae cortex	Frangula bark	*Rhamnus frangula* L. (syn.: *Frangula alnus* Mill.)	Bark
Fritillariae thunbergii bulbus	Thunberg fritillary bulb	*Fritillaria thunbergii* Miq.	Bulb
Gentianae radix	Gentian	*Gentiana lutea* L.	Root
Ginkgonis folium	Ginkgo leaf	*Ginkgo biloba* L.	Leaf
Ginseng radix	Ginseng	*Panax ginseng* C.A. Mey.	Root
Guaranae semen	Guarana	*Paullinia cupana* Kunth	Seed
Hamamelidis cortex	Hamamelis bark	*Hamamelis virginiana* L.	Bark
Hamamelidis folium	Hamamelis leaf		Leaf
Harpagophyti radix	Devil's claw root	*Harpagophytum procumbens* DC. ex Meisn., *H. zeyheri* Decne.	Root
Hederae folium	Ivy leaf	*Hedera helix* L.	Leaf
Hibisci sabdariffae flos	Roselle	*Hibiscus sabdariffa* L.	Flower
Hippocastani semen	Horse-chestnut fruit	*Aesculus hippocastanum* L.	Seed
Houttuyniae herba	Houttuynia herb (Fish mint herb)	*Houttuynia cordata* Thunb.	Herb
Hyperici herba	St John's wort	*Hypericum perforatum* L.	Herb
Hydrastis rhizoma	Goldenseal root	*Hydrastis canadensis* L.	Rhizome
Ipecacuanhae radix	Ipecacuanha	*Carapichea ipecacuanha* (Brot.) L. Andersson	Root
Isatidis radix	Isatis root	*Isatis tinctoria* L.	Root
Juniperi pseudofructus	Juniper cone ('Berry')	*Juniperus communis* L.	Cone
Lavandulae flos	Lavender flower	*Lavandula angustifolia* Mill.	Flower
Leonuri cardiacae herba	Motherwort	*Leonurus cardiaca* L.	Herb
Levistici radix	Lovage root	*Levisticum officinale* W.D.J. Koch	Root
Lichen islandicus	Iceland moss	*Cetraria islandica* (L.) Ach.	Thallus
Ligustici radix et rhizoma	Ligusticum root and rhizome	*Ligusticum sinense* Olive, *L. jeholense* (Nakai & Kitag.) Nakat & Kitak	Root and rhizome
Lini semen	Linseed	*Linum usitatissimum* L.	Seed
Liquiritiae radix	Liquorice root	*Glycyrrhiza glabra* L., *G. inflata* Batalin, *G. uralensis* Fisch.	Root and stolon
Lupuli flos	Hops	*Humulus lupulus* L.	Flower
Lycii fructus	Barbary wolfberry fruit	*Lycium barbarum* L.	Fruit
Lycopi herba	Lycopus lucidus herb	*Lycopus lucidus* var. *hirtus* (Regel) Makino & Nemoto	Herb

Continued

TABLE A.1   Herbal Drug Names and Definitions Focusing on Botanical Drugs Available on European Markets—cont'd

Latin Pharmaceutical Name	English Monograph Name	Accepted Botanical Name of Species	Part of Plant Used
Lythri herba	Loosestrife	*Lythrum salicaria* L.	Herb
Magnolia cortex	Magnolia bark	*Magnolia officinalis* Rehder & E.H. Wilson	Bark
Malvae folium	Mallow leaf	*Malva sylvestris* L. and *M. neglecta* Wallr.	Leaf
Malvae sylvestris flos	Mallow flower		Flower
Marrubii herba	White horehound	*Marrubium vulgare* L.	Herb
Mate folium	Mate leaf	*Ilex paraguariensis* A. St-Hil.	Leaf
Matricariae flos	Matricaria flowers	*Matricaria recutita* L.	Flowerhead
Meliloti herba	Melilot	*Melilotus officinalis* (L.) Pall.	Herb
Melaleucae atheroleum	Tea tree oil	*Melaleuca alternifolia* (Maiden & Betch) Cheel., and other species	Essential oil
Melissae folium	Lemon balm	*Melissa officinalis* L.	Leaf
Menthae piperitae folium	Peppermint	*Mentha* × *piperita* L.	Leaf
Millefolii herba	Yarrow	*Achillea millefolium* L.	Herb
Moutan cortex	Moutan bark	*Paeonia* × *suffruticosa* Andrews	Bark
Myrrha	Myrrh	*Commiphora myrrha* (Nees) Engl. and others	Oleoresin
Myrtilli fructus recens	Bilberry fruit, fresh	*Vaccinium myrtillus* L.	Fruit, fresh
Myrtilli fructus siccus	Bilberry fruit, dried		Fruit, dried
Notoginseng radix	Notoginseng root	*Panax notoginseng* (Burkill) F.H. Chen	Root
Oleae folium	Olive leaf	*Olea europaea* L.	Leaf
Olibanum indicum	Indian frankincense	*Boswellia serrata* Roxb. ex Colebr.	Gum resin
Oenothera oleum	Evening primrose oil	*Oenothera biennis* L., *O. lamarckiana* Ser.	
Ononidis radix	Restharrow root	*Ononis spinosa* L.	Root
Origani herba	Oregano	*Origanum onites* L., *O. vulgare* L.	Herb
Orthosiphonis folium	Java tea	*Orthosiphon aristatus* (Blume) Miq.	Leaf
Opium crudum/Opii pulvatus normatus	Opium, raw/prepared	*Papaver somniferum* L.	Latex from unripe fruit
Ophiopogonis radix	Dwarf lilyturf tuber	*Ophiopogon japonicus* (Thunb.) Ker. Gawl.	Root
Paeoniae radix alba	White peony root	*Paeonia lactiflora* Pall., processed	Root
Paeoniae radix rubra	Red peony root	*P. lactiflora* Pall. and/or *P. veitchii* Lynch, untreated	
Papaveris rhoeados flos	Red poppy petals	*Papaver rhoeas* L.	Flower petals
Passiflorae herba	Passionflower	*Passiflora incarnata* L.	Herb
Pelargonii radix	Pelargonium	*Pelargonium sidoides* DC., *P. reniforme* (Andrews) Curtis	Root
Piperis fructus	Pepper	*Piper nigrum* L.	Fruit
Piperis longi fructus	Long pepper	*Piper longum* L.	Fruit spike
Plantaginis lanceolatae folium	Plantain, ribwort plantain	*Plantago lanceolata* L. s.l.	Leaf
Plantaginis ovatae semen	Ispaghula	*Plantago ovata* Forssk.	Seed/seed husk
Platycodonis radix	Platycodon root	*Platycodon grandiflorus* (Jacq.) A. DC.	Root
Poria	Poria	*Wolfiporia extensa* (Peck) Ginns (syn.: *Poria cocos* (Schw.) Wolf) (a fungus)	Sclerotium
Psyllii semen	Psyllium	*Plantago indica* L., *P. afra* L.	Seed
Polygalae radix	Senega root	*Polygala senega* L., *P. tenuifolia* Willd.	Root
Polygoni avicularis herba	Knotgrass	*Polygonum aviculare* L. s.l.	Herb
Polygoni cuspidata rhizome et radix	Polygonum cuspidatum rhizome and root	*Reynoutria japonica* Houtt. (syn.: *Polygonum cuspidatum* Siebold & Zucc.)	Rhizome and root
Polygoni multiflora radix	Fleeceflower root	*Fallopia multiflora* (Thunb.) Haraldson (syn.: *Polygonum multiflorum* Thunb.)	Root
Prunellae spica	Selfheal fruit spike	*Prunella vulgaris* L.	Fruit spike
Pruni africanae cortex	Pygeum bark	*Prunus africana* (Hook. f) Kalkman (syn.: *Pygeum africanum* Hook. f)	Bark
Puerariae lobatae radix	Kudzu vine	*Pueraria montana* var. *lobata* (Willd.) Sanjappa & Pradeep	Root
Puerariae thomsonii radix	Thomson kudzu vine	*Pueraria montana* var. *thomsonii* Wiersema ex D.B. Ward	Root
Quercus cortex	Oak bark	*Quercus robur* L., *Q. petraea* (Matt.) Liebl., *Q. pubescens* Will.	Bark
Quillajae cortex	Quillaia bark	*Quillaja saponaria* Molina s.l.	Bark
Rehmanniae radix	Rehmannia root	*Rehmannia glutinosa* (Gaertn.) DC.	Root
Rhamni purshianae cortex	Cascara	*Frangula purshiana* (DC.) A. Gray ex J.G. Cooper	Bark
Rhei radix	Rhubarb	*Rheum palmatum* L.	Root
Ribis nigri folium	Blackcurrant leaf	*Ribes nigrum* L.	Leaf

Continued

TABLE A.1   Herbal Drug Names and Definitions Focusing on Botanical Drugs Available on European Markets—cont'd

Latin Pharmaceutical Name	English Monograph Name	Accepted Botanical Name of Species	Part of Plant Used
Rosae pseudofructis	Dog rose, rosehip	*Rosa canina* L. and others	(False fruit)
Rusci rhizoma	Butcher's broom	*Ruscus aculeatus* L.	Rhizome
Rosmarini folium	Rosemary	*Rosmarinus officinalis* L.	Leaf
Sabalis serrulatae fructus	Saw palmetto	*Serenoa repens* (W. Bartram) Small	Fruit
Salicis cortex	Willow bark	Salix spp.	Bark
Salviae miltiorrhizae radix et rhizoma	Salvia miltiorrhiza root and rhizome	*Salvia miltiorrhiza* Bunge	Root and rhizome
Salviae officinalis folium	Sage leaf	*Salvia officinalis* L.	Leaf
Salviae trilobae folium	Three-lobed sage leaf	*Salvia fruticosa* Mill. (syn.: *S. triloba* L.)	Leaf
Sambuci flos	Elderflower	*Sambucus nigra* L.	Flower
Sambuci fructus	Elderberry		Fruit
Sanguisorbae radix	Greater burnet root	*Sanguisorba officinalis* L.	Root
Schisandrae chinensis fructus	Schisandra fruit	*Schisandra chinensis* (Turcz.) Baill.	Fruit
Scutellariae baicalensis radix	Baical skullcap root	*Scutellaria baicalensis* Georgi	Root
Sinomenii caulis	Orientvine stem	*Sinomenium acutum* (Thunb.) Rehder & H. Wilson	Stem
Sennae folium	Senna leaf	*Cassia senna* L.	Leaf
Sennae fructus acutifoliae	Senna fruit	*C. senna* (syn.: *C. acutifolia* Delile)	Fruit ('pods')
Sennae fructus angustifoliae		*C. senna* (syn.: *C. angustifolia* Vahl)	
Serpylli herba	Wild thyme	*Thymus serpyllum* L.	Herb
Solidaginis herba	Goldenrod	*Solidago gigantea* Aiton, *S. canadensis* L.	Herb
Solidaginis virgaureae herba	European goldenrod	*Solidago virgaurea* L.	Herb
Sophorae flavescentis radix	Lightyellow sophora root	*Sophora flavescens* Aiton	Root
Sophorae japonicae flos	Sophora flower	*Styphnolobium japonicum* (L.) Schott (syn.: *Sophora japonica* L.)	Open flower
Sophorae japonicae flos immaturus	Sophora flower bud		Flower bud
Stephaniae tetrandrae radix	Fourstamen stephania root	*Stephania tetrandra* S. Moore	Root
Stramonii folium	Stramonium leaf	*Datura stramonium* L.	Leaf
Tanaceti parthenii herba	Feverfew	*Tanacetum parthenium* (L.) Sch.Bip.	Herb
Taraxaci officinalis herba cum radice	Dandelion herb with root	*Taraxacum officinale* F.H. Wigg	Herb with root
Taraxaci officinalis radix	Dandelion root		Root
Thymi herba	Thyme	*Thymus vulgaris* L.	Herb
Tiliae flos	Lime flower	*Tilia cordata* Mill., *T. platyphyllos* Scop., *T. xvulgaris* Hayne.	Flower
Tormentillae rhizoma	Tormentil	*Potentilla erecta* (L.) Raeusch. (syn.: *P. tormentilla* Stokes)	Rhizome
Trigonellae foenugraeci semen	Fenugreek	*Trigonella foenum-graecum* L.	Seed
Uncariae rhynchophylla ramulus cum uncis	Uncaria stem with hooks	*Uncaria rhynchophylla* Miq.	Stems
Urticae folium	Nettle leaf	*Urtica dioica* L.	Leaf
Urticae radix	Nettle root		Root
Uva-ursi folium	Bearberry	*Arctostaphylos uva-ursi* (L.) Spreng.	Leaf
Valerianae radix	Valerian	*Valeriana officinalis* L.	Root
Verbasci flos	Mullein flower	*Verbascum thapsus* L., *V. densiflorum* Bertol., *V. phlomoides* L.	Flower
Verbenae citriodorae folium	Lemon verbena leaf	*Aloysia citriodora* Paláu (syn.: *Verbena triphylla* L'Hér.	Leaf
Verbenae herba	Verbena herb	*Verbena officinalis* L.	Herb
Violae herba cum flore	Wild pansy	*Viola arvensis* Murray, *V. tricolor* L.	Herb with flower
Zanthoxylli bungeani pericarpium	Zanthoxylum bungeanum pericarp	*Zanthoxylum bungeanum* Maxim.	Peel of ripe fruit
Zingiberis rhizoma	Ginger	*Zingiber officinale* Roscoe	Rhizome

FURTHER READING

Allkin, B., Patmore, K., 2022. Botanical nomenclature for herbal medicines and natural products: its significance for pharmacovigilance. In: Barnes, J. (Ed.), Pharmacovigilance for Herbal and Traditional Medicines: Advances, Challenges and Perspectives. Springer, Cham.

Chan, K., Shaw, D., Simmonds, M.S., Leon, C.J., Xu, Q., Lu, A., et al., 2012. Good practice in reviewing and publishing studies on herbal medicine, with special emphasis on traditional Chinese medicine and Chinese materia medica. J. Ethnopharmacol. 140 (3), 469–475.

Rivera, D., Allkin, R., Obón, C., Alcaraz, F., Verpoorte, R., Heinrich, M., 2014. What is in a name? The need for accurate scientific nomenclature for plants. J. Ethnopharmacol. 152, 393–402. doi.org/10.1016/j.jep.2013.12.022.

INDEX

Note: Page numbers followed by *b* indicate boxes, *f* indicate figures and *t* indicate tables.